CW00825906

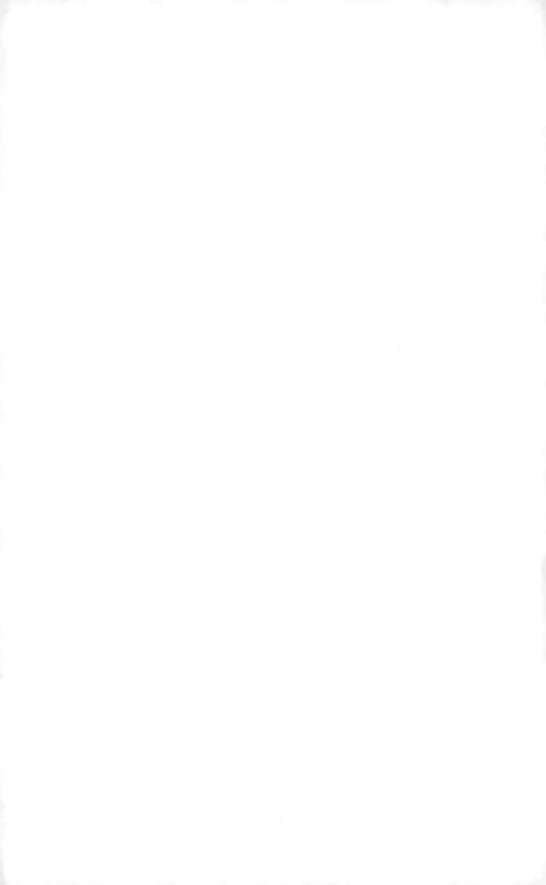

THE HUMAN AMYGDALA

THE HUMAN AMYGDALA

EDITED BY
PAUL J. WHALEN
ELIZABETH A. PHELPS

THE GUILFORD PRESS
New York   London

© 2009 The Guilford Press
A Division of Guilford Publications, Inc.
72 Spring Street, New York, NY 10012
www.guilford.com

All rights reserved

No part of this book may be reproduced, translated, stored in a retrieval system,
or transmitted, in any form or by any means, electronic, mechanical, photocopying,
microfilming, recording, or otherwise, without written permission from
the Publisher.

Printed in the United States of America

This book is printed on acid-free paper.

Last digit is print number: 9 8 7 6 5 4 3 2

Library of Congress Cataloging-in-Publication Data

The human amygdala / edited by Paul J. Whalen, Elizabeth A. Phelps.
  p. ; cm.
  Includes bibliographical references and index.
  ISBN 978-1-60623-033-6 (hardcover : alk. paper)
  1. Amygdaloid body. 2. Neuropsychology. I. Whalen, Paul J., 1963–
II. Phelps, Elizabeth A.
  [DNLM: 1. Amygdala—physiology. 2. Emotions—physiology.
3. Neuropsychology. WL 314 H918 2009]
  QP376.H86 2009
  612.8′2—dc22

                                                                    2008032099

About the Editors

Paul J. Whalen, PhD, is Professor in the Department of Psychological and Brain Sciences at Dartmouth College. The focus of his research is to better understand the neural substrates of biologically relevant learning in humans. To this end, Dr. Whalen's laboratory studies the human amygdala as a model system for such learning. Specifically, he studies the response of the human amygdala to facial expressions of emotion to assess normal amygdala–prefrontal function, as well as aberrations in this circuitry in psychopathology.

Elizabeth A. Phelps, PhD, is Silver Professor of Psychology and Neural Science at New York University. Her laboratory has earned widespread acclaim for its groundbreaking research on how the human brain processes emotion, particularly as it relates to learning, memory, and decision making. Dr. Phelps is the recipient of the 21st Century Scientist Award from the James S. McDonnell Foundation and a Fellow of the American Association for the Advancement of Science. She has served on the Board of Directors of the Association for the Psychological Sciences and the Society for Neuroethics, was President of the Society for Neuroeconomics, and is the current Editor of the journal *Emotion*.

Contributors

Ralph Adolphs, PhD, Division of Humanities and Social Sciences, California Institute of Technology, Pasadena, California, and Department of Neurology, University of Iowa, Iowa City, Iowa

David G. Amaral, PhD, The M.I.N.D. Institute, University of California, Davis, California

Tony W. Buchanan, PhD, Department of Psychology, St. Louis University, St. Louis, Missouri

Turhan Canli, PhD, Graduate Program in Genetics and Department of Psychology, Stony Brook University, Stony Brook, New York

B. J. Casey, PhD, Sackler Institute for Developmental Psychobiology, Weill Cornell Medical College, New York, New York

F. Caroline Davis, BA, Department of Psychological and Brain Sciences, Dartmouth College, Hanover, New Hampshire

Michael Davis, PhD, Center for Behavioral Neuroscience, Yerkes National Primate Research Center, and Department of Psychiatry and Behavioral Sciences, Emory University, Atlanta, Georgia

Erica J. Duncan, MD, Center for Behavioral Neuroscience and Department of Psychiatry and Behavioral Sciences, Emory University, Atlanta, Georgia, and Mental Health Service, Atlanta Veterans Affairs Medical Center, Decatur, Georgia

Jennifer L. Freese, PhD, Department of Neurology, University of California at San Francisco, San Francisco, California

Stephan Hamann, PhD, Department of Psychology, Emory University, Atlanta, Georgia

Todd A. Hare, PhD, Sackler Institute for Developmental Psychobiology, Weill Cornell Medical College, New York, New York

Ahmad R. Hariri, PhD, Departments of Psychiatry and Psychology, University of Pittsburgh Medical Center, Pittsburgh, Pennsylvania

Daphne J. Holt, MD, PhD, Department of Psychiatry, Massachusetts General Hospital, Harvard Medical School, Boston, Massachusetts

Alicia Izquierdo, PhD, Department of Psychology, California State University, Los Angeles, California

Tanja Jovanovic, PhD, Center for Behavioral Neuroscience and Department of Psychiatry and Behavioral Sciences, Emory University, Atlanta, Georgia, and Mental Health Service, Atlanta Veterans Affairs Medical Center, Decatur, Georgia

Hackjin Kim, PhD, Department of Psychology, Korea University, Seoul, Korea

M. Justin Kim, MA, Department of Psychological and Brain Sciences, Dartmouth College, Hanover, New Hampshire

Kevin S. LaBar, PhD, Center for Cognitive Neuroscience, Duke University, Durham, North Carolina

Joseph E. LeDoux, PhD, Center for Neural Science, New York University, New York, New York

Ludise Malkova, PhD, Department of Pharmacology, Georgetown University, Washington, DC

Elisabeth A. Murray, PhD, Laboratory of Neuropsychology, National Institute of Mental Health, Bethesda, Maryland

Karyn M. Myers, PhD, Behavioral Genetics Laboratory, Mailman Research Center, McLean Hospital, Harvard Medical School, Belmont, Massachusetts

Maital Neta, BS, Department of Psychological and Brain Sciences, Dartmouth College, Hanover, New Hampshire

Seth D. Norrholm, PhD, Center for Behavioral Neuroscience and Department of Psychiatry and Behavioral Sciences, Emory University, Atlanta, Georgia, and Mental Health Service, Atlanta Veterans Affairs Medical Center, Decatur, Georgia

Arne Öhman, PhD, Psychology Section, Department of Clinical Neuroscience, Karolinska Institute, Karolinska University Hospital, Stockholm, Sweden

Jonathan A. Oler, PhD, Department of Psychiatry, University of Wisconsin, Madison, Wisconsin

Elizabeth A. Phelps, PhD, Department of Psychology, New York University, New York, New York

Mary L. Phillips, MD, Department of Psychiatry, Western Psychiatric Institute and Clinic, University of Pittsburgh School of Medicine, Pittsburgh, Pennsylvania

Roger K. Pitman, MD, Department of Psychiatry, Massachusetts General Hospital, Harvard Medical School, Boston, Massachusetts

Scott L. Rauch, MD, Department of Psychiatry, McLean Hospital, Harvard Medical School, Boston, Massachusetts

Daniela Schiller, PhD, Center for Neural Science and Department of Psychology, New York University, New York, New York

Cynthia Mills Schumann, PhD, Department of Neurosciences, University of California at San Diego, La Jolla, California

Lisa M. Shin, PhD, Department of Psychology, Tufts University, Medford, Massachusetts, and Department of Psychiatry, Massachusetts General Hospital, Harvard Medical School, Boston, Massachusetts

Nim Tottenham, PhD, Sackler Institute for Developmental Psychobiology, Weill Cornell Medical College, New York, New York

Donna J. Toufexis, PhD, Department of Psychology, University of Vermont, Burlington, Vermont

Daniel Tranel, PhD, Department of Neurology, University of Iowa, Iowa City, Iowa

Patrik Vuilleumier, MD, Laboratory for Neurology and Imaging of Cognition, Department of Neuroscience and Clinic of Neurology, University Medical Center, and Swiss National Center for Affective Sciences, University of Geneva, Geneva, Switzerland

Lauren H. Warren, PhD, Center for Cognitive Neuroscience, Duke University, Durham, North Carolina

Daniel R. Weinberger, MD, Genes, Cognition, and Psychosis Program, Intramural Research Program, National Institute of Mental Health, Bethesda, Maryland

Paul J. Whalen, PhD, Department of Psychological and Brain Sciences, Dartmouth College, Hanover, New Hampshire

James T. Winslow, PhD, Intramural Research Program, National Institute of Mental Health, Bethesda, Maryland

Christopher I. Wright, MD, PhD, Laboratory of Aging and Emotion, Massachusetts General Hospital–East, Charlestown, Massachusetts, and Division of Cognitive and Behavioral Neurology, Department of Neurology, Brigham and Women's Hospital, Harvard Medical School, Boston, Massachusetts

Preface

The anatomist K. F. Burdach is credited as the first to use the term "amygdala" in the 19th century to describe the subcortical gray matter found rostral to the hippocampus in the medial temporal lobe. Several contemporary anatomists have noted that Burdach probably chose this name because the shape of the basolateral amygdala resembled that of an almond. J. B. Johnstone is credited in the early 1920s with the formal recognition of the contemporary partition of the amygdala into its basolateral, centromedial, and cortical divisions. As in other animals, these divisions of the human amygdala can be justified on both functional and anatomical grounds. Over 80 years later, we continue to use this conceptualization of the amygdala to guide the questions we ask about the role of this structure in affective information processing.

This volume presents the latest information available about the structure and function of the human amygdala, as well as the animal models that have offered a theoretical framework for understanding the role of the amygdala in human behavior. Part I begins with an examination of the nonhuman primate amygdala as it relates to the human structure. Subsequent chapters in this part of the book detail influential animal models assessing the role of the amygdala in associative learning paradigms, such as fear conditioning, extinction, and reward conditioning.

Part II addresses healthy human amygdala function. Many of the investigators whose work is described here use functional brain imaging as a means to study the human amygdala. Much of this work is influenced by the animal studies detailed in Part I, demonstrating human amygdala responses during fear conditioning and extinction in humans that parallel the animal data. Though the spatial resolution of human neuroimaging limits our present ability to make strong claims about localization of function for different amygdala subdivisions, work with animals detailing different roles for various amygdala subnuclei clearly influences the hypotheses driving much of this human neuroimaging work. Thus Part II provides a blueprint for research using the technological advances of the future (e.g., neuroimaging with higher spatial resolution) to elucidate different functions for the subnuclei of the human amygdala.

Part III of this volume links the work described in Parts I and II with the field of psychiatry. Here leaders in psychiatric research document human amygdala dysfunction in psychopathological disorders. Many of these findings converge with findings from the animal literature. For example, studies show that the amygdala is implicated in emotional disorders, such as anxiety and depression. These studies also suggest that these disorders involve a breakdown in communication between the medial prefrontal cortex and the amygdala. Such findings were predicted by studies in rats by LeDoux and colleagues showing a deficit in extinction learning following medial prefrontal cortex lesions. Additional data show that the amygdala has been implicated in more pervasive disorders, such as schizophrenia and autism. Part III concludes with data demonstrating the promise for identifying genes that might predict amygdala function and, in turn, its dysfunction in pathological anxiety.

This volume reflects a long and distinguished research tradition: the anatomists of the 1800s; the lesion studies in nonhuman primates of Klüver and Bucy in the 1930s; the human lesion work by Weiskrantz in the 1950s; Kaada and Ursin's amygdala stimulation and simultaneous EEG studies in cats and the electrical stimulation studies of the human amygdala by Gloor in the 1960s; the Blanchards' work on fear states in the 1970s; Kapp, LeDoux, McGaugh, and Davis's establishment of a field based on Pavlovian fear conditioning in the 1980s; and further human amygdala lesion work and nonhuman primate amygdala anatomical studies, together with human functional neuroimaging of the amygdala, in the 1990s. All this research is responsible for the still-growing interest in understanding the role of this relatively small brain structure in emotional learning and memory. These studies offer a vast amount of data from which to derive testable predictions concerning human amygdala function; this volume documents this field's modest initial efforts at addressing these predictions. To date, it is clear that the human amygdala and the nonhuman animal amygdala have much in common. The goal for the future will be to elucidate some of the important differences—differences that might explain the complexity of individual differences in normal human emotions and their aberrances in psychopathology.

PAUL J. WHALEN
ELIZABETH A. PHELPS

Contents

Part III. Human Amygdala Dysfunction

THE HUMAN AMYGDALA

PART I

From Animal Models
to Human Amygdala Function

CHAPTER 1

Neuroanatomy of the Primate Amygdala

Jennifer L. Freese and David G. Amaral

The amygdala[1] has historically been considered to be part of the limbic system, with connections mainly to the hypothalamus and brainstem. However, neuroanatomical studies carried out over the last 30 years clearly demonstrate that the amygdala has a wide-reaching network of connections with a diverse array of brain regions (Aggleton, Burton, & Passingham, 1980; Aggleton & Mishkin, 1984; Amaral & Price, 1984; Amaral, Price, Pitkänen, & Carmichael, 1992; Amaral, Veazey, & Cowan, 1982; Carmichael & Price, 1995; Cheng et al., 1997; Freese & Amaral, 2005; Fudge, Kunishio, Walsh, Richard, & Haber, 2002; Iwai & Yukie, 1987; Mehler, 1980; Mizuno, Takahashi, Satoda, & Matsushima, 1985; Norita & Kawamura, 1980; Russchen, Bakst, Amaral, & Price, 1985). Moreover, it is also clear that the amygdala has undergone an evolutionary reorganization; for example, the lateral nucleus of the amygdala occupies a much larger proportion of the nonhuman primate and human amygdala than of the rodent or carnivore amygdala (Barger, Stefanacci, & Semendeferi, 2007; Stephan, Frahm, & Baron, 1987). This makes sense, given that the lateral nucleus is the major recipient of neocortical inputs, and the neocortex has undergone the greatest elaboration in the primate brain (Gloor, 1997; McDonald, 1998; Stephan et al., 1987).

The neuroanatomy of the amygdaloid complex has been reviewed on a number of occasions over the last 30 years (Aggleton et al., 1980; Amaral et al., 1992; McDonald, 1992; Price, Russchen, & Amaral, 1987). In this short chapter, we focus on a description of the subdivisions and patterns of connectivity of the nonhuman primate amygdaloid complex. Available evidence indicates that the macaque monkey amygdala is a reasonable proxy for the human amygdala. Where comparisons have been made—for example, in the cytoarchitectonic organization (Pitkänen & Kemppainen, 2002; Sorvari, Soininen, Palijarvi, Karkola, & Pitkänen, 1995; Sorvari, Soininen, & Pitkänen, 1996a; Sorvari, Soininen, & Pitkänen, 1996b)—there is almost complete homology between the two species. There is, however, virtually no available information on the connectivity of the human amygdala. Thus findings from the nonhuman primate provide the most reasonable estimate of the neuroanatomical relationships in which the human amygdala is involved.

CYTOARCHITECTONIC ORGANIZATION

The amygdaloid complex is a heterogeneous group of nuclei and cortical regions located in the medial temporal lobe just rostral to the hippocampal formation. The nonhuman primate amygdaloid complex can be divided into 13 nuclei and cortical areas (Amaral & Bassett, 1989; Amaral et al., 1992; Gloor, 1997; Pitkänen & Amaral, 1998; Price et al., 1987) (Figure 1.1). For convenience, these often are classified as "deep nuclei" (the lateral nucleus [abbreviated as L in Figure 1.1], basal nucleus [B in Figure 1.1], accessory basal nucleus [AB], and paralaminar nucleus [PL]); "superficial nuclei" (the medial nucleus [M], the anterior cortical nucleus [COa], the posterior cortical nucleus [COp], the nucleus of the lateral olfactory tract [NLOT], and the periamygdaloid cortex [PAC]); and "remaining nuclei" (the anterior amygdaloid area [AAA], the central nucleus [CE], the amygdalohippocampal area [AHA], and the intercalated nuclei [I]) (Table 1.1). We have provided a series of coronal sections (Figures 1.1A–1.1G) in which the locations and rostrocaudal extents of each of these nuclei and cortical areas are indicated. It is important to provide this full series of sections, since some nuclei are only located at certain rostrocaudal levels. The central nucleus, for example, is only found within the caudal half of the amygdaloid complex. We now provide a bit more detail on the organization and intrinsic connections of each of these regions. The intrinsic connections are summarized in Figure 1.2.

SUBDIVISIONS, CYTOARCHITECTURE, AND INTRA-AMYGDALOID CONNECTIVITY

Deep Nuclei

Lateral Nucleus

The lateral nucleus is subdivided into dorsal, dorsal intermediate, ventral intermediate, and ventral divisions (Pitkänen & Amaral, 1998; Price et al., 1987) on the basis of cell density, size, and chemoarchitechtonics. Neurons in the dorsal divisions are less densely packed and stain weakly for acetylcholin-

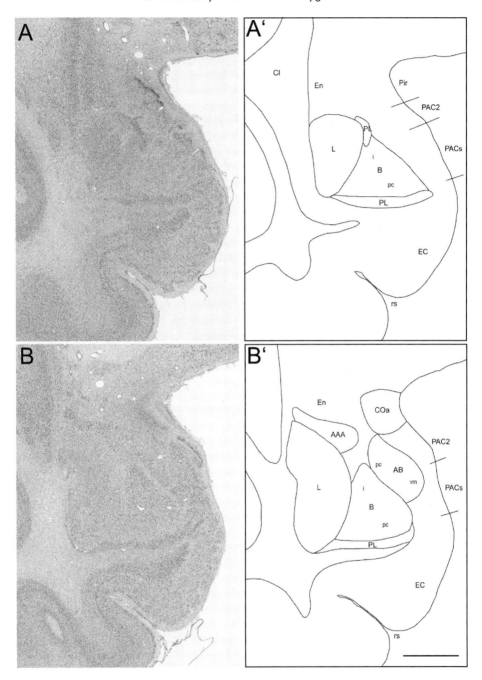

FIGURE 1.1.

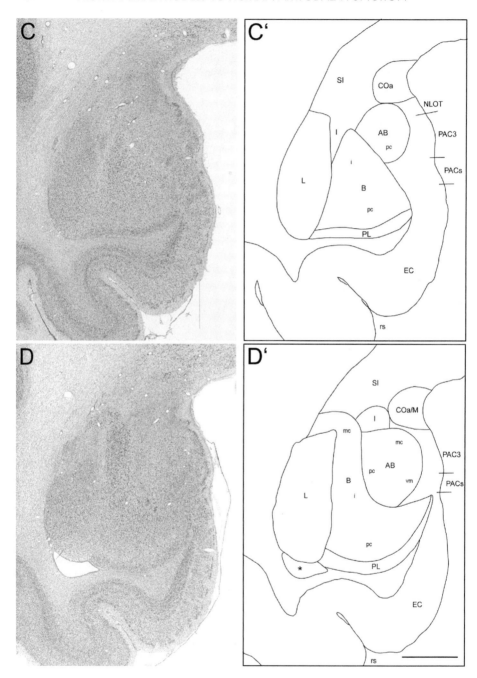

FIGURE 1.1.

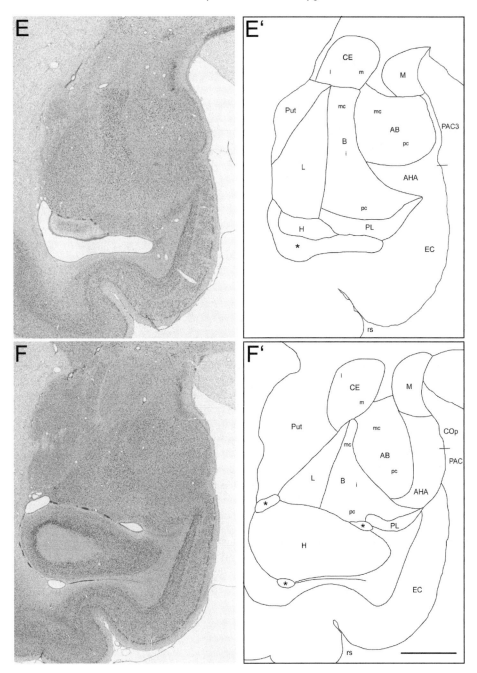

FIGURE 1.1.

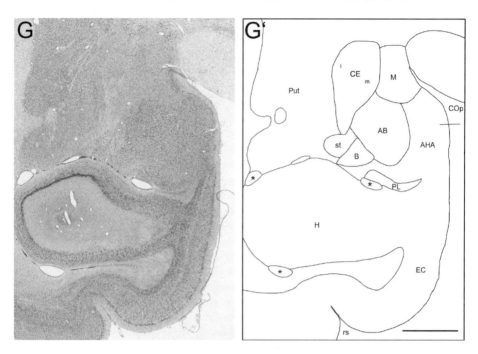

FIGURE 1.1. *Nuclei of the amygdala.* Nissl images of the primate amygdala from rostral (A) to caudal (G), sectioned in the coronal plane. The sections are 720 μm apart. Line drawings (A′–G′) representing the borders of nuclei and subdivisions accompany each Nissl section. Scale bar = 2 mm. AAA, anterior amygdaloid area; ABmc, accessory basal nucleus, magnocellular division; ABpc, accessory basal nucleus, parvicellular division; ABvm, accessory basal nucleus, ventromedial division; AHA, amygdalohippocampal area; Bi, basal nucleus, intermediate division; Bmc, basal nucleus, magnocellular division; Bpc, basal nucleus, parvicellular division; CEl, central nucleus, lateral division; CEm, central nucleus, medial division; COa, anterior cortical nucleus; COp, posterior cortical nucleus; EC, entorhinal cortex; En, endopiriform nucleus; H, hippocampus; I, intercalated nucleus; Ld, lateral nucleus, dorsal division; Ldi, lateral nucleus, dorsal intermediate division; Lv, lateral nucleus, ventral division; Lvi, lateral nucleus, ventral intermediate division; *, lateral ventricle; M, medial nucleus; NLOT, nucleus of the lateral olfactory tract; PAC, periamygdaloid cortex; Pir, piriform cortex; PL, paralaminar nucleus; Put, putamen; rs, rhinal sulcus; SI, substantia innominata; st, stria terminalis.

TABLE 1.1. Nuclei of the Amygdaloid Complex

Deep nuclei

Lateral nucleus (L)
   Dorsal division (Ld)
   Dorsal intermediate division (Ldi)
   Ventral intermediate division (Lvi)
   Ventral division (Lv)
Basal nucleus (B)
   Magnocellular division (Bmc)
   Intermediate division (Bi)
   Parvicellular division (Bpc)
Accessory basal nucleus (AB)
   Magnocellular division (ABmc)
   Parvicellular (ABpc)
   Ventromedial (ABvm)
Paralaminar nucleus (PL)

Superficial nuclei

Medial nucleus (M)
Anterior cortical nucleus (COa)
Posterior cortical nucleus (COp)
Nucleus of the lateral olfactory tract (NLOT)
Periamygdaloid cortex (PAC)
   PAC2
   PAC3
   PACs

Remaining nuclei

Anterior amygdaloid area (AAA)
Central nucleus (CE)
   Medial division (CEm)
   Lateral division (CEl)
Amygdalohippocampal area (AHA)
Intercalated nuclei (I)

esterase (AChE), whereas cells in the ventral divisions are more densely packed and stain more strongly for AChE. Additional details on the cytoarchitectonic organization are provided in Pitkänen and Amaral (1998).

Connections within the lateral nucleus originate mainly in the three dorsal divisions and terminate in the ventral division (Pitkänen & Amaral, 1998). As we note later in this chapter, the dorsal parts of the lateral nucleus receive inputs from sensory neocortex that are at least partially segregated. Since these in turn project onto the most ventral portion of the lateral nucleus, it can be thought of as the "polysensory" portion of the lateral nucleus. The lateral nucleus receives few and light projections from other amygdaloid nuclei; only the basal, accessory basal, and central nuclei send meager projections to the lateral nucleus (Aggleton, 1985; Price & Amaral, 1981).

In the primate, the lateral nucleus projects to all other nuclei of the amygdaloid complex, although the projections vary in magnitude. It has strong

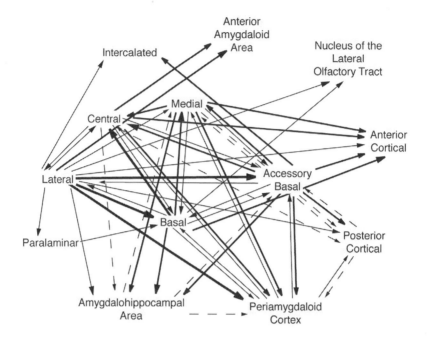

FIGURE 1.2. *Intra-amygdaloid connections.* The 13 nuclei of the primate amygdala are heavily interconnected, allowing for extensive processing of incoming information. Stronger connections are represented with a thicker line, and weaker connections with a thinner line. Tentative connections, complicated by injections that include additional nuclei, are indicated by a dashed line. The nuclei are drawn in their approximate relative locations. In general, information within the amygdala flows from lateral to medial.

projections to all subdivisions of the basal and accessory basal nuclei and the periamygdaloid cortex (Aggleton, 1985; Amaral & Insausti, 1992; Pitkänen & Amaral, 1991, 1998). Lighter projections are directed at the paralaminar nucleus, the medial nucleus, the anterior and posterior cortical nuclei, the nucleus of the lateral olfactory tract, the anterior amygdaloid area, the central nucleus, the amygdalohippocampal area, and the intercalated nuclei (Aggleton, 1985; Pitkänen & Amaral, 1998; Price & Amaral, 1981). It is important to emphasize that the projections to the central nucleus are fairly weak from the lateral nucleus, certainly in comparison to the major projections from the basal nucleus.

Basal Nucleus

Based on cytoarchitectonics, the basal nucleus is parceled into magnocellular, intermediate, and parvicellular divisions (Amaral & Bassett, 1989; Price et al., 1987). The magnocellular division, the most dorsal and caudal of the three divisions, was named for the large, darkly stained neurons observed in Nissl preparations. Dorsoventrally and rostrocaudally, the intermediate division is situated between the magnocellular and parvicellular divisions. Neurons of this division are also quite large, but are more lightly stained and less densely packed than those of the magnocellular division. The most ventrally and rostrally positioned parvicellular division is composed of the smallest cells of the basal nucleus.

Different dorsoventral positions within the basal nucleus are reciprocally connected. However, the strongest projections are from dorsal aspects of the magnocellular division to ventral aspects of the magnocellular division and the intermediate division, and from these areas to the parvicellular division (Price et al., 1987). Hence, similar to that in the lateral nucleus, the flow of information within the basal nucleus is mainly from dorsal to ventral. All three subdivisions of the basal nucleus receive a strong projection from the lateral nucleus (Aggleton, 1985; Pitkänen & Amaral, 1991, 1998). As we describe later, the basal nucleus sends projections to many cortical areas that project to the lateral nucleus, and hence completes the loop of sensory information flow between the amygdala and neocortex. Additional but lighter inputs originate in the accessory basal nucleus, the paralaminar nucleus, the medial nucleus, the periamygdaloid cortex, and the central nucleus (Aggleton, 1985; Amaral & Insausti, 1992; Pitkänen & Amaral, 1991, 1998; Price & Amaral, 1981; Van Hoesen, 1981).

The major intrinsic efferent projections of the basal nucleus are directed at the medial nucleus, the central nucleus, the anterior cortical nucleus, and the amygdalohippocampal area. Lighter projections innervate the lateral nucleus, the accessory basal nucleus, the nucleus of the lateral olfactory tract, and the periamygdaloid cortex (Aggleton, 1985; Price & Amaral, 1981).

Accessory Basal Nucleus

The most medial of the deep nuclei is the accessory basal nucleus. It is subdivided into magnocellular, parvicellular, and ventromedial divisions (Price et al., 1987). The magnocellular division is dorsolaterally located in caudal levels and contains medium- to large-sized neurons with moderate to high levels of AChE. The parvicellular division is apparent through most of the rostrocaudal extent of the accessory basal nucleus and is the major component of rostral aspects of this nucleus. Neurons in this division are small and lightly stained; the nucleus is characterized as having low levels of AChE. The ventromedial division is the most medial division and is positioned at middle rostrocaudal levels. It contains elongated, strongly AChE-positive cells that are more densely packed than those of the parvicellular division.

The magnocellular and parvicellular divisions of the accessory basal nucleus are interconnected (Amaral et al., 1992; Price et al., 1987). The major intrinsic input to the accessory basal nucleus comes from the lateral nucleus. The accessory basal nucleus also receives projections from the basal nucleus, the medial nucleus, the periamygdaloid cortex, and the central nucleus (Aggleton, 1985; Pitkänen & Amaral, 1998; Price & Amaral, 1981).

The strongest projection from the accessory basal nucleus terminates in the central nucleus, primarily in its medial division (Price & Amaral, 1981). The accessory basal nucleus sends a moderate projection to the medial nucleus, the anterior and posterior cortical nuclei, the periamygdaloid cortex, the amygdalohippocampal area, and the intercalated nuclei, and it returns a light projection to the lateral and basal nuclei (Aggleton, 1985; Gloor, 1997).

Paralaminar Nucleus

The paralaminar nucleus is a narrow band of densely packed, darkly Nissl-stained cells along the ventral and rostral limits of the amygdala. It also contains a large number of glial cells that distinguish it from other amygdaloid nuclei. Scant information is available concerning the connections of the paralaminar nucleus with the other amygdaloid nuclei. It receives a projection from lateral aspects of the lateral nucleus (Pitkänen & Amaral, 1998), and it projects to the basal nucleus (Amaral & Insausti, 1992; Pitkänen & Amaral, 1991).

Superficial Nuclei

Medial Nucleus

The medial nucleus is located in caudal aspects of the amygdala and is characterized by a dense, narrow band of darkly stained layer II cells. The medial nucleus is also composed of a cell-free layer I and a less dense, lightly stained layer III. Interestingly, a large portion of these neurons are gamma-aminobutyric acid-ergic (GABAergic). The strongest projections to the medial nucleus originate in the lateral nucleus (Pitkänen & Amaral, 1998). The medial nucleus also receives projections from the basal nucleus, the accessory basal nucleus, and the periamygdaloid cortex (Aggleton, 1985; Price & Amaral, 1981; Van Hoesen, 1981).

Efferents of the medial nucleus include the anterior cortical nucleus, the periamygdaloid cortex, the central nucleus, and the amygdalohippocampal area (Aggleton, 1985). The medial nucleus generates a light projection to the basal and accessory basal nuclei (Aggleton, 1985; Gloor, 1997).

Anterior Cortical Nucleus

The anterior cortical nucleus is rostrally continuous with the medial nucleus and includes a wide, cell-free layer I; a thick, diffuse, lightly stained layer II;

and an even less dense layer III. The anterior cortical nucleus is differentiated from the medial nucleus because its layers II and III form nearly a continuous mass, whereas the medial nucleus has a distinct layer II. The anterior cortical nucleus receives projections from the lateral nucleus, the accessory basal nucleus, the medial nucleus, and the central nucleus (Pitkänen & Amaral, 1998; Price & Amaral, 1981; Price et al., 1987). There are no reports that it gives rise to projections to other amygdaloid nuclei.

Posterior Cortical Nucleus

The posterior cortical nucleus is caudally positioned and contains only two cell layers. Layer I is quite thin, while layer II is slightly thicker and consists of medium-sized, lightly stained neurons. The posterior cortical nucleus receives projections from the lateral nucleus, the accessory basal nucleus, and the periamygdaloid cortex (Pitkänen & Amaral, 1998; Price & Amaral, 1981; Van Hoesen, 1981). Evidence from horseradish peroxidase injections raises the possibility that the posterior cortical nucleus receives input from the medial and central nuclei, but these data are complicated by involvement of other nuclei in the injections (Aggleton, 1985).

A projection from the posterior cortical nucleus to the accessory basal nucleus, the medial nucleus, and the periamygdaloid cortex may exist, but this conclusion is tentative. Thus far, all neuroanatomical tracer injections of this nucleus have also included the amygdalohippocampal area, so it is unclear which projections are solely from the posterior cortical nucleus (Amaral et al., 1992; Price et al., 1987).

Nucleus of the Lateral Olfactory Tract

The nucleus of the lateral olfactory tract is located in the rostral half of the amygdaloid complex and is identifiable by the moderately dense layer II and an overall intense staining for AChE. Although it is a prominent nucleus in the rat and cat, it is often difficult to discern its borders in primates (Price et al., 1987). The nucleus of the lateral olfactory tract does not appear to be interconnected heavily with the other nuclei of the amygdaloid complex. The only reported connection is a light projection from the lateral and basal nuclei (Pitkänen & Amaral, 1998).

Periamygdaloid Cortex

The periamygdaloid cortex is located on the medial surface of the amygdala and extends through much of its rostrocaudal extent. It is a heterogeneous region that has been given many different names and subdivided in a number of ways (Jimenez-Castellanos, 1949; Johnston, 1923; Price et al., 1987). Our laboratory has divided it into PAC2, PAC3, and PACs subdivisions (Amaral &

Bassett, 1989). In PAC2, layer II is thin and dense and contains darkly stained cells in Nissl material, whereas layer III contains scattered lightly stained cells. The two layers are often separated by a cell-free zone. PAC3 is located caudal to PAC2. Layer II is wide, with lighter stained cells as well as lighter AChE staining than in layer II of PAC2. PACs is the most rostrally positioned division, and layers II and III are not easily distinguished. The periamygdaloid cortex receives projections from the lateral nucleus, the basal nucleus, the accessory basal nucleus, the medial nucleus, and the central nucleus (Aggleton, 1985; Pitkänen & Amaral, 1998; Price & Amaral, 1981). It projects to the basal nucleus, the accessory basal nucleus, the medial nucleus, the posterior cortical nucleus, and the central nucleus (Price & Amaral, 1981; Price et al., 1987; Van Hoesen, 1981).

Remaining Nuclei

Anterior Amygdaloid Area

Like the nucleus of the lateral olfactory tract, the anterior amygdaloid area is less prominent in monkeys than in rats and cats. It is located in the rostral half of the amygdala and contains small and medium-sized cells that have low levels of AChE but are darkly stained in Nissl preparations.

Projections from the lateral nucleus and the central nucleus terminate in the region of the anterior amygdaloid area (Aggleton, 1985; Pitkänen & Amaral, 1998). However, no studies have reported intrinsic amygdaloid projections from the anterior amygdaloid area.

Central Nucleus

The central nucleus is located in the caudal half of the primate amygdala. It is typically subdivided into medial and lateral divisions, based on its cytoarchetecture (Price et al., 1987). The medial division contains a heterogeneous mixture of lightly stained small and medium-sized cells. Neurons in the lateral division are more homogeneous in appearance, more densely packed, and more darkly stained in Nissl preparations.

The central nucleus is one of the primary recipients of intrinsic amygdaloid connections. The medial division receives strong projections from the basal nucleus and the accessory basal nucleus; it receives lighter projections from the lateral nucleus, the medial nucleus, and the periamygdaloid cortex (Aggleton, 1985; Pitkänen & Amaral, 1998; Price & Amaral, 1981; Price et al., 1987; Van Hoesen, 1981).

The central nucleus generates projections to the anterior cortical nucleus, the periamygdaloid cortex, the anterior amygdaloid area, and the amygdalohippocampal area (Aggleton, 1985; Price & Amaral, 1981). In addition, it sends light projections to the lateral, basal, and accessory basal nuclei. A distinguishing feature of the central nucleus is its strong immunoreactivity for

GABA and glutamic acid decarboxylase (GAD), a precursor to GABA. This suggests that many projections of the central nucleus are GABAergic.

Amygdalohippocampal Area

The amygdalohippocampal area forms the caudal pole of the amygdala. Rostrally, neurons of this nucleus are lightly packed and pale in Nissl-stained material. In contrast, cells in caudal portions are densely packed and darkly stained. Intrinsic connections to the amygdalohippocampal area originate in the lateral nucleus, the basal nucleus, the accessory basal nucleus, the medial nucleus, and the central nucleus (Aggleton, 1985; Pitkänen & Amaral, 1998; Price & Amaral, 1981). The amygdalohippocampal area may send a projection to the accessory basal nucleus, the medial nucleus, and the periamygdaloid cortex (Amaral et al., 1992). However, all tracer injections to date have also included the posterior cortical nucleus, so the exact projections of the amygdalohippocampal area remain unknown.

Intercalated Nuclei

The intercalated nuclei are small, separated cell masses located in different areas of the amygdala. There has been enormous interest in these nuclei in the rodent brain (Paré, Quirk, & LeDoux, 2004; Royer, Martina, & Paré, 1999; Royer & Paré, 2002). However, much less is known about their organization in the nonhuman primate brain. In general, they tend to be relatively less prominent in the primate brain than in the rodent brain. Some are located between the basal and accessory basal nuclei; others are located between the basal and lateral nuclei; and still others are found in the fibers just ventral to the central nucleus. They receive projections from the lateral and accessory basal nuclei (Aggleton, 1985; Pitkänen & Amaral, 1998).

EXTRINSIC CONNECTIONS OF THE AMYGDALA

The amygdaloid complex projects to, and receives projections from, many other structures of the brain. Its various nuclei have the potential of influencing regions of the nervous system ranging from the spinal cord, brainstem, and hypothalamus to cortical regions in the frontal, cingulate, insular, temporal, and occipital cortices.

Major Pathways

The amygdala is reciprocally interconnected with a variety of subcortical regions through the ventral amygdalofugal pathway and the stria terminalis (Amaral et al., 1992; Price et al., 1987). The ventral amygdalofugal pathway fibers collect along the dorsomedial edge at the rostrocaudal extent of the amygdala, whereas those of the stria terminalis gather at ventromedial aspects of the caudal amygdala. These two pathways do not carry distinct fibers; fibers travel from one bundle to join the other (Price & Amaral, 1981; Russchen et al., 1985), or use both bundles to reach the same destination. Although the stria terminalis and ventral amygdalofugal pathways are classically described as the major pathways of the amygdala, the reality is that many of the amygdaloid inputs and outputs do not follow either of these pathways. Many of the projections between the amygdala and the neocortex, for example, form fascicles that travel within the subcortical white matter. We have described some of these fascicles that distribute fibers to the temporal and occipital cortices as the "temporo-occipital amygdalocortical pathway" (TOACP) (Freese & Amaral, 2005), although most of these bundles do not have distinct names.

Subcortical Connectivity

The amygdaloid complex has widespread connectivity with many subcortical regions. These are summarized in Figure 1.3.

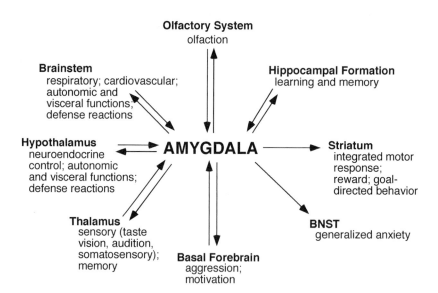

FIGURE 1.3. *Amygdaloid connections with subcortical structures.* The amygdala receives projections from numerous subcortical structures. These areas convey information concerning external stimuli and the animal's internal state to the amygdala. The amygdaloid complex integrates this incoming information and sends a return projection to each area, providing an emotional influence over behaviors mediated by these subcortical structures. BNST, bed nucleus of the stria terminalis.

Striatum

Although the striatum does not project to the amygdala, the amygdala provides a substantial projection to both the neostriatum (the caudate and putamen) and the ventral striatum (Fudge et al., 2002; Nauta, 1962; Parent, Mackey, & De Bellefeville, 1983; Russchen, Bakst, Amaral, & Price, 1985). The basal and accessory basal nuclei originate most of these projections, while the lateral nucleus, medial nucleus, periamygdaloid cortex, anterior and posterior cortical nuclei, amygdalohippocampal area, and central nucleus all make minor contributions. The amygdalostriatal projections are topographically organized, such that the parvicellular division of the basal nucleus projects to the medial part of the nucleus accumbens, whereas the magnocellular basal nucleus projects to the tail and body of the caudate and the rostroventral putamen (Russchen, Bakst, et al., 1985). Beyond the basal nucleus, neurons in the periamygdaloid cortex and amygdalohippocampal area (medial aspects of the amygdala) project mainly to the most medial and ventral parts of the caudate and putamen, whereas the lateral nucleus projections are directed to more caudal parts of the ventral putamen and the tail of the caudate nucleus (Fudge et al., 2002).

Bed Nucleus of the Stria Terminalis

In many ways, the bed nucleus of the stria terminalis (BNST) is an extension of the amygdala proper and is sometimes considered to be a portion of the so-called "extended amygdala."[2] Certain terminologies group the medial and intermediate aspects of the BNST with the medial nucleus of the amygdala, and include lateral and ventral aspects of the BNST with the central nucleus (Alheid & Heimer, 1988; De Olmos & Heimer, 1999). These extensions are based on the physical continuity observed in lower mammals, as well as on connectional and chemoarchitectonic evidence that indicates similarities between the BNST and the medial and central nuclei of the amygdala (Alheid & Heimer, 1988; De Olmos & Heimer, 1999; Grove, 1988; Holstege, Meiners, & Tan, 1985; McDonald, Shammah-Lagnado, Shi, & Davis, 1999; Moga et al., 1990; Schwanzel-Fukuda, Morrell, & Pfaff, 1984). As found in the striatum, the central and medial nuclei contain a higher proportion of GABAergic neurons than do the lateral and basal nuclei (McDonald, 1992). However, in primates the BNST is physically separated from the amygdala by the internal capsule, and studies in the rat have revealed differences in connectivity between the amygdala and BNST (Canteras, Simerly, & Swanson, 1995; Dong, Petrovich, & Swanson, 2001). Therefore, we consider this structure to be separate from the amygdala.

Studies have not reported projections from the BNST to the amygdaloid complex in the primate. However, the BNST receives projections from almost all of the amygdaloid nuclei, including the basal nucleus, the accessory basal nucleus, the medial nucleus, the posterior cortical nucleus, the amygdalohippocampal area, and the central nucleus (Price & Amaral, 1981; Price et al., 1987). These are arranged topographically, such that more medial amygdaloid nuclei (the medial nucleus, the posterior cortical nucleus, and the amygdalohippocampal area) project to more medial areas of the BNST, and a more lateral amygdaloid area (the magnocellular division of the basal nucleus) projects to more lateral areas of the BNST (Price et al., 1987). The accessory basal nucleus, the central nucleus, and the parvicellular division of the basal nucleus project to both divisions of the BNST (Price & Amaral, 1981; Price et al., 1987).

Basal Forebrain

The basal forebrain is a heterogeneous set of structures including the basal nucleus of Meynert, the diagonal band of Broca, the ventral pallidum, and the septal nuclei. The basal nucleus of Meynert originates a heavy projection to the amygdala, and the vertical and horizontal nuclei of the diagonal band each contribute slightly to the amygdaloid projection (Aggleton et al., 1980; Mesulam, Mufson, Levey, & Wainer, 1983). Most of these projections terminate in the magnocellular division of the basal nucleus and the nucleus of the lateral olfactory tract, but the ventral intermediate division of the lateral nucleus, the parvicellular division of the basal nucleus, the magnocellular and ventromedial divisions of the accessory basal nucleus, the periamygdaloid cortex, and the central nucleus also receive minor projections (Amaral & Bassett, 1989; Price et al., 1987). Lateral aspects of the basal nucleus of Meynert receive projections from and originate projections to the amygdala (Mesulam et al., 1983; Price & Amaral, 1981). However, this projection is not perfectly reciprocal. Although the magnocellular division of the basal nucleus and the nucleus of the lateral olfactory tract receive the heaviest projection from the basal nucleus of Meynert, they provide a very small return projection to the basal forebrain areas (Price, 1986).

Many of the amygdaloid nuclei project to the basal forebrain, with the parvicellular and the caudal magnocellular divisions of the basal nucleus, the magnocellular division of the accessory basal nucleus, and the central nucleus originating most of these projections (Price & Amaral, 1981; Russchen, Amaral, & Price, 1985). The basal nucleus of Meynert and the horizontal nucleus of the diagonal band receive a substantial projection from the amygdaloid complex, with the more lateral aspects of these areas receiving a heavier projection (Price & Amaral, 1981; Russchen, Amaral, & Price, 1985). Light projections extend through the vertical nucleus of the diagonal band and the ventral pallidum, but the septal nuclei do not appear to receive any amygdaloid fibers (Price & Amaral, 1981; Russchen, Amaral, & Price, 1985). Although the same fibers that project to the basal forebrain regions continue to other subcortical areas, these do not appear to be simply fibers of passage. Studies using the neuroanatomical tracer *Phaseolus vulgaris*-leucoagglutinin (PHA-L) reveal that the fibers contain varicosities, which are probably synaptic boutons (Russchen, Amaral, & Price, 1985).

Thalamus

Typically, the amygdala shares reciprocal connections with subcortical areas. Connections between the amygdala and the thalamus are distinctive, in that amygdaloid afferents are not specifically reciprocated by the thalamus. The nucleus paraventricularis, the nucleus subparafascicularis, the nucleus centralis complex of Olszewski, the nucleus paracentralis, the nucleus rotundis, and the nucleus reuniens send a projection to the amygdaloid complex; this terminates in the magnocellular division of the basal nucleus, the medial nucleus, and the central nucleus (Aggleton et al., 1980; Aggleton & Mishkin, 1984; Mehler, 1980). Portions of the medial geniculate complex also originate a projection to the lateral nucleus, the accessory basal nucleus, the medial nucleus, and the central nucleus of the amygdala (Amaral et al., 1992; Mehler, 1980). Finally, a modest projection from the medial nucleus of the pulvinar to the lateral nucleus has also been reported (Aggleton et al., 1980; Jones & Burton, 1976).

The most substantial amygdalothalamic projection originates in the parvicellular division of the basal nucleus of the amygdala and terminates in the rostral third of the magnocellular portion of the nucleus medialis dorsalis (Aggleton & Mishkin, 1984; Russchen, Amaral, & Price, 1987). The lateral nucleus, the magnocellular division of the basal nucleus, the accessory basal nucleus, the periamygdaloid cortex, and the amygdalohippocampal area also contribute to this projection (Aggleton & Mishkin, 1984). These projections terminate in distinct patches with a high degree of specificity. In particular, the parvicellular division of the basal nucleus and the periamygdaloid cortex project to different patches within the ventromedial region of the magnocellular portion of the mediodorsal nucleus, while the magnocellular division of the basal nucleus, the accessory basal nucleus, and the lateral nucleus all project to specific patches within the ventrolateral region of the magnocellular portion of the mediodorsal nucleus (Russchen et al., 1987). Although this thalamic nucleus is the main recipient of amygdalothalamic projections, it does not reciprocate these connections. A second amygdalothalamic connection extends from the medial nucleus, the central nucleus, and the amygdalohippocampal area to the nucleus reuniens and the nucleus centralis complex of Olszewski (Aggleton & Mishkin, 1984; Price & Amaral, 1981). The central nucleus of the amygdala sends an additional projection to the pulvinar (Price & Amaral, 1981).

Hypothalamus

Extensive connections with the hypothalamus have historically placed the amygdaloid complex in the "limbic system," and for many years the most widely recognized roles of the amygdala was related to visceral and autonomic functions (MacLean, 1970). The strongest projection from the hypothalamus to the amygdaloid complex originates in the ventromedial nucleus and terminates in the medial division of the central nucleus (Amaral et al., 1982; Mehler, 1980). The ventromedial nucleus of the hypothalamus also sends a heavy projection to the parvicellular division of the basal nucleus, the parvicellular division of the accessory basal nucleus, and the medial nucleus. And it sends a lighter projection to the periamygdaloid cortex, the nucleus of the lateral olfactory tract, and the anterior amygdaloid area (Amaral et al., 1982; Mehler, 1980). These projections are bilateral, but the contralateral projection is considerably weaker (Amaral et al., 1982). Caudal regions of the lateral hypothalamic area have a similar projection pattern, with fibers terminating in the medial nucleus, the cortical nuclei, the anterior amygdaloid area, and the medial division of the central nucleus (Amaral et al., 1982; Mehler, 1980). Whereas the lateral division of the central nucleus receives a light projection from the lateral mammillary nucleus (Amaral et al., 1982; Mehler, 1980), the medial nucleus of the amygdala receives projections from the supramammillary region (Amaral et al., 1982; Mehler, 1980). The medial portion of the substantia nigra has a small projection to both divisions of the central nucleus, but the ventral tegmental area has a very limited projection to only the lateral division of the central nucleus (Amaral et al., 1982; Mehler, 1980).

In the primate, the preoptic area and the anterior hypothalamus receive projections from the medial nucleus and the anterior cortical nucleus (Price, 1986; Price et al., 1987). Projections to the ventromedial nucleus of the hypothalamus have a distinct termination pattern. The accessory basal nucleus, the medial nucleus, and the anterior cortical nucleus target the central region, whereas the amygdalohippocampal area fibers are directed to the outer shell region (Price, 1986; Price et al., 1987). Further caudally, projections from the accessory basal nucleus, the medial nucleus, and the anterior and posterior cortical nuclei terminate in the dorsal and ventral premammillary nuclei and the supramammillary nuclei (Price et al., 1987). The basal nucleus projects to the lateral tuberal nucleus and appears to have a projection to the perifornical region (Price et al., 1987). Finally, a substantial number of amygdalohypothalamic projections flow from the central nucleus of the amygdala to regions in the lateral hypothalamus, including the dorsomedial nucleus, the perifornical region, the supramammillary area, the tuberomammillary, and (most heavily) the caudal regions of the paramammillary nucleus (Price & Amaral, 1981).

Midbrain

The peripeduncular nucleus of the midbrain sends a projection to the lateral nucleus and to the medial nucleus of the amygdala (Aggleton et al., 1980; Amaral & Insausti, 1992; Jones, Burton, Saper, & Swanson, 1976; Mehler, 1980). Rostral and caudal subdivisions of the nucleus linearis and the dorsal raphe nucleus also project to the amygdala (Mehler, 1980; Price et al., 1987), and the periaqueductal gray originates a projection that appears to focus on the accessory basal nucleus (Aggleton et al., 1980). In addition, a dopaminergic input to the central nucleus originates in the ventral tegmental area; the substantia nigra, pars compacta; and the A8 and A10 cell groups (Aggleton et al., 1980; Mehler, 1980).

The central nucleus of the amygdaloid complex sends a significant number of fibers to the substantia nigra (especially to the substantia nigra, pars compacta), the peripeduncular nuclei, the ventral tegmental area, and the mesencephalic reticular formation (Hopkins, 1975; Price, 1986; Price & Amaral, 1981; Price et al., 1987). Projections also terminate in and around the A8 and A10 dopaminergic cell groups (Price, 1986; Price et al., 1987). In more rostral aspects of the periaqueductal gray, projections are diffuse, but focus on the ventrolateral and dorsomedial regions in caudal aspects of the periaqueductal gray (Price, 1986; Price & Amaral, 1981). Finally, the central nucleus also sends heavy projections to the nucleus of the posterior commissure, the raphe nuclei, and the cuneiform nucleus (Price & Amaral, 1981).

Pons, Medulla, and Spinal Cord

To facilitate its role in autonomic response, the central nucleus has substantial reciprocal connections with the hindbrain. The lateral parabrachial nucleus of the pons sends a projection to the central nucleus of the amygdala (Mehler, 1980). Substantial projections from the locus coeruleus, the nucleus subcoeruleus, and the pars dorsalis of the nucleus subcoeruleus terminate not only in the central nucleus, but also in the basal nucleus (Mehler, 1980; Price et al., 1987).

Only the central nucleus of the amygdala projects to the pons and medulla. These fibers terminate heavily in the medial and lateral parabrachial nuclei of the pons around the superior cerebellar peduncle (Price, 1986; Price & Amaral, 1981). In more rostral sections of the brainstem, central nucleus fibers are found in the ventral region of the locus coeruleus, the dorsal aspect of the motor nucleus of the vagus, the mesencephalic nucleus of the trigeminal nerve, the nucleus subcoeruleus, and the lateral portion of the pontine reticular formation (Price, 1986; Price & Amaral, 1981; Price et al., 1987). Caudally, projections terminate in the nucleus ambiguus and the nucleus of the solitary tract (Price, 1986; Price & Amaral, 1981). Almost all subdivisions of rostral aspects of the nucleus of the solitary tract receive fibers from the central nucleus, but caudally the fibers focus on the parvocellular component (Price & Amaral, 1981). Fibers also run through the pontine nucleus and descend along the dorsolateral edge of the pyramidal tract (Price & Amaral, 1981). More central nucleus fibers are added as this bundle extends caudally until it ends at the spinomedullary border (Price & Amaral, 1981). In addition, some fibers have been observed in the cervical spinal cord (Mizuno et al., 1985). At least 30% of the cells from the central nucleus that originate these projections are immunoreactive for GAD, a marker for GABAergic cells (Jongen-Relo &

Amaral, 1998). Hence many of the long amygdaloid projections to brainstem regions are GABAergic.

Connections with the Olfactory System

Connections between the amygdala and the olfactory system have been well described in the rat (De Olmos, Hardy, & Heimer, 1978; Luskin & Price, 1983; Ottersen, 1982; Price, 1973), an animal that relies heavily on olfaction. Although connections with the olfactory system have not been studied as thoroughly in the monkey, significant afferent and efferent projections of the amygdala with the olfactory system also exist in the primate.

The primate olfactory bulb sends a strong, direct projection to the anterior cortical nucleus, the nucleus of the lateral olfactory tract, and the periamygdaloid cortex (Turner, Gupta, & Mishkin, 1978). The piriform cortex also sends a projection to those same divisions of the amygdala (Amaral et al., 1992). The nucleus of the lateral olfactory tract and the periamygdaloid cortex send a projection to the olfactory bulb (Amaral et al., 1992).

Connections with the Hippocampal Formation

The amygdaloid complex is connected with the entire hippocampal formation, including the hippocampus proper (the CA3, CA2, and CA1 fields and the dentate gyrus), the entorhinal cortex, and the subiculum (Amaral, 1986; Amaral & Cowan, 1980; Rosene & Van Hoesen, 1977; Van Hoesen, 1981).

Hippocampus

Hippocampoamygdaloid projections are significantly lighter than amygdalohippocampal projections (Aggleton, 1986; Saunders, Rosene, & Van Hoesen, 1988). Projections to the amygdaloid complex originate mainly in rostral areas of the hippocampus (Aggleton, 1986; Saunders et al., 1988). The CA1 field generates a projection to the basal nucleus, the accessory basal nucleus, the paralaminar nucleus, the periamygdaloid cortex, and the cortical nuclei (Aggleton, 1986; Rosene & Van Hoesen, 1977; Saunders et al., 1988; Van Hoesen, 1981). Anterograde and retrograde experiments suggest that the CA2 and CA3 fields of the hippocampus do not project to the amygdaloid complex in the primate (Saunders et al., 1988).

Projections to the hippocampus originate primarily in the accessory basal nucleus and the posterior cortical nucleus of the amygdala (Aggleton, 1986; Amaral, 1986; Saunders et al., 1988). These projections extend through the rostrocaudal extent of the CA1, CA2, and CA3 fields and terminate most heavily in the stratum lacunosum–moleculare. A substantial projection from the parvicellular division of the basal nucleus, joined by fewer projections from the periamygdaloid cortex, provides innervation to the subiculum–CA1 border region (Amaral, 1986; Amaral & Cowan, 1980; Saunders et al., 1988).

The monkey amygdala does not appear to share afferent or efferent connections with the dentate gyrus.

Remaining Hippocampal Formation Structures

The full rostrocaudal extent of the subiculum sends projections to the amygdaloid complex (Aggleton, 1986; Saunders et al., 1988). These projections originate in neurons along the CA1–subiculum border. The parvicellular division of the basal nucleus and the periamygdaloid cortex are the main recipients of these projections, but the lateral nucleus, the intermediate and magnocellular divisions of the basal nucleus, and the cortical nucleus receive a light projection as well. In addition, the entorhinal cortex projects to the lateral nucleus, the basal nucleus, and the periamygdaloid cortex (Aggleton, 1986; Stefanacci & Amaral, 2000; Van Hoesen, 1981).

The parvicellular division of the basal nucleus sends a robust projection to the subiculum, and the magnocellular division of the basal nucleus, the accessory basal nucleus, and the cortical nucleus make minor contributions (Aggleton, 1986; Saunders et al., 1988). Unlike the projections to the hippocampus, projections to the subiculum terminate in both the molecular and the pyramidal cell layers. Projections from the parvicellular division of the basal nucleus and the lateral nucleus terminate in the plexiform and cellular layers of the parasubiculum, whereas only the parvicellular division of the basal nucleus sends projections to the presubiculum (Aggleton, 1986; Amaral, 1986).

The amygdaloid complex generates a robust projection to the entorhinal cortex, particularly to rostral levels (Aggleton, 1986; Amaral, 1986; Insausti, Amaral, & Cowan, 1987; Pitkänen et al., 2002; Saunders & Rosene, 1988). This constitutes a second pathway by which the amygdala can influence the hippocampus proper, as the entorhinal cortex projects to all hippocampal fields via the perforant path (Witter & Amaral, 1991). The lateral nucleus provides the strongest input to the entorhinal cortex (Aggleton, 1986; Amaral, 1986; Amaral & Price, 1984; Insausti et al., 1987; Pitkänen et al., 2002; Saunders & Rosene, 1988). It projects to all levels of the entorhinal cortex, but the projections are strongest to more rostral levels and tend to focus on the superficial layers, particularly layer III. The basal nucleus projects to rostral fields of the entorhinal cortex, but does not project to the more caudal fields (Aggleton, 1986; Amaral, 1986; Amaral & Price, 1984; Insausti et al., 1987; Pitkänen et al., 2002; Saunders & Rosene, 1988). Projections from the accessory basal nucleus extend throughout the rostrocaudal extent of the entorhinal cortex and are particularly strong to layers I and III (Aggleton, 1986; Amaral, 1986; Insausti et al., 1987; Pitkänen et al., 2002; Saunders & Rosene, 1988). Finally, the magnocellular division of the basal nucleus, the medial nucleus, the anterior cortical nucleus, the periamygdaloid cortex, and the anterior amygdaloid area contribute a minor projection to more rostral fields of the entorhinal cortex, and the paralaminar nucleus gives rise to a light projection to the entire entorhinal cortex (Amaral, 1986; Insausti et al., 1987; Saunders & Rosene, 1988).

Connections between the Amygdala and the Neocortex

Most early studies of the amygdala focused on its strong connections with olfactory structures, the hypothalamus, the pons, and the medulla (Adey & Meyer, 1952; Cowan, Raisman, & Powell, 1965; Hilton & Zbrozyna, 1963; Ishikawa, Kawamura, et al., 1969). Accordingly, during this time and for years thereafter, the amygdala was thought to be involved primarily in more primitive functions such as initiating autonomic responses (MacLean, 1970). It was not until the 1970s and early 1980s, when more extensive lesion studies were completed and improved neuroanatomical tracers were developed, that the widespread connectivity of the amygdaloid complex and the neocortex was appreciated. Interestingly, many of these pioneering studies were completed in monkeys, leading to our current understanding of the connections between the amygdala and the neocortex.

The amygdaloid complex receives projections from numerous cortical areas in the frontal, insular, cingulate, and temporal lobes. Amygdalocortical projections are more widespread, encompassing even more areas than the afferent connections and including areas in the occipital lobe. In general, the deep nuclei—specifically the lateral, basal, and accessory basal—are the main recipients and originators of neocortical–amygdaloid connections.

Frontal Cortex

Leichnetz and colleagues (Leichnetz & Astruc, 1976, 1977; Leichnetz, Povlishock, & Astruc, 1976) were among the first to describe the prefrontal cortical projections to the amygdaloid complex in monkeys, which were confirmed and refined by later tracing studies. Afferents to the amygdala arise mainly from the orbitofrontal (including areas 11, 13, and parts of areas 10, 12, 14, and 24) and medial prefrontal (area 32 and parts of areas 9, 10, 14, and 24) cortices (Figure 1.4) (Aggleton et al., 1980; Amaral & Insausti, 1992; Carmichael & Price, 1995; Cavada, Compañy, Tejedor, Cruz-Rizzolo, & Reinoso-Suarez, 2000; Ghashghaei & Barbas, 2002; Leichnetz & Astruc, 1976, 1977; Leichnetz et al., 1976; Stefanacci & Amaral, 2000, 2002; Van Hoesen, 1981). Rostral aspects of the orbitofrontal cortex send a very light projection to the amygdala, directed primarily at the magnocellular division of the basal nucleus, and secondarily at the other divisions of the basal nucleus and the lateral and accessory basal nuclei (Carmichael & Price, 1995; Ghashghaei & Barbas, 2002; Stefanacci & Amaral, 2000, 2002). Projections from caudal aspects of the orbotifrontal cortex are heavier, more widespread, and most dense in caudal aspects of the amygdala (Ghashghaei & Barbas, 2002; Stefanacci & Amaral, 2002). Both orbitofrontal and medial prefrontal cortex

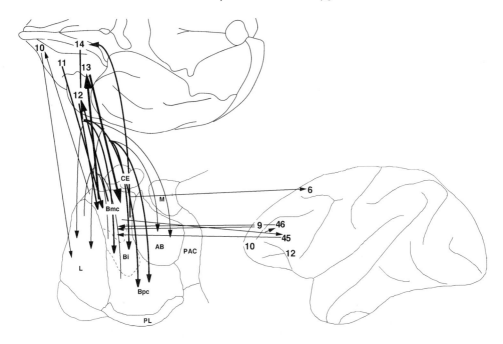

FIGURE 1.4. *Amygdaloid connections with frontal cortex.* The amygdala is heavily interconnected with orbital prefrontal and mediodorsal frontal cortices. These areas provide important social cues to the amygdala, which sends return projections to provide an emotional influence over social behavior. The density of projections is indicated by the thickness of the line. A ventral view of the brain is on the top of the figure; a lateral view is on the right-hand side of the figure. Abbreviations as in Figure 1.1.

projections are moderate in density and are focused on the lateral nucleus, the basal nucleus, the accessory basal nucleus, the medial nucleus, the anterior and posterior cortical nuclei, the periamygdaloid cortex, and the central nucleus. The caudal orbitofrontal cortex sends additional projections to the nucleus of the lateral olfactory tract, the anterior amygdaloid area, and the intercalated masses, whereas the medial prefrontal cortex projects to the amygdalohippocampal area (Aggleton et al., 1980; Amaral & Insausti, 1992; Carmichael & Price, 1995; Cavada et al., 2000; Ghashghaei & Barbas, 2002; Stefanacci & Amaral, 2000, 2002; Van Hoesen, 1981).

The lateral prefrontal cortical areas (8, 45, and 46, and parts of 9 and 12) send a sparse projection to the basal nucleus (Amaral & Insausti, 1992; Ghashghaei & Barbas, 2002). The amygdala also receives a light projection from the premotor cortex, which primarily terminates in the basal nucleus (Avendaño, Price, & Amaral, 1983).

Projections from the prefrontal cortex are organized along a rostrocaudal gradient, such that the most rostral prefrontal areas generate a light projection to the lateral nucleus, the basal nucleus, and the accessory basal nucleus.

More caudal regions send heavier projections, which terminate in more of the amygdaloid nuclei (Ghashghaei & Barbas, 2002; Stefanacci & Amaral, 2002). Most of these projections originate in the superficial layers, although projections from the orbital prefrontal cortex also arise in layer V (Aggleton et al., 1980; Stefanacci & Amaral, 2002). A similar topographical and laminar pattern is seen among corticoamygdaloid projections from many different areas.

Amygdaloid fibers terminate widely within areas of the frontal cortex (Figure 1.4) (Amaral & Price, 1984; Barbas & De Olmos, 1990; Carmichael & Price, 1995; Ghashghaei & Barbas, 2002; Porrino, Crane, & Goldman-Rakic, 1981). The orbitofrontal and mediolateral cortices are the major recipients of these projections, with the dorsolateral prefrontal cortex receiving a much lighter projection (Amaral & Price, 1984; Barbas & De Olmos, 1990; Baylis, Rolls, & Baylis, 1995; Carmichael & Price, 1995; Ghashghaei & Barbas, 2002; Morecraft, Geula, & Mesulam, 1992; Porrino et al., 1981). Projections from the frontal cortex to the amygdala are more extensive and include more amygdaloid nuclei than the return projections (Cavada et al., 2000).

Most of the projections to the orbitofrontal cortical areas arise predominantly in the basal nucleus, with lesser projections arising from the lateral nucleus and the accessory basal nucleus (Amaral & Price, 1984; Barbas & De Olmos, 1990; Baylis et al., 1995; Carmichael & Price, 1995; Cavada et al., 2000; Ghashghaei & Barbas, 2002; Morecraft et al., 1992; Porrino et al., 1981). The projections are heaviest in caudal aspects of the orbitofrontal cortex; they do extend to the frontal pole, but are much less dense in this region (Amaral & Price, 1984; Carmichael & Price, 1995).

The basal nucleus also generates most of the projections to the medial prefrontal cortex (Amaral & Price, 1984; Barbas & De Olmos, 1990; Carmichael & Price, 1995; Ghashghaei & Barbas, 2002; Porrino et al., 1981). Small contributions to this projection are made by the accessory basal nucleus, the medial nucleus, and the anterior and posterior cortical nuclei as well (Barbas & De Olmos, 1990; Carmichael & Price, 1995; Ghashghaei & Barbas, 2002).

The dorsolateral prefrontal cortex receives a very light projection from the basal nucleus of the amygdala (Amaral & Price, 1984; Barbas & De Olmos, 1990; Ghashghaei & Barbas, 2002). The termination pattern is quite sparse and generally follows the arcuate and principal sulci (Amaral & Price, 1984).

In addition, the amygdala sends a projection to the premotor cortex (Amaral & Price, 1984; Avendaño et al., 1983). It is a much lighter projection than the other amygdaloid projections to the frontal cortex, and it only originates in caudal aspects of the magnocellular division of the basal nucleus.

Amygdalocortical projections are denser to caudal than to rostral frontal cortices, and heavier projections arise from caudal levels of the amygdaloid complex (Amaral & Price, 1984; Barbas & De Olmos, 1990; Carmichael & Price, 1995). Projections to the orbitofrontal and medial prefrontal cortices terminate along the border between layers I and II and in layers V and VI. At the frontal pole and in dorsolateral prefrontal cortex—areas that receive lighter projections—the termination pattern is restricted to the superficial layers (Amaral & Price, 1984). As with corticoamygdaloid connections, this pattern is repeated in several other amygdalocortical projections.

Insular Cortex

The insular cortex projects to almost all the nuclei of the amygdala (Amaral & Insausti, 1992; Carmichael & Price, 1995; Friedman, Murray, O'Neill, & Mishkin, 1986; Mufson, Mesulam, & Pandya, 1981; Stefanacci & Amaral, 2002; Van Hoesen, 1981). Indeed, it provides one of the strongest cortical inputs to the primate amygdaloid complex. Most of these projections originate in the rostral insular cortices, specifically the agranular (Ia) and rostral aspects of the dysgranular (Id) divisions (Aggleton et al., 1980; Amaral & Insausti, 1992; Carmichael & Price, 1995; Friedman et al., 1986; Mufson et al., 1981; Stefanacci & Amaral, 2000, 2002; Van Hoesen, 1981). The densest projections are to the dorsal intermediate division of the lateral nucleus, the parvicellular division of the basal nucleus, and the central nucleus (Aggleton et al., 1980; Amaral & Insausti, 1992; Carmichael & Price, 1995; Friedman et al., 1986; Mufson et al., 1981; Stefanacci & Amaral, 2000, 2002; Turner, Mishkin, & Knapp, 1980; Van Hoesen, 1981). Ia and Id also provide projections to the other divisions of the lateral and basal nuclei, the accessory basal nucleus, the medial nucleus, the anterior cortical nucleus, the nucleus of the lateral olfactory tract, the periamygdaloid cortex, and the anterior amygdaloid area (Aggleton et al., 1980; Amaral & Insausti, 1992; Carmichael & Price, 1995; Friedman et al., 1986; Mufson et al., 1981; Stefanacci & Amaral, 2000, 2002; Turner et al., 1980; Van Hoesen, 1981).

Projections from more caudal divisions of the insular cortex (caudal divisions of Id and the granular insular cortex [Ig]) are less dense and less widespread; they focus on the dorsal intermediate subdivision of the lateral nucleus and the central nucleus (Aggleton et al., 1980; Amaral & Insausti, 1992; Friedman et al., 1986; Mufson et al., 1981; Stefanacci & Amaral, 2000, 2002; Van Hoesen, 1981). The parainsular cortex sends projections to the lateral nucleus, the basal nucleus, and the accessory basal nucleus (Aggleton et al., 1980; Amaral & Insausti, 1992; Stefanacci & Amaral, 2000). The frontoparietal operculum, a cortical taste area, projects to the dorsomedial part of the lateral nucleus (Van Hoesen, 1981).

Most of the insular projections are directed toward middle to caudal aspects of the amygdala and originate predominantly in layers II and III, with a lesser contribution from layer V (Aggleton et al., 1980; Friedman et al., 1986; Mufson et al., 1981; Stefanacci & Amaral, 2002).

The amygdaloid complex returns projections throughout the insular cortex and to superficial and deep layers. Rostral aspects, namely area Ia and rostral regions of area Id, receive the heaviest projections (Amaral & Price, 1984; Carmichael & Price, 1995; Mufson et al., 1981). These connections are generated by the lateral nucleus, the basal nucleus, the accessory basal nucleus, the medial nucleus, the anterior cortical nucleus, the periamygdaloid cortex, and the anterior amygdaloid area (Amaral & Price, 1984; Friedman et al., 1986; Carmichael & Price, 1995; Mufson et al., 1981).

Caudal regions of area Id and area Ig receive fewer projections from the amygdaloid complex (Amaral & Price, 1984; Mufson et al., 1981). Most of these originate in the basal nucleus and the accessory basal nucleus, with a small contribution from the lateral nucleus (Amaral & Price, 1984; Mufson et al., 1981). Weak projections from the basal nucleus and the accessory basal nucleus also terminate in the frontoparietal operculum and the peri-insular cortex (Amaral & Price, 1984).

The insular cortex has been implicated in the mediation of heart rate and in taste and gustatory processing. Given the role of the amygdaloid complex in identifying dangers in the environment, these connections may be a route for gustatory and autonomic information to be processed by the amygdala.

Cingulate Cortex

Moderate projections from the rostral cingulate cortex—particularly areas 24 and 25—terminate in the amygdala (Amaral & Insausti, 1992; Pandya, Van Hoesen, & Domesick, 1973; Stefanacci & Amaral, 2000, 2002; Van Hoesen, 1981). The lateral nucleus and basal nucleus are the main recipients of these projections, but the accessory basal nucleus, the anterior amygdaloid area, and the central nucleus also receive minor projections (Amaral & Insausti, 1992; Pandya et al., 1973; Stefanacci & Amaral, 2000, 2002; Van Hoesen, 1981). The projections mainly originate in the deep layers of the anterior cingulate cortex with a lesser projections from superficial layers (Stefanacci & Amaral, 2000). Caudal aspects of the cingulate cortex do not appear to project to the amygdala (Amaral & Insausti, 1992; Pandya et al., 1973; Stefanacci & Amaral, 2000, 2002; Van Hoesen, 1981).

The amygdala sends a robust projection to rostral, but not caudal, cingulate cortical areas (Amaral & Price, 1984; Porrino et al., 1981; Vogt & Pandya, 1987). The projections originate mainly in the basal nucleus, with a weaker contribution from the lateral nucleus and the accessory basal nucleus, and they target superficial and deep layers (Amaral & Price, 1984; Porrino et al., 1981; Vogt & Pandya, 1987).

Parietal Cortex

There is no evidence of projections to the amygdala from the parietal cortex (Aggleton et al., 1980; Stefanacci & Amaral, 2000, 2002; Turner et al., 1980), and the primate amygdaloid complex does not project extensively to the parietal cortex (Figure 1.5). A very small projection from the basal nucleus and the accessory basal nucleus extends into area 7 (Amaral & Price, 1984), and the magnocellular division of the basal nucleus projects to the medial superior temporal (MST) visual area, which is located in caudal aspects of the parietal lobe (Iwai & Yukie, 1987).

Temporal Cortex

The amygdala has substantial connections with the unimodal and multimodal cortical areas that make up the temporal lobe. Projections from TE, a high-level visual cortical area, terminate mainly in the lateral nucleus of the amygdala, with lighter projections to the basal nucleus, the accessory basal nucleus, and the anterior amygdaloid area (Figure 1.6) (Aggleton et al., 1980; Amaral & Insausti, 1992; Cheng et al., 1997; Ghashghaei & Barbas, 2002; Herzog & Van Hoesen, 1976; Iwai & Yukie, 1987; Iwai, Yukie, Suyama, & Shirakawa, 1987; Jones & Powell, 1970; Stefanacci & Amaral, 2000, 2002; Turner et al., 1980; Van Hoesen, 1981; Van Hoesen & Pandya, 1975; Webster, Ungerleider, & Bachevalier, 1991). The lateral nucleus and the basal nucleus also receive a modest projection from visual area TEO (Stefanacci & Amaral, 2000, 2002; Webster et al., 1991). Only the most rostral subdivisions of auditory area TA project to the amygdala, specifically to the lateral part of middle and caudal aspects of the lateral nucleus (Kosmal, Malinowska, & Kowalska, 1997; Yukie, 2002).

The amygdala also receives projections from multimodal areas of the temporal cortex. Fibers from the perirhinal cortex terminate in the lateral nucleus, the basal nucleus, the magnocellular division of the accessory basal nucleus, the medial nucleus, the anterior cortical nucleus, the posterior cortical nucleus, and the periamygdaloid cortex (Aggleton et al., 1980; Amaral & Insausti, 1992; Iwai & Yukie, 1987; Ghashghaei & Barbas, 2002; Herzog & Van Hoesen, 1976; Stefanacci & Amaral, 2000, 2002; Stefanacci, Suzuki, & Amaral, 1996; Turner et al., 1980; Van Hoesen, 1981; Van Hoesen & Pandya, 1975). A weak projection to the lateral nucleus originates in the parahippocampal cortex (Amaral & Insausti, 1992; Stefanacci & Amaral, 2000; Stefanacci et al., 1996). The polysensory region in the superior temporal gyrus and the dorsal bank of the superior temporal sulcus projects to all divisions of the lateral and basal nuclei. The most rostral aspects of the superior temporal gyrus send additional fibers to the accessory basal nucleus, the anterior amygdaloid area, the central nucleus, the anterior and posterior cortical nuclei, the nucleus of the lateral olfactory tract, the periamygdaloid cortex, and the medial nucleus (Aggleton et al., 1980; Amaral & Insausti, 1992; Ghashghaei & Barbas, 2002; Herzog & Van Hoesen, 1976; Stefanacci & Amaral, 2000, 2002; Turner et al., 1980; Van Hoesen, 1981).

Projections from the amygdala to areas of the temporal cortex are much more widespread than amygdalopetal projections from these areas. The magnocellular and intermediate divisions of the basal nucleus generate heavy projections to temporal cortical areas, and lighter projections arise from the parvicellular division of the basal nucleus, the lateral nucleus, and the accessory

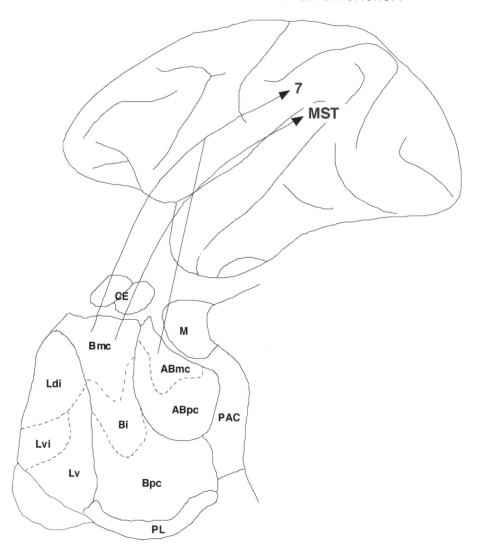

FIGURE 1.5. *Amygdaloid connections with parietal cortex.* The amygdala does not receive projections from any parietal cortical areas. It does send a projection to area 7, a somatosensory area, and the medial superior temporal (MST) visual area, which responds selectively to visual motion. Other abbreviations as in Figure 1.1.

basal nucleus, all via the TOACP to area TE (Figure 1.6) (Amaral, Behniea, & Kelly, 2003; Amaral & Price, 1984; Freese & Amaral, 2005; Webster et al., 1991). These connections are very strong ipsilaterally, but the amygdala does generate a light projection to area TE in the contralateral hemisphere as well (Iwai & Yukie, 1987; Webster et al., 1991). Projections to area TEO originate in the magnocellular and intermediate divisions of the basal nucleus, and terminate only in the ipsilateral hemisphere (Amaral et al., 2003; Amaral & Price, 1984; Freese & Amaral, 2005; Iwai & Yukie, 1987; Webster et al., 1991). The lateral nucleus, basal nucleus, and accessory basal nucleus project to the anterior auditory area TA (Yukie, 2002). In contrast, only the magnocellular and intermediate portions of the basal nucleus send projections to the more caudal areas TC and TAc (Amaral & Price, 1984; Yukie, 2002).

Projections to the perirhinal cortex originate mainly in the lateral nucleus, the basal nucleus, the accessory basal nucleus, and the periamygdaloid cortex, and a lesser projection extends from the medial nucleus and the anterior and posterior cortical nuclei (Amaral & Price, 1984; Iwai & Yukie, 1987; Morán, Mufson, & Mesulam, 1987; Stefanacci et al., 1996; Yukie, 2002). Fibers from the magnocellular division of the basal nucleus terminate in ventral aspects of the parahippocampal cortex, and a minor projection arises from the intermediate and parvicellular divisions of the basal nucleus, the lateral nucleus, the accessory basal nucleus, the periamygdaloid cortex, and the anterior amygdaloid area (Amaral & Price, 1984; Stefanacci et al., 1996). The multimodal areas in the superior temporal gyrus are also strongly connected with the amygdala (Amaral & Price, 1984). These connections with visual, auditory, and multimodal sensory areas are yet another pathway by which the amygdala can participate in sensory processing.

Occipital Cortex

No evidence exists of projections to the amygdala from any area in the occipital lobe (Aggleton et al., 1980; Iwai & Yukie, 1987; Stefanacci & Amaral, 2000; Turner et al., 1980).

The magnocellular division of the basal nucleus is the only part of the amygdala to generate projections to areas of the occipital cortex, including areas V1, V2, V3, and V4 and the middle temporal visual area (Figure 1.6) (Amaral et al., 2003; Amaral & Price, 1984; Freese & Amaral, 2005; Iwai & Yukie, 1987; Mizuno et al., 1981; Tigges et al., 1982; Tigges, Walker, & Tigges, 1983; Weller, Steele, & Kaas, 2002). The projections follow a rostrocaudal topographic organization: Only caudal levels of the magnocellular division project to area V1, while more rostral visual cortices such as area V4 receive projections from middle to caudal levels of the basal nucleus (Amaral et al., 2003; Amaral & Price, 1984; Freese & Amaral, 2005; Iwai & Yukie, 1987). Hence the amygdala maintains significant connections with different levels of visual cortical areas.

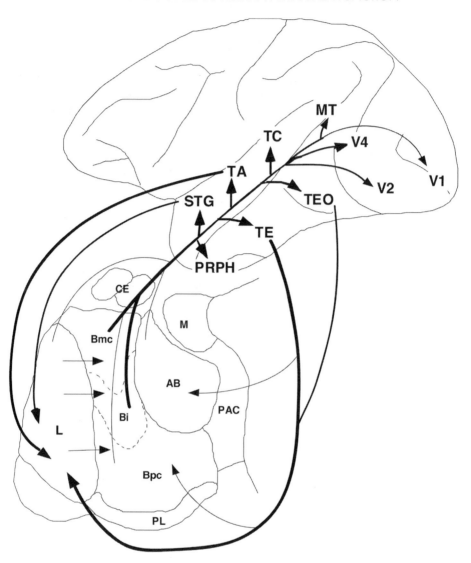

FIGURE 1.6. *Amygdaloid connections with temporal and occipital cortices.* The amygdala receives and sends projections to a variety of unimodal and multimodal areas of the temporal and occipital cortices. Visual inputs to the amygdala arise primarily from rostral areas TEO and area TE. These terminate predominantly in the dorsal half of the lateral nucleus. The lateral nucleus gives rise to a short intrinsic projection to the basal nucleus. The basal nucleus, in turn, gives rise to projections back to the visual cortex. These distribute not only to areas TE and TEO but to essentially all portions of the ventral stream visual pathway and even primary visual cortex (V1). A similar situation applies to the auditory cortex of the superior temporal region. Projections arise from high-end unimodal auditory processing areas (e.g., TA), whereas amygdaloid projections terminate in earlier stages of auditory processing (TC). Abbreviations as in Figure 1.1.

Synaptic Organization of Amygdaloid Connections

Few studies have examined the ultrastructural organization of intrinsic amygdaloid connections, and to date none have been completed in the primate. In cats and rodents, most intra-amygdaloid connections form asymmetric synapses onto spines and shafts, although symmetric synapses are also sometimes observed (Paré, Smith, & Paré, 1995; Savander, Miettinen, LeDoux, & Pitkänen, 1997; Smith & Paré, 1994; Smith, Paré, & Paré, 2000; Stefanacci et al., 1992).

As with intrinsic connections, the details of synaptic connectivity between the amygdala and neocortex in the primate are largely unknown. The only corticoamygdaloid pathway to be examined at the ultrastructural level in the primate is from the frontal cortex. Projections from this area form asymmetric synapses onto spines and distal shafts of amygdaloid neurons (Leichnetz et al., 1976; Smith et al., 2000).

Approximately 84% of amygdalocortical projections to the entorhinal cortex form asymmetric axospinous synapses, and the remaining amygdaloid boutons form asymmetric axodendritic synapses (Pitkänen et al., 2002). Projections from the amygdala to areas TE and V1 form exclusively asymmetric synapses (Freese & Amaral, 2006). Again, spines are the major targets of these fibers.

THE HUMAN AMYGDALA

The human amygdala is not as well studied and characterized as that of the nonhuman primate. In general, the nomenclature of the monkey (Amaral et al., 1992; Price et al., 1987) has been adapted to the human amygdala (Gloor, 1997; Schumann & Amaral, 2005; Sorvari et al., 1995). Like that of the nonhuman primate, the human amygdaloid complex can be divided into 13 nuclei and cortical areas (some of which are illustrated in Figure 1.7). However, the subdivisions of some of these nuclei vary between species. For example, in the monkey, the lateral nucleus is divided into four subdivisions: the dorsal, dorsal intermediate, ventral intermediate, and ventral regions. In the human, this same nucleus contains only two subdivisions, the lateral and medial (Pitkänen & Kemppainen, 2002; Sorvari et al., 1995). Likewise, the calcium-binding proteins parvalbumin, calretinin, and calbindin maintain a similar distribution in the monkey and human amygdala, but also reveal subtle differences in the frequency of cell types (Sorvari et al., 1995, 1996a, 1996b).

For technical reasons, the connectivity of the human amygdala is largely unknown. Diffusion tensor magnetic resonance imaging has confirmed connections between the amygdala and visual cortical areas of the occipital lobe (Catani, Jones, Donato, & Ffytche, 2003). We hope that with the advent of new noninvasive imaging techniques, other intrinsic and extrinsic connections of the human amygdala will be confirmed and uncovered.

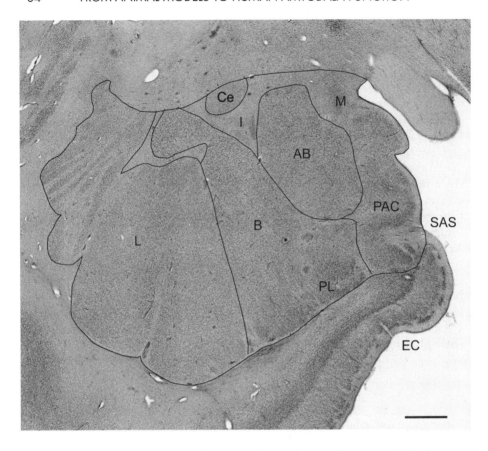

FIGURE 1.7. *The human amygdala.* Nissl-stained coronal section of the human amygdala. Line drawings indicate the borders of nuclei. Scale bar = 2 mm.

WHAT WE THINK

The primate amygdala is privy to sensory information arising from all modalities. In the primate (and presumably in the human), however, it is most heavily influenced by the visual system. The amygdala receives most visual input from the ventral "what" visual pathway, and this information terminates mainly in the lateral nucleus. Our behavioral studies in the rhesus monkey indicate that the amygdala is in large part a danger detector. Sensory information arriving at the lateral nucleus is evaluated in order to determine whether an environmental stimulus is a known or potential danger. This evaluation can also take place via sensory information arriving from other modalities. For example, one can detect a rattlesnake both visually and through the sound of the rattle. Interestingly, visual and auditory information is topographically segregated within the lateral nucleus. Perhaps this allows for a more rapid response to a unimodally defined danger stimulus. There is also the possibility for multimodal convergence within the lateral nucleus. Thus, when a stimulus is particularly subtle, the ventral portion of the lateral nucleus has the potential of integrating across several modalities to disambiguate the stimulus. Of course, this is at the expense of one or more synaptic processing delays.

Once the amygdala has determined that a danger is present, it can orchestrate a whole-body response, which often takes the form of escape. Connections to the neocortex may mediate selective attention to the danger stimulus, whereas projections to the cholinergic basal forebrain may enhance generalized arousal. Projections to the hypothalamus and brainstem, particularly from the central nucleus, can mobilize visceral and autonomic components of an escape response. Projections from the amygdala to the hippocampal formation may enhance memories of particular life episodes that lead to a dangerous event, in order to preclude similar episodes in the future.

One curious component of this scenario is why the evaluation nucleus (the lateral nucleus) does not project heavily to the effector nucleus (the central nucleus); the basal nucleus is interposed. We believe that this may be the case because whether or not a potentially dangerous stimulus elicits an escape response depends on the context in which the stimulus is perceived. The major cortical input to the basal nucleus is from the orbitofrontal cortex, which could provide the context signal. Thus a snake may elicit a fear response if it is encountered along a walk in the forest, but should not elicit the same fear response if it is encountered behind thick Plexiglas at the zoo. The basal nucleus, therefore, gets inputs both from the lateral nucleus and from the orbitofrontal cortex, and potentially acts as a coincidence detector. If a potential danger is detected *and* the individual is in a dangerous situation, the basal nucleus activates the central nucleus, which is the first stage in the fear response. If on the other hand, the context is not dangerous, the fear signal is filtered from reaching the central nucleus. This system is probably subject to both genetic and environmental determinants of a set point. So, for some individuals (e.g., bungee jumpers), typically fearful stimuli do not evoke an escape response; for other individuals (e.g., persons with social phobia), a normally benign stimulus such as another person may be fear-provoking. This scenario also implies that stimuli of all emotional valences must interact with amygdaloid neurons, at least at the level of the lateral nucleus, where evaluation of possible dangers takes place. This may explain why negative stimuli such as fearful faces have a much more powerful effect on the bold signal in the amygdala than neutral or happy faces, since the latter will get no further than the lateral nucleus, whereas the former will activate several synapses throughout the amygdala. Thus, although it is likely that the amygdala participates in a number of other behaviors (e.g., maternal and sexual behavior), we believe that a fundamental and essential role of the amygdala is danger detection.

ACKNOWLEDGMENTS

Original work described in this chapter was supported by Grant No. MH 41479 from the National Institutes of Health.

NOTES

1. We use the terms "amygdala" and "amygdaloid complex" synonymously.
2. We have not adopted the use of the "extended amygdala" concept, but the interested reader is referred to Heimer and Van Hoesen (2006) for a historical overview.

REFERENCES

Adey, W. R., & Meyer, M. (1952). Hippocampal and hypothalamic connexions of the temporal lobe in the monkey. *Brain, 75,* 358–384.

Aggleton, J. P. (1985). A description of intra-amygdaloid connections in Old World monkeys. *Experimental Brain Research, 57,* 390–399.

Aggleton, J. P. (1986). A description of the amygdalo-hippocampal interconnections in the macaque monkey. *Experimental Brain Research, 64,* 515–526.

Aggleton, J. P., Burton, M. J., & Passingham, R. E. (1980). Cortical and subcortical afferents to the amygdala of the rhesus monkey (*Macaca mulatta*). *Brain Research, 190*(2), 347–368.

Aggleton, J. P., & Mishkin, M. (1984). Projections of the amygdala to the thalamus in the cynomolgus monkey. *Journal of Comparative Neurology, 222,* 56–68.

Alheid, G. F., & Heimer, L. (1988). New perspectives in basal forebrain organization of special relevance for neuropsychiatric disorders: The striatopallidal, amygdaloid, and corticopetal components of substantia innominata. *Neuroscience, 27,* 1–39.

Amaral, D. G. (1986). Amygdalohippocampal and amygdalocortical projections in the primate brain. *Advances in Experimental Medicine and Biology, 203,* 3–17.

Amaral, D. G., & Bassett, J. L. (1989). Cholinergic innervation of the monkey amygdala: An immunohistochemical analysis with antisera to choline acetyltransferase. *Journal of Comparative Neurology, 281*(3), 337–361.

Amaral, D. G., Behniea, H., & Kelly, J. L. (2003). Topographic organization of projections from the amygdala to the visual cortex in the macaque monkey. *Neuroscience, 118,* 1099–1120.

Amaral, D. G., & Cowan, W. M. (1980). Subcortical afferents to the hippocampal formation in the monkey. *Journal of Comparative Neurology, 189,* 573–591.

Amaral, D. G., & Insausti, R. (1992). Retrograde transport of D-[³H]-aspartate injected into the monkey amygdaloid complex. *Experimental Brain Research, 88,* 375–388.

Amaral, D. G., & Price, J. L. (1984). Amygdalo-cortical projections in the monkey (*Macaca fascicularis*). *Journal of Comparative Neurology, 230,* 465–496.

Amaral, D. G., Price, J. L., Pitkänen, A., & Carmichael, T. (1992). Anatomical organization of the primate amygdaloid complex. In J. Aggleton (Ed.), *The amygdala: Neurobiological aspects of emotion, memory, and mental dysfunction* (pp. 1–66). New York: Wiley-Liss.

Amaral, D. G., Veazey, R. B., & Cowan, W. M. (1982). Some observations on hypothalamo-amygdaloid connections in the monkey. *Brain Research, 252,* 13–27.

Avendaño, C., Price, J. L., & Amaral, D. G. (1983). Evidence for an amygdaloid projection to premotor cortex but not to motor cortex in the monkey. *Brain Research, 264*(1), 111–117.

Barbas, H., & De Olmos, J. (1990). Projections from the amygdala to basoventral and mediodorsal prefrontal regions in the rhesus monkey. *Journal of Comparative Neurology, 300*(4), 549–571.

Barger, N., Stefanacci, L., & Semendeferi, K. (2007). A comparative volumetric analysis of the amygdaloid complex and basolateral division in the human and ape brain. *American Journal of Physical Anthropology, 134*, 392–402.

Baylis, L. L., Rolls, E. T., & Baylis, G. C. (1995). Afferent connections of the caudolateral orbitofrontal cortex taste area of the primate. *Neuroscience, 64*, 801–812.

Canteras, N. S., Simerly, R. B., & Swanson, L. W. (1995). Organization of projections from the medial nucleus of the amygdala: A PHA-L study in the rat. *Journal of Comparative Neurology, 360*, 213–245.

Carmichael, S. T., & Price, J. L. (1995). Limbic connections of the orbital and medial prefrontal cortex in macaque monkeys. *Journal of Comparative Neurology, 363*(4), 615–641.

Catani, M., Jones, D. K., Donato, R., & Ffytche, D. H. (2003). Occipito-temporal connections in the human brain. *Brain, 126*(Pt. 9), 2093–2107.

Cavada, C., Compañy, T., Tejedor, J., Cruz-Rizzolo, R. J., & Reinoso-Suarez, F. (2000). The anatomical connections of the macaque monkey orbitofrontal cortex. A review. *Cerebral Cortex, 10*(3), 220–242.

Cheng, K., Saleem, K. S., & Tanaka, K. (1997). Organization of corticostriatal and corticoamygdalar projections arising from the anterior inferotemporal area TE of the macaque monkey: A *Phaseolus vulgaris*-leucoagglutinin study. *Journal of Neuroscience, 17*, 7902–7925.

Cowan, W. M., Raisman, G., & Powell, T. P. (1965). The connexions of the amygdala. *Journal of Neurology, Neurosurgery, and Psychiatry, 28*, 137–151.

De Olmos, J., Hardy, H., & Heimer, L. (1978). The afferent connections of the main and the accessory olfactory bulb formations in the rat: An experimental HRP-study. *Journal of Comparative Neurology, 181*(2), 213–244.

De Olmos, J. S., & Heimer, L. (1999). The concepts of the ventral striatopallidal system and extended amygdala. *Annals of the New York Academy of Sciences, 877*, 1–32.

Dong, H. W., Petrovich, G. D., & Swanson, L. W. (2001). Topography of projections from amygdala to bed nuclei of the stria terminalis. *Brain Research Reviews, 38*, 192–246.

Freese, J. L., & Amaral, D. G. (2005). The organization of projections from the amygdala to visual cortical areas TE and V1 in the macaque monkey. *Journal of Comparative Neurology, 486*, 295–317.

Freese, J. L., & Amaral, D. G. (2006). Synaptic organization of projections from the amygdala to visual cortical areas TE and V1 in the macaque monkey. *Journal of Comparative Neurology, 496*(5), 655–667.

Friedman, D. P., Murray, E. A., O'Neill, J. B., & Mishkin, M. (1986). Cortical connections of the somatosensory fields of the lateral sulcus of macaques: Evidence for a corticolimbic pathway for touch. *Journal of Comparative Neurology, 252*(3), 323–347.

Fudge, J. L., Kunishio, K., Walsh, P., Richard, C., & Haber, S. N. (2002). Amygdaloid projections to ventromedial striatal subterritories in the primate. *Neuroscience, 110*(2), 257–275.

Ghashghaei, H. T., & Barbas, H. (2002). Pathways for emotion: Interactions of prefrontal and anterior temporal pathways in the amygdala of the rhesus monkey. *Neuroscience, 115*(4), 1261–1279.

Gloor, P. (1997). The amygdaloid system. In P. Gloor (Ed.), *The temporal lobe and limbic system* (pp. 591–721). New York: Oxford University Press.

Grove, E. A. (1988). Efferent connections of the substantia innominata in the rat. *Journal of Comparative Neurology, 277,* 347–364.

Heimer, L., & Van Hoesen, G. W. (2006). The limbic lobe and its output channels: Implications for emotional functions and adaptive behavior. *Neuroscience and Biobehavioral Reviews, 30*(2), 126–147.

Herzog, A. G., & Van Hoesen, G. W. (1978). Temporal neocortical afferent connections to the amygdala in the rhesus monkey. *Brain Research, 115,* 57–69.

Hilton, S. M., & Zbrozyna, A. W. (1963). Amygdaloid region for defense reactions and its efferent pathway to the brain stem. *Journal of Physiology, 165,* 160–173.

Holstege, G., Meiners, L., & Tan, K. (1985). Projections of the bed nucleus of the stria terminalis to the mesencephalon, pons, and medulla oblongata in the cat. *Experimental Brain Research, 58,* 379–391.

Hopkins, D. A. (1975). Amygdalotegmental projections in the rat, cat and rhesus monkey. *Neuroscience Letters, 1,* 263–270.

Insausti, R., Amaral, D. G., & Cowan, W. M. (1987). The entorhinal cortex of the monkey: III. Subcortical afferents. *Journal of Comparative Neurology, 264,* 396–408.

Ishikawa, I., Kawamura, S., & Tanaka, O. (1969). An experimental study on the efferent connections of the amygdaloid complex in the cat. *Acta Medica Okayama, 23,* 519–539.

Iwai, E., & Yukie, M. (1987). Amygdalofugal and amygdalopetal connections with modality-specific visual cortical areas in macaques (*Macaca fuscata, M. mulatta,* and *M. fascicularis*). *Journal of Comparative Neurology, 261*(3), 362–387.

Iwai, E., Yukie, M., Suyama, H., & Shirakawa, S. (1987). Amygdalar connections with middle and inferior temporal gyri of the monkey. *Neuroscience Letters, 83,* 25–29.

Jimenez-Castellanos, J. (1949). The amygdaloid complex in monkey studies by reconstructional methods. *Journal of Comparative Neurology, 91*(3), 507–526.

Johnston, J. B. (1923). Further contributions to the study of the evolution of the forebrain. *Journal of Comparative Neurology, 35,* 337–481.

Jones, E. G., & Burton, H. (1976). A projection from the medial pulvinar to the amygdala in primates. *Brain Research, 104,* 142–147.

Jones, E. G., Burton, H., Saper, C. B., & Swanson, L. W. (1976). Midbrain, diencephalic and cortical relationships of the basal nucleus of Meynert and associated structures in primates. *Journal of Comparative Neurology, 167,* 385–419.

Jones, E. G., & Powell, T. P. (1970). An anatomical study of converging sensory pathways within the cerebral cortex of the monkey. *Brain, 93,* 793–820.

Jongen-Relo, A. L., & Amaral, D. G. (1998). Evidence for a GABAergic projection from the central nucleus of the amygdala to the brainstem of the macaque monkey: A combined retrograde tracing and *in situ* hybridization study. *European Journal of Neuroscience, 10*(9), 2924–2933.

Kosmal, A. Malinowski, M., & Kowalska, D. M. (1997). Thalamic and amygdaloid connections of the auditory association cortex of the superior temporal gyrus in rhesus monkey (*Macaca mulatta*). *Acta Neurobiologiae Experimentalis (Wars), 57,* 165–188.

Leichnetz, G. R., & Astruc, J. (1976). The efferent projections of the medial pre-frontal cortex in the squirrel monkey (*Saimiri sciureus*). *Brain Research, 109*(3), 455–472.

Leichnetz, G. R., & Astruc, J. (1977). The course of some prefrontal corticofugals to the pallidum, substantia innominata, and amygdaloid complex in monkeys. *Experimental Neurology, 54*, 104–109.

Leichnetz, G. R., Povlishock, J. T., & Astruc, J. (1976). A prefronto-amygdaloid pro-jection in the monkey: Light and electron microscopic evidence. *Neuroscience Letters, 2*, 261–265.

Luskin, M. B., & Price, J. L. (1983). The topographic organization of associational fibers of the olfactory system in the rat, including centrifugal fibers to the olfac-tory bulb. *Journal of Comparative Neurology, 216*, 264–291.

MacLean, P. D. (1970). The triune brain, emotion, and scientific bias. In F. O. Schmitt (Ed.), *Neurosciences: Second study program* (pp. 336–349). New York: Rock-efeller University Press.

McDonald, A. J. (1992). Cell types and intrinsic connections of the amygdala. In J. Aggleton (Ed.), *The amygdala: Neurobiological aspects of emotion, memory, and mental dysfunction* (pp. 67–96). New York: Wiley-Liss.

McDonald, A. J. (1998). Cortical pathways to the mammalian amygdala. *Progress in Neurobiology, 55*, 257–332.

McDonald, A. J., Shammah-Lagnado, S. J., Shi, C., & Davis, M. (1999). Cortical afferents to the extended amygdala. *Annals of the New York Academy of Sci-ences, 877*, 309–338.

Mehler, W. R. (1980). Subcortical afferent connections of the amygdala in the mon-key. *Journal of Comparative Neurology, 190*, 733–762.

Mesulam, M. M., Mufson, E. J., Levey, A. I., & Wainer, B. H. (1983). Cholinergic innervation of cortex by the basal forebrain: Cytochemistry and cortical con-nections of the septal area, diagonal band nuclei, nucleus basalis (substantia innominata), and hypothalamus in the rhesus monkey. *Journal of Comparative Neurology, 214*(2), 170–197.

Mizuno, N., Takahashi, O., Satoda, T., & Matsushima, R. (1985). Amygdalospinal projections in the macaque monkey. *Neuroscience Letters, 53*(3), 327–330.

Mizuno, N., Uchida, K., Nomura, S., Nakamura, Y., Sugimoto, T., & Uemura-Sumi, M. (1981). Extrageniculate projections to the visual cortex in the macaque mon-key: An HRP study. *Brain Research, 212*, 454–459.

Moga, M. M., Herbert, H., Hurley, K. M., Yasui, Y., Gray, T. S., & Saper, C. B. (1990). Organization of cortical, basal forebrain, and hypothalamic afferents to the parabrachial nucleus in the rat. *Journal of Comparative Neurology, 295*, 624–661.

Morán, M. A., Mufson, E. J., & Mesulam, M. M. (1987). Neural inputs into the temporopolar cortex of the rhesus monkey. *Journal of Comparative Neurology, 256*, 88–103.

Morecraft, R. J., Geula, C., & Mesulam, M. M. (1992). Cytoarchitecture and neural afferents of orbitofrontal cortex in the brain of the monkey. *Journal of Compara-tive Neurology, 323*, 341–358.

Mufson, E. J., Mesulam, M. M., & Pandya, D. N. (1981). Insular interconnections with the amygdala in the rhesus monkey. *Neuroscience, 6*, 1231–1248.

Nauta, W. J. H. (1962). Neural associations of the amygdaloid complex in the mon-key. *Brain, 85*, 505–520.

Norita, M., & Kawamura, K. (1980). Subcortical afferents to the monkey amygdala: An HRP study. *Brain Research, 190*, 225–230.

Ottersen, O. P. (1982). Connections of the amygdala of the rat: IV. Corticoamygdaloid and intraamygdaloid connections as studied with axonal transport of horseradish peroxidase. *Journal of Comparative Neurology, 205*(1), 30–48.

Pandya, K. N., Van Hoesen, G. W., & Domesick, V. B. (1973). A cingulo-amygdaloid projection in the rhesus monkey. *Brain Research, 61*, 369–373.

Paré, D., Quirk, G. J., & LeDoux, J. E. (2004). New vistas on amygdala networks in conditioned fear. *Journal of Neurophysiology, 92*(1), 1–9.

Paré, D., Smith, Y., & Paré, J. F. (1995). Intra-amygdaloid projections of the basolateral and basomedial nuclei in the cat: *Phaseolus vulgaris*-leucoagglutinin anterograde tracing at the light and electron microscopic level. *Neuroscience, 69*, 567–583.

Parent, A., Mackey, A., & De Bellefeuille, L. (1983). The subcortical afferents to caudate nucleus and putamen in primate: A fluorescent retrograde double labeling study. *Neuroscience, 10*, 1137–1150.

Pitkänen, A., & Amaral, D. G. (1991). Demonstration of projections from the lateral nucleus to the basal nucleus of the amygdala: A PHA-L study in the monkey. *Experimental Brain Research, 83*, 465–470.

Pitkänen, A., & Amaral, D. G. (1998). Organization of the intrinsic connections of the monkey amygdaloid complex: Projections originating in the lateral nucleus. *Journal of Comparative Neurology, 398*(3), 431–458.

Pitkänen, A., Kelly, J. L., & Amaral, D. G. (2002). Projections from the lateral, basal, and accessory basal nuclei of the amygdala to the entorhinal cortex in the macaque monkey. *Hippocampus, 12*(2), 186–205.

Pitkänen, A., & Kemppainen, S. (2002). Comparison of the distribution of calcium-binding proteins and intrinsic connectivity in the lateral nucleus of the rat, monkey, and human amygdala. *Pharmacology, Biochemistry, and Behavior, 71*, 369–377.

Porrino, L. J., Crane, A. M., & Goldman-Rakic, P. S. (1981). Direct and indirect pathways from the amygdala to the frontal lobe in the rhesus monkey. *Journal of Comparative Neurology, 198*, 121–136.

Price, J. L. (1973). An autoradiographic study of complementary laminar patterns of termination of afferent fibers to the olfactory cortex. *Journal of Comparative Neurology, 150*(1), 87–108.

Price, J. L. (1986). Subcortical projections from the amygdaloid complex. In Y. Ben-Air & R. Schwartz (Eds.), *Excitatory amino acids and epilepsy* (pp. 19–33). New York: Plenum Press.

Price, J. L., & Amaral, D. G. (1981). An autoradiographic study of the projections of the central nucleus of the monkey amygdala. *Journal of Neuroscience, 1*(11), 1242–1259.

Price, J. L., Russchen, F. T., & Amaral, D. G. (1987). The limbic region: II. The amygdaloid complex. In A. Bjorklund, T. Hokfelt, & L. W. Swanson (Eds.), *Handbook of chemical neuroanatomy: Vol. 5. Integrated systems of the CNS* (Part I, pp. 279–388). Amsterdam: Elsevier Science.

Rosene, D. L., & Van Hoesen, G. W. (1977). Hippocampal efferents reach widespread areas of cerebral cortex and amygdala in the rhesus monkey. *Science, 198*, 315–317.

Royer, S., Martina, M., & Paré, D. (1999). An inhibitory interface gates impulse traffic between the input and output stations of the amygdala. *Journal of Neuroscience, 19*(23), 10575–10583.

Royer, S., & Paré, D. (2002). Bidirectional synaptic plasticity in intercalated amygdala neurons and the extinction of conditioned fear responses. *Neuroscience, 115*(2), 455–462.

Russchen, F. T., Amaral, D. G., & Price, J. L. (1985). The afferent connections of the substantia innominata in the monkey, *Macaca fascicularis. Journal of Comparative Neurology, 242*(1), 1–27.

Russchen, F. T., Amaral, D. G., & Price, J. L. (1987). The afferent input to the magnocellular division of the mediodorsal thalamic nucleus in the monkey, *Macaca fascicularis. Journal of Comparative Neurology, 256*(2), 175–210.

Russchen, F. T., Bakst, I., Amaral, D. G., & Price, J. L. (1985). The amygdalostriatal projections in the monkey: An anterograde tracing study. *Brain Research, 329*(1–2), 241–257.

Saunders, R. C., Rosene, D. L., & Van Hoesen, G. W. (1988). Comparison of the efferents of the amygdala and the hippocampal formation in the rhesus monkey: II. Reciprocal and non-reciprocal connections. *Journal of Comparative Neurology, 271*(2), 185–207.

Savander, V., Miettinen, R., LeDoux, J. E., & Pitkänen, A. (1997). Lateral nucleus of the rat amygdala is reciprocally connected with basal and accessory basal nuclei: A light and electron microscopic study. *Neuroscience, 77*, 767–781.

Schumann, C. M., & Amaral, D. G. (2005). Stereological estimation of the number of neurons in the human amygdaloid complex. *Journal of Comparative Neurology, 491*, 320–329.

Schwanzel-Fukuda, M., Morrell, J. I., & Pfaff, D. W. (1984). Localization of forebrain neurons which project directly to the medulla and spinal cord of the rat by retrograde tracing with wheat germ agglutinin. *Journal of Comparative Neurology, 226*, 1–20.

Smith, Y., & Paré, D. (1994). Intra-amygdaloid projections of the lateral nucleus in the cat: PHA-L anterograde labeling combined with postembedding GABA and glutamate immunocytochemistry. *Journal of Comparative Neurology, 342*, 232–248.

Smith, Y., Paré, J. F., & Paré, D. (2000). Differential innervation of parvalbumin-immunoreactive interneurons of the basolateral amygdaloid complex by cortical and intrinsic inputs. *Journal of Comparative Neurology, 416*, 496–508.

Sorvari, H., Soininen, H., Paljarvi, L., Karkola, K., & Pitkänen, A. (1995). Distribution of parvalbumin-immunoreactive cells and fibers in the human amygdaloid complex. *Journal of Comparative Neurology, 360*, 185–212.

Sorvari, H., Soininen, H., & Pitkänen, A. (1996a). Calbindin-D28K-immunoreactive cells and fibres in the human amygdaloid complex. *Neuroscience, 75*, 421–443.

Sorvari, H., Soininen, H., & Pitkänen, A. (1996b). Calretinin-immunoreactive cells and fibers in the human amygdaloid complex. *Journal of Comparative Neurology, 369*, 188–208.

Stefanacci, L., & Amaral, D. G. (2000). Topographic organization of cortical inputs to the lateral nucleus of the macaque monkey amygdala: A retrograde tracing study. *Journal of Comparative Neurology, 421*(1), 52–79.

Stefanacci, L., & Amaral, D. G. (2002). Some observations on cortical inputs to the macaque monkey amygdala: An anterograde tracing study. *Journal of Comparative Neurology, 451*(4), 301–323.

Stefanacci, L., Farb, C. R., Pitkänen, A., Go, G., LeDoux, J. E., & Amaral, D. G. (1992). Projections from the lateral nucleus to the basal nucleus of the amygdala: A light and electron microscopic PHA-L study in the rat. *Journal of Comparative Neurology, 323,* 586–601.

Stefanacci, L., Suzuki, W. A., & Amaral, D. G. (1996). Organization of connections between the amygdaloid complex and the perirhinal and parahippocampal cortices in macaque monkeys. *Journal of Comparative Neurology, 375,* 552–582.

Stephan, H., Frahm, H. D., & Baron, G. (1987). Comparison of brain structure volumes in Insectivora and primates: VII. Amygdaloid components. *Journal für Hirnforsch, 28*(5), 571–584.

Tigges, J., Tigges, M., Cross, N. A., McBride, R. L., Letbetter, W. D., & Anschel, S. (1982). Subcortical structures projecting to visual cortical areas in squirrel monkey. *Journal of Comparative Neurology, 209,* 29–40.

Tigges, J., Walker, L. C., & Tigges, M. (1983). Subcortical projections to the occipital and parietal lobes of the chimpanzee brain. *Journal of Comparative Neurology, 220,* 106–115.

Turner, B. H., Gupta, K. C., & Mishkin, M. (1978). The locus and cytoarchitecture of the projection areas of the olfactory bulb in *Macaca mulatta. Journal of Comparative Neurology, 177,* 381–396.

Turner, B. H., Mishkin, M., & Knapp, M. (1980). Organization of the amygdalopetal projections from modality-specific cortical association areas in the monkey. *Journal of Comparative Neurology, 191,* 515–543.

Van Hoesen, G. W. (1981). The differential distribution, diversity and sprouting of cortical projections to the amygdala in the rhesus monkey. In Y. Ben-Ari (Ed.), *The amygdaloid complex* (pp. 77–90). Amsterdam: Elsevier/North Holland.

Van Hoesen, G. W., & Pandya, D. N. (1975). Some connections of the entorhinal (area 28) and perirhinal (area 35) cortices of the rhesus monkey. III. Efferent connections. *Brain Research, 95,* 3959.

Vogt, B. A., & Pandya, D. N. (1987). Cingulate cortex of the rhesus monkey: II. Cortical efferents. *Journal of Comparative Neurology, 262,* 271–289.

Webster, M. J., Ungerleider, L. G., & Bachevalier, J. (1991). Connections of inferior temporal areas TE and TEO with medial temporal-lobe structures in infant and adult monkeys. *Journal of Neuroscience, 11,* 1095–1116.

Weller, R. E., Steele, G. E., & Kaas, J. H. (2002). Pulvinar and other subcortical connections of dorsolateral visual cortex in monkeys. *Journal of Comparative Neurology, 450,* 215–240.

Witter, M. P., & Amaral, D. G. (1991). Entorhinal cortex of the monkey: V. Projections to the dentate gyrus, hippocampus, and subicular complex. *Journal of Comparative Neurology, 307*(3), 437–459.

Yukie, M. (2002). Connections between the amygdala and auditory cortical areas in the macaque monkey. *Neuroscience Research, 42*(3), 219–229.

CHAPTER 2

The Human Amygdala
INSIGHTS FROM OTHER ANIMALS

Joseph E. LeDoux and Daniela Schiller

Research on the human brain is often based on findings from studies in experimental animals, where the nervous system can be explored in greater detail. This was especially true before the advent of functional imaging, which has greatly enhanced the ability to study the human brain. However, even functional imaging is more limited than animal research in the level of precision at which the brain can be examined. Research on the amygdala provides an excellent example of this point. The basic findings regarding the functions of the amygdala obtained from studies of animals have been found to apply, at least in a first approximation, to the human amygdala. However, whereas the animal studies have revealed that different nuclei and even subnuclei of the amygdala contribute uniquely to certain functions, studies of the human amygdala have mainly been at the level of the whole region—that is, at the level of "the amygdala." Human researchers hope that technical advances, such as high-resolution imaging and other approaches yet to be developed, will also allow explorations of subareas within the amygdala. In this chapter, we therefore give an overview, based on animal research, of the anatomical organization of the amygdala, including its nuclei and subnuclei and their connectivity, and then discuss certain functions associated with these anatomical entities.

ANATOMICAL ORGANIZATION AND NOMENCLATURE

The amygdaloid region of the brain (the amygdala) was identified in the early 19th century (Burdach, 1819–1822). The name "amygdala," derived from the Greek, was meant to denote an almond-shaped structure in the medial temporal lobe. The almond-shaped area is now recognized to be a subdivision of the amygdala rather than the whole region (Swanson & Petrovich, 1998). Nevertheless, the term "amygdala" refers to the larger area (Plate 2.1 in color insert).

Traditionally, the amygdala has been thought of as consisting of two broad subdivisions (Johnston, 1923). This partition was based on evolutionary criteria that identified a phylogenetically primitive division associated with the olfactory system (the central, medial, and cortical nuclei) and an evolutionarily newer division associated with the neocortex (the lateral, basal, and accessory basal nuclei) (Plate 2.2 in color insert). These can be called the centrocorticomedial and the basolateral divisions. Each of these in turn is composed of several distinct nuclei.

Nuclei within brain areas like the amygdala are typically distinguished on the basis of histological criteria, such as the density, configuration, shape, and size of stained cells; the trajectory of fibers passing through; and/or chemical signatures (Plate 2.3 in color insert). On the basis of such criteria, a dozen or so distinct nuclear divisions have been identified (e.g., Alheid & Heimer, 1988; Amaral, Price, Pitkänen, & Carmichael, 1992; McDonald, 1998; Pitkänen, Savander, & LeDoux, 1997). Thus the centrocorticomedial region is made up of the cortical, medial, and central nuclei, whereas the basolateral region consists of the lateral, basal, and accessory basal nuclei. Other nuclei, such as the intercalated nuclei or the intra-amygdala nucleus of the stria terminalis, are situated between the main nuclei.

It is easy to be confused by the terminology used to describe the amygdala nuclei, as different sets of terms are used. This problem is especially acute with regard to the basolateral region of the amygdala. One popular scheme refers to the basolateral region as consisting of the "lateral," "basal," and "accessory basal" nuclei. Another scheme uses the terms "basolateral" and "basomedial" nuclei to refer to the regions named as the "basal" and "accessory basal" nuclei in the first scheme. Particularly confusing is the use of the term "basolateral" to refer both to a specific nucleus (the basal or basolateral nucleus) and to the larger region that includes the lateral, basal, and accessory basal nuclei (the basolateral complex).

In the interest of facilitating cross-species comparisons, since the field is attempting to use findings about amygdala nuclei in animals to understand the functions of amygdala nuclei in humans, it is important that the nuclei be labeled similarly in different species. In rats, the species in which much work has been conducted, the "lateral," "basolateral," and "basomedial" terminology was used to label the basolateral complex. However, for consistency with primates, including humans, the terms "lateral," "basal," and "accessory basal" are now more often used in rats (Amaral et al., 1992; Pitkänen, 2000; Pitkänen et al., 1997).

Each of the amygdala nuclei can be further partitioned into subnuclei (Amaral et al., 1992; Pitkänen, 2000; Pitkänen et al., 1997). For example, in rats and monkeys, the lateral nucleus has three major divisions: dorsal, ventro-lateral, and medial (Plate 2.4 in color insert). Further division is also possible: In rats, the dorsal subdivision has been divided into a superior and an inferior region, based on physiological results showing that cells in the superior and inferior parts are involved in different aspects of fear memory (the superior part in learning, and the inferior part in long-term storage) (Repa et al., 2001).

Given that the nuclei can be grouped, and that the resolution of imaging studies is still at the level of the whole amygdala, why bother with nuclei, much less subnuclei? The short answer is that if it is likely that the nuclear and subnuclear organization of the rat and monkey brain is likely to apply to the human brain, the information may therefore be highly relevant for interpretation of human results, even when the human studies themselves cannot parse the amygdala at the finer level.

In recent years, several researchers have attempted to rethink the organization of the amygdala. One view is that the central and medial amygdala extend into the basal forebrain to form a continuum with the lateral and medial nuclei of the bed nucleus of the stria terminals (Heimer, 2003). Another recent proposal argues that the amygdala is neither a structural nor a functional unit, and instead consists of regions that belong to other regions or systems of the brain (Swanson & Petrovich, 1998). For example, in this scheme, the nuclei of the basolateral complex are viewed as nuclear extensions of the cortex (rather than as amygdala regions related to the cortex), whereas the central, medial, and cortical amygdala are said to be ventral extensions of the striatum. This scheme has merit, but the present chapter focuses on the organization and function of the nuclei and subnuclei that are traditionally said to be part of the amygdala, since most of the functions of the amygdala are understood in these terms. For example, the lateral nucleus will continue to be an important region in fear learning (see below) even if the concept of the amygdala is eliminated.

CONNECTIONS

Each nucleus of the amygdala has unique inputs and outputs. Given that the connectivity of a region defines its functions, differences in connectivity are an important way of identifying functional entities. A thorough discussion of all the connections of the various amygdala nuclei is beyond the present scope; instead, a few key examples are given. The emphasis is on connections of the rat amygdala (Pitkänen, 2000; Pitkänen et al., 1997). The primate, including human, amygdala has similar connectivity (Amaral et al., 1992), though some differences also exist (Petrovich, Risold, & Swanson, 1996).

The lateral amygdala is generally viewed as the sensory interface of the amygdala (Amaral et al., 1992; Heimer & Van Hoesen, 2006; LeDoux, Cicchetti, Xagoraris, & Romanski, 1990; McDonald, 1998; Turner & Herkenham, 1991). It is the major site receiving inputs from the visual, auditory, somatosensory (including pain), olfactory, and taste systems (olfactory and taste information is also transmitted by other nuclei as well). Other amygdala regions receive inputs from other brain areas, allowing diverse kinds of information to be processed by the amygdala (Plate 2.5 in color insert).

Because the auditory input connections of the amygdala have been studied most thoroughly, these are described in detail (Plate 2.6 in color insert). The auditory thalamus and cortex both project to the lateral nucleus, where the inputs converge onto single cells (LeDoux, Ruggiero, & Reis, 1985; LeDoux, Farb, & Ruggiero, 1990; Romanski, Clugnet, Bordi, & LeDoux, 1993; Romanski & LeDoux, 1993). The thalamic neurons that project directly to the lateral amygdala are in extralemniscal areas that weakly encode frequency properties of the auditory stimulus (Bordi & LeDoux, 1994a). These provide a rapid but imprecise auditory signal to the amygdala (LeDoux, Farb, & Romanski, 1991). Cortical inputs from the auditory and other sensory systems arise from the association areas rather than from the primary cortical regions (McDonald, 1998; Romanski & LeDoux, 1993; Turner, Mishkin, & Knapp, 1980). These provide the amygdala with a more elaborate representation than the thalamic inputs, but are slower because more numerous synaptic connections are involved (thalamus to primary cortex, primary cortex to association cortex, intra-association cortex connections, and ultimately association cortex to amygdala).

The sensory inputs to the lateral amygdala terminate most extensively in the dorsal subregion (Romanski et al., 1993). The dorsal subregion communicates with the ventrolateral and medial areas, which then connect with other amygdala areas (Pitkänen et al., 1997). Particularly important are connections from lateral amygdala subnuclei to the central and basal nuclei.

The central nucleus is believed to be an important output region for the expression of innate emotional responses and associated physiological responses (Kapp, Whalen, Supple, & Pascoe, 1992). Connections between the lateral and central nuclei are thus important (Plate 2.7 in color insert). There are some direct connections from the lateral nucleus to the central nucleus, but these are relatively sparse (Pitkänen et al., 1997; Smith & Paré, 1994). The main channels of communication between the lateral and the central nuclei are thus thought to involve connections from the medial part of the lateral nucleus to other amygdala nuclei, which then connect with the central nucleus (Pitkänen et al., 1997). For example, the lateral nucleus projects to the basal nucleus, which projects to the central nucleus. In addition, both the lateral and basal nuclei project to the intercalated cells, which then connect with the central nucleus (Paré, Royer, Smith, & Lang, 2003). The expression of emotional responses via outputs of the central amygdala involves connections from the medial subdivision of the central nucleus to brainstem areas that control specific behavioral and physiological control systems. Output connections are shown in Plate 2.8 (in color insert).

Another important set of output connections of the amygdala arises from the basal nucleus (Plate 2.8 in color insert). In addition to connecting with the central nucleus, the basal nucleus connects with striatal areas involved in the control of instrumental behaviors (Everitt & Robbins, 1992; Fudge, Kunishio, Walsh, Richard, & Haber, 2002; Pitkänen et al., 1997; Russchen, Bakst, Amaral, & Price, 1985). Thus, while the output connections of the central amygdala to the brainstem are involved in controlling emotional reactions (e.g., freezing in the presence of a predator), connections from the basal amygdala to the striatum are involved in controlling actions (e.g., running to safety or toward food) (Amorapanth, LeDoux, & Nader, 2000; Cardinal, Parkinson, Hall, & Everitt, 2002; Everitt et al., 1999; Killcross, Robbins, & Everitt, 1997; Nader, Majidishad, Amorapanth, & LeDoux, 2001).

Before we end this discussion of connectivity, it is important to consider a potential source of confusion in cross-species comparisons, especially as we attempt to build functional bridges between the rat and human amygdala. As noted above, an important step is to use the same terminology to describe the nuclei in rats and primates. Fortunately, the primate amygdala terminology is being used more and more often in studies of rats. But brain regions that provide inputs to the amygdala are not always consistently labeled across species. For example, studies of rats have shown in great detail that the posterior intralaminar nucleus is adjacent to and is functionally part of the auditory thalamus (Bordi & LeDoux, 1994b; LeDoux, Farb, & Ruggiero, 1990); that its cells send auditory inputs to the lateral amygdala (Bordi & LeDoux, 1994a; LeDoux, Farb, & Ruggiero, 1990); and that these projections play an important role in the conditioning of fear responses to auditory stimuli (LeDoux, 2000; LeDoux, Cicchetti, et al., 1990). In primates, there is also a region that projects to the lateral amygdala and that is adjacent to the auditory thalamus, but it is called the peripenduncluar region and is usually considered a nonspecific brainstem nucleus (Aggleton, Burton, & Passingham, 1980). It is likely, though, that this region is functionally equivalent to the posterior intralaminar nucleus. As such, it probably provides the lateral amygdala with subcortical auditory inputs. This digression is important, because the existence of subcortical sensory inputs to the amygdala has been questioned in primates (Pessoa & Ungerleider, 2004). Although much of the debate in primates has been about the visual modality, the lesson from the auditory system is that terminological and empirical issues need to be very carefully addressed before any conclusions are drawn. A further reason to pursue this issue empirically, especially physiologically, in primates is that the lateral amygdala receives inputs from various thalamic areas that are loosely associated with the visual system, the way the posterior intralaminar nucleus is loosely associated with the auditory system (Doron & LeDoux, 1999; LeDoux et al., 1985). Included are regions of the posterior thalamus such as the suprageniculate nucleus and pulvinar, as well as some cells in the dorsal division of the medial geniculate body, which is traditionally auditory in nature but is believed to subserve some visual functions as well.

CELLULAR ACTIVITY

Anatomical organization and connectivity suggest functions, but cellular activity in a region begins to reveal exactly what functions the region participates in. Although the amygdala has been studied far less at the cellular level than regions such as the hippocampus, neocortex, or cerebellum, some progress has been made.

Cells in the amygdala are known to be relatively "silent." That is, the cells have low baseline levels of activity (Ben-Ari, Le Galla Salle, & Champagnat, 1974; Bordi, LeDoux, Clugnet, & Pavlides, 1993; Clugnet, LeDoux, & Morrison, 1990; Paré & Gaudreau, 1996). Novel stimuli elicit responses, but these rapidly habituate if the stimulus is repeated (Ben-Ari et al., 1974; Clugnet et al., 1990). As we discuss later, this inhibition can be overcome when a novel stimulus is presented in association with a significant event. In this case, rather than dissipating, the responses are potentiated.

Most of the inputs to the amygdala involve excitatory pathways that use glutamate as a transmitter (Farb & LeDoux, 1999; Li, Stutzmann, & LeDoux, 1996; McDonald, 1994). These inputs form synaptic connections on the dendrites of excitatory principal neurons that transmit signals to other regions or subregions of the amygdala or to extrinsic regions. Principal neurons are thus also called projection neurons, since they project out. However, axons of principal neurons also give rise to local connections to inhibitory interneurons, which then provide feedback inhibition to the principal neurons (Muller, Mascagni, & McDonald, 2006). In addition to terminating on projection neurons, some of the excitatory inputs to the amygdala terminate on local inhibitory interneurons, which in turn connect with principal neurons; this sequence gives rise to feedforward inhibition (Bissière, Humeau, & Lüthi, 2003; Li, Armony, & LeDoux, 1996; Woodson, Farb, & LeDoux, 2000). These connections allow stimulus-driven inhibition to build up and account for the decrease in responses when stimuli are repeated.

The so-called "silence" of the amygdala observed in animal studies refers to the activity of excitatory projection neurons. These are strongly inhibited by gamma-aminobutyric acid-ergic (GABAergic) interneurons (Bauer & LeDoux, 2004; Bissière et al., 2003; McDonald, 1985; Paré & Gaudreau, 1996; Woodruff, Monyer, & Sah, 2006). The interneurons are thus not silent, but are more difficult to record from because they are smaller.

The inhibition of excitation by interneurons prevents projection cells from firing action potentials to irrelevant stimuli. Only significant stimuli get past the inhibitory gate. Significance can come from innate wiring (i.e., from so-called "prepared" stimuli that elicit fear or other emotional responses with no or limited prior exposure) or from associative learning (see below). Functional magnetic resonance imaging (fMRI) blood-oxygen-level-dependent (BOLD) signals do not distinguish inhibitory from excitatory activity. The relation between projection and inhibitory interneurons may therefore be more difficult to assess in human imaging studies.

The scheme of inputs and connections just described applies more closely to the neurons of the basolateral region (especially the lateral and basal nuclei) than to neurons within the centrocorticomedial group. For example, the projection neurons in the central nucleus tend to be inhibitory in nature (Paré & Smith, 1993; Sun & Cassell, 1993). Thus excitation of these leads to inhibition of output activity, whereas inhibition of these gives rise to increased output activity. How then might these inhibitory outputs lead to the expression of emotional responses? One possibility is that activation of the inhibitory intercalated cells by the lateral and basal amygdala may inhibit the central amygdala output cells, thus disinhibiting their targets and leading to the expression of responses (Royer & Paré, 2002).

Although fMRI techniques, including high-resolution approaches, have limited spatial resolution and cannot provide information about the cellular organization of the amygdala, recent studies using another approach have made some progress in exploring cellular activity in the human brain. Depth electrode recordings from single cells have been obtained in patients with epilepsy as part of their presurgical screening (Fried, Cameron, Yashar, Fong, & Morrow, 2002). When combined with structural MRI, such recordings can be isolated to at least gross partitions of the amygdala. Though obviously limited by practical and ethical considerations, such recordings can be used to at least verify that human amygdala cells have basic response functions similar to those observed in animals. But such studies also offer the opportunity to examine unique aspects of the function of human amygdala cells.

NEUROCHEMICAL MODULATION
OF CELLULAR ACTIVITY

The flow of information through amygdala circuits is modulated by a variety of chemical systems. There are three categories of so-called "neuromodulators": peptides, released locally from axons in the amygdala; amine transmitters, which are released widely in the brain from distal areas; and hormones, which reach the amygdala via the bloodstream.

The amines norepinephrine, dopamine, serotonin, and acetylcholine are all released in the amygdala and influence how excitatory and inhibitory neurons interact. Importantly, output connections of the central nucleus terminate on these cells' modulatory networks in the brainstem. Thus activation of the amygdala leads to the release of these modulatory chemicals in the amygdala and throughout other forebrain areas. Various peptides (including receptors for opioid peptides, oxytocin, vasopressin, corticotropin-releasing factor, and neuropeptide Y, to name a few) and hormones (including glucocorticoid and estrogen, among others) are also released in the amygdala.

The various neuromodulators have more diffuse effects than excitatory and inhibitory transmitters, which mostly act at specific synaptic junctions. However, specificity comes from the fact that the receptors for the various modulators are differentially distributed in the amygdala. Thus, for example, glucocorticoids may bathe large areas of the amygdala, but will only affect neurons that have glucocorticoid receptors.

An important challenge for the future is to understand how the various chemical systems interact to set the overall tone of the amygdala. For example, it is known that release of serotonin inhibits cellular activity in the lateral nucleus. However, this is achieved by serotonin-exciting GABAergic cells that inhibit projection neurons. Furthermore, the adrenal glucocorticoid hormone corticosterone is necessary for these effects of serotonin. Many possible interactions are likely to exist among the various chemical systems in the amygdala.

Techniques for exploring the neurochemistry of the human brain are in their infancy. Some progress has been made in using positron emission tomography to measure levels of certain chemical systems, such as glutamate and dopamine, but more work is needed. An exciting indirect approach has involved using fMRI to measure functional activity in relation to variation in neurotransmitter-related genes, such as the serotonin transporter gene (Hariri et al., 2002). Such studies show that genetic variation predicts fMRI signal activity elicited by emotional stimuli in the amygdala.

BEHAVIORAL FUNCTIONS

In the late 1930s, researchers observed that damage to the temporal lobe resulted in profound changes in fear reactivity, feeding, and sexual behavior (Klüver & Bucy, 1937). In the middle of the 20th century, it was determined that damage to the amygdala accounted for these changes in emotional processing (Weiskrantz, 1956). Numerous investigators subsequently attempted to understand the role of the amygdala in emotional functions (Goddard, 1964; Sarter & Markowitsch, 1985; Spiegler & Mishkin, 1981). The result was a large and confusing body of knowledge about the functions of the amygdala, partly because much of the research ignored the nuclear and subnuclear organization of the amygdala (which was not fully appreciated), and partly because the functions measured by behavioral tasks were not well understood.

Fear has been the function most associated with the amygdala. Early studies following up on the Klüver–Bucy syndrome used fear-motivated avoidance conditioning tasks (Goddard, 1964; Maren, Poremba, & Gabriel, 1991; Sarter & Markowitsch, 1985; Weiskrantz, 1956). These measured fear in terms of how well an animal learns to avoid shock. However, avoidance is a two-stage process in which (1) Pavlovian conditioning establishes fear responses to stimuli that predict the occurrence of the shock; and then (2) new behaviors that allow escape from or avoidance of the shock, and thus that reduce the fear elicited by the stimuli, are learned (Mowrer, 1939). In the 1980s, researchers began to use tasks that isolated the Pavlovian from the instrumental components of the task to study the brain mechanisms of fear.

In Pavlovian fear conditioning, a neutral conditioned stimulus (CS) that is paired with a painful shock (an unconditioned stimulus, or US) comes to elicit fear responses, such as freezing behavior and related changes in body physiology (Plate 2.9 in color insert). Studies in rodents have mapped the inputs to and outputs of amygdala nuclei and subnuclei that mediate fear conditioning (e.g., LeDoux, 2000; Maren, 2001; Schafe, Nader, Blair, & LeDoux, 2001). In particular, it is widely accepted that convergence of the CS and US leads to synaptic plasticity in the lateral amygdala. When the CS then occurs alone later, it flows through these potentiated synapses to the other amygdala targets and ultimately to the medial part of the central nucleus, outputs of which control conditioned fear responses (Plate 2.10 in color insert).

Single-unit recording studies have shown that cells in the dorsal subnucleus of the lateral amygdala have the kinds of properties needed to be involved in fear conditioning (LeDoux, 2000; Maren & Quirk, 2004; Quirk, Armony, & LeDoux, 1997; Quirk & Mueller, 2008). These cells receive convergent CS inputs from the auditory thalamus and cortex. The same cells also receive inputs about the footshock US. After the CS and US are paired, the cellular response to the CS is greatly enhanced (more action potentials are elicited; Plate 2.11 in color insert). Two kinds of responses occur within the dorsal lateral amygdala (Repa et al., 2001). Initially, cells in the superior part of the dorsal lateral amygdala rapidly undergo plasticity. Over several trials, they reset their responses back to the starting point. However, cells in the inferior dorsal lateral nucleus have slowly changed by this point, and these then maintain the plasticity over time. Even when the animal has fully extinguished the fear and is no longer responding behaviorally, these inferior cells retain the memory. Such cells may be responsible for the well-known phenomenon that fear in people and animals can be successfully eliminated by treatment but then brought back by stress.

Much has been learned about the cellular and molecular mechanisms within lateral amygdala cells that underlie the plastic changes in fear conditioning (Blair, Schafe, Bauer, Rodrigues, & LeDoux, 2001; Maren, 2001; Rogan, Stäubli, & LeDoux, 1997; Sah & Lopez De Armentia, 2003; Schafe et al., 2001; Shin, Tsvetkov, & Bolshakov, 2006). This has been achieved in part by conducting studies of long-term potentiation (LTP), a cellular model of synaptic plasticity, in the lateral amygdtala in parallel with studies of fear conditioning. Because the input synapses in the amygdala involved in fear conditioning are known, it is possible to induce LTP in pathways that play an established role in this form of learning. Because in vitro studies of LTP allow detailed analysis of cellular and molecular mechanisms, these make possible an understanding of the molecular basis of amygdala plasticity. The molecules involved can then be tested in vivo by infusion in the amygdala in conjunction with studies of fear conditioning. Such studies have found striking parallels between LTP and fear conditioning (Rodrigues, Schafe, & LeDoux, 2004; Schafe et al., 2001).

The overall molecular mechanisms involved in fear conditioning are summarized in Plate 2.12 (in color insert) (Rodrigues et al., 2004). In brief, during conditioning, glutamate released from sensory fibers in the lateral amygdala binds to excitatory amino acid receptors (in particular, alpha-amino-3-hydroxy-5-methyl-4-isoxazolepropionic acid [AMPA] and N-methyl-D-aspartate

[NMDA] receptors). AMPA binding leads to depolarizations that come to be inhibited with repetition. Binding to NMDA receptors is inconsequential, since the level of depolarization produced by AMPA binding is insufficient to remove the magnesium block on NMDA receptors. If the cell is strongly depolarized by another input (such as an electric shock) at about the same time, the magnesium block is removed, and calcium is allowed to enter the cell. This calcium is sufficient to maintain temporary plasticity and thus short-term memory. However, enduring plasticity underlying long-term memory requires additional calcium entering through voltage-gated calcium channels that are also opened by the shock stimulus. The combined level of calcium activates protein kinases (such as mitogen-activated protein kinase), which then translocate to the cell nucleus and trigger gene expression and protein synthesis. The synthesized proteins are then trafficked back to the plastic synapses and stabilize the connection with the presynaptic input. Particularly important may be AMPA receptor protein synthesis, because AMPA trafficking has been implicated in the memory of fear conditioning (Rumpel, LeDoux, Zador, & Malinow, 2005).

Although fear is the emotion best understood in terms of brain mechanisms, the amygdala has also been implicated in a variety of other emotional functions. A relatively large body of research has focused on the role of the amygdala in processing of rewards and the use of rewards to motivate and reinforce behavior (Cardinal et al., 2002; Everitt et al., 1999; Holland & Gallagher, 2004). As with aversive conditioning, the lateral, basal, and central amygdala have been implicated in different aspects of reward learning and motivation, as well as drug addiction. The amygdala has also been implicated in emotional states associated with aggressive, maternal, sexual, and ingestive (eating and drinking) behaviors (Bahar, Samuel, Hazvi, & Dudai, 2003; Galaverna, De Luca, Schulkin, Yao, & Epstein, 1992; Miczek et al., 2007; Pfaff, 2005; Siegel & Edinger, 1983). Less is known about the detailed circuitry involved in these emotional states than is known about fear circuitry, however.

The amygdala is also involved in the regulation or modulation of various cognitive functions, such as attention, perception, and explicit memory (McGaugh, 2000; Phelps, 2006; Phelps & LeDoux, 2005). The amygdala, in fact, has extensive connectivity with cortical areas involved in cognitive functions (Amaral, Behniea, & Kelly, 2003; Barbas, 2000; McDonald, 1998). Interestingly, although the amygdala mainly receives inputs from the late stages of sensory processing, it projects back to the earlier stages. Once the amygdala has detected an emotional stimulus, its activity can then influence the cortical processing of that stimulus. In addition, the amygdala projects to higher-order association areas in the temporal and frontal lobes, including prefrontal areas. However, some of the prefrontal areas involved in higher cognitive functions (such as working memory, executive control, and attention) do not project to the amygdala. Thus, whereas the amygdala can influence cognitive functions directly, higher cognitive functions are less directly capable of influencing the amygdala. At the same time, there are connections between amygdala areas and medial prefrontal cortex, which provide an indirect channel for cortical executive control decisions to influence amygdala activity. This is important to note, given that recent studies have shown that cognitive strategies such as reappraisal can alter functional activity in the amygdala during the processing of emotional stimuli (Ochsner, Bunge, Gross, & Gabrieli, 2002; Phelps, 2006).

In addition to its direct connections with cortical areas, the amygdala can influence cortical functions indirectly. When the amygdala detects an emotionally significant stimulus, its outputs direct the release neuromodulators (norepinephrine, dopamine, serotonin, acetylcholine) in the brain that then alter cognitive processing in cortical areas. Moreover, amygdala activity leads to the release of hormones into the bloodstream that feed back to the brain (McGaugh, 2000). For example, glucocorticoid hormone released into the bloodstream from the adrenal cortex, via outputs of the amygdala to the pituitary gland, travels to the brain and then binds to neurons in the basal amygdala. Norepinephrine is released from the adrenal medulla following amygdala activity, but does not cross the blood–brain barrier. It nevertheless has indirect effects that ultimately alter processing in the basal amygdala. Activity in the basal amygdala then influences the hippocampal processing of explicit memory. The ability of emotional stimuli to enhance the storage and retrieval of explicit memories is likely to depend on these central and peripheral consequences of amygdala activity.

SUMMARY AND CONCLUSIONS

In this chapter, we have reviewed the detailed anatomy of the amygdala, the connectivity among its subdivisions, and their related functions. The amygdala consists of two major subdivisions defined based on evolutionary criteria, the basolateral and centrocorticomedial divisions, which are further divided into subnuclei. The lateral, basal, and accessory basal nuclei belong to the basolateral group, and the cortical, medial, and central nuclei are in the centrocorticomedial group. The lateral nucleus is considered the sensory interface of the amygdala, as it receives inputs from a wide range of sensory areas. The auditory input connections have been studied most thoroughly and reach the lateral nucleus via two major routes: Direct thalamic inputs provide rapid but imprecise (weakly tuned) auditory information, and a thalamocorticoamygdala route originating from the auditory association cortex provides more elaborate information but does so more slowly. Two key output regions of the amygdala are the central nucleus, which controls emotional reactions and associated physiological responses via connections to the brainstem; and the basal nucleus, which influences instrumental behaviors and actions through connections with other forebrain regions, mostly notably the striatum. The basal nucleus is also one of the channels of communication between the lateral and the central nuclei. Connections from both lateral and basal nuclei to the central nucleus are in part gated through an intermediate mass of inhibitory cells called the intercalated neurons.

At the cellular level, amygdala excitatory projection neurons in the lateral and basal nuclei have a relatively low level of baseline activity. These neurons are routinely "silenced" by inhibitory GABAergic interneurons, which prevent the excitatory cells from firing in response to insignificant stimuli. Only meaningful stimuli, transmitted to the amygdala through excitatory glutamatergic sensory inputs, bypass the inhibitory gate. These sensory inputs also terminate on local inhibitory interneurons, which in turn connect with amygdala projection neurons. Such wiring gives rise to feedforward inhibition, allowing the gradual development of amygdala inhibition, and thus habituation, when stimuli are presented repeatedly. The centrocorticomedial division occupies a different wiring scheme. Here, the projection neurons tend to be inhibitory in nature. Thus inhibiting them (e.g., by way of excitatory connections from the lateral nucleus to the inhibitory intercalated neurons) removes the inhibitory effects of inhibitory output cells in the central amygdala on target areas in the brainstem, allowing emotional reactions to emerge.

Three types of neuromodulators manage the flow of information within amygdala pathways: amine transmitters, peptides, and hormones. Amine transmitters (such as dopamine and norepinephrine) modulate widespread areas in the brain, including the amygdala. Outputs of the central nucleus terminate on regions in the brainstem where these neuromodulatory systems originate. Various peptides are released locally within the amygdala, and hormones are transported there via the bloodstream. Although these neuromodulators are released in a diffuse manner, their effects are specific to locations within the amygdala containing the corresponding receptors.

Research on the behavioral function goes back to the late 1930s with the initial observation that temporal lobe damage leads to profound changes in emotional function, termed the Klüver–Bucy syndrome. During the 1950s, the amygdala was pinpointed as the locus of this damage. This triggered abundant research, initially investigating instrumental avoidance learning and later focusing on Pavlovian fear conditioning. The principal region underlying the latter type of learning is the dorsal subdivision of the lateral nucleus where CS and US inputs converge. The superior part of this subdivision initially undergoes rapid plasticity, but after several CS–US pairings resets to the starting point. The inferior part undergoes slower plasticity that is maintained over time. These processes correspond to short- and long-term fear memory storage, respectively.

The amygdala is implicated in a variety of emotional functions and states such as aggressive, maternal, sexual, and reward-driven behaviors. Fear, which is the emotion most studied, provides the best-understood example of emotion processing in the amygdala. Beyond this, the amygdala also interacts extensively with cortical and subcortical areas, through which it regulates attention, perception, memory, and other cognitive processes. Cortical inputs to the amygdala originate from the final stages of sensory processing, but the amygdala projects back to initial stages, thus influencing subsequent processing of sensory stimuli. The amygdala's outputs induce neuromodulator release, and are thus an indirect means by which the amygdala can modulate cortical functions as well.

The meticulous knowledge on the anatomy and function of the amygdala described above is based on extensive animal research conducted in the last several decades. In contrast, studies of the human amygdala have so far only been able to probe this region as a whole. Because there are obvious restrictions on using invasive methodology in human brain research, much of this research relies on noninvasive imaging techniques. But the current resolution of existing techniques imposes limitations on the ability to resolve functional activity in small areas of the brain over time. Some promising novel techniques aimed at improving temporal and spatial resolution may permit more detailed study of the human amygdala in the future. In addition to demonstrating cross-species similarities, such developments would be valuable in increasing the ability to investigate the amygdala in a broader context. For example, examining interactions between amygdala subregions and other areas in real time would shed light on emotional processing at the network level. We hope that these techniques will develop rapidly, because there are some areas of research that are best done in humans rather than animal models, such as studies of social interactions in healthy individuals or psychiatric disease states.

WHAT WE THINK

Research on the amygdala in nonhuman animals goes back to the first half of the 20th century, but especially rapid progress took place during the 1980s when Pavlovian fear conditioning became a key research paradigm for studying amygdala functions. As a result, much is known about the anatomical organization and taxonomy of the various compartments of the animal amygdala. Moreover, the cellular processes and, in some cases, molecular mechanisms that give rise to particular functions of the amygdala have been described in great detail. Figuring out how this information applies to the human amygdala is currently one of the major challenges of research on the neural basis of emotion. In contrast to animal research, human research relies heavily on state-of-the-art noninvasive techniques such as functional magnetic resonance imaging. Further developments in spatial and temporal resolution will make it possible to build further on the animal work in understanding the human amygdala in more detail. Another exciting avenue in human work involves correlations between imaging measurements and genetic factors or with electrophysiological measurements using depth electrodes implanted for therapeutic purposes in patients. Such developments may not only confirm what is known from nonhuman animals, but also may reveal human-specific functions, especially for behaviors that are more complex and perhaps unique to humans, such as those involving social interactions. Finally, while animal research is not very informative on its own regarding the neurobiology of feelings, we have the advantage of being able to integrate information about feelings from human studies with very detailed knowledge of emotional processing that has been gained from studies of nonhuman animals. The future is thus bright for research on human emotions in the brain.

ACKNOWLEDGMENTS

The original work described in this chapter was supported by Grant Nos. MH038774, MH046516, MH058911, and MH067048 from the National Institutes of Health to Joseph LeDoux.

REFERENCES

Aggleton, J. P., Burton, M. J., & Passingham, R. E. (1980). Cortical and subcortical afferents to the amygdala of the rhesus monkey (*Macaca mulatta*). *Brain Research, 190*(2), 347–368.

Alheid, G. F., & Heimer, L. (1988). New perspectives in basal forebrain organization of special relevance for neuropsychiatric disorders: The striatopallidal, amygdaloid, and corticopetal components of substantia innominata. *Neuroscience, 27*(1), 1–39.

Amaral, D. G., Behniea, H., & Kelly, J. L. (2003). Topographic organization of projections from the amygdala to the visual cortex in the macaque monkey. *Neuroscience, 118*(4), 1099–1200.

Amaral, D. G., Price, J. L., Pitkänen, A., & Carmichael, T. (1992). Anatomical organization of the primate amygdaloid complex. In J. P. Aggleton (Ed.), *The amygdala: Neurobiological aspects of emotion, memory, and mental dysfunction* (pp. 1–66). New York: Wiley-Liss.

Amorapanth, P., LeDoux, J. E., & Nader, K. (2000). Different lateral amygdala outputs mediate reactions and actions elicited by a fear-arousing stimulus. *Nature Neuroscience, 3*(1), 74–79.

Bahar, A., Samuel, A., Hazvi, S., & Dudai, Y. (2003). The amygdalar circuit that acquires taste aversion memory differs from the circuit that extinguishes it. *European Journal of Neuroscience, 17*(7), 1527–1530.

Barbas, H. (2000). Connections underlying the synthesis of cognition, memory, and emotion in primate prefrontal cortices. *Brain Research Bulletin, 52*(5), 319–330.

Bauer, E. P., & LeDoux, J. E. (2004). Heterosynaptic long-term potentiation of inhibitory interneurons in the lateral amygdala. *Journal of Neuroscience, 24*, 9507–9512.

Ben-Ari, Y., Le Galla Salle, G., & Champagnat, J. (1974). Lateral amygdala unit activity: I. Relationship between spontaneous and evoked activity. *Electroencephalography and Clinical Neurophysiology, 37*(5), 449–461.

Bissière, S., Humeau, Y., & Lüthi, A. (2003). Dopamine gates LTP induction in lateral amygdala by suppressing feedforward inhibition. *Nature Neuroscience, 6*(6), 587–592.

Blair, H. T., Schafe, G. E., Bauer, E. P., Rodrigues, S., & LeDoux, J. E. (2001). Synaptic plasticity in the lateral amygdala: A cellular hypothesis of fear conditioning. *Learning and Memory, 8*(5), 229–242.

Bordi, F., LeDoux, J., Clugnet, M. C., & Pavlides, C. (1993). Single-unit activity in the lateral nucleus of the amygdala and overlying areas of the striatum in freely behaving rats: Rates, discharge patterns, and responses to acoustic stimuli. *Behavioral Neuroscience, 107*(5), 757–769.

Bordi, F., & LeDoux, J. E. (1994a). Response properties of single units in areas of rat auditory thalamus that project to the amygdala: I. Acoustic discharge patterns and frequency receptive fields. *Experimental Brain Research, 98*(2), 261–274.

Bordi, F., & LeDoux, J. E. (1994b). Response properties of single units in areas of rat auditory thalamus that project to the amygdala: II. Cells receiving convergent auditory and somatosensory inputs and cells antidromically activated by amygdala stimulation. *Experimental Brain Research, 98*(2), 275–286.

Burdach, K. F. (1819–1822). *Vom Baue und Leben des Gehirns.* Leipzig.

Cardinal, R. N., Parkinson, J. A., Hall, J., & Everitt, B. J. (2002). Emotion and motivation: The role of the amygdala, ventral striatum, and prefrontal cortex. *Neuroscience and Biobehavioral Reviews, 26*(3), 321–352.

Clugnet, M. C., LeDoux, J. E., & Morrison, S. F. (1990). Unit responses evoked in the amygdala and striatum by electrical stimulation of the medial geniculate body. *Journal of Neuroscience, 10*(4), 1055–1061.

Doron, N. N., & LeDoux, J. E. (1999). Organization of projections to the lateral amygdala from auditory and visual areas of the thalamus in the rat. *Journal of Comparative Neurology, 412*(3), 383–409.

Everitt, B. J., Parkinson, J. A., Olmstead, M. C., Arroyo, M., Robledo, P., & Robbins, T. W. (1999). Associative processes in addiction and reward: The role of amygdala–ventral striatal subsystems. *Annals of the New York Academy of Sciences, 877*, 412–438.

Everitt, B. J., & Robbins, T. W. (1992). Amygdala–ventral striatal interactions and reward-related processes. In J. P. Aggleton (Ed.), *The amygdala: Neurobiological aspects of emotion, memory, and mental dysfunction* (pp. 401–430). New York: Wiley-Liss.

Farb, C. R., & LeDoux, J. E. (1999). Afferents from rat temporal cortex synapse on lateral amygdala neurons that express NMDA and AMPA receptors. *Synapse, 33*(3), 218–229.

Fried, I., Cameron, K. A., Yashar, S., Fong, R., & Morrow, J. W. (2002). Inhibitory and excitatory responses of single neurons in the human medial temporal lobe during recognition of faces and objects. *Cerebral Cortex, 12*(6), 575–584.

Fudge, J. L., Kunishio, K., Walsh, P., Richard, C., & Haber, S. N. (2002). Amygdaloid projections to ventromedial striatal subterritories in the primate. *Neuroscience, 110*(2), 257–275.

Galaverna, O., De Luca, L. A., Jr., Schulkin, J., Yao, S. Z., & Epstein, A. N. (1992). Deficits in NaCl ingestion after damage to the central nucleus of the amygdala in the rat. *Brain Research Bulletin, 28*(1), 89–98.

Goddard, G. V. (1964). Functions of the amygdala. *Psychological Bulletin, 62*, 89–109.

Hariri, A. R., Mattay, V. S., Tessitore, A., Kolachana, B., Fera, F., Goldman, D., et al. (2002). Serotonin transporter genetic variation and the response of the human amygdala. *Science, 297*, 400–403.

Heimer, L. (2003). A new anatomical framework for neuropsychiatric disorders and drug abuse. *American Journal of Psychiatry, 160*, 1726–1739.

Heimer, L., & Van Hoesen, G. W. (2006). The limbic lobe and its output channels: Implications for emotional functions and adaptive behavior. *Neuroscience and Biobehavioral Reviews, 30*(2), 126–147.

Holland, P. C., & Gallagher, M. (2004). Amygdala–frontal interactions and reward expectancy. *Current Opinion in Neurobiology, 14*(2), 148–155.

Johnston, J. B. (1923). Further contribution to the study of the evolution of the forebrain. *Journal of Comparative Neurology, 35*, 337–481.

Kapp, B. S., Whalen, P. J., Supple, W. F., & Pascoe, J. P. (1992). Amygdala contributions to conditioned arousal and sensory information processing. In J. P. Aggleton (Ed.), *The amygdala: Neurobiological aspects of emotion, memory, and mental dysfunction* (pp. 229–254). New York: Wiley-Liss.

Killcross, S., Robbins, T. W., & Everitt, B. J. (1997). Different types of fear-conditioned behaviour mediated by separate nuclei within amygdala. *Nature, 388*, 377–380.

Klüver, H., & Bucy, P. C. (1937). "Psychic blindness" and other symptoms following bilateral temporal lobectomy in rhesus monkeys. *American Journal of Physiology, 119,* 352–353.

LeDoux, J. E. (2000). Emotion circuits in the brain. *Annual Review of Neuroscience, 23,* 155–184.

LeDoux, J. E., Cicchetti, P., Xagoraris, A., & Romanski, L. M. (1990). The lateral amygdaloid nucleus: Sensory interface of the amygdala in fear conditioning. *Journal of Neuroscience, 10*(4), 1062–1069.

LeDoux, J. E., Farb, C., & Ruggiero, D. A. (1990). Topographic organization of neurons in the acoustic thalamus that project to the amygdala. *Journal of Neuroscience, 10*(4), 1043–1054.

LeDoux, J. E., Farb, C. R., & Romanski, L. M. (1991). Overlapping projections to the amygdala and striatum from auditory processing areas of the thalamus and cortex. *Neuroscience Letters, 134*(1), 139–144.

LeDoux, J. E., Ruggiero, D. A., & Reis, D. J. (1985). Projections to the subcortical forebrain from anatomically defined regions of the medial geniculate body in the rat. *Journal of Comparative Neurology, 242*(2), 182–213.

Li, X. F., Armony, J. L., & LeDoux, J. E. (1996a). GABAA and GABAB receptors differentially regulate synaptic transmission in the auditory thalamo-amygdala pathway: An *in vivo* microiontophoretic study and a model. *Synapse, 24*(2), 115–124.

Li, X. F., Stutzmann, G. E., & LeDoux, J. E. (1996b). Convergent but temporally separated inputs to lateral amygdala neurons from the auditory thalamus and auditory cortex use different postsynaptic receptors: *In vivo* intracellular and extracellular recordings in fear conditioning pathways. *Learning and Memory, 3*(2–3), 229–242.

Maren, S. (2001). Neurobiology of Pavlovian fear conditioning. *Annual Review of Neuroscience, 24,* 897–931.

Maren, S., Poremba, A., & Gabriel, M. (1991). Basolateral amygdaloid multi-unit neuronal correlates of discriminative avoidance learning in rabbits. *Brain Research, 549,* 311–316.

Maren, S., & Quirk, G. J. (2004). Neuronal signalling of fear memory. *Nature Reviews Neuroscience, 5*(11), 844–852.

McDonald, A. J. (1985). Immunohistochemical identification of gamma-aminobutyric acid-containing neurons in the rat basolateral amygdala. *Neuroscience Letters, 53*(2), 203–207.

McDonald, A. J. (1994). Neuronal localization of glutamate receptor subunits in the basolateral amygdala. *NeuroReport, 6*(1), 13–16.

McDonald, A. J. (1998). Cortical pathways to the mammalian amygdala. *Progress in Neurobiology, 55*(3), 257–332.

McGaugh, J. L. (2000). Memory—a century of consolidation. *Science, 287,* 248–251.

Miczek, K. A., de Almeida, R. M., Kravitz, E. A., Rissman, F. F., de Boer, S. F., & Raine, A. (2007). Neurobiology of escalated aggression and violence. *Journal of Neuroscience, 27,* 11803–11806.

Mowrer, O. H. (1939). A stimulus–response analysis of anxiety and its role as a reinforcing agent. *Psychological Review, 46,* 553–565.

Muller, J. F., Mascagni, F., & McDonald, A. J. (2006). Pyramidal cells of the rat basolateral amygdala: Synaptology and innervation by parvalbumin-immunoreactive interneurons. *Journal of Comparative Neurology, 494*(4), 635–650.

Nader, K., Majidishad, P., Amorapanth, P., & LeDoux, J. E. (2001). Damage to the lateral and central, but not other, amygdaloid nuclei prevents the acquisition of auditory fear conditioning. *Learning and Memory, 8*(3), 156–163.

Ochsner, K. N., Bunge, S. A., Gross, J. J., & Gabrieli, J. D. (2002). Rethinking feelings: An FMRI study of the cognitive regulation of emotion. *Journal of Cognitive Neuroscience, 14*(8), 1215–1229.

Paré, D., & Gaudreau, H. (1996). Projection cells and interneurons of the lateral and basolateral amygdala: Distinct firing patterns and differential relation to theta and delta rhythms in conscious cats. *Journal of Neuroscience, 16*(10), 3334–3350.

Paré, D., Royer, S., Smith, Y., & Lang, E. J. (2003). Contextual inhibitory gating of impulse traffic in the intra-amygdaloid network. *Annals of the New York Academy of Sciences, 985*, 78–91.

Paré, D., & Smith, Y. (1993). Distribution of GABA immunoreactivity in the amygdaloid complex of the cat. *Neuroscience, 57*(4), 1061–1076.

Pessoa, L., & Ungerleider, L. G. (2004). Neuroimaging studies of attention and the processing of emotion-laden stimuli. *Progress in Brain Research, 144*, 171–182.

Petrovich, G. D., Risold, P. Y., & Swanson, L. W. (1996). Organization of projections from the basomedial nucleus of the amygdala: A PHAL study in the rat. *Journal of Comparative Neurology, 374*(3), 387–420.

Pfaff, D. (2005). Hormone-driven mechanisms in the central nervous system facilitate the analysis of mammalian behaviours. *Journal of Endocrinology, 184*(3), 447–453.

Phelps, E. A. (2006). Emotion and cognition: Insights from studies of the human amygdala. *Annual Review of Psychology, 57*, 27–53.

Phelps, E. A., & LeDoux, J. E. (2005). Contributions of the amygdala to emotion processing: From animal models to human behavior. *Neuron, 48*(2), 175–187.

Pitkänen, A. (2000). Connectivity of the rat amygdaloid complex. In J. P. Aggleton (Ed.), *The amygdala: A functional analysis* (pp. 31–116). Oxford, UK: Oxford University Press.

Pitkänen, A., Savander, V., & LeDoux, J. E. (1997). Organization of intra-amygdaloid circuitries in the rat: An emerging framework for understanding functions of the amygdala. *Trends in Neurosciences, 20*(11), 517–523.

Quirk, G. J., Armony, J. L., & LeDoux, J. E. (1997). Fear conditioning enhances different temporal components of tone-evoked spike trains in auditory cortex and lateral amygdala. *Neuron, 19*(3), 613–624.

Quirk, G. J., & Mueller, D. (2008). Neural mechanisms of extinction learning and retrieval. *Neuropsychopharmacology, 33*(1), 56–72.

Repa, J. C., Muller, J., Apergis, J., Desrochers, T. M., Zhou, Y., & LeDoux, J. E. (2001). Two different lateral amygdala cell populations contribute to the initiation and storage of memory. *Nature Neuroscience, 4*(7), 724–731.

Rodrigues, S. M., Schafe, G. E., & LeDoux, J. E. (2004). Molecular mechanisms underlying emotional learning and memory in the lateral amygdala. *Neuron, 44*(1), 75–91.

Rogan, M. T., Stäubli, U. V., & LeDoux, J. E. (1997). Fear conditioning induces associative long-term potentiation in the amygdala. *Nature, 390*, 604–607.

Romanski, L. M., Clugnet, M. C., Borid, F., & LeDoux, J. E. (1993). Somatosensory and auditory convergence in the lateral nucleus of the amygdala. *Behavioral Neuroscience, 107*(3), 444–450.

Romanski, L. M., & LeDoux, J. E. (1993). Information cascade from primary auditory cortex to the amygdala: Corticocortical and corticoamygdaloid projections of temporal cortex in the rat. *Cerebral Cortex, 3*(6), 515–532.

Royer, S., & Paré, D. (2003). Conservation of total synaptic weight through balanced synaptic depression and potentiation. *Nature, 422*, 518–522.

Rumpel, S., LeDoux, J., Zador, A., & Malinow, R. (2005). Postsynaptic receptor trafficking underlying a form of associative learning. *Science, 308*, 83–88.

Russchen, F. T., Bakst, I., Amaral, D. G., & Price, J. L. (1985). The amygdalostriatal projections in the monkey: An anterograde tracing study. *Brain Research, 329*(1–2), 241–257.

Sah, P., & Lopez De Armentia, M. (2003). Excitatory synaptic transmission in the lateral and central amygdala. *Annals of the New York Academy of Sciences, 985*, 67–77.

Sarter, M., & Markowitsch, H. J. (1985). Involvement of the amygdala in learning and memory: A critical review, with emphasis on anatomical relations. *Behavioral Neuroscience, 99*(2), 342–380.

Schafe, G. E., Nader, K., Blair, H. T., & LeDoux, J. E. (2001). Memory consolidation of Pavlovian fear conditioning: A cellular and molecular perspective. *Trends in Neurosciences, 24*(9), 540–546.

Shin, R. M., Tsvetkov, E., & Bolshakov, V. Y. (2006). Spatiotemporal asymmetry of associative synaptic plasticity in fear conditioning pathways. *Neuron, 52*(5), 883–896.

Siegel, A., & Edinger, H. M. (1983). Role of the limbic system in hypothalamically elicited attack behavior. *Neuroscience and Biobehavioral Reviews, 7*(3), 395–407.

Smith, Y., & Paré, D. (1994). Intra-amygdaloid projections of the lateral nucleus in the cat: PHA-L anterograde labeling combined with postembedding GABA and glutamate immunocytochemistry. *Journal of Comparative Neurology, 342*(2), 232–248.

Spiegler, B. J., & Mishkin, M. (1981). Evidence for the sequential participation of inferior temporal cortex and amygdala in the acquisition of stimulus–reward associations. *Behavioural Brain Research, 3*(3), 303–317.

Sun, N., & Cassell, M. D. (1993). Intrinsic GABAergic neurons in the rat central extended amygdala. *Journal of Comparative Neurology, 330*(3), 381–404.

Swanson, L. W., & Petrovich, G. D. (1998). What is the amygdala? *Trends in Neurosciences, 21*(8), 323–331.

Turner, B. H., & Herkenham, M. (1991). Thalamoamygdaloid projections in the rat: A test of the amygdala's role in sensory processing. *Journal of Comparative Neurology, 313*(2), 295–325.

Turner, B. H., Mishkin, M., & Knapp, M. (1980). Organization of the amygdalopetal projections from modality-specific cortical association areas in the monkey. *Journal of Comparative Neurology, 191*(4), 515–543.

Weiskrantz, L. (1956). Behavioral changes associated with ablation of the amygdaloid complex in monkeys. *Journal of Comparative and Physiological Psychology, 49*(4), 381–391.

Woodruff, A. R., Monyer, H., & Sah, P. (2006). GABAergic excitation in the basolateral amygdala. *Journal of Neuroscience, 26*, 11881–11887.

Woodson, W., Farb, C. R., & LeDoux, J. E. (2000). Afferents from the auditory thalamus synapse on inhibitory interneurons in the lateral nucleus of the amygdala. *Synapse, 38*(2), 124–137.

CHAPTER 3

Measurement of Fear Inhibition in Rats, Monkeys, and Humans with or without Posttraumatic Stress Disorder, Using the AX+, BX– Paradigm

Karyn M. Myers, Donna J. Toufexis, James T. Winslow,
Tanja Jovanovic, Seth D. Norrholm, Erica J. Duncan,
and Michael Davis

A great deal is now known about the behavioral characteristics and neural substrates of fear acquisition, thanks in large part to the study of Pavlovian fear conditioning. In this paradigm, an organism is exposed to pairings of an initially neutral stimulus such as a light or tone (the conditioned stimulus, or CS) with an aversive event such as a mild footshock or air blast (the unconditioned stimulus, or US); the organism thus comes to exhibit a fear conditioned response (CR) in the presence of the CS. "Fear" is defined operationally in several ways—including freezing and ultrasonic vocalization in rodents, and an increase in the amplitude of an acoustic startle response in rodents, nonhuman primates, and humans—and is observable following a single CS–US pairing under some circumstances (Paschall & Davis, 2002). Fear conditioning is thus an extremely robust form of learning, and as a model system it has lent itself well to neural analyses on the systemic, cellular, and molecular levels (Davis, 2000; Phelps & LeDoux, 2005; Rodrigues, Schafe, & LeDoux, 2004).

In contrast to the extensive literature on fear acquisition, relatively little is known about the mechanisms of fear suppression or inhibition, although the question is receiving increasing interest because of its clear clinical relevance (Bouton, 2000). The slow progress in understanding fear inhibition may be attributable in part to the fact that paradigms for the study of inhibition are not particularly well developed. The most common inhibitory fear-learning paradigm is extinction, in which a feared CS is presented repeatedly in the absence of the US, leading to a reduction or elimination of the fear CR (Myers & Davis, 2007). Extinction is an important paradigm, and one that we have used extensively in our own work; however, we believe that certain attendant difficulties limit its usefulness, the most prominent among them being the difficulty in distinguishing mechanisms of fear inhibition from those of fear expression. Considerable evidence indicates that a CS undergoing extinction retains the ability to generate a CR (i.e., controls an "excitatory" association), but develops a secondary, overriding propensity to suppress CR generation (an "inhibitory" association) (Bouton, 2004). Thus after extinction a CS is both a fear elicitor and a fear inhibitor, making it difficult to determine whether the effect of a manipulation is on one or the other of these processes, or on some combination of the two.

In our laboratories, we have sought to develop an alternative paradigm for the study of fear inhibition that circumvents this problem by endowing CSs with exclusively excitatory or inhibitory associations. Borrowing from the extensive animal literature on conditioned inhibition, we have explored discrimination training procedures in which certain cues or cue compounds are paired with an aversive event and others are not, with the result that some of the cues become fear-eliciting and others become fear-inhibiting. In this chapter, we describe this work, which was begun with rats and has since been expanded to nonhuman primates as well as humans (including both nondisordered and psychiatric populations). We conclude by discussing how these paradigms might be used to study the neurobiology of fear inhibition, including the role of the amygdala.

CONDITIONED INHIBITION: THE A+, BA− DISCRIMINATION

Pavlov (1927) noted that a cue (B) could be trained to inhibit a salivary response elicited by another, separately reinforced cue (A), if A and B were presented together and the meat powder reinforcer that typically followed A was omitted. This was called "A+, BA−" training, where A and B represent discriminable cues such as a light and a tone, and "+" and "−" indicate the presence and absence, respectively, of reinforcement. Pavlov referred to this phenomenon as "conditioned inhibition," to emphasize that the B cue inhibited the CR occasioned by A, and that this inhibitory property developed through training. Other investigators have shown that a conditioned inhibitor is capable of inhibiting the CR not only to the cue with which it was trained, but also to other cues paired separately with the same US, and that the phenomenon extends to aversive as well as appetitive conditioning paradigms (Rescorla, 1969).

Mathematical models of Pavlovian conditioning, such as the Rescorla–Wagner model (Rescorla & Wagner, 1972; Wagner & Rescorla, 1972), represent the learning that occurs during conditioned inhibition training as shown in the top panel of Figure 3.1. During A+, BA– training, the organism learns to respond to the A cue and to withhold responding in the presence of BA. The discrimination is solved when A becomes "excitatory," meaning that it has achieved positive associative strength or is fear-eliciting, and B becomes

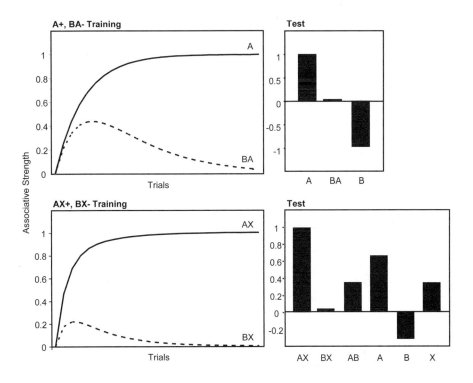

FIGURE 3.1. *Top panel:* Conditioned responding during the acquisition of an A+, BA– discrimination (left) and to A, B, and BA test cues following the completion of discrimination learning (right) as predicted by a computer simulation of the Rescorla–Wagner model (Rescorla & Wagner, 1972; Wagner & Rescorla, 1972). Discrimination learning proceeds as A acquires positive associative strength and B acquires negative associative strength (i.e., becomes a conditioned inhibitor). Comparison of responding on A and BA test trials reveals the inhibition that has accrued to B. *Bottom panel:* Conditioned responding during the acquisition of an AX+, BX– discrimination (left) and to AX, BX, AB, A, B, and X test cues following the completion of discrimination learning (right) as predicted by a computer simulation of the Rescorla–Wagner model. For both simulations, parameter values were set as follows: $\alpha\beta$ = 0.25 and λ = 1 on reinforced trials, and $\alpha\beta$ = 0.15 and λ = 0 on nonreinforced trials.

"inhibitory," meaning that it has achieved negative associative strength or is fear-inhibiting. When A and B are presented in compound, these two tendencies summate, producing a zero or near-zero associative value for the BA compound. B is able to inhibit responding to any other cue with a positive associative value through this same summative mechanism.

In the interest of using this procedure to study the neural basis of fear inhibition, Falls and Davis (1997) explored the possibility of adapting the A+, BA– discrimination to the rat fear-potentiated startle paradigm. In this paradigm, a rat is presented with a CS paired with a mild footshock, and as a result exhibits an increased amplitude of the acoustic startle response when startle is elicited in the presence versus the absence of the CS (Brown, Kalish, & Farber, 1951; Davis & Astrachan, 1978). Startle elicited by a loud sound is measured in a specially designed cage. Movement of the cage by the startle reaction displaces an accelerometer that puts out a voltage proportionate to the magnitude of the startle reflex (Figure 3.2, top panel). Falls and Davis presented rats with two phases of training; the first involved simple A+ training (where A was a 3.7-sec light or a white noise, counterbalanced, and the reinforcer was a 0.5-sec footshock), and the second involved A+, BA– training (where B was whichever of the light and noise cues did not serve as A). After such training, animals were tested for responding to A, B, and BA. Although Pavlov (1927) noted that overlapping presentation of A and B cues was most effective in endowing B with inhibitory properties, Falls and Davis used a serial compound presentation in which the offset of B coincided with the onset of A (Figure 3.3). This choice was motivated by a desire to avoid "external inhibition," defined as an unconditioned decrement in responding to an excitatory CS when a second CS is presented just before or at the same time as the excitatory CS. That is, it was critical in these experiments that the inhibition of responding to A on BA test trials occurred only after A+, BA– training (conditioned inhibition) and not in untrained animals or animals trained under control conditions (external inhibition). External inhibition was a persistent problem in experiments in which A and B overlapped, but was avoided when A and B were presented such that the B cue turned off as soon as the A cue came on, as shown in Figure 3.3.

Falls and Davis (1997) found that rats were able to learn the A+, BA– discrimination; that is, rats exhibited fear-potentiated startle in the presence of A, and significantly less fear-potentiated startle in the presence of BA. Unexpectedly, however, the rats also exhibited potentiation in the presence of B, the putative conditioned inhibitor, but then this excitatory effect was replaced by an inhibitory effect once the B cue went off. For example, in one experiment, startle magnitude was probed at various points during the BA test trial following the completion of A+, BA– training: 0.5 sec prior to the offset of B, and 1.2, 2.2, and 3.2 sec after the onset of A (Figure 3.3), with the different time points being tested on separate trials. Additional test trials involved startle probes 1.2, 2.2, and 3.2 sec after the onset of A when A was not preceded by B. Finally, startle magnitude in the absence of any cue was

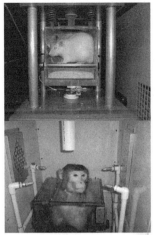

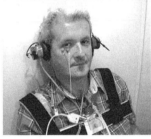

FIGURE 3.2. *Top panel:* In the rat fear-potentiated startle paradigm, a rat is confined to a wire mesh cage suspended between compression springs and housed within a sound-attenuating chamber. Cues including lights, tones, white noises, and a stream of air from a computer fan mounted to the top of the cage are available as CSs. The US is a mild (0.4- or 0.6-mA), 500-msec footshock. A whole-body startle response is elicited via a 95-dB, 50-msec white noise burst. Startle responses are detected by an accelerometer affixed to the bottom of the cage, which produces a voltage output proportional to the velocity of cage movement that is detected and quantified by a computer. *Middle panel:* In the monkey fear-potentiated startle paradigm, a rhesus macaque is confined to a custom-built restraint box and placed inside a sound-attenuating testing chamber. Cues including lights, tones, white noises, and a stream of air from a computer fan mounted overhead and directed through a plastic tube are available as CSs. The US is a 500-msec air blast directed to the face of the monkey. A whole-body startle response is elicited via a 40-msec white noise burst of varying intensities (90–120 dB). Startle responses are detected by an accelerometer mounted on a platform assembly underneath the restraint box, which produces a voltage output proportional to the velocity of cage movement that is detected and quantified by a computer. *Bottom panel:* In the human fear-potentiated startle paradigm, a participant is seated in a sound-attenuating chamber facing a display of colored light bulbs mounted to the opposite wall that serve as CSs. The US is a 100-msec air blast directed to the larynx. A startle response is elicited via a 40-msec noise burst (104 or 108 dB) delivered binaurally through earphones. The eyeblink component of the startle response is measured by electromyography of the right orbicularis oculi muscle.

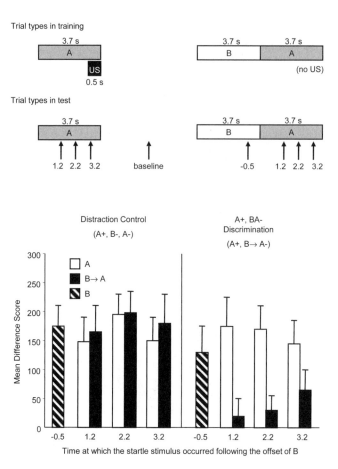

Trial types in training

3.7 s
A
US
0.5 s

3.7 s   3.7 s
B   A
(no US)

Trial types in test

3.7 s
A
1.2 2.2 3.2   baseline

3.7 s   3.7 s
B   A
-0.5   1.2 2.2 3.2

Distraction Control
(A+, B-, A-)

A+, BA-
Discrimination
(A+, B→ A-)

□ A
■ B→ A
◧ B

Mean Difference Score

Time at which the startle stimulus occurred following the offset of B

FIGURE 3.3. *Top panel:* Schematic representation of the trial types used by Falls and Davis (1997) during training on the A+, BA– discrimination in rats. A and B were 3.7-sec light and white noise cues, counterbalanced, and the US was a 0.5-sec mild footshock. The BA compound cue was presented in a serial fashion (i.e., the onset of A co-occurred with the offset of B). *Middle panel:* Schematic representation of the trial types used by Falls and Davis (1997) in test following training on the A+, BA– discrimination. Startle magnitude was assessed 1.2, 2.2, and 3.2 sec after the onset of A, both when A was presented in isolation and when it was preceded by B; 0.5 sec prior to the onset of A when A was preceded by B; and in the absence of any other cue, as a baseline startle measure. The different placements of the startle probe relative to the cue(s) occurred on separate trials, such that only one startle stimulus occurred per presentation of A or BA. *Bottom panel:* Mean startle difference scores (startle in the presence of a cue minus baseline startle) on the various test trial types, in two groups of animals: a distraction control group trained on A+, B–, A– (which was included to assess the contribution of external inhibition to responding on BA test trials), and a feature-negative group trained on the A+, BA– discrimination. No inhibition of fear-potentiated startle was observed in the distraction control group, whereas the feature-negative group exhibited robust, time-dependent inhibition on BA test trials. From Falls and Davis (1997). Copyright 1997 by the American Psychological Association. Reprinted by permission.

assessed throughout the session as a measure of baseline startle magnitude. In animals trained on the A+, BA− discrimination, startle magnitude was elevated significantly in the presence of B and at all time points probed during the duration of A when A was presented in isolation (Figure 3.3). By contrast, when A was preceded by B, the elevation of startle magnitude was lower than that observed when A was presented alone. The most profound inhibition occurred 1.2 and 2.2 sec after the onset of A, and more modest inhibition occurred 3.2 sec after the onset of A. By comparison, there was no inhibition of potentiated startle on BA test trials in a distraction control group that was not trained on the A+, BA− discrimination, indicating that the inhibition observed in the A+, BA− group was due to conditioned inhibition and not to external inhibition.

The observation that startle was both potentiated in the presence of B and inhibited in the presence of A when A was preceded by B, indicated that B had been endowed with both excitatory (fear-eliciting) and inhibitory (fear-inhibiting) properties that were expressed sequentially, one after the other. Hence the A+, BA− discrimination was, under these conditions, not entirely successful in endowing the cues involved with purely excitatory or inhibitory tendencies; in fact, it could be argued that the outcome was only somewhat better than that observed following extinction in terms of being able to study these associative properties separately, since a single cue still controlled both tendencies. However, the temporal separation between the two made it possible to observe an effect of a manipulation upon one or the other, and indeed the A+, BA− discrimination has been used successfully in several studies of the neural mechanisms of conditioned inhibition (Campeau et al., 1997; Falls, Bakken, & Heldt, 1997; Falls & Davis, 1995; Gewirtz, Falls, & Davis, 1997; Heldt, Coover, & Falls, 2002; Heldt & Falls, 1998, 2003, 2006; Josselyn, Falls, Gewirtz, Pistell, & Davis, 2005; Waddell, Heldt, & Falls, 2003).

THE AX+, BX− DISCRIMINATION

Nevertheless, we were eager to develop a paradigm that would achieve more completely the goal of separating excitatory and inhibitory tendencies for separate neural analysis. To this end, we conducted a number of pilot studies on external inhibition of fear-potentiated startle, with the goal of understanding the conditions under which external inhibition is observed and identifying any procedures that could be used to eliminate it from experiments on conditioned inhibition. We do not describe these experiments in any detail here; interested readers are referred to Myers and Davis (2004) for a full account. We concluded that external inhibition is a very potent factor in fear-potentiated startle whenever an excitor is presented in compound with a neutral stimulus, particularly when the two cues occur as a simultaneous compound (i.e., with concurrent onsets and offsets), but that external inhibition can be minimized or even eliminated altogether (even with simultaneous compound stimulus presentations) if animals have experience with the excitor and the external inhibitor as parts of compounds involving other cues prior to testing.

A simple modification of the A+, BA– discrimination fulfills this requirement. By adding a third cue, X, to obtain AX+, BX–, one would expect external inhibition on the crucial AB test trials to be minimized, because both the excitor (A) and the putative external inhibitor (B) have been experienced as parts of compounds (AX and BX) before being compounded with one another (AB) in testing. As shown in the lower panel of Figure 3.1, the Rescorla–Wagner model (Rescorla & Wagner, 1972; Wagner & Rescorla, 1972) predicts that the acquisition of the discrimination should proceed similarly to the A+, BA– discrimination, and that the discrimination is solved by much the same mechanism. Here, both A and X become excitors (fear elicitors), and B becomes a conditioned inhibitor. The inhibitory property of B is evident on BA test trials, in which responding to BA is lower than that to A alone.[1]

The AX+, BX– Discrimination in Rats

Myers and Davis (2004) adapted the AX+, BX– discrimination for use in the rat fear-potentiated startle paradigm. A, B, and X were represented by 3.7-sec cues (light, white noise, and quiet fan, counterbalanced), and the reinforcer was a 0.5-sec mild footshock. Compounded cues were presented simultaneously. As shown in the top panel of Figure 3.4, rats tested following several sessions of training on the AX+, BX– discrimination exhibited reliably greater fear-potentiated startle to AX than to BX, indicating successful discrimination, as well as reliably lower fear-potentiated startle to AB than to A, indicating that B functioned as a conditioned inhibitor. This pattern of responding is in close accord with that predicted by the Rescorla–Wagner model (Rescorla & Wagner, 1972; Wagner & Rescorla, 1972) and observed by other investigators using different experimental paradigms (Rickert, Lorden, Dawson, Smyly, & Callahan, 1979; Wagner, Logan, Haberlandt, & Price, 1968). Importantly, the difference in responding to AB and A was evident from the first presentations of these cues during the test session (data not shown), indicating that it was not something that developed over the course of the test session, but rather occurred as a result of learning during discrimination training. Separate experiments confirmed that the lower responding to AB than to A was due to conditioned rather than external inhibition: When a fourth cue, C, was preexposed (nonreinforced) prior to training as many times as B was presented in training, animals exhibited no decrement in responding on AC test trials (external inhibition), whereas they showed a robust decrement in responding on AB test trials (conditioned inhibition), relative to responding on A test trials (Myers, Toufexis, Bowser, & Davis, 2007; Toufexis, Myers, Bowser, & Davis, 2007). As shown in the lower panel of Figure 3.4, acquisition of the AX+, BX– discrimination proceeded as predicted by the Rescorla–Wagner model, with responding to BX– following an up-and-down pattern character-

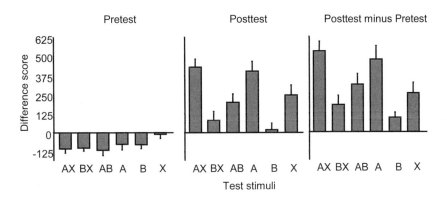

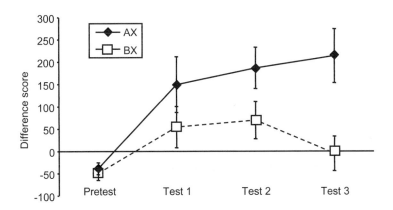

FIGURE 3.4. *Top panel:* Mean startle difference scores obtained on AX, BX, AB, A, B, and X trial types in a pretest conducted prior to training (left) and in a posttest conducted after the completion of training (middle) on the AX+, BX− discrimination in rats. The rightmost panel presents the same data, transformed by subtracting the mean difference score of each rat on each trial type in the pretest from its corresponding mean difference score in the posttest. *Bottom panel:* Mean startle difference scores obtained on AX and BX test trial types in tests conducted prior to training (pretest) and following the completion of one, two, or three sessions of AX+, BX− training, in separate groups of rats. From Myers and Davis (2004a). Copyright 2004 by the Cold Spring Harbor Laboratory Press. Reprinted by permission.

istic of situations in which conditioned inhibition develops over trials. In this experiment, separate groups of animals were given one, two, or three sessions of AX+, BX– training, each involving 5 AX+ and 5 BX– presentations, and then were tested to AX and BX (as well as AB, A, B, and X) 24 hours following their final training session (Myers & Davis, 2004).

The original experiments reported by Myers and Davis (2004) were conducted with male rats, but since then Toufexis and colleagues (2007) have shown that the discrimination proceeds in much the same manner with female rats and is sensitive to manipulations of gonadal steroids. That is, gonadectomized male and female rats, and gonadectomized male rats treated chronically with estrogen, exhibit lower responding to AB than to A after training on the AX+, BX– discrimination. By contrast, gonadectomized female rats treated chronically with estrogen respond equally highly to A and to AB, suggesting that estrogen interferes with the use of safety signals in female rats specifically. This may be consistent with reports that estrogen interferes with emotional inhibition under a variety of circumstances in women (Goldstein et al., 2005; Milad, Rauch, Pitman, & Quirk, 2006; Protopopescu et al., 2005). Interestingly, estrogen receptor alpha and beta modulators disrupted discrimination learning in rats of both sexes, in opposite directions: The estrogen receptor alpha agonist propyl-pyrazole-triol enhanced, and the estrogen receptor beta agonist diarylpropionitrile suppressed, responding to all cues (relative to responding in sham-treated controls). These findings suggest that the effect of estrogen is mediated by opposing actions at these two receptor subtypes.

We (Myers & Davis, 2004b) also have used the AX+, BX– discrimination to examine the role of the medial prefrontal cortex in the development and expression of conditioned inhibition. Consistent with earlier work from our laboratory examining extinction and conditioned inhibition with the A+, BA– discrimination (Gewirtz et al., 1997), we have found no evidence to support a role of this region in inhibition of fear-potentiated startle.

The AX+, BX– Discrimination in Nonhuman Primates

Our interest in the role of higher cortical areas, including the medial prefrontal cortex, in conditioned inhibition led us and our colleague Pam Noble to consider the possibility of adapting the AX+, BX– discrimination to the nonhuman primate fear-potentiated startle paradigm (Winslow, Noble, & Davis, 2008; Winslow, Parr, & Davis, 2002). Startle was measured in monkeys basically the same way as in rats, but with a larger cage (Figure 3.2, center panel). This paradigm is very similar to the rodent fear-potentiated startle paradigm. It involves presenting rhesus macaques with cues including lights, tones, and fans paired with an aversive event (in this case, a 100-p.s.i., 500-msec air blast directed at the face, rather than a footshock), and then measuring the amplitude of a whole-body acoustic startle response when startle is elicited in the presence versus the absence of these cues.

Whereas the AX+, BX– discrimination can be learned by rats in a single session of training under some circumstances, Winslow and colleagues (2008) found that rhesus macaques required a more complex sequence of training. Because in pilot studies they found that some monkeys showed an unconditioned increase in startle amplitude to some of the cues or cue combinations, they first preexposed all monkeys (12 male rhesus macaques) to each of the three cues and cue combinations, to habituate these unconditioned facilitatory effects. There were two or three sessions of pretraining to A, B, X, AX, BX, and AB, where A, B, and X were represented by 4-sec light, tone, and fan cues, counterbalanced, and AX, BX, and AB compound cues were presented simultaneously (i.e., with concurrent onsets and offsets of the component cues). Each session involved eight presentations of each cue or cue combination with a startle stimulus (a 40-msec, 90- to 120-dB broadband noise burst) occurring 3.5 sec after cue onset, as well as additional startle stimuli occurring in the absence of any cue. Pretraining continued until each monkey exhibited less than 20% potentiation on any trial type.

After this, there were three stages of training. The first was A+ training, in which there were three sessions each involving four pairings of the A cue with an air blast. The A+ trials were embedded among 36 presentations of the startle stimulus—half of which occurred in the presence of 18 additional, unreinforced A presentations, and half of which occurred in the absence of any other cue—for the purpose of assessing fear acquisition to A. The second stage of training was A+, B–, which was structured similarly to A+ training except that the four pairings of A with the air blast were embedded among 36 startle stimuli—12 of which occurred in the presence of 12 additional, unreinforced A presentations, 12 of which occurred in the presence of 12 unreinforced B presentations, and 12 of which occurred in the absence of any other cue. The third stage of training was AX+, BX–, which was structured exactly like A+, B– except that the X cue was presented simultaneously with every presentation of A and B. Finally, the monkeys were given a posttest of fear-potentiated startle to AX, BX, AB, A, B, and X, which involved two presentations of each of these cues with a startle stimulus and four presentations of the startle stimulus in the absence of any cue.

The results are shown in Figure 3.5. After the habituation procedures, none of the cues or cue combinations produced any potentiation of startle prior to training (not shown). However, upon introduction of A+ trials, the monkeys showed potentiated startle in the presence of A that increased in magnitude across sessions of training. When B– trials were added, the monkeys came quickly to discriminate between A and B. Finally, when an X cue was added to create simultaneous AX+ and BX– compounds, the monkeys learned quickly to discriminate between AX and BX. In testing, responding to AX was significantly greater than responding to BX—and, importantly, responding to AB was significantly less than responding to A alone from the first presentation of these cues, suggesting that B was a conditioned inhibitor

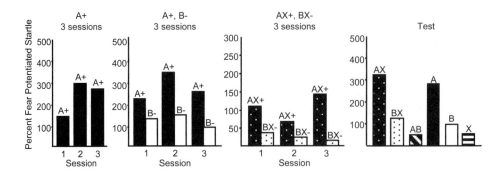

FIGURE 3.5. Mean percentage of fear-potentiated startle across several stages of training and test in the AX+, BX− discrimination in the nonhuman primate fear-potentiated startle paradigm. Monkeys were exposed to several sessions of A+ training, then to several sessions of A+, B− training, and finally to several sessions of AX+, BX− training. In testing, monkeys exhibited significantly less fear-potentiated startle to AB than to A, suggesting that B was a conditioned inhibitor. From Winslow, Noble, and Davis (2008). Copyright 2008 by the Cold Spring Harbor Laboratory Press. Reprinted by permission.

that suppressed the startle potentiation occasioned by A. Overall, the pattern of responding on the AX, BX, AB, A, B, and X test trials looked very similar to that seen in rats in the Myers and Davis (2004) study (compare with Figure 3.4).

This represents the first study to demonstrate transfer of a safety signal in a discrimination learning experiment with fear-potentiated startle in nonhuman primates under conditions in which external inhibition (as well as other complications, including second order conditioning and configural learning) are minimized. Because the AX+, BX− paradigm permits an independent analysis of fear potentiation and fear inhibition in the same subject in the same session, it should provide a unique opportunity to look at neural processes associated with modulation of fear, such as cortical regulation of the amygdala. Currently underway are experiments in which repeated AX+, BX− training and testing in the same set of monkeys, using pictures as cues, will allow within-subject comparisons of amygdalar and cortical inactivation or pharmacological treatments on both the acquisition and expression of inhibitory learning.

The AX+, BX− Discrimination in Healthy Humans

The ultimate aim of all of this work, obviously, is to understand the mechanisms of conditioned fear acquisition and inhibition in humans, as well as the ways in which these processes go awry with psychopathology. To this end, Tanja Jovanovic, Seth Norrholm, and Erica Duncan translated the AX+, BX− procedure into a human fear-potentiated startle paradigm (Figure 3.2, lower panel), to allow for the most direct translation possible from animal to human studies (Jovanovic et al., 2005, 2006, in press). They began by studying healthy humans and more recently have begun to examine psychiatric populations as well, focusing in particular on people suffering from posttraumatic stress disorder (PTSD).

One of the difficulties in translating animal paradigms to situations involving human participants is that humans tend to perceive a compound stimulus as a unique, single stimulus rather than as a collection of separate stimulus elements (Williams, Sagness, & McPhee, 1995). Such configural processing would allow humans to solve the AX+, BX− discrimination by treating AX as one stimulus and BX as another. As a result, they would not learn that stimulus B signaled safety but rather that stimulus BX did, making it unlikely that B would inhibit A in an AB test trial. In an effort to encourage participants to process each cue as a separate element, several modifications from the rodent protocol were incorporated into the human protocol. First, only compound cues (AX, BX, and AB, and not A, B, and X) were used, to avoid having people see single cues as categorically different from compound cues. Second, compound cues were presented in a sequential manner, and the order in which the component cues appeared in the sequence varied across trials. Finally, a response keypad was used during the session to assess "contingency awareness" (defined as a participant's knowledge of the reinforcement contingencies in the experiment; Lovibond & Shanks, 2002) for lights A, X, and B separately. Participants rated each cue as it appeared in sequence as reinforced (threat), nonreinforced (safe), or unclear by pressing different buttons on the keypad.

In the initial study in this series, Jovanovic and colleagues (2005) tested 41 healthy participants (16 women and 25 men; age range = 20–74 years; no current or lifetime Axis I disorders; no auditory or visual impairment). Participants were seated in a sound-attenuating chamber directly across from a display of green, purple, orange, and blue light bulbs that served as the cues (counterbalanced). They were given a single session of training involving multiple phases: habituation, conditioning, test phase 1, reconditioning, and test phase 2. During habituation, the participants were exposed to six startle probes (104- to 108-dB, 40-msec broadband noise burst) in the absence of any cue for the purpose of habituating the startle response to a stable baseline. Next, during conditioning, participants were presented with two blocks of trials, each including three pairings of AX with an air blast (100 msec, 140 p.s.i.) directed to the larynx, three presentations of BX without an air blast, and three startle probes in the absence of any other cue. The AX and BX trials were structured as described above, with an alternating sequential presentation of the component cues across trials (represented schematically in the top panel of Figure 3.6). A startle probe was presented on each occurrence of AX and BX and preceded the onset of the US on AX+ trials. Hence, unlike the rodent and nonhuman primate paradigms, startle potentiation was assessed "online" to AX and BX during training rather than in separate test trials.[2]

After conditioning, the participants were given two phases of testing, the order of which was counterbalanced across subjects. The first test phase involved six presentations of either AB or AC (where C was a novel cue) together with a startle stimulus, and six presentations of the startle stimulus in the absence of any cue. The AB test trial, as before, assessed the ability of B to inhibit startle potentiation occasioned by A, and the AC test trial was included to assess whether B's inhibitory power was conditioned (in which case no suppression of potentiation would be expected in the presence of C) or unconditioned (in which case responding in the presence of AC should be similarly low as in the presence of AB). After test phase 1, there was a brief reconditioning phase involving three AX+ trials and three startle stimuli in the absence of any cue. Finally, participants were exposed to test phase 2, which was structured exactly like test phase 1 except that each participant received whichever of the AB or AC cues they did not experience in test phase 1. On each cued trial throughout training and test, participants were instructed to use the response keypad to respond to each light separately by pressing one of three buttons: "+" when they expected a light to be followed by the air blast; "–" when they did not expect the light to be followed by the air blast; and "0" when they were uncertain of what to expect.

The lower panel of Figure 3.6 presents the startle potentiation observed to AX and BX in the second block of conditioning and to AB and AC in testing. As expected, the subjects discriminated between AX and BX—and, importantly, they exhibited less potentiation to AB than to AX or to AC. This indicates that, similar to rats and rhesus macaques, humans are able to learn the AX+, BX– discrimination and do so by acquiring conditioned inhibition to B. Interestingly, on the response keypad, B (when presented as part of an AB compound) was labeled as nonreinforced 94.7% of the time, whereas C (when presented as part of an AC compound) was labeled as unknown 68.4% of the time, corroborating the difference in startle responding to these cues. In a separate study with a different cohort of participants, Jovanovic and colleagues (2006) found that participants who were aware of the experimental contingencies showed fear potentiation to AX, discrimination between AX and BX, and inhibition of fear potentiation on AB trials; participants who were unaware showed fear potentiation to AX, but no discrimination between AX and BX, and no inhibition on AB trials. This study suggests that different processes underlie fear acquisition and fear inhibition, such that fear acquisition may occur through a low-level mechanism that does not require cognitive input, whereas fear inhibition processes may be based on a cognitive model and require contingency awareness (Lovibond, 2004).

Trial types in training

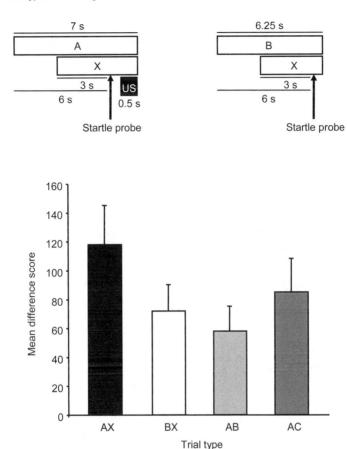

FIGURE 3.6. *Top panel:* Schematic representation of the trial types used by Jovanovic et al. (2005, 2006, in press) during training on the AX+, BX– discrimination in humans. A, B, and X were represented by the illumination of colored light bulbs. Compound cues were presented sequentially as shown. The order of the two cues varied across trials; hence in some AX+ trials, A came on first and was followed by X, and in other trials, X came on first and was followed by A. On all trials, a startle probe occurred 6 sec after the onset of the first cue. On AX+ trials, the startle probe was followed 0.5 sec later by an air blast US, and on BX– trials, the lights coterminated 0.5 sec after the startle probe and the air blast was omitted. AB and AC test trials were structured similarly to the BX– training trial. *Bottom panel:* Mean startle difference scores to AX, BX, AB, and AC in nondisordered human participants following training on the AX+, BX– discrimination. Participants discriminated between AX and BX and showed less inhibition of fear-potentiated startle to AB than to AC. From Jovanovic et al. (2005). Copyright 2005 by the Society of Biological Psychiatry. Reprinted by permission.

The AX+, BX– Discrimination in Patients with PTSD

One of the central problems in PTSD is an inability to suppress fear even under safe conditions (Rothbaum & Davis, 2003), and it has been hypothesized that impairments in fear suppression mechanisms are a risk factor for the development of PTSD (Guthrie & Bryant, 2006). Jovanovic and her colleagues (in press) hypothesized that these deficits might be manifested as a failure of inhibition on AB test trials after training on the AX+, BX– discrimination, and that those patients with the greatest current symptom severity would exhibit the most pronounced deficits on the task. To evaluate this, Jovanovic et al. tested 31 healthy volunteers and 33 Vietnam and Iraq War veterans seeking treatment for PTSD at the Atlanta Veterans Affairs Medical Center; the same protocol as that described above was used. The patients with PTSD were divided into low- and high-symptom groups according to the symptoms they experienced in the preceding month, as assessed by the Clinician-Administered PTSD Scale (Blake et al., 1990), but the two subgroups with PTSD did not otherwise differ in age, race, or severity of combat exposure.

The data are presented in Figure 3.7, which shows the mean percentage of startle potentiation observed to AX, BX, AB, and AC in each of the three groups. In this experiment, unlike the previous one (Jovanovic et al., 2005), there was no evidence that B was a conditioned as opposed to an external

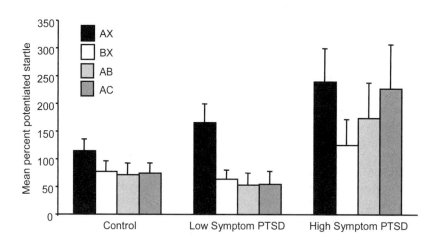

FIGURE 3.7. Mean percentage of fear-potentiated startle to AX, BX, AB, and AC after training on the AX+, BX– discrimination in controls as well as in low- and high-symptom participants with PTSD drawn from a population of Vietnam and Iraq War veterans seeking treatment for PTSD at the Atlanta Veterans Affairs Medical Center in Atlanta, Georgia. High-symptom patients did not discriminate significantly between AX and BX, nor did they exhibit lower responding to AB than to AX, unlike low-symptom patients or controls. From Jovanovic et al. (in press). Copyright by Elsevier. Reprinted by permission.

inhibitor, because responding on AC test trials was just as low as on AB test trials in the control group. Nevertheless, an interesting pattern emerged when the low- and high-symptom groups with PTSD were compared: Whereas the low-symptom group behaved very similarly to the control group, the high-symptom group exhibited a deficit in inhibition to both AB and AC. That is, in the high-symptom group, neither AB nor AC was significantly lower than AX. Interestingly, contingency awareness as assessed via the response keypad was similar in all three groups: Both the controls and the low- and high-symptom patients indicated that they expected the air blast following AX, but not following BX, AB, or AC. This is consistent with the hypothesis that explicit and implicit learning of fear and fear inhibition may proceed by different neural mechanisms (Jovanovic et al., 2006), and suggests that awareness of safety may be *necessary* to inhibit fear-potentiated startle but is not always *sufficient*.

The deficit in fear inhibition in the presence of AB fits nicely with clinical perspectives of PTSD as a fundamental lack of fear suppression or moderation in circumstances in which safety might reasonably be expected. Hence we believe that the AX+, BX− paradigm will prove to be useful in evaluating potential treatments for PTSD in terms of their ability to mitigate the difficulty in suppressing fear on AB test trials. It is possible that this test may be able to measure a biological marker of PTSD, which would be an extremely helpful diagnostic and research tool.

CONCLUSIONS AND FUTURE DIRECTIONS

In this chapter, we have described a body of work geared toward developing a paradigm for the investigation of fear inhibition, translating that paradigm across species, and verifying its validity in animals and humans (including both healthy and psychiatric populations). We have provided evidence that the AX+, BX− discrimination may be used to examine the neurobiology of fear inhibition and to detect specific deficiencies in fear inhibition processes in psychiatric populations.

Still on the horizon is a systematic analysis of the neural mechanisms of fear inhibition, although it is not difficult to imagine how the AX+, BX− paradigm might be used to this end. We have mentioned some work that has already been done, including examinations of the role of gonadal steroids (Toufexis et al., 2007) and the medial prefrontal cortex (Myers & Davis, 2004b) in the development and expression of fear inhibition, but clearly much more remains to be accomplished. In humans in particular, relatively little is known about the circuitry of fear inhibition. As we have described, the AX+, BX− discrimination is particularly beneficial in that it allows fear elicitation and fear inhibition processes to be examined separately, because each of these tendencies is controlled by a different stimulus. For this reason, the discrimination is likely to prove very useful in a variety of neurobiological investigations, including imaging studies in humans.

ACKNOWLEDGMENTS

We thank Michael E. Bowser, Pamela L. Noble, Kevin Hertzberg, Jennifer Fennell, Megan Keyes, and Ana M. Fiallos for their assistance with several of the experiments described in this chapter. This work was supported by Kirchstein National Research Service Award Individual Fellowships No. 1F32 MH77420 to Karyn M. Myers and No. 1F32 MH070129 to Tanja Jovanovich; National Institute of Mental Health (NIMH) Grant Nos. MH47840, MH57250, MH52384, MH58922, and MH59906 to Michael Davis and Grant No. MH76869 to Donna J. Toufexis; a grant from the Intramural Program of the National Institutes of Health and the NIMH to James T. Winslow; National Institute on Drug Abuse Grant No. 1R01 DA018294-01A2 to Erica J. Duncan; an American Psychiatric Association GlaxoSmithKline Award to Erica J. Duncan; the National Science Foundation under Agreement No. IBN-9876754 (Venture Grant) to Erica J. Duncan; the Woodruff Foundation; the Science and Technology Center (the Center for Behavioral Neuroscience of the National Science Foundation under Agreement No. IBN-9876754); the Yerkes Base Grant; and the Mental Health Service, Atlanta Veterans Affairs Medical Center.

NOTES

1. Note that B is predicted to become less inhibitory after training on the AX+, BX– discrimination than after training on the A+, BA– discrimination. This is because conditioned inhibition develops to B to the extent that the cue with which it is compounded has developed excitatory associative strength. Hence, because X becomes a somewhat weak excitor due to compound cue overshadowing on AX+ trials, B becomes less inhibitory after AX+, BX– training than after A+, BA– training. This incomplete inhibition that develops to B with AX+, BX– training is less than ideal, but was considered acceptable in light of the other benefits afforded by the AX+, BX– discrimination over the A+, BA– discrimination, including the mitigation of external inhibition, second order conditioning, and configural learning.
2. The trials were designed in this way because humans habituate very quickly and profoundly to the startle stimulus, and hence it was considered desirable to keep the experimental session as brief as possible. Rats can be trained under a similar protocol in which the startle stimulus is embedded within the training trials, and they behave very similarly to what is seen when they are given a separate test session (Toufexis et al., 2007).

REFERENCES

Blake, D. D., Weather, F. W., Nagy, L. M., Kaloupek, D. G., Klauminker, G., Charney, D. S., et al. (1990). A clinical rating scale for assessing current and lifetime PTSD: The CAPS-1. *The Behavior Therapist, 18,* 187–188.

Bouton, M. E. (2000). A learning theory perspective on lapse, relapse, and the maintenance of behavior change. *Health Psychology, 19,* 57–63.

Bouton, M. E. (2004). Context and behavioral processes in extinction. *Learning and Memory, 11,* 485–494.

Brown, J. S., Kalish, H. I., & Farber, I. E. (1951). Conditional fear as revealed by magnitude of startle response to an auditory stimulus. *Journal of Experimental Psychology, 41,* 317–328.

Campeau, S., Falls, W. A., Cullinan, W. E., Helmreich, D. L., Davis, M., & Watson, S. J. (1997). Elicitation and reduction of fear: Behavioral and neuroendocrine indices and brain induction of the immediate-early gene *c-fos. Neuroscience, 78,* 1087–1104.

Davis, M. (2000). The role of the amygdala in conditioned and unconditioned fear and anxiety. In J. P. Aggleton (Ed.), *The amygdala: A functional analysis* (2nd ed., pp. 213–287). Oxford, UK: Oxford University Press.

Davis, M., & Astrachan, D. I. (1978). Conditioned fear and startle magnitude: Effects of different footshock or backshock intensities used in training. *Journal of Experimental Psychology: Animal Behavior Processes, 4,* 95–103.

Falls, W. A., Bakken, S., & Heldt, S. A. (1997). Lesions of the perirhinal cortex block conditioned excitation but not conditioned inhibition of fear. *Behavioral Neuroscience, 111,* 476–486.

Falls, W. A., & Davis, M. (1995). Lesions of the central nucleus of the amygdala block conditioned excitation, but not conditioned inhibition of fear as measured with the fear-potentiated startle effect. *Behavioral Neuroscience, 109,* 379–387.

Falls, W. A., & Davis, M. J. (1997). Inhibition of fear-potentiated startle can be detected after the offset of a feature trained in a serial feature negative discrimination. *Journal of Experimental Psychology: Animal Behavior Processes, 23,* 3–14.

Gewirtz, J. C., Falls, W. A., & Davis, M. (1997). Normal conditioned inhibition and extinction of freezing and fear potentiated startle following electrolytic lesions of medial prefrontal cortex. *Behavioral Neuroscience, 111,* 712–726.

Goldstein, J. M., Jerram, M., Poldrack, R., Ahern, T., Kennedy, D. N., Seidman, L. J., et al. (2005). Hormonal cycle modulates arousal circuitry in women using functional magnetic resonance imaging. *Journal of Neuroscience, 25,* 9309–9316.

Guthrie, R. M., & Bryant, R. A. (2006). Extinction learning before trauma and subsequent posttraumatic stress. *Psychosomatic Medicine, 68,* 307–311.

Heldt, S. A., Coover, G. D., & Falls, W. A. (2002). Posttraining but not pretraining lesions of the hippocampus interfere with feature-negative discrimination of fear-potentiated startle. *Hippocampus, 12,* 774–786.

Heldt, S. A., & Falls, W. A. (1998). Destruction of the auditory thalamus disrupts the production of fear but not the inhibition of fear conditioned to an auditory stimulus. *Brain Research, 813,* 274–282.

Heldt, S. A., & Falls, W. A. (2003). Destruction of the inferior colliculus disrupts the production and inhibition of fear conditioned to an acoustic stimulus. *Behavioural Brain Research, 144,* 175–185.

Heldt, S. A., & Falls, W. A. (2006). Posttraining lesions of the auditory thalamus, but not cortex, disrupt the inhibition of fear conditioned to an auditory stimulus. *European Journal of Neuroscience, 23,* 765–779.

Josselyn, S. A., Falls, W. A., Gewirtz, J. C., Pistell, P., & Davis, M. (2005). The nucleus accumbens is not critically involved in mediating the effects of a safety signal on behavior. *Neuropsychopharmacology, 30,* 17–26.

Jovanovic, T., Keyes, M., Fiallos, A., Myers, K. M., Davis, M., & Duncan, E. J. (2005). Fear potentiation and fear inhibition in a human fear-potentiated startle paradigm. *Biological Psychiatry, 57,* 1559–1564.

Jovanovic, T., Norrholm, S. D., Fennell, J. E., Keyes, M., Fiallos, A. M., Myers, K. M., et al. (in press). Posttraumatic stress disorder may be associated with impaired fear inhibition: Relation to symptom severity. *Psychiatry Research.*

Jovanovic, T., Norrholm, S. D., Keyes, M., Fiallos, A., Jovanovic, S., Myers, K. M., et al. (2006). Contingency awareness and fear inhibition in a human fear-potentiated startle paradigm. *Behavioral Neuroscience, 120,* 995–1004.

Lovibond, P. F. (2004). Cognitive processes in extinction. *Learning and Memory, 11,* 495–500.

Lovibond, P. F., & Shanks, D. R. (2002). The role of awareness in Pavlovian conditioning: Empirical evidence and theoretical implications. *Journal of Experimental Psychology: Animal Behavior Processes, 28,* 3–26.

Milad, M. R., Rauch, S. L., Pitman, R. K., & Quirk, G. J. (2006). Fear extinction in rats: Implications for human brain imaging and anxiety disorders. *Biological Psychiatry, 73,* 61–71.

Myers, K. M., & Davis, M. (2004a). AX+, BX– discrimination learning in the fear-potentiated startle paradigm: Possible relevance to inhibitory fear learning in extinction. *Learning and Memory, 11,* 464–475.

Myers, K. M., & Davis, M. (2004b). [Inactivation of the infralimbic region of medial prefrontal cortex does not impair extinction or conditioned inhibition of fear-potentiated startle]. Unpublished raw data.

Myers, K. M., & Davis, M. (2007). Mechanisms of fear extinction. *Molecular Psychiatry, 12,* 120–150.

Myers, K. M., Toufexis, D. J., Bowser, M. E., & Davis, M. (2007). [External inhibition does not account for the reduction in responding to A in the presence of B in the AX+, BX– paradigm]. Unpublished raw data.

Paschall, G. Y., & Davis, M. (2002). Olfactory mediated fear potentiated startle. *Behavioral Neuroscience, 116,* 4–12.

Pavlov, I. P. (1927). *Conditioned reflexes.* Oxford, UK: Oxford University Press.

Phelps, E. A., & LeDoux, J. E. (2005). Contributions of the amygdala to emotion processing: From animal models to human behavior. *Neuron, 48,* 175–187.

Protopopescu, X., Pan, H., Altemusu, M., Tuescher, O., Polanecsky, M., McEwen, B., et al. (2005). Orbitofrontal cortex activity related to emotional processing changes across the menstrual cycle. *Proceedings of the National Academy of Sciences USA, 102,* 16060–16065.

Rescorla, R. A. (1969). Pavlovian conditioned inhibition. *Psychological Bulletin, 72,* 77–94.

Rescorla, R. A., & Wagner, A. R. (1972). A theory of Pavlovian conditioning: Variations in the effectiveness of reinforcement and nonreinforcement. In A. H. Black & W. F. Prokasy (Eds.), *Classical conditioning II: Current research and theory* (pp. 64–99). New York: Appleton-Century-Crofts.

Rickert, E. J., Lorden, J. F., Dawson, R., Jr., Smyly, E., & Callahan, M. F. (1979). Stimulus processing and stimulus selection in rats with hippocampal lesions. *Behavioral and Neural Biology, 27,* 454–465.

Rodrigues, S. M., Schafe, G. E., & LeDoux, J. E. (2004). Molecular mechanisms underlying emotional learning and memory in the lateral amygdala. *Neuron, 44,* 75–91.

Rothbaum, B. O., & Davis, M. (2003). Applying learning principles to the treatment of post-trauma reactions. *Annals of the New York Academy of Sciences, 1008,* 112–121.

Toufexis, D. J., Myers, K. M., Bowser, M. E., & Davis, M. (2007). Estrogen disrupts the inhibition of fear in female rats, possibly through antagonistic effects of ERα and ERβ. *Journal of Neuroscience, 27,* 9729–9735.

Waddell, J., Heldt, S., & Falls, W. A. (2003). Posttraining lesion of the superior colliculus interferes with feature-negative discrimination of fear-potentiated startle. *Behavioural Brain Research, 142,* 115–124.

Wagner, A. R., Logan, F. A., Haberlandt, K., & Price, T. (1968). Stimulus selection in animal discrimination learning. *Journal of Experimental Psychology, 76,* 177–186.

Wagner, A. R., & Rescorla, R. A. (1972). Inhibition in Pavlovian conditioning: application of a theory. In R. A. Boakes & M. S. Halliday (Eds.), *Inhibition and learning* (pp. 301–336). London: Academic Press.

Williams, D. A., Sagness, K. E., & McPhee, J. E. (1995). Configural and elemental strategies in predictive learning. *Journal of Experimental Psychology: Learning, Memory, and Cognition, 20,* 694–709.

Winslow, J. T., Noble, P. L., & Davis, M. (2008). AX+/BX– discrimination learning in the fear-potentiated startle paradigm in monkeys. *Learning and Memory, 15,* 63–66.

Winslow, J. T., Parr, L. A., & Davis, M. (2002). Acoustic startle, prepulse inhibition and fear-potentiated startle measured in rhesus monkeys. *Biological Psychiatry, 51,* 859–866.

CHAPTER 4

Amygdala Function in Positive Reinforcement
CONTRIBUTIONS FROM STUDIES OF NONHUMAN PRIMATES

Elisabeth A. Murray, Alicia Izquierdo, and Ludise Malkova

A role for the amygdala in *negative* reinforcement and *negative* affect has received considerable attention in contemporary neuroscience. The conditioned fear paradigm, including fear-potentiated startle, has been so extensively studied that the literature as a whole sometimes gives the impression that the amygdala functions primarily in negatively valenced emotion. Indeed, as conditioned fear studies have shown, the amygdala is essential for linking initially neutral sensory cues (e.g., a light or a tone) with a naturally aversive stimulus (e.g., an electrical shock) that by itself produces an array of defensive responses. An animal need only experience a few presentations of an originally neutral cue (the conditioned stimulus, or CS) and an aversive stimulus (the unconditioned stimulus, or US) to learn that the former predicts the latter. As a result of amygdala-dependent learning, exposure to the CS alone comes to produce the defensive responses originally elicited by the aversive US, including freezing, reflex potentiation, tachycardia and other aspects of autonomic arousal, hypoalgesia, and a stress response, among others. This widely studied aspect of amygdala function has led to the idea that the amygdala serves primarily to process negative reinforcement and to produce negative affect.

Much of the emphasis on negative reinforcement and negative emotions comes from research on rodents, but some primate researchers have also adopted this perspective. For example, Amaral and his colleagues have likened the primate amygdala to a "protection device." In this view, amygdala function "is expected to be most clearly manifested as a cautious response to novelty, ambiguity, and perceived danger and should diminish as exposures are repeated, assuming adverse consequences do not ensue" (Mason, Capitanio, Machado, Mendoza, & Amaral, 2006, p. 79). Although the notion that the amygdala functions only in *negative* emotions and reinforcement has the attraction of simplicity, it rests on a narrow selection of the relevant data rather than on a comprehensive analysis of amygdala function. Early neuroimaging work on the amygdala likewise appeared to give credence to this narrow view of amygdala function (e.g., Morris et al., 1996). Although more recent research has contradicted some of those early results, some of the impressions left by the earlier findings have proven difficult to dispel.

Notwithstanding the popularity of this "negative" view of amygdala function, experimental work in rodents and nonhuman primates has indicated that the amygdala's role in learning about potentially valuable "good things" via positive reinforcement is as important as its role in learning about potentially damaging "bad things" via negative reinforcement. Much of the literature on this topic has been reviewed previously (Baxter & Murray, 2002; Everitt, Cardinal, Parkinson, & Robbins, 2003; Holland & Gallagher, 1999) and is not reexamined here. Instead, this chapter broadens the discussion to address *why* the amygdala contributes to both positive and negative reinforcement. "Why" questions, as is well known, depend on a comparative and evolutionary perspective for their answers, and we attempt to put the amygdala and its function in such a perspective.

We first address the nature of positive reinforcement in experimental neuropsychology. The concept of reward and reinforcement is not as simple as it is sometimes portrayed, and the next section explains the diverse ways in which positive reinforcement can be used by advanced mammals, such as nonhuman primates and humans. Then we show that the amygdala contributes crucially to positive reinforcement. The amygdala is not, however, involved in all aspects of positive reinforcement, and we also identify important behaviors that depend on positive reinforcement, but for which the amygdala is not needed. Finally, we place the primate amygdala in a comparative perspective, presenting the idea that the amygdala endows cognitive constructs (including words, rules, concepts, and conclusions) with emotional valence.

Throughout this chapter, we develop three major themes. First, as noted above, the amygdala contributes as much to positive reinforcement and positive affect as it does to the negative. Second, it does so in part by linking initially neutral neural representations with innate response mechanisms. And, third, two distinct parts of the amygdala—typified by the basolateral amygdala and the central nucleus of the amygdala, respectively—contribute to amygdala function differently and in parallel. As proposed by Balleine and

Killcross (2006), the basolateral amygdala links initially neutral representations with specific aspects of reinforcement, such as the tastes, smells, and visceral sensory signals associated with a given kind of food or fluid, whereas the central nucleus performs a similar linkage for general aspects of reinforcement.

HOW DO ADVANCED ANIMALS USE POSITIVE REINFORCEMENT?

A key problem in understanding the role of the amygdala in positive reinforcement is that neither "reinforcement" nor "reward" is an uncomplicated concept. Reward has many aspects, including hedonic (liking) and incentive (wanting and seeking) value. In addition, reward is conditional, varying in terms of probability, timing, quantity and quality, consistency over time, effort required to obtain it, and so forth. For example, a given reinforcer could be always rewarding, more rewarding recently, or usually rewarding but not as much recently; it could be "worth the effort" required to obtain it now, but not an hour ago; and, in humans at least, it could be wanted, yet at the same time not *wanted* to be wanted.

Many tasks previously used to probe the role of the amygdala (and other structures) in positive reinforcement in nonhuman primates have depended on some version of object discrimination and reversal learning. These and related tasks are taken up again below (see "What the Amygdala Does Not Do"), because it turns out that the reputed role of the amygdala in such tasks was incorrect. Object discrimination and reversal learning, however, serve to illustrate some of the many problems inherent in an oversimplified view of reinforcement and reward. In these tasks, one object is designated as correct, and choice of this object produces a reward—for example, a peanut. Another object is designated as incorrect, and choice of this object yields nothing. This task has been the "coin of the realm" in primate neuropsychology since the 1950s, and remains so to an astonishing extent. On the surface, object discrimination tasks seem simple, even elegant. As Gaffan (1985) has observed, however, this surface simplicity is deceptive. Beneath the surface are cognitive processes of enormous complexity, and, especially in advanced mammals, several different mechanisms can be used to perform discrimination and reversal tasks. Although they all in some way involve learning by and about positive reinforcement, such tasks can be solved by several means:

- Object–outcome associations: Choosing the object that is predicted to produce the outcome with the highest biological value.
- Action–outcome associations: Choosing the action that is predicted to produce the outcome with the highest biological value.
- Habits: Choosing a certain object whenever it appears, without reference to predicted outcome.

- Selective behavioral inhibition: Avoiding a certain object whenever it appears, with or without reference to predicted outcome.
- Performance rules or strategies: Choosing the object that occurred in proximity to food reward (i.e., the one that is associated in memory with the appearance of a peanut). In this example, the food reward plays two roles. First, it provides a signal to guide object selection; second, it serves to reinforce the performance rule (see Gaffan, 1985).
- Conditional associations: When one object is to the right and another to the left, choosing the one at left, and vice versa. In this case, what is reinforced is the conditional association of a configuration of objects with a particular spatially directed action.

And all of the foregoing can apply to both positive reinforcement as a general proposition and to each and every sensory aspect of the reinforcer in particular (e.g., the olfactory, gustatory, tactile, and visceral aspects of a food reinforcer). Naturally occurring rewards include food, water, salt, and sex, among other things, and environmental stimuli linked to these types of rewards can themselves become reinforcing. Given this diversity of cognitive processes, it should not be surprising that the amygdala—or a part of the amygdala—plays a role in some, but not all, of the foregoing processes. But which ones, and why?

WHAT THE AMYGDALA DOES

One answer to the "why" question posed immediately above is that the amygdala is essential for the formation of several types of associations that are central to survival, including associations guiding food-seeking, ingestive, reproductive, parental, and defensive behaviors, among others. In many instances, the amygdala appears to link sensory inputs with neural circuits mediating instinctive behaviors, such as autonomic reflexes (Braesicke et al., 2005) and orienting responses (Gallagher, Graham, & Holland, 1990). In other instances, the amygdala acts to enhance the processing of unexpected ("surprising") sensory events (Holland & Gallagher, 1993), perhaps because unexpected inputs trigger innate responses. And in yet other instances, the amygdala acts to assign positive or negative value to neural representations of sensory inputs, and other representations as well. Thus the amygdala plays a key role in connecting external sensory information to the instinctive processes that underlie the most fundamental aspects of vertebrate behavior.

Neuropsychology in Rodents

Although this chapter emphasizes work in nonhuman primates, we briefly discuss the amygdala's contributions to positive reinforcement in rodents, to provide a broader perspective. What follows is by no means an exhaustive account, which can be found elsewhere (Balleine, 2005; Balleine & Killcross, 2006; Everitt et al., 2003). Although various reinforcers (such as water and other fluids, sex, and drugs) have been investigated, the examples cited below use food as the reinforcer, for simplicity's sake.

Central Nucleus of the Amygdala

PAVLOVIAN APPROACH

One major effect of pairing an initially neutral cue—that is, a CS—with a food is that presentation of the CS leads to the production of the same set of responses occurring in the presence of the food. Specifically, in the presence of the CS alone, an animal will exhibit conditioned responses that anticipate the upcoming reward delivery, in a way that is often specific to the reward type. For example, if the reward is a fluid, a CS may elicit licking, whereas if the reward is food, a CS may elicit biting movements or salivation. CSs also elicit approach responses. All these kinds of learning promote the likelihood of obtaining nutrients and fluids, and several studies have shown that the amygdala is essential for such learning. For example, in Pavlovian-approach conditioning, the presentation of one visual stimulus on a monitor screen precedes food delivery in a different location. As a control procedure, presentation of a second visual stimulus occurs independently of food delivery. In these circumstances, rats will selectively approach the CS (i.e., the stimulus that has been paired with food delivery), even though there is no requirement to do so.

The amygdala, or at least a part of the amygdala, plays a crucial role in learning about such positive reinforcement. Contrary to the idea that the amygdala is mainly involved in negative reinforcement and affect, lesions of the central nucleus of the amygdala disrupt the acquisition of these conditioned approach responses (Parkinson, Robbins, & Everitt, 2000). Note that the central nucleus is also a key structure for conditioned fear learning, so not even this small part of the amygdala has a function confined to negative reinforcement (see also Killcross, Robbins, & Everitt, 1997). Note also that there is no requirement for the animal to approach the CS, nor is this behavior instrumental in producing any outcome. Why then does it occur? We do not know the complete answer to this question, but it seems likely that Pavlovian approach occurs, at least in part, because of the innate responses (biting movements, salivation, etc.) elicited by the CS and by the instinctive food-seeking behavior incidentally triggered by those responses. As Gaffan (1985, pp. 90–91) has explained, "any stimulus that is associated in memory with food . . . operates via a fixed translation rule . . . to elicit approach." This rule is considered a "fixed, unlearned effect" (i.e., an innate performance rule).

Two additional factors need to be kept in mind. First, the amygdala is not essential for all forms of Pavlovian conditioning. And second, the basolateral amygdala does not need to be intact for Pavlovian-approach learning to take place. According to a recent theory by Balleine and Killcross (2006), the central nucleus of the amygdala functions in general reinforcement mechanisms and arousal, whereas the basolateral amygdala operates on specific aspects of different types of reinforcement. Accordingly, we turn now to aspects of positive reinforcement mediated by the basolateral amygdala.

Basolateral Amygdala

Recent work suggests that the basolateral complex of the amygdala is important for associating stimuli with the specific sensory features of a reinforcer, such as the visual, gustatory, and olfactory properties of a particular foodstuff (Balleine, 2005; Blundell, Hall, & Killcross, 2001). To preview the conclusions presented below, it is thought that the basolateral amygdala allows the CS to evoke a representation of the specific and updated value of a given positive reinforcer, which provides CSs with the ability to support new learning. Evidence in support of this idea is provided by tests of second-order conditioning, conditioned cue preference, reinforcer devaluation, and Pavlovian-instrumental transfer, among others. The need for an intact basolateral amygdala in these four types of tests further demonstrates the importance of the amygdala in positive reinforcement.

SECOND-ORDER CONDITIONING

Second-order conditioning studies ask whether a CS can support new learning. Such a CS is often called a "secondary reinforcer." This test is carried out in two steps. First (in the first-order conditioning), animals learn that a given cue (CS_1) signals a food reward. In a second step (the second-order conditioning), a second cue, CS_2, is paired with CS_1 in the absence of food. Intact animals show new learning based on presentation of CS_2, even though there is no delivery of a primary reinforcer at this stage. In one example, presentation of a light (CS_1) is paired with food delivery, and intact rats learn to approach and enter a food cup in anticipation of food delivery. In a second stage, a tone (CS_2) is paired with the light (CS_1); after this additional experience, control rats—in the presence of the tone (CS_2) alone—display the same kind of approach to the food cup as in the first stage, even though food is not available.

Although rats with pretraining lesions of the basolateral amygdala acquire the first-order conditioning as quickly as controls, they fail to show new learning in the second stage (Hatfield, Han, Conley, Gallagher, & Holland, 1996). Damage to the basolateral amygdala also prevents new learning if the second phase involves an operant response rather than a Pavlovian pairing (Everitt & Robbins, 1992). Recently it has been shown that once the first-order conditioning has taken place, rats do not need the amygdala to acquire the second-order conditioning (Setlow, Gallagher, & Holland, 2002). Consequently, the contribution of the amygdala to this kind of learning appears to be limited to the cue–food association that was acquired in the first stage of learning, but only to support second-order conditioning, not to support first-order conditioning (Hatfield et al., 1996).

These findings on second-order conditioning accord with the idea that the amygdala links initially neutral stimuli with innate mechanisms—in this case, the ability of initially neutral objects (secondary reinforcers) to support learning in a manner like the one that works instinctively for primary reinforcers.

CONDITIONED CUE PREFERENCE

The amygdala is also essential for conditioned cue preference, which involves Pavlovian pairing of one set of cues with food and, on a separate occasion, pairing of another set of cues with nothing (nonreinforced). The cues can be either locations (conditioned place preference) or objects (conditioned object preference). Rats are later given the opportunity to choose between the two sets of cues, and the experimenter records how much time is spent in proximity with one or the other. Intact animals tend to spend more time near the set of cues that was originally paired with food than they do with the set of cues that was not paired with food.

Lesions of the basolateral amygdala disrupt the rat's ability to express a preference for the cues that were paired with food, presumably because the basolateral amygdala is mediating the association of the cue(s) with reward value (Everitt, Morris, O'Brien, & Robbins, 1991; McDonald & White, 1993). The mechanisms underlying this behavior resemble those for Pavlovian approach: linking an initially neutral sensory representation with an innate response rule.

REINFORCER DEVALUATION

Another way that the amygdala's role in positive reinforcement has been assessed is through experiments that devalue the food paired with a CS. In an example involving Pavlovian conditioning, rats are first given paired presentations of a light CS and food. As a result, the rats approach the food cup (a conditioned response) in the presence of the CS. In a second step, conducted outside the test apparatus, the food is devalued in some of the rats by pairing food ingestion with injection of lithium chloride, which produces malaise. Eventually, these rats develop an aversion to eating the food. Later, when the rats are given the opportunity to exhibit food cup approach in the presence of the light CS, rats for which the food was devalued show many fewer approaches than do rats in which the value of the food was undisturbed.

This phenomenon is disrupted by lesions of the basolateral amygdala, but not by lesions of the central nucleus (Hatfield et al., 1996). Beyond strengthening the conclusion that the amygdala contributes crucially to positive reinforcement, this finding also supports the idea that it does so by linking initially neutral representations with innate processes and, in the case of basolateral amygdala function, eliciting a representation of the updated value of a specific reinforcer. Similar to the case for second-order conditioning described above, once the CS–food associations have been made, the amygdala is no longer needed to mediate the reinforcer devaluation effects (Pickens et al., 2003).

PAVLOVIAN-INSTRUMENTAL TRANSFER

Pavlovian-instrumental transfer (PIT) is a phenomenon through which reward-related cues influence actions. Experiments that reveal this phenomenon are carried out in three stages. First, CS–food pairings are learned in a Pavlovian manner. Second, animals learn that an action—for example, pressing a lever—produces the same kind of food. Third, the influence of the CS on instrumental responding is evaluated. As the animals perform the lever press in the presence of the CS for the first time, intact rats perform more instrumental responses than they do in the absence of the CS, revealing an excitatory influence of the CS on actions.

PIT is disrupted by lesions of the amygdala. Although early work suggested that the central nucleus alone is essential for PIT (Hall, Parkinson, Connor, Dickinson, & Everitt, 2001; Holland & Gallagher, 2003), more recent work has demonstrated that both the central nucleus and basolateral amygdala contribute, albeit in somewhat different ways. Whereas the central nucleus is essential for the CS to produce a general excitatory effect on actions, one independent of the particular foodstuff, the basolateral amygdala is essential for mediating effects specific to the primary reinforcer (Corbit & Balleine, 2005). In general, then, the basolateral amygdala appears to be important for linking cues with specific sensory properties of reward, whereas the central nucleus of the amygdala appears to link cues to reward in a more general way, perhaps by increasing arousal (Balleine & Killcross, 2006). In both cases, the amygdala seems to function by endowing initially neutral stimulus representations with the ability to invoke innate responses, such as arousal, and to mediate innate mechanisms, such as those driven by primary reinforcement.

Neuropsychology in Nonhuman Primates

Work in nonhuman primates has historically employed predominantly instrumental conditioning techniques rather than Pavlovian ones. In addition, the work capitalizes on the fact that vision is the sensory modality through which primates gather most information about the external world. Accordingly, to assess whether the primate amygdala contributes to assignment of value to a CS, Malkova, Gaffan, and Murray (1997) adapted a reinforcer devaluation procedure used with rats (Hatfield et al., 1996) for use with monkeys. Rather than employing Pavlovian-conditioned food cup approach, the task used in monkeys evaluates instrumental responses to objects. And rather than pairing food ingestion with malaise (produced by lithium chloride injection), the task employs a selective satiation procedure to devalue the food. In practice, monkeys learn about a large number of objects—some of which are associated with one kind of food, designated Food 1, and some associated with a different food, designated Food 2. The vehicle for acquiring these associations is a concurrent object discrimination task, in which 60 object pairs, each consisting of one baited object (S+) and one unbaited object (S−), are presented for choice each day, until each monkey learns to approach and displace the S+ to obtain the food reward hidden underneath.

Following the learning phase, monkeys are for the first time given the opportunity to choose between objects associated with either Food 1 or Food 2 in a series of critical test sessions carried out on separate days. There are three conditions: (1) baseline sessions to assess each monkey's relative preference for the different classes of objects; (2) sessions preceded by feeding to satiety of Food 1; and (3) sessions preceded by feeding to satiety of Food 2. In each condition, the monkeys are given the opportunity to choose between the two classes of objects, and their choices are recorded. In the baseline condition, the choices presumably reflect the monkeys underlying food preferences, although they express these preferences by the choice of objects. In the two other conditions, the ones employing the selective satiation procedure, intact monkeys avoid choosing the objects overlying the devalued food. The sensitivity to changes in reinforcer value is quantified by calculating a "difference score." For tests conducted with Food 1, for example, the difference score is the number of Food 1 objects chosen during the baseline condition minus the number of Food 1 objects chosen in the Food 1 devaluation condition. For simplicity, the two scores (one for Food 1 and one for Food 2) are summed to yield a cumulative difference score. Thus the higher the difference score, the greater the response to changes in reinforcer value.

Recently, we (Izquierdo & Murray, 2007) have reinvestigated the role of the amygdala in CS–value association, and have confirmed and extended the findings of Malkova and colleagues (1997). In this experiment, as in the earlier one, we used a magnetic-resonance-guided stereotaxic surgical approach combined with the injection of the excitotoxin ibotenic acid into the amygdala in rhesus monkeys. This procedure is intended to produce complete cell loss in the amygdala, but to spare axons arising from neighboring structures that might pass nearby or through the amygdala. The experimental design involved two stages of surgery, with injections of excitotoxin in the left amygdala in the first stage followed by injections in the right amygdala in the second stage or vice versa, with training and testing after each stage. Control monkeys remained unoperated. Although monkeys with unilateral amygdala lesions acquired the discrimination problems at the same rate as controls, they obtained lower difference scores than controls; that is, they failed to shift their choices of objects to the same extent as controls following reinforcer devaluation (Figure 4.1, Test 1). After the second-stage surgery, the operated monkeys—now under the influence of bilateral amygdala lesions— obtained even lower difference scores (Figure 4.1, Test 2). Yet another test (Test 3), carried out about 18 months after surgery with a new set of objects,

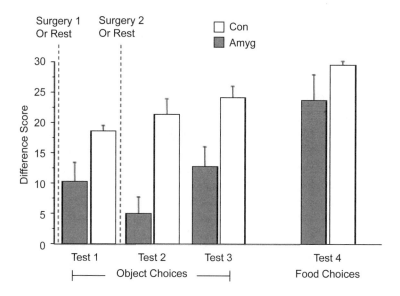

FIGURE 4.1. Effects of selective excitotoxic amygdala lesions on choices of objects (left) and foods (right) after reinforcer devaluation produced via selective satiation. Tests 1–3: Control monkeys avoided choosing objects overlying the devalued food, thereby achieving high difference scores. Monkeys with unilateral (Test 1) or bilateral (Tests 2 and 3) amygdala lesions were less efficient than controls at avoiding objects overlying devalued foods, achieving low difference scores. The groups differed significantly on this measure. Food choices: Both controls and operated monkeys alike were sensitive to selective satiation. When faced with visual choices of two foods, both groups avoided choosing the devalued food, and they did so to the same degree. Con: Unoperated control monkeys ($n = 4$). Amyg: Monkeys with selective excitotoxic amygdala lesions made with ibotenic acid ($n = 5$). Data from Izquierdo and Murray (2007).

gave the same result. The three tests together indicated a significant, detrimental effect of amygdala lesions on the ability of monkeys to make adaptive responses. During the critical sessions, whereas intact monkeys avoided choosing objects overlying the devalued food, thereby obtaining high difference scores, monkeys with selective amygdala lesions continued to choose just as they had in the baseline condition, thereby obtaining low difference scores. We argue that this deficit in the monkeys with amygdala lesions results from their inability to link objects with the current value of the food reinforcer. Because monkeys with amygdala lesions perform just as well as controls on many tests of visual discrimination learning and visual memory (Malkova et al., 1997; Murray, Gaffan, & Mishkin, 1993; Murray & Mishkin, 1998), changes in visual-perceptual abilities cannot account for their deficit. In addition, although one might wonder whether monkeys with amygdala lesions are insensitive to food value, or have altered satiety mechanisms, control procedures have shown that monkeys with amygdala lesions continue to show distinct preferences among familiar foods (Aggleton & Passingham, 1982; Murray, Gaffan, & Flint, 1996). Furthermore, when presented with choices between the two foods directly, they avoid choosing a devalued food to the same extent as the intact monkeys (Figure 4.1, Test 4). Thus monkeys with selective amygdala lesions can discriminate foods and appear to have intact selective satiety mechanisms.

Precisely how objects are linked to food value, and how this information translates to shifts in response selection, has not been determined. The reinforcer devaluation task has several components: forming object representations, linking those representations with the incentive value of the associated food, registering and encoding a change in the reward value due to selective satiation, linking object representations with those updated values, and using these changed representations in object choices.

To better understand the precise manner in which the amygdala contributes to reinforcer devaluation effects, Wellman, Gale, and Malkova (2005) used, instead of permanent lesions, a method of transient inactivation of the amygdala by focal infusion of the gamma-aminobutyric acid (GABA) agonist muscimol. Specifically, they examined whether the amygdala is necessary during the registration of the change in the reinforcer value (i.e., during the time when the reinforcer is devalued by selective satiation). These investigators inactivated the amygdala during two different stages of the experiment: either during the selective satiation procedure (muscimol infusion *before* satiation) or during the subsequent choice test (muscimol infusion *after* satiation). Monkeys received infusions of either saline or muscimol, bilaterally, via cannulae lowered to the basolateral amygdala (defined as the lateral, lateral basal, medial basal, and accessory basal nuclei), either before or after satiation. Each infusion treatment was followed by a probe session like the critical sessions described above.

As expected, saline infusions yielded a pattern of difference scores like that observed in intact monkeys (Figure 4.2). In the saline infusion condition, monkeys showed a significant shift in object choices after reinforcer devaluation; on average, they chose 30% fewer objects covering the devalued food relative to baseline. Nearly identical results (29%) were obtained when the basolateral amygdala was inactivated *after* the selective satiation procedure (labeled "MUS After Satiation" in Figure 4.2). By contrast, inactivation of the basolateral amygdala *before* the satiation procedure ("MUS Before Satiation" in Figure 4.2) prevented the shift in object choices; the monkeys chose only 3% fewer objects covering the devalued food relative to baseline.

The amount of food consumed during the selective satiation procedures did not differ across conditions. This ruled out the possibility that the lack of reinforcer devaluation effects when the basolateral amygdala was inactivated resulted from the monkeys' lower consumption of the food during the selective satiation procedure. An additional procedure controlled for another interpretation of the data. Perhaps the muscimol infused *after* selective satia-

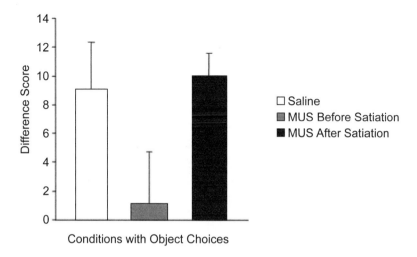

FIGURE 4.2. Effect of temporary inactivation of the basolateral amygdala—produced by infusion of the GABA agonist muscimol—on object choices. Tissue was inactivated either during the selective satiation procedure (muscimol infusion *before* satiation) or during the subsequent choice test (muscimol infusion *after* satiation). Inactivation of the basolateral amygdala during the selective satiation procedure led to a significant reduction in difference scores. Saline: Saline infused bilaterally into the basolateral amygdala. MUS Before Satiation: Muscimol infused bilaterally into the basolateral amygdala before the selective satiation procedure. MUS After Satiation: Muscimol infused bilaterally into the basolateral amygdala after the selective satiation procedure had been completed. From Wellman, Gale, and Malkova (2005). Copyright 2005 by the Society for Neuroscience. Reprinted by permission.

tion (i.e., before the choice tests) failed to have an effect because there was insufficient time for the drug to diffuse over the same extent of the basolateral amygdala, compared to when the drug was infused *before* satiation. To test this possibility, in the control procedure muscimol was infused immediately after the selective satiation procedure as before, but now the probe session was delayed by 30 minutes. This condition matched the one in which muscimol was infused before satiation in the amount of time between the end of infusion and the beginning of the probe session. This yielded the same result as before (i.e., reinforcer devaluation effects were intact). Thus the basolateral amygdala needs to be functionally intact for registration of a change in the incentive value of the food reward and for the subsequent adjustment in the monkey's choices of objects during the probe session. Apparently, once the value of the primary reinforcer has been updated, basolateral amygdala activity is not required for these functions.

Although this section emphasizes our own work in macaque monkeys, other researchers have identified amygdala contributions to processing of primary reinforcement in primates that support the findings described above for rats and monkeys. For example, Roberts and her colleagues (Parkinson et al., 2001) have found that lesions of the amygdala in marmoset monkeys disrupt the ability of a CS to support responding in a conditioned reinforcement paradigm.

Neurophysiology

Physiological studies in monkeys have shown that the activity of many neurons in the amygdala reflects some aspect of reinforcement. For example, neurons show responses to visual stimuli, including foodstuffs, that have been associated with reinforcement (Nishijo, Ono, & Nishino, 1988; Sanghera, Rolls, & Roper-Hall, 1979; Sugase-Miyamoto & Richmond, 2005). Some studies have been carried out in the context of a visual discrimination task involving reversal of the stimulus–reinforcement associations, so that the activity of single neurons can be related to either positive or negative reinforcement per se. In this paradigm, very few amygdala neurons exhibit activity that follows a reversal—in other words, activity that is linked specifically to the positive or negative value of the reinforcer (Sanghera et al., 1979; Wilson & Rolls, 2005).

Recently Paton, Belova, Morrison, and Salzman (2006) recorded from single neurons in the amygdala of monkeys while visual stimuli presented on a monitor acquired a positive or negative valence through Pavlovian conditioning. In their experiment, presentation of individual complex two-dimensional images was consistently paired with either a small liquid reward (positive reinforcement), a brief air puff directed at the face (negative reinforcement), or nothing (no reinforcement). It was evident that the monkeys learned the image–valence association, because they licked or blinked after viewing the images that had been paired with positive and negative reinforcement, respectively. To understand the contribution of individual neurons to representing valence, as opposed to representing image identity, the reinforcer assignments were reversed after monkeys had learned about the images. Paton and colleagues found that the activity of many neurons in the amygdala coded for either positive or negative valence, independently of both image identity and motor responses. Importantly, activity patterns reflecting positive and negative valence were found in different populations of neurons. The activity of other neurons reflected both valence and image identity. Some neurons represented valence exclusively during a limited period—for example, during the presentation of the image or during the unfilled interval between image presentation and reinforcement—whereas other neurons exhibited sustained activity across both intervals. Interestingly, after a reversal, indices of significant shifts in behavior (i.e., learning to lick or blink) were highly correlated with significant changes in the neural activity.

Thus, in the study by Paton and colleagues (2006), unlike earlier studies that had employed instrumental conditioning paradigms (e.g., visual discrimination and reversals) in monkeys, the neuronal activity during image presentation closely followed the type of reinforcer (positive or negative). The differences between the Paton and colleagues study and earlier ones are numerous, and future studies will need to assess the impact of each one on how neuronal signals in the amygdala come to reflect the learned value of visual stimuli. The use by Paton and colleagues of new stimuli every day—in contrast to earlier studies, which often used a single well-learned pair of stimuli—probably accentuated the role of the amygdala in learning about CS–reinforcer associations. For single, familiar stimulus pairs, occurrence (or nonoccurrence) of reward on just one trial is sufficient to trigger a switch between two well-learned states (i.e., to allow response selection via a performance rule), and learning per se is unnecessary. Regardless of the reasons, Paton and colleagues' work demonstrates conclusively that the amygdala processes signals related to positive reinforcement, as well as negative reinforcement.

WHAT THE AMYGDALA DOES NOT DO

There is abundant evidence that the amygdala is not necessary for all reward-based learning. Perhaps the fact that the amygdala is involved in some, but not all, aspects of positive reinforcement has contributed to the idea that it does not function in positive reinforcement at all. It is easy to understand how, by examining only one or a few types of behaviors and finding no effect of amygdala removals or inactivations, one would be tempted to overgeneralize the result to all behaviors reliant on positive reinforcement. We therefore begin this section by considering some of the cognitive processes for which the amygdala is *not* essential, even though the learning relies on receipt of positive reinforcement in the form of food or fluids.

One such example of amygdala-independent learning is conditional motor learning, in which monkeys must learn to associate a stimulus with a motor or spatial response. Typically, complex visual stimuli guide responses, such that CS_1 instructs the monkey to move a joystick to the right, whereas CS_2 instructs a movement to the left. This procedure is often called a "conditional discrimination task." The monkey's only feedback about the accuracy of responses is the delivery (or nondelivery) of food reward. In this task, complete bilateral removal of the amygdala has no effect on either the learning or recall of these associations (Murray & Wise, 1996).

A more widely used form of instrumental learning is visual discrimination learning, mentioned earlier in this chapter. Monkeys are presented with a choice between two objects on a test tray. The same two objects are presented in pairwise fashion over a series of trials; one of the objects of the pair (S+) is always baited (i.e., covers a small food reward, such as a peanut), whereas the other is always unbaited (S−). Through trial and error, the monkeys learn to displace the baited object, regardless of its location. Like the negative results obtained for conditional motor learning, complete, selective amygdala removal does not affect the rate at which visual discrimination problems are acquired (Izquierdo & Murray, 2007; Malkova et al., 1997). Although some minor amygdala contribution to these kinds of learning cannot be ruled out, evidently structures outside the amygdala can mediate these types of learning. In addition, some examples of amygdala-independent learning can be categorized as easy and others as difficult, as defined by the number of trials required to learn a task, so difficulty also does not seem to be an important factor in determining whether the amygdala makes an essential contribution to this form of learning based on positive reinforcement.

Although older findings based on aspirative or radiofrequency lesions of the amygdala in monkeys suggested that the amygdala plays a fairly general role in associating stimuli with reward, findings based on more selective lesions of the amygdala have overturned these ideas (see Baxter & Murray, 2002, for a review). Specifically, recent studies have reassessed the contribution of the amygdala to two types of tasks that have been extremely influential in linking the amygdala with the process of stimulus–reward association in monkeys: (1) win–stay/lose–shift and (2) object reversal learning. In one version of win–stay/lose–shift, on the basis of a single acquisition trial, animals must return to an object that led to success and avoid one that led to failure in producing rewards. Gaffan (1985) has referred to this procedure as a "congruent recall" performance rule. In object reversal learning, animals must rapidly make and break stimulus–reward associations; after a "reversal," the S+ becomes the S–, and vice versa. Remarkably, although both tasks are severely disrupted by aspirative lesions of the amygdala in monkeys (Jones & Mishkin, 1972; Schwartzbaum & Poulos, 1965; Spiegler & Mishkin, 1981), the more selective, excitotoxic amygdala lesions lead to only a mild, transient impairment on a win–stay/lose–shift task (Stefanacci, Clark, & Zola, 2003) and have no effect on object reversal learning (Izquierdo & Murray, 2007). The long-standing misconception of these tasks as amygdala-dependent derived from use of nonselective lesion techniques; inadvertent damage to either the inferior temporal cortex or its connections with prefrontal cortex was the likely source of the impairments.

These findings thus accord with the general picture outlined above—namely, that the amygdala is not essential for many types of visual learning, including many that require the use of information provided by positive reinforcement. Contrary to current doctrine, the amygdala is not necessary even when monkeys must link objects with the delivery of food reward to choose correctly. As discussed in the preceding section, a plausible explanation for the lack of an amygdala contribution to these behaviors is that monkeys quickly learn a visually based performance rule (Murray & Izquierdo, 2007) and treat the positive reinforcement much as they would treat any other sensory signal. According to this idea, the occurrence (or nonoccurrence) of food guides the selection of a performance rule, and this function is independent of the amygdala. On this view, once a performance rule has been learned, the role of food in such tasks is largely limited to its informational value as opposed to its reinforcing value, and is not dramatically affected by an affective response generated by its appearance. Supporting this idea is the finding that intact monkeys can learn a performance rule of the win–stay/lose–shift type (congruent recall) no faster than the opposite performance rule (win–shift/lose–stay, or incongruent recall), despite the fact that they must reject their most recent reinforcement history for the latter rule (Gaffan, 1985).

SUMMARY, CONCLUSIONS, AND SPECULATION

Up to this point, we have provided evidence that the amygdala plays a role in positive reinforcement (although not all aspects of positive reinforcement), along with its more generally accepted role in negative reinforcement. We have developed two additional themes as well. One is that the amygdala performs its functions by linking initially neutral neural representations with innate responses (such as autonomic reflexes) and performance rules (such as "Approach stimuli of positive valence"). The other, following the work of Killcross and colleagues in rodents (Blundell et al., 2001; see also Balleine, 2005), is that the basolateral amygdala plays a crucial role in eliciting updated representations of value for specific aspects of each reinforcer or reinforcer type, whereas the central nucleus of the amygdala functions for general aspects of reinforcement (Balleine & Killcross, 2006).

But why would the amygdala in particular be so closely linked with innate behavior? And why would the central nucleus and basolateral amygdala have such distinct and parallel functions? As noted above, answering "why" questions requires a comparative and evolutionary perspective. As we have seen, the amygdala provides a link between simple stimuli such as tones, lights, and objects on the one hand, and innate processes that lead to affective responses on the other hand. We propose that the amygdala provides the same function for the highest aspects of cognition. This idea is supported by (1) the amygdala's long evolutionary history, stretching back to the earliest land animals and perhaps beyond to the earliest vertebrates; (2) its relatively direct connections with the hypothalamus; and (3) its reciprocal anatomical relations with higher-order cortical areas such as the granular prefrontal cortex—a cortical region that evolved uniquely in primates.

But many readers, especially those familiar with the evolutionary writings of MacLean (1985, 1990), may find it surprising to hear that the amygdala has such a long evolutionary history. In addition, many readers may be surprised by the notion that the prefrontal cortex evolved uniquely in primates. Although an in-depth treatment of these topics is beyond the scope of this chapter, we briefly discuss them below. Then we conclude with a consideration of prefrontal–amygdala interactions as a key to understanding amygdala function.

Does the Amygdala Have a Long Evolutionary History?

A major and common misconception about amygdala evolution stems from the popular and much-cited writings of MacLean (1985, 1990). He proclaimed, in his theory of the triune brain, that the amygdala, like other parts of the limbic system, was part of the primitive mammalian brain. However, MacLean's idea that the amygdala evolved with the advent of mammals has no meaningful support from comparative neuroanatomy (Martínez-García, Novejarque, & Lanuza, 2007; Striedter, 2005). The amygdala has clear homologues in the brains of all amniotes—a group that includes all reptiles, mammals, and birds—and thus almost certainly evolved by the advent of the earliest amniotes. An even earlier origin is likely, because there is fairly good evidence for a homologue of the amygdala in modern amphibians, which suggests an origin in early land animals.

Does the Rodent Amygdala Have Genuine Prefrontal Inputs?

Several areas that are called "prefrontal" in rodent brains have clear homologues in primate brains. Among these areas are the infralimbic and prelimbic cortex, the anterior cingulate cortex, and the agranular insular cortex. However, according to Preuss (1995), rodents do not have a homologue of the granular prefrontal cortex in primates. Because rodents lack these areas, their amygdala cannot receive projections from, or send projections to, the granular prefrontal cortex. Consequently, research on the rodent amygdala may not provide a complete representation of amygdala function in primate brains. The idea that input from the granular prefrontal cortex to the amygdala provides a key to understanding amygdala function in humans is taken up below.

Prefrontal–Amygdala Interactions in Monkeys

We propose that one function of the amygdala is to act as a link between information processed by higher-order "association" cortex on the one hand, and instinctive behavior and value assignment on the other. It is nearly a truism that incentive learning involves the interaction between motivational changes in reward value and the internal state of the animal (Balleine & Dickinson, 1994; Cechetto, 1987), but the reliance of these processes on innate mechanisms has received scant attention. In fact, little is known about how higher cognitive functions (ideas, abstract concepts, analogical and inferential reasoning, etc.) acquire emotional significance.

Current opinion emphasizes an important role for amygdalocortical projections in representing the relative value of objects and actions, which is held to be stored in orbitofrontal cortex (e.g., Holland & Gallagher, 2004). Indeed, studies in rodents have found that the neural activity in orbital prefrontal cortex that reflects the value of expected outcomes—especially the activity evident during the presentation of a CS—depends on the integrity of the amygdala (Schoenbaum, Setlow, Saddoris, & Gallagher, 2003). Consequently, the prevailing view is that CS–value associations mediated by the basolateral amygdala are represented in orbital prefrontal cortex and serve as the basis of reward expectancy.

The findings from the reinforcer devaluation paradigms described earlier are consistent with this general view. The sight of an object (CS) elicits activity in orbital prefrontal cortex that reflects the value of the expected outcome (Padoa-Schioppa & Assad, 2006; Roesch & Olson, 2004; Tremblay & Schultz, 2000; Wallis & Miller, 2003), and surgical disconnection of the amygdala from the orbital prefrontal cortex disrupts reinforcer devaluation effects (Baxter, Parker, Lindner, Izquierdo, & Murray, 2000). The amygdala's contribution is thought to be in updating or otherwise altering the representation of value, not in acting as a site of storage of that representation or in maintaining the representation, once stored.

According to the view espoused here, the amygdala serves as a key link between the recently evolved granular prefrontal cortex and innate response mechanisms. This linkage could account for the emotional correlates of abstractions such as cognitive constructs, including emotionally laden words, images, and ideas. If the amygdala is important for linking object representations with value (see "What the Amygdala Does," above), then why would it not also be important for linking other types of representations with value? In our species, with our profoundly derived capacities for abstract thought and language, perhaps the amygdala provides the key link between ideas and emotions. It may mediate aesthetics and the valuation of abstract goals, such as climbing Mount Everest or hitching a ride on a UFO. Combined with mental time travel, the ability of the amygdala to link the products of cognition to value may serve as the basis for images of ourselves as positive (or negative) entities moving through time. The amygdala does not play an essential role in all aspects of positive reinforcement, but the ones that it does underlie may get to the heart of what it means to a person to be a person—or to a monkey to be a monkey.

WHAT WE THINK

One function of the amygdala is to assign value to object representations, at least in certain circumstances. We have proposed that the amygdala also assigns value to ideas and abstract concepts, thereby providing a basis for aesthetics and valuation of abstract goals. But much remains to be understood. Perhaps the most important element missing from the experimental work is an understanding of just how central the capacity of value assignment is in the lives of humans and other primates. Does this value assignment capacity strongly influence our everyday behavior, or does it affect our activities only under rare circumstances? Studies of adult humans with amygdala damage reveal fairly selective deficits, including deficits in recognizing facial expressions of fear (Adolphs, Tranel, Damasio, & Damasio, 1994); in judging from facial expressions whether others are trustworthy (Adolphs, Tranel, & Damasio, 1998); in fear conditioning (LaBar, LeDoux, Spencer, & Phelps, 1995); and, in accord with the thesis of this chapter, in assigning positive values to pictures associated with food reward (Johnsrude, Owen, White, Zhao, & Bohbot, 2000). Although the relatively narrow selectivity of these findings suggests a fairly modest role for the amygdala in human behavior, the amygdala could have a profound impact on human behavior in at least two ways:

1. The amygdala could act to assign value to conspecifics and to rules regarding social behavior that would guide social interactions. The amygdala has been proposed to be important in human development for socialization—for instance, in acquiring social conventions such as learning to avoid actions that will harm others (Blair, Peschardt, Budhani, Mitchell, & Pine, 2006). Although the role of the amygdala in social behavior has been investigated in monkeys (Bachevalier, Malkova, & Mishkin, 2001; Bauman, Lavenex, Mason, Capitanio, & Amaral, 2004; Emery et al., 2001), this complex and complicated aspect of behavior deserves much additional study.

2. The value assignments mediated by the amygdala could be inaccessible to conscious awareness, at least in any direct way. Johnsrude and colleagues (2000) employed a test design pairing individual pictures with a high, medium, or low probability of food reward. They found that a control group acquired and expressed picture preferences (high > low) that were clearly due to learning, although they were unaware of the relationship between picture presentation and probability of food rewards. Patients with amygdala damage did not display such preferences. Thus the amygdala-damaged subjects failed to acquire the unconscious bias, or preference, for particular objects. The potential contribution of the amygdala to unconscious bias and preference not only of objects, but of conspecifics, ideas, abstract concepts, and beliefs, should be investigated further.

ACKNOWLEDGMENT

This work was supported by the Intramural Research Program of the National Institute of Mental Health. Because this chapter was prepared by employees of a U.S. government agency, it is in the public domain.

REFERENCES

Adolphs, R., Tranel, D., & Damasio, A. R. (1998). The human amygdala in social judgment. *Nature, 393,* 470–474.

Adolphs, R., Tranel, D., Damasio, H., & Damasio, A. (1994). Impaired recognition of emotion in facial expressions following bilateral damage to the human amygdala. *Nature, 372,* 669–672.

Aggleton, J. P., & Passingham, R. E. (1982). An assessment of the reinforcing properties of foods after amygdaloid lesions in rhesus monkeys. *Journal of Comparative and Physiological Psychology, 96,* 71–77.

Bachevalier, J., Malkova, L., & Mishkin, M. (2001). Effects of selective neonatal temporal lobe lesions on socioemotional behavior in infant rhesus monkeys (*Macaca mulatta*). *Behavioral Neuroscience, 115*, 545–559.

Balleine, B. W. (2005). Neural bases of food-seeking: Affect, arousal and reward in corticostriatolimbic circuits. *Physiology and Behavior, 86*, 717–730.

Balleine, B. W., & Dickinson, A. (1994). Role of cholecystokinin in the motivational control of instrumental action in rats. *Behavioral Neuroscience, 108*, 590–605.

Balleine, B. W., & Killcross, S. (2006). Parallel incentive processing: An integrated view of amygdala function. *Trends in Neurosciences, 29*, 272–279.

Bauman, M. D., Lavenex, P., Mason, W. A., Capitanio, J. P., & Amaral, D. G. (2004). The development of social behavior following neonatal amygdala lesions in rhesus monkeys. *Journal of Cognitive Neuroscience, 16*, 1388–1411.

Baxter, M. G., & Murray, E. A. (2002). The amygdala and reward. *Nature Reviews Neuroscience, 3*, 563–573.

Baxter, M. G., Parker, A., Lindner, C. C., Izquierdo, A. D., & Murray, E. A. (2000). Control of response selection by reinforcer value requires interaction of amygdala and orbital prefrontal cortex. *Journal of Neuroscience, 20*, 4311–4319.

Blair, R. J., Peschardt, K. S., Budhani, S., Mitchell, D. G., & Pine, D. S. (2006). The development of psychopathy. *Journal of Child Psychology and Psychiatry, 47*, 262–276.

Blundell, P., Hall, G., & Killcross, S. (2001). Lesions of the basolateral amygdala disrupt selective aspects of reinforcer representation in rats. *Journal of Neuroscience, 21*, 9018–9026.

Braesicke, K., Parkinson, J. A., Reekie, Y., Man, M.-S., Hopewell, L., Pears, A., et al. (2005). Autonomic arousal in an appetitive context in primates: A behavioural and neural analysis. *European Journal of Neuroscience, 21*, 1733–1740.

Cechetto, D. F. (1987). Central representation of visceral function. *Federation Proceedings, 46*, 17–23.

Corbit, L. H., & Balleine, B. W. (2005). Double dissociation of basolateral and central amygdala lesions on the general and outcome-specific forms of Pavlovian-instrumental transfer. *Journal of Neuroscience, 25*, 962–970.

Emery, N. J., Capitanio, J. P., Mason, W. A., Machado, C. J., Mendoza, S. P., & Amaral, D. G. (2001). The effects of bilateral lesions of the amygdala on dyadic social interactions in rhesus monkeys (*Macaca mulatta*). *Behavioral Neuroscience, 115*, 515–544.

Everitt, B. J., Cardinal, R. N., Parkinson, J. A., & Robbins, T. W. (2003). Appetitive behavior, impact of amygdala-dependent mechanisms of emotional learning. *Annals of the New York Academy of Sciences, 985*, 233–250.

Everitt, B. J., Morris, K. A., O'Brien, A., & Robbins, T. W. (1991). The basolateral amygdala–ventral striatal system and conditioned place preference: Further evidence of limbic–striatal interaction underlying reward-related processes. *Neuroscience, 42*, 1–18.

Everitt, B. J., & Robbins, T. W. (1992). Amygdala–ventral striatal interactions and reward-related processes. In J. P. Aggleton (Ed.), *The amygdala: Neurobiological aspects of emotion, memory, and mental dysfunction* (pp. 401–429). New York: Wiley-Liss.

Gaffan, D. (1985). Hippocampus, memory, habit and voluntary movement. *Philosophical Transactions of the Royal Society of London, Series B, 308*, 87–99.

Gallagher, M., Graham, P. W., & Holland, P. C. (1990). The amygdala central nucleus and appetitive Pavlovian conditioning: Lesions impair one class of conditioned behavior. *Journal of Neuroscience, 10,* 1906–1911.

Hall, J., Parkinson, J. A., Connor, T. M., Dickinson, A., & Everitt, B. J. (2001). Involvement of the central nucleus of the amygdala and nucleus accumbens core in mediating Pavlovian influences on instrumental behaviour. *European Journal of Neuroscience, 13,* 1984–1992.

Hatfield, T., Han, J. S., Conley, M., Gallagher, M., & Holland, P. C. (1996). Neurotoxic lesions of basolateral, but not central, amygdala interfere with Pavlovian second-order conditioning and reinforcer devaluation effects. *Journal of Neuroscience, 16,* 5256–5265.

Holland, P. C., & Gallagher, M. (1993). Amygdala central nucleus lesions disrupt increments, but not decrements, in conditioned stimulus processing. *Behavioral Neuroscience, 107,* 246–253.

Holland, P. C., & Gallagher, M. (1999). Amygdala circuitry in attentional and representational processes. *Trends in Cognitive Sciences, 3,* 65–73.

Holland, P. C., & Gallagher, M. (2003). Double dissociation of the effects of lesions of basolateral and central amygdala on conditioned stimulus-potentiated feeding and Pavlovian-instrumental transfer. *European Journal of Neuroscience, 17,* 1680–1694.

Holland, P. C., & Gallagher, M. (2004). Amygdala–frontal interactions and reward expectancy. *Current Opinion in Neurobiology, 14,* 148–155.

Izquierdo A., & Murray, E. A. (2007). Selective bilateral amygdala lesions in rhesus monkeys fail to disrupt object reversal learning. *Journal of Neuroscience, 27,* 1054–1062.

Johnsrude, I. S., Owen, A. M., White, N. M., Zhao, W. V., & Bohbot, V. (2000). Impaired preference conditioning after anterior temporal lobe resection in humans. *Journal of Neuroscience, 20,* 2649–2656.

Jones, B., & Mishkin, M. (1972). Limbic lesions and the problem of stimulus–reinforcement associations. *Experimental Neurology, 36,* 362–377.

Killcross, S., Robbins, T. W., & Everitt, B. J. (1997). Different types of fear-conditioned behaviour mediated by separate nuclei within amygdala. *Nature, 388,* 377–380.

LaBar, K., LeDoux, J., Spencer, D., & Phelps, E. (1995). Impaired fear conditioning following unilateral temporal lobectomy in humans. *Journal of Neuroscience, 15,* 6846–6855.

MacLean, P. D. (1985). Evolutionary psychiatry and the triune brain. *Psychological Medicine, 15,* 219–221.

MacLean, P. D. (1990). *The triune brain in evolution.* New York: Plenum Press.

Malkova, L., Gaffan, D., & Murray, E. A. (1997). Excitotoxic lesions of the amygdala fail to produce impairment in visual learning for auditory secondary reinforcement but interfere with reinforcer devaluation effects in rhesus monkeys. *Journal of Neuroscience, 17,* 6011–6020.

Martínez-García, F., Novejarque, A., & Lanuza, E. (2007). Evolution of the amygdala in vertebrates. In J. H. Kaas (Ed.), *Evolution of nervous systems* (Vol. 2, pp. 255–334). Amsterdam: Elsevier.

Mason, W. A., Capitanio, J. P., Machado, C. J., Mendoza, S. P., & Amaral, D. G. (2006). Amygdalectomy and responsiveness to novelty in rhesus monkeys (*Macaca mulatta*): Generality and individual consistency of effects. *Emotion, 6,* 73–81.

McDonald, R. J., & White, N. M. (1993). A triple dissociation of memory systems:

Hippocampus, amygdala, and dorsal striatum. *Behavioral Neuroscience, 107*, 3–22.

Morris, J. S., Frith, C. D., Perrett, D. I., Rowland, D., Young, A. W., Calder, A. J., et al. (1996). A differential neural response in the human amygdala to fearful and happy facial expressions. *Nature, 383*, 812–815.

Murray, E. A., Gaffan, E. A., & Flint, R. W. (1996). Anterior rhinal cortex and amygdala: Dissociation of their contributions to memory and food preference in rhesus monkeys. *Behavioral Neuroscience, 110*, 30–42.

Murray, E. A., Gaffan, D., & Mishkin, M. (1993). Neural substrates of visual stimulus–stimulus association in rhesus monkeys. *Journal of Neuroscience, 13*, 4549–4561.

Murray, E. A., & Izquierdo, A. (2007). Orbitofrontal cortex and amygdala contributions to affect and action in primates. In G. Schoenbaum, J. A. Gottfried, E. A. Murray, & S. J. Ramus (Eds.), *Linking affect to action: Critical contributions of the orbitofrontal cortex* (pp. 273–296). Boston: Blackwell.

Murray, E. A., & Mishkin, M. (1998). Object recognition and location memory in monkeys with excitotoxic lesions of the amygdala and hippocampus. *Journal of Neuroscience, 18*, 6568–6582.

Murray, E. A., & Wise, S. P. (1996). Role of the hippocampus plus subjacent cortex but not amygdala in visuomotor conditional learning in rhesus monkeys. *Behavioral Neuroscience, 110*, 1261–1270.

Nishijo, H., Ono, T., & Nishino, H. (1988). Single neuron responses in amygdala of alert monkey during complex sensory stimulation with affective significance. *Journal of Neuroscience, 8*, 3570–3583.

Padoa-Schioppa, C., & Assad, J. A. (2006). Neurons in the orbitofrontal cortex encode economic value. *Nature, 441*, 223–226.

Parkinson, J. A., Crofts, H. S., McGuigan, M., Tomic, D. L, Everitt, B. J., & Roberts, A. C. (2001). The role of the primate amygdala in conditioned reinforcement. *Journal of Neuroscience, 21*, 7770–7780.

Parkinson, J. A., Robbins, T. W., & Everitt, B. J. (2000). Dissociable roles of the central and basolateral amygdala in appetitive emotional learning. *European Journal of Neuroscience, 12*, 405–413.

Paton, J. J., Belova, M. A., Morrison, S. E., & Salzman, C. D. (2006). The primate amygdala represents the positive and negative value of visual stimuli during learning. *Nature, 439*, 865–870.

Pickens, C. L., Saddoris, M. P., Setlow, B., Gallagher, M., Holland, P. C., & Schoenbaum, G. (2003). Different roles for orbitofrontal cortex and basolateral amygdala in a reinforcer devaluation task. *Journal of Neuroscience, 23*, 11078–11084.

Preuss, T. M. (1995). Do rats have prefrontal cortex?: The Rose–Woolsey–Akert program reconsidered. *Journal of Cognitive Neuroscience, 7*, 1–24.

Roesch, M. R., & Olson, C. R. (2004). Neuronal activity related to reward value and motivation in primate frontal cortex. *Science, 304*, 307–310.

Sanghera, M. K., Rolls, E. T., & Roper-Hall, A. (1979). Visual responses of neurons in the dorsolateral amygdala of the alert monkey. *Experimental Neurology, 63*, 610–626.

Schoenbaum, G., Setlow, B., Saddoris, M. P., & Gallagher, M. (2003). Encoding predicted outcome and acquired value in orbitofrontal cortex during cue sampling depends upon input from basolateral amygdala. *Neuron, 39*, 855–867.

Schwartzbaum, J. S., & Poulos, D. A. (1965). Discrimination behavior after amygdalectomy in monkeys, learning set and discrimination reversals. *Journal of Comparative and Physiological Psychology, 60*, 320–328.

Setlow, B., Gallagher, M., & Holland, P. C. (2002). The basolateral complex of the amygdala is necessary for acquisition but not expression of CS motivational value in appetitive Pavlovian second-order conditioning. *European Journal of Neuroscience, 15*, 1841–1853.

Spiegler, B. J., & Mishkin, M. (1981). Evidence for the sequential participation of inferior temporal cortex and amygdala in the acquisition of stimulus–reward associations. *Behavioural Brain Research, 3*, 303–317.

Stefanacci, L., Clark, R. E., & Zola, S. M. (2003). Selective neurotoxic amygdala lesions in monkeys disrupt reactivity to food and object stimuli and have limited effects on memory. *Behavioral Neuroscience, 117*, 1029–1043.

Striedter, G. F. (2005). *Principles of brain evolution.* Sunderland, MA: Sinauer.

Sugase-Miyamoto, Y., & Richmond, B. J. (2005). Neuronal signals in the monkey basolateral amygdala during reward schedules. *Journal of Neuroscience, 25*, 11071–11083.

Tremblay, L., & Schultz, W. (2000). Modifications of reward expectation-related neuronal activity during learning in primate orbitofrontal cortex. *Journal of Neurophysiology, 83*, 1877–1885.

Wallis, J. D., & Miller, E. K. (2003). Neuronal activity in primate dorsolateral and orbital prefrontal cortex during performance of a reward preference task. *European Journal of Neuroscience, 18*, 2069–2081.

Wellman, L. L., Gale, K., & Malkova, L. (2005). GABAA-mediated inhibition of basolateral amygdala blocks reward devaluation in macaques. *Journal of Neuroscience, 25*, 4577–4586.

Wilson, F. A., & Rolls, E. T. (2005). The primate amygdala and reinforcement: A dissociation between rule-based and associatively-mediated memory revealed in neuronal activity. *Neuroscience, 133*, 1061–1072.

PART II
Human Amygdala Function

CHAPTER 5

A Developmental Perspective on Human Amygdala Function

Nim Tottenham, Todd A. Hare, and B. J. Casey

The amygdala has been implicated in learning about the emotional significance of stimuli. Having a mechanism to determine the relative safety or danger of situations is adaptive at any age, although the emotional significance of information may vary as a function of developmental stage. Children typically have caregivers in close proximity to help guide their actions, but they must learn to navigate emotional situations and eventually make decisions about the relative safety or danger on their own. In this chapter, we explore the development of amygdala functioning during childhood and adolescence, in the context of learning about the emotional significance of environmental stimuli.

The process of learning through pairing an initially neutral stimulus with an emotionally significant stimulus is the basis of classical conditioning. Fear conditioning, a form of classical conditioning, involves repeated pairing of a conditioned stimulus with an aversive stimulus (e.g., shock) until the conditioned stimulus itself elicits the fear response, and this type of learning is dependent on the amygdala (LeDoux, 1993). A classical conditioning framework is useful in examining the development of amygdala-dependent learning, because conditioning paradigms reduce learning to its most basic components (Maren, 2001). The amygdala is particularly engaged by these learning paradigms when the association is ambiguous. As defined by Whalen (1998), ambiguity in learning contexts exists when "stimuli have more than one possible interpretation, leading to more than one prediction of subsequent biologically relevant events" (p. 181). Such ambiguity is generally greater when associations are first being learned, and likewise, it is during this initial period of learning in experimental settings that the amygdala is most strongly recruited (LaBar, Gatenby, Gore, LeDoux, & Phelps, 1998).

Analogous learning occurs in the developing system. Development is a period when there tends to be more ambiguity, as emotionally neutral stimuli become associated with emotionally significant situations through experience. Over the course of development, such pairings establish representations of safety or danger associated with these cues. It is our view that early in life, when less is known about the relative safety or danger of different cues, the amygdala plays a key role in assigning valence to stimuli through learning processes like those observed in fear conditioning paradigms. We present findings from developmental lesion and imaging studies that support this view and are consistent with (1) continued development of amygdala function throughout childhood and adolescence, and (2) the importance of the amygdala in helping an individual learn about the emotional significance of stimuli as social and emotional contexts change across development.

LESION STUDIES

Lesion studies provide a useful means of understanding the role of a given brain region in producing a behavior. The most relevant lesion studies of the amygdala in the context of development are those in which the timing of the lesion (i.e., the age of the animal) is manipulated. Amygdala lesions that occur in either neonatal or adult macaques result in the animals' showing less fear of nonsocial items. However, these lesions produce distinct responses to social stimuli that vary as a function of the timing of the lesion. Amygdala lesions in adult animals result in an increase in affiliative social behaviors (e.g., less distance from peers, more affiliative vocalization coos, more walk-bys; Emery & Amaral, 1999), but when they occur in infancy, these lesions result in exaggerated fear responses during social interactions (e.g., decreased exploration, increased fear grimaces, more screams; Bauman, Lavenex, Mason, Capitanio, & Amaral, 2004; Emery & Amaral, 1999; Prather et al., 2001). Prather and colleagues (2001) suggest that the exaggerated social fear in monkeys with early amygdala lesions is the result of these monkeys never having the capacity to appropriately learn any social signal from conspecifics, and therefore being left unable to recognize social cues that signal safety.

Neuropsychological studies of amygdala lesions in humans support the important role of the amygdala in establishing an understanding of social and emotional signals. The literature suggests that amygdala lesions early in life (i.e., congenitally or during early childhood) dramatically impair processing of facial expressions, particularly fearful ones (Adolphs, Tranel, Damasio, & Damasio, 1994). However, amygdala lesions later in life (i.e., during adulthood) appear to have less of an effect on processing these expressions (Hamann & Adolphs, 1999). These developmental differences are most apparent in nonverbal tasks (e.g., judgments of perceived similarity between expressions). Presumably, the amygdala is important during developmental periods when learning about the meaning of relevant social stimuli (such as facial expressions) is occurring, but may be less critical once these associations have been formed.

These lesion studies in both humans and nonhuman primates add support to the notion that the amygdala is involved in learning about the meaning of emotionally relevant stimuli during development, consistent with its role in fear conditioning (Davis & Whalen, 2001; LeDoux, 2003). Lesion studies alone, however, provide only one view into the functional organization and development of the amygdala.

FUNCTIONAL NEUROIMAGING STUDIES

Functional neuroimaging techniques allow us to examine the development of human brain function within the context of an intact, typically developing brain. Only recently have neuroimaging studies of amygdala function and development been conducted. Findings from these studies suggest that throughout childhood and adolescence, neural processes in the amygdala support learning about the emotional significance of stimuli of both positive and negative valence. Fear conditioning experiments with adolescents (e.g., pairing a neutral cue with an air blast directed at the larynx) have shown that adolescents can learn to associate a neutral stimulus with a negative one, and that this learning is accompanied by increased amygdala activity in response to the conditioned stimulus (Monk, Grillon, et al., 2003). This type of amygdala-dependent fear conditioning seems to be a similar process to the one identified in adults (Critchley, Mathias, & Dolan, 2002; Knight, Nguyen, & Bandettini, 2005; LaBar et al., 1998; Phelps et al., 2001).

The acquisition of fear is not the only form of learning used to examine the functional development of the amygdala. Experiments that incorporate safety cues have also been informative. In these studies, the amygdala is recruited for cues that signal safety in addition to those that signal danger. For instance, learning that certain cues are *not* associated with aversive puffs of air to the eye (i.e., safe conditions) is paralleled by recruitment of the amygdala in adolescents (Monk, Grillon, et al., 2003), similar to what is observed during extinction trials in adults (i.e., when subjects are learning that a cue will no longer predict a shock) (LaBar et al., 1998). Thus, as in adulthood (Breiter et al., 1996; Hennenlotter et al., 2005; Somerville, Kim, Johnstone, Alexander, & Whalen, 2004), the amygdala supports learning about the emotional significance of stimuli beyond aversive ones, and also responds to positive stimuli during childhood and adolescence. Other categories of positively valenced stimuli that recruit the amygdala during adolescence include food (Holsen et al., 2005) and positive facial expressions (Yang, Menon, Reid, Gotlib, & Reiss, 2003). A system that helps the organism learn about positive and negative valence enables it to learn signals of both threat and safety across development. For humans, these signals will be particularly relevant in social domains.

Studies on the developmental course of amygdala activity in response to facial expressions show many consistencies in such activity among adults, adolescents, and children. Imaging studies suggest that children and adolescents reliably recruit the amygdala when processing emotion from facial expressions. Greater amygdala activity in response to fearful faces than to fixation is observed in both adolescents (Baird et al., 1999; Killgore, Oki, & Yurgelun-Todd, 2001) and children (Thomas, Drevets, Whalen, et al., 2001). This pattern of response is consistent with the pattern observed in adults (Breiter et al., 1996), indicating that the amygdala is sensitive to emotional faces across development.

However, children and adults differ in which emotional expressions most strongly recruit the amygdala. When fearful faces are contrasted with neutral expressions, striking developmental differences emerge, and children's pattern of amygdala activity looks different from that observed in adults. Older adolescents (Monk, Grillon, et al., 2003; Monk, McClure, et al., 2003) and adults (Breiter et al., 1996) show more amygdala activity in response to fearful facial expressions than to neutral expressions. Children, however, show the opposite pattern, with neutral faces resulting in greater amygdala recruitment than fearful faces (Thomas, Drevets, Dahl, et al., 2001) and other facial expressions (Lobaugh, Gibson, & Taylor, 2006). This difference may reflect different interpretations of neutral faces that result from different experiences with faces across age. These data support the notion that emotional interpretations of facial expressions are not static, but instead are shaped by learning and experiences, as has been suggested by others (Adolphs, Tranel, Damasio, & Damasio, 1995; Davis & Whalen, 2001).

The imaging data suggest that a neutral face is interpreted as more emotionally significant by children than it is by adults. How does this changing pattern of amygdala activity across development relate to behavior? Recent work in our laboratory has identified a behavioral correlate of amygdala recruitment to neutral faces in children. On a task requiring participants to identify the object category of the presented image (face or house) and *not* the emotion category (although the faces expressed different emotions), children made more errors than adults and adolescents in responding to neutral faces, but not to other expressions (see Figure 5.1). These errors are interpreted as resulting from the interference caused by the emotional distraction of neutral faces for children. Similar interference effects of facial expressions on task performance have been reported in adults by Hare, Tottenham, Davidson, Glover, and Casey (2005) and McClure and colleagues (2004) (e.g., slower responses to negative expressions relative to positive ones), and these effects are paralleled by increased recruitment of the amygdala. We view these data as evidence that emotionally relevant information can affect behavior throughout development, but that interpretations of the information will change as a result of experiences and learning.

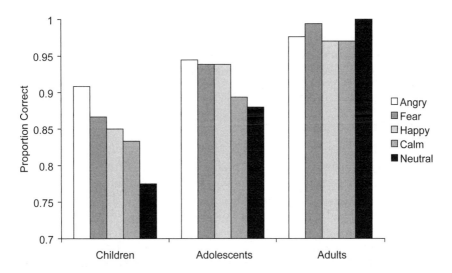

FIGURE 5.1. Neutral faces result in more errors for children. On a task requiring subjects to indicate whether an object was a face or a house, children made more errors than adults and adolescents, but their errors were specific to neutral faces.

How might experiences shape interpretations of facial expressions? What researchers call a "neutral" face may actually be experienced as having a more negative valence in childhood than in adulthood. For example, an adult's neutral face may be interpreted as a "mean" or "strict" face by a child. A caregiver's disappointment is more likely to be associated with a stern or serious face (i.e., neutral) than with a caricatured threat face, thereby establishing an association between neutral faces and punishment.

An aspect of the neutral face that can potentiate the amygdala response is its ambiguous nature. The exact outcome of seeing a neutral face is uncertain for children, in the same way that has been described of fear faces for adult observers (see Whalen, 1998). Therefore, neutral faces may increase amygdala activity in children because of their associative ambiguity (i.e., they require more information from the environment to deduce outcome). Whether amygdala activity for neutral faces in children reflects its association with punishment, a neutral face's associative ambiguity, or both (since these two factors are not orthogonal to each other) cannot be disentangled by the existing literature. Consistent with any of these possibilities, neutral faces may have more emotional relevance than fearful faces for the child viewer, as evidenced by increased amygdala response and disruption of behavior with neutral faces, which results from experience.

The findings presented above suggest that the meaning of facial expressions is learned through experience, which contrasts with the notion that this knowledge is unlearned or "prewired" (see the "What We Think" box). Amygdala activity for neutral faces decreases with age as humans see more of them in emotionally neutral contexts, which perhaps reflects new learning about the expression as experience changes. Understanding these mechanisms that support experience-dependent change over the course of development requires an understanding of the brain regions with which the amygdala interacts over the course of development.

Amygdala-Related Circuitry

The amygdala does not function in isolation, but is part of complex neural circuits. Developmental changes in emotion processing are likely to involve developmental changes not only in amygdala function, but also in the function of other brain regions within this circuitry. Reciprocal connections exist between the amygdala and prefrontal regions involved in top-down modulation of behavior (e.g., Amaral, 1986; Ghashghaei & Barbas, 2002; McDonald, 1987). Neuroimaging studies of affective control in adults suggest prefrontal modulation of subcortical regions during emotion processing (Hariri, Mattay, Tessitore, Fera, & Weinberger, 2003; Hatfield, Graham, & Gallagher, 1992; Keightley et al., 2003; Lange et al., 2003; Nomura et al., 2004; Ochsner, Bunge, Gross, & Gabrieli, 2002; Ochsner et al., 2004). Animal studies corroborate these findings and show the importance of prefrontal connections with the amygdala in emotional (e.g., fear) conditioning (Cardinal, Parkinson, Hall, & Everitt, 2002; Corcoran & Quirk, 2007; Garcia, Vouimba, Baudry, & Thompson, 1999; Morgan & LeDoux, 1995). Given the protracted development of the prefrontal cortex (Alexander & Goldman, 1978; Casey, Giedd, & Thomas, 2000; Fuster, 2002; Giedd, 2004; Sowell, Thompson, Holmes, Jernigan, & Toga, 1999), prefrontal–amygdala interactions are likely to play an important role in developmental changes in emotion processing. Emerging evidence indicates that emotion processing early in life relies more heavily on subcortical structures, and that increasing maturity involves a shift from subcortical to cortical processing during adolescence and adulthood (Casey, Galvan, & Hare, 2005; Casey, Tottenham, Liston, & Durston, 2005), as has been shown empirically (Galvan et al., 2006; Killgore et al., 2001; Levesque et al., 2004; Monk, McClure, et al., 2003). Therefore, a complete understanding of the development of amygdala function requires investigation of the strengthening connections among those cortical systems with which it interacts (Hare & Casey, 2005).

CONCLUSION

Although the basic neuroanatomical architecture of the amygdala is present at birth (Humphrey, 1968; Ulfig, Setzer, & Bohl, 2003), fine-tuning of amygdala function continues throughout childhood and adolescence. Part of this fine-tuning is the result of changes in the interactions between the amygdala and other brain regions. In addition, the functional imaging data suggest that *what* associations are formed between a stimulus and its emotional significance change as the emotional and/or social environment changes. The changing amygdala response to emotional stimuli throughout life may reflect these changes in environments, which are correlated with age.

Both functional neuroimaging studies and lesion studies suggest that the amygdala plays a critical role in learning associations between a stimulus and its emotional significance. Amygdala lesions very early in life appear to cause an inability to learn about safety signals. The effects of these lesions in altering social-emotional behavior may extend beyond the amygdala, since these early lesions will also disrupt the normal development of other regions with which the amygdala interacts in dynamic ways, as has been described in other developing systems (Karmiloff-Smith, 2006). The striking behavioral deficits seen after early amygdala lesions highlight the hierarchical nature of development. Therefore, developmental approaches offer a unique opportunity to examine changing dynamics between subcortical regions (such as the amygdala) and top-down cortical ones across development (Galvan et al., 2006). Such an approach may be the very tool that will allow us to best address the questions regarding the functional role of the amygdala in emotional development.

WHAT WE THINK

The framework presented in this chapter, in which we argue that facial expressions are a class of conditioned stimuli, does not preclude the possibility that some genetic preparedness makes fear faces more likely to be associated with negative events, resulting in the pattern of activity observed in adults. In other words, the reliability with which fearful faces recruit the amygdala in adults may result from loose genetic constraints that make fearful faces more readily associated with aversive outcomes. Evidence for such stimulus specificity in amygdala-dependent learning comes from conditioning paradigms that show better conditioning for phylogenetically fear-relevant than for irrelevant stimuli. Cook, Mineka, Wolkenstein, and Laitsch (1985) have shown that nonhuman primates can acquire fear responses for snakes, but not flowers, by observing conspecifics respond fearfully to snakes or flowers. Furthermore, greater resistance to extinction for fear-relevant stimuli (e.g., snakes) than for ontogenetically fear-relevant stimuli (Mineka & Öhman, 2002) has also been demonstrated. Although there may be certain classes of stimuli with which there is increased readiness for learning, it is nevertheless our view that experience is critical in establishing interpretations of facial expressions of emotion.

Evidence that processing of facial expressions is learned would present a challenge to evolutionary theories of such processing, but it would also have powerful implications for intervention and altering interpretations in cases of atypical face-processing skills. The response to neutral faces in childhood suggests that activity seen in response to faces reflects learning about the meaning of a face, making facial expressions a class of conditioned stimuli, as has been suggested by others (Adolphs et al., 1995; Davis & Whalen, 2001). If facial expressions are conditioned stimuli, then the types of experience that shape social perception systems must be considered. Training paradigms will be useful to determine the role of experience in altering associations between a facial expression and its emotional meaning through development. The results from such studies can be applied to atypical populations with altered social-emotional perception (Thomas, Drevets, Dahl, et al., 2001; Wang, Dapretto, Hariri, Sigman, & Bookheimer, 2004). Establishing the efficacy of conditioning paradigms in altering emotional interpretations would form a short bridge between basic research into emotion processing and clinical applications for altering the trajectories of developmental disorders.

REFERENCES

Adolphs, R., Tranel, D., Damasio, H., & Damasio, A. R. (1994). Impaired recognition of emotion in facial expressions following bilateral damage to the human amygdala. *Nature, 372,* 669–672.

Adolphs, R., Tranel, D., Damasio, H., & Damasio, A. R. (1995). Fear and the human amygdala. *Journal of Neuroscience, 15*(9), 5879–5891.

Alexander, G. E., & Goldman, P. S. (1978). Functional development of the dorsolateral prefrontal cortex: An analysis utilizing reversible cryogenic depression. *Brain Research, 143*(2), 233–249.

Amaral, D. G. (1986). Amygdalohippocampal and amygdalocortical projections in the primate brain. *Advances in Experimental Medicine and Biology, 203,* 3–17.

Baird, A. A., Gruber, S. A., Fein, D. A., Maas, L. C., Steingard, R. J., Renshaw, P. F., et al. (1999). Functional magnetic resonance imaging of facial affect recognition in children and adolescents. *Journal of the American Academy of Child and Adolescent Psychiatry, 38*(2), 195–199.

Bauman, M. D., Lavenex, P., Mason, W. A., Capitanio, J. P., & Amaral, D. G. (2004). The development of social behavior following neonatal amygdala lesions in rhesus monkeys. *Journal of Cognitive Neuroscience, 16*(8), 1388–1411.

Breiter, H., Etcoff, N. L., Whalen, P. J., Kennedy, W. A., Rauch, S., Buckner, R. L., et al. (1996). Response and habituation of the human amygdala during visual processing of facial expression. *Neuron, 17,* 875–887.

Cardinal, R. N., Parkinson, J. A., Hall, J., & Everitt, B. J. (2002). Emotion and motivation: The role of the amygdala, ventral striatum, and prefrontal cortex. *Neuroscience and Biobehavioral Reviews, 26*(3), 321–352.

Casey, B. J., Galvan, A., & Hare, T. A. (2005). Changes in cerebral functional organization during cognitive development. *Current Opinion in Neurobiology, 15*(2), 239–244.

Casey, B. J., Giedd, J. N., & Thomas, K. M. (2000). Structural and functional brain development and its relation to cognitive development. *Biological Psychology, 54*(1–3), 241–257.

Casey, B. J., Tottenham, N., Liston, C., & Durston, S. (2005). Imaging the developing brain: What have we learned about cognitive development? *Trends in Cognitive Sciences, 9*(3), 104–110.

Cook, M., Mineka, S., Wolkenstein, B., & Laitsch, K. (1985). Observational conditioning of snake fear in unrelated rhesus monkeys. *Journal of Abnormal Psychology, 94*(4), 591–610.

Corcoran, K. A., & Quirk, G. J. (2007). Activity in prelimbic cortex is necessary for the expression of learned, but not innate, fears. *Journal of Neuroscience, 27*(4), 840–844.

Critchley, H. D., Mathias, C. J., & Dolan, R. J. (2002). Fear conditioning in humans: The influence of awareness and autonomic arousal on functional neuroanatomy. *Neuron, 33*(4), 653–663.

Davis, M., & Whalen, P. J. (2001). The amygdala: Vigilance and emotion. *Molecular Psychiatry, 6*(1), 13–34.

Emery, N. J., & Amaral, D. G. (1999). The role of the amygdala in primate social cognition. In R. D. Lane & L. Nadel (Eds.), *Cognitive neuroscience of emotion* (pp. 156–191). Oxford, UK: Oxford University Press.

Fuster, J. M. (2002). Frontal lobe and cognitive development. *Journal of Neurocytology, 31*(3–5), 373–385.

Galvan, A., Hare, T. A., Parra, C. E., Penn, J., Voss, H., Glover, G., et al. (2006). Earlier development of the accumbens relative to orbitofrontal cortex might underlie risk-taking behavior in adolescents. *Journal of Neuroscience, 26*(25), 6885–6892.

Garcia, R., Vouimba, R. M., Baudry, M., & Thompson, R. F. (1999). The amygdala modulates prefrontal cortex activity relative to conditioned fear. *Nature, 402,* 294–296.

Ghashghaei, H. T., & Barbas, H. (2002). Pathways for emotion: Interactions of prefrontal and anterior temporal pathways in the amygdala of the rhesus monkey. *Neuroscience, 115*(4), 1261–1279.

Giedd, J. N. (2004). Structural magnetic resonance imaging of the adolescent brain. *Annals of the New York Academy of Sciences, 1021,* 77–85.

Hamann, S. B., & Adolphs, R. (1999). Normal recognition of emotional similarity between facial expressions following bilateral amygdala damage. *Neuropsychologia, 37*(10), 1135–1141.

Hare, T. A., & Casey, B. J. (2005). The neurobiology and development of cognitive and affective control. *Cognition, Brain, and Behavior, 9,* 273–285.

Hare, T. A., Tottenham, N., Davidson, M. C., Glover, G. H., & Casey, B. J. (2005). Contributions of amygdale and striatal activity in emotion regulation. *Biological Psychiatry, 57*(6), 624–632.

Hariri, A. R., Mattay, V. S., Tessitore, A., Fera, F., & Weinberger, D. R. (2003). Neocortical modulation of the amygdala response to fearful stimuli. *Biological Psychiatry, 53*(6), 494–501.

Hatfield, T., Graham, P. W., & Gallagher, M. M. (1992). Taste-potentiated odor aversion learning: Role of the amygdaloid basolateral complex and central nucleus. *Behavioral Neuroscience, 106,* 286–293.

Hennenlotter, A., Schroeder, U., Erhard, P., Castrop, F., Haslinger, B., Stoecker, D., et al. (2005). A common neural basis for receptive and expressive communication of pleasant facial affect. *NeuroImage, 26*(2), 581–591.

Holsen, L. M., Zarcone, J. R., Thompson, T. I., Brooks, W. M., Anderson, M. F., Ahluwalia, J. S., et al. (2005). Neural mechanisms underlying food motivation in children and adolescents. *NeuroImage, 27*(3), 669–676.

Humphrey, T. (1968). The development of the human amygdala during early embryonic life. *Journal of Comparative Neurology, 132*(1), 135–165.

Karmiloff-Smith, A. (2006). The tortuous route from genes to behavior: A neuroconstructivist approach. *Cognitive, Affective, and Behavioral Neuroscience, 6*(1), 9–17.

Keightley, M. L., Winocur, G., Graham, S. J., Mayberg, H. S., Hevenor, S. J., & Grady, C. L. (2003). An fMRI study investigating cognitive modulation of brain regions associated with emotional processing of visual stimuli. *Neuropsychologia, 41*(5), 585–596.

Killgore, W. D., Oki, M., & Yurgelun-Todd, D. A. (2001). Sex-specific developmental differences in amygdala responses to affective faces. *NeuroReport, 12*(2), 427–433.

Knight, D. C., Nguyen, H. T., & Bandettini, P. A. (2005). The role of the human amygdala in the production of conditioned fear responses. *NeuroImage, 26*(4), 1193–1200.

LaBar, K. S., Gatenby, J. C., Gore, J. C., LeDoux, J. E., & Phelps, E. A. (1998). Human amygdala activation during conditioned fear acquisition and extinction: A mixed-trial fMRI study. *Neuron, 20*, 937–945.

Lange, K., Williams, L. M., Young, A. W., Bullmore, E. T., Brammer, M. J., Williams, S. C., et al. (2003). Task instructions modulate neural responses to fearful facial expressions. *Biological Psychiatry, 53*(3), 226–232.

LeDoux, J. E. (1993). Emotional memory systems in the brain. *Behavioural Brain Research, 58*(1–2), 69–79.

LeDoux, J. E. (2003). The emotional brain, fear, and the amygdala. *Cellular and Molecular Neurobiology, 23*(4–5), 727–738.

Levesque, J., Joanette, Y., Mensour, B., Beaudoin, G., Leroux, J. M., Bourgouin, P., et al. (2004). Neural basis of emotional self-regulation in childhood. *Neuroscience, 129*(2), 361–369.

Lobaugh, N. J., Gibson, E., & Taylor, M. J. (2006). Children recruit distinct neural systems for implicit emotional face processing. *NeuroReport, 17*(2), 215–219.

Maren, S. (2001). Neurobiology of Pavlovian fear conditioning. *Annual Review of Neuroscience, 24*, 897–931.

McClure, E. B., Monk, C. S., Nelson, E. E., Zarahn, E., Leibenluft, E., Bilder, R. M., et al. (2004). A developmental examination of gender differences in brain engagement during evaluation of threat. *Biological Psychiatry, 55*(11), 1047–1055.

McDonald, A. J. (1987). Organization of amygdaloid projections to the mediodorsal thalamus and prefrontal cortex: A fluorescence retrograde transport study in the rat. *Journal of Comparative Neurology, 262*(1), 46–58.

Mineka, S., & Öhman, A. (2002). Phobias and preparedness: The selective, automatic, and encapsulated nature of fear. *Biological Psychiatry, 52*(10), 927–937.

Monk, C. S., Grillon, C., Baas, J. M., McClure, E. B., Nelson, E. E., Zarahn, E., et al. (2003). A neuroimaging method for the study of threat in adolescents. *Developmental Psychobiology, 43*(4), 359–366.

Monk, C. S., McClure, E. B., Nelson, E. E., Zarahn, E., Bilder, R. M., Leibenluft, E., et al. (2003). Adolescent immaturity in attention-related brain engagement to emotional facial expressions. *NeuroImage, 20*(1), 420–428.

Morgan, M. A., & LeDoux, J. E. (1995). Differential contribution of dorsal and ventral medial prefrontal cortex to the acquisition and extinction of conditioned fear in rats. *Behavioral Neuroscience, 109*(4), 681–688.

Nomura, M., Ohira, H., Haneda, K., Iidaka, T., Sadato, N., Okada, T., et al. (2004). Functional association of the amygdala and ventral prefrontal cortex during cognitive evaluation of facial expressions primed by masked angry faces: An event-related fMRI study. *NeuroImage, 21*(1), 352–363.

Ochsner, K. N., Bunge, S. A., Gross, J. J., & Gabrieli, J. D. (2002). Rethinking feelings: An FMRI study of the cognitive regulation of emotion. *Journal of Cognitive Neuroscience, 14*(8), 1215–1229.

Ochsner, K. N., Ray, R. D., Cooper, J. C., Robertson, E. R., Chopra, S., Gabrieli, J. D., et al. (2004). For better or for worse: Neural systems supporting the cognitive down- and up-regulation of negative emotion. *NeuroImage, 23*(2), 483–499.

Phelps, E. A., O'Connor, K. J., Gatenby, J. C., Gore, J. C., Grillon, C., & Davis, M. (2001). Activation of the left amygdala to a cognitive representation of fear. *Nature Neuroscience, 4*(4), 437–441.

Prather, M. D., Lavenex, P., Mauldin-Jourdain, M. L., Mason, W. A., Capitanio, J. P., Mendoza, S. P., et al. (2001). Increased social fear and decreased fear of objects in monkeys with neonatal amygdala lesions. *Neuroscience, 106*(4), 653–658.

Somerville, L. H., Kim, H., Johnstone, T., Alexander, A. L., & Whalen, P. J. (2004). Human amygdala responses during presentation of happy and neutral faces: Correlations with state anxiety. *Biological Psychiatry, 55*(9), 897–903.

Sowell, E. R., Thompson, P. M., Holmes, C. J., Jernigan, T. L., & Toga, A. W. (1999). *In vivo* evidence for post-adolescent brain maturation in frontal and striatal regions. *Nature Neuroscience, 2*(10), 859–861.

Thomas, K. M., Drevets, W. C., Dahl, R. E., Ryan, N. D., Birmaher, B., Eccard, C. H., et al. (2001). Amygdala response to fearful faces in anxious and depressed children. *Archives of General Psychiatry, 58*(11), 1057–1063.

Thomas, K. M., Drevets, W. C., Whalen, P. J., Eccard, C. H., Dahl, R. E., Ryan, N. D., et al. (2001). Amygdala response to facial expressions in children and adults. *Biological Psychiatry, 49*(4), 309–316.

Ulfig, N., Setzer, M., & Bohl, J. (2003). Ontogeny of the human amygdala. *Annals of the New York Academy of Sciences, 985*, 22–33.

Wang, A. T., Dapretto, M., Hariri, A. R., Sigman, M., & Bookheimer, S. Y. (2004). Neural correlates of facial affect processing in children and adolescents with autism spectrum disorder. *Journal of the American Academy of Child and Adolescent Psychiatry, 43*(4), 481–490.

Whalen, P. J. (1998). Fear, vigilance, and ambiguity: Initial neuroimaging studies of the human amygdale. *Current Directions in Psychological Science, 7*(6), 177–188.

Yang, T. T., Menon, V., Reid, A., Gotlib, I., & Reiss, A. L. (2003). Amygdalar activation associated with happy facial expressions in adolescents: A 3-T functional MRI study. *Journal of the American Academy of Child and Adolescent Psychiatry, 42*(8), 979–985.

CHAPTER 6

Human Fear Conditioning
and the Amygdala

Arne Öhman

There is strong evidence from animal studies that the amygdala is the critical nexus of the brain network for fear conditioning (e.g., Davis, 2000; Fanselow & Poulus, 2005; Kim & Jung, 2006; LeDoux, 2000). The primary purpose of the present chapter is to examine the role of the amygdala in human fear conditioning. I start out by situating fear conditioning in two distinct research traditions: one focusing on associations connecting the conditioned stimulus (CS) and the unconditioned stimulus (US), and the other focusing on the functional role of the conditioned response (CR) in a biological perspective. The chapter then provides an overview of definitions and control procedures in fear conditioning before the human literature on the role of the amygdala in this type of learning is reviewed. Next, several sections review brain imaging and neuropsychological studies of human fear conditioning. The chapter terminates with a review and a discussion of a topic not dealt with in animal fear conditioning: the relationship between conditioned changes in the amygdala and human cognition, as manifested in explicit knowledge about stimulus relationships.

PERSPECTIVES ON PAVLOVIAN FEAR CONDITIONING

The basic procedure of human Pavlovian fear conditioning is to let a relatively neutral stimulus (the CS) precede an aversive event (the US) in some regular temporal arrangement. The US may be a potentially painful or otherwise threatening stimulus, such as a loud noise or a mild electric shock. Pavlovian conditioning has several important effects. First, an association is formed between the CS and the US, such that the CS prompts retrieval of the US from memory. Second, the retrieval of US from memory before its actual occurrence allows the organism to expect and prepare for the delivery of the US. Third, in humans, the CS–US contingency becomes stored not only in implicit memory but also in declarative memory, which makes it represented in awareness, and thus an object for verbal commentary.

The Associative Tradition

Even though they are mutually dependent, the associative and preparatory effects of a Pavlovian contingency between a CS and a US have historically been embedded in two different research traditions. The dominating tradition has chartered the principles for forming associations between CSs and USs. For example, one of its most important discoveries is that the effectiveness of a US in incrementing the associative bond between the CS and the US is inversely related to its predictability from the sum total of available stimuli (Rescorla & Wagner, 1972). In other words, the degree to which a US is surprising determines its capacity to support conditioning (Kamin, 1969). A surprising event represents a failure of prediction; that is, it can be taken as an error signal that may be used to adjust the weight of available stimuli, in order to predict future USs more accurately. Thus, because it emphasizes the role of the CS as a signal predicting the US, the focus of the associative tradition is on the *contingency* between, rather than on the number of *pairings* of, the CS and the US. Indeed, with the number of CS–US pairings held constant, strength of conditioning is inversely related to the number of unsignaled USs presented between the conditioning trials, because the unsignaled USs dilute the CS–US contingency, making the US less predictable from the CS (Rescorla, 1968). From this perspective, the function of Pavlovian conditioning is to help disentangle the causal structure of the environment by finding out what events lead to other important events (Rescorla, 1988).

The Functional Tradition

The other tradition takes an explicit biological perspective by focusing on the functional consequences of Pavlovian conditioning (Domjan, 2005; Hollis, 1997; Öhman & Wiens, 2003). Whereas the focus of the associative tradition is on *learning*, the focus in the functional tradition has been on the principles of how associations are *expressed* in behavior. An important goal of the functionalist tradition is to understand how the CS, by signaling biologically important events (USs), enables animals to prepare functionally for, and respond adaptively to, these events. From this perspective, Pavlovian conditioning involves changes in integrated behavioral systems rather than changes in the amplitude or probability of isolated responses.

Fear conditioning results in a state of conditioned fear associated with species-specific defense responses (Bolles, 1970), the expression of which is determined by the actual situation. The imminence of threat provided by the US (e.g., a predator) is a major determinant of how the CR is expressed. A distant threat merely results in interference with foraging; for example, a gazelle may continue grazing, but will keep an eye on a lion resting in the distance. When the threat is closer but not imminent (the lion is moving), the likely CRs are freezing and scanning of the environment for evaluating the threat and potential escape routes (Blanchard & Blanchard, 1988). When the lion is approaching, suggesting that it may be preparing for attack, the likely CRs are flight and (if necessary) fight (Fanselow, 1994). These different behavioral responses are associated with different patterning of autonomic and somatic responses, which may be used to index different aspects of fear conditioning (Lang, Bradley, & Cuthbert, 1997).

For example, to human participants wired up to a polygraph in a psychophysiological laboratory for a Pavlovian conditioning experiment (not to speak of those being inserted into a brain scanner!), the only available defense response is immobility (freezing). Consequently, they are likely to show autonomic responses associated with freezing and environmental scanning, such as skin conductance responses (SCRs) and heart rate deceleration, rather than the heart rate acceleration associated with active defenses such as flight and fight (Lang et al., 1997; Öhman, Hamm, & Hugdahl, 2000; Öhman & Wiens, 2003).

In the natural environment, the CS and the US tend to be nonrandomly connected, which is likely to facilitate conditioning. Not just any faint sounds or odors are likely to become associated with an 'attack by a predator, but sounds and odors that may forebode an attack because they are produced by the predator itself (e.g., Domjan, 2005; Öhman & Mineka, 2001). Thus evolutionary pressures not only have shaped the mammalian defense repertoire, but are also likely to have biased the associative apparatus of animals to pick up systematic ecological relationships between stimuli (Seligman, 1970, 1971). This hypothesis, known as the "preparedness hypothesis" (Seligman, 1970), suggests that human fears and phobias may be related to a large but still limited set of objects and events, which tend to cluster on situations that in themselves involve some degree of danger, particularly in an evolutionary perspective (Öhman, Dimberg, & Öst, 1985; Öhman & Mineka, 2001; Olsson, Ebert, Banaji, & Phelps, 2005). For example, common phobic objects and events such as snakes, enclosed (as well as wide-open) spaces, heights, and mutilated conspecifics have been related to recurrent survival threats in mammalian evolution, and this relationship has put a premium on learning easily to fear and avoid them. My colleagues and I (Öhman et al., 1985) have argued that signals of dominant social threat (e.g., angry faces) have served a similar function in evolution within the context of dominance conflicts, thus incorporating social phobia into the preparedness argument (see Öhman & Mineka, 2001, for an extensive review).

Implications of the Two Traditions

The two traditions of Pavlovian conditioning have honored different methodological approaches and emphases. If the focus is on the forming of associations between the CS and the US, then it makes sense to work with stimuli that are arbitrarily related to each other, to assure that the emerging principles are general. Investigators adhering to the functional tradition, on the other hand, are likely to favor CSs and USs that are ecologically related. If they want to understand these types of processes, they may be better off with evolutionarily shaped principles for specific situations than with general principles of associating arbitrary stimuli (e.g., Fanselow, 1994; Öhman & Mineka, 2001). Similarly, for associationists, the choice of which CR to study is one of mere convenience: They should use whatever easily measured index tracks the conditioning process. Functionists, on the other hand, are more likely to be interested in the organism in its natural environment and the functional role of the CR in this context.

The two traditions also provide different perspectives on the neural substrates of fear conditioning. Of course, both traditions share the core of an apparatus for forming and storing learned relationships between the CS and the US, but whereas this is the central focus of the associationists, it is necessary but not sufficient for the functionalists. From the functionalist perspective, on the other hand, the focus is the neural underpinning of conditioned behavior directed at adaptive coping with the US. It should be obvious that a primary motivation for an interest in the neural architecture of fear conditioning—its potential as a key to anxiety disorders—is closer to the functionalist than to the associationist perspective on Pavlovian conditioning.

METHODOLOGICAL ISSUES
IN HUMAN FEAR CONDITIONING

Pavlovian Fear Conditioning and Its Control Procedures

At the level of behavioral and peripheral psychophysiological changes, "Pavlovian conditioning" can be defined as any modification in response to the CS that can be attributed to repeated exposures to contingent presentations of the CS and the US (see, e.g., Öhman, 1983). This operational definition is applicable to functional magnetic resonance imaging (fMRI) research in which brain activation is indexed by regional hemodynamic activation, as assessed by blood-oxygenation-level-dependent (BOLD) changes.

For an investigator to be able to attribute a putative CR to the CS–US contingency, control procedures are necessary (see Prokasy, 1977; Rescorla, 1967). The inference that a response results from this contingency requires the demonstration that the putative CR is stronger than responses produced by similar stimuli lacking a history of contingent CS–US presentations. This can be accomplished in a "single-cue conditioning" procedure, in which an experimental group of subjects is given a sequence of trials where the CS reliably predicts the occurrence of the US. For conditioning to be inferred, responding to the CS in this group has to exceed responding to the CS in a control group with noncontingent (unpaired or random) presentation of the CS and the US during the training trials. Alternatively, a "differential conditioning" procedure may be used to assess conditioning. In this type of procedure, subjects are exposed to two different CSs that initially do not induce different responses. One of them, the CS+, is then followed by the US, whereas the other stimulus, the CS–, serves as a control stimulus never presented with the US. If, as training proceeds, subjects start to show larger responses to the CS+ than to the CS–, differential Pavlovian conditioning has been demonstrated. (See Öhman, 1983, for a thorough discussion of control procedures in human fear conditioning.)

Problems with Control Procedures in a Brain Imaging Context

With the single-cue procedure, the conditioning contrast must be between subjects in order to achieve experimental control of order effects. Given that the dependent variable in brain imaging research is typically based on contrasts between relative blood flow changes in experimental and control conditions presented to the same participant, the between-subject nature of control procedures for single-cue conditioning provides an important limitation by requiring an absolute measure of changes in brain activity at various brain areas. In principle, it is possible to assess single-cue conditioning on a within-subject basis, but only at the price of inevitably confounding order effects when the contingent and noncontingent CS and US procedures are presented in blocks, or at different sessions, to the same group of participants. Several problems complicate within-subject versions of controls for single-cue conditioning. First, if the control condition is given at the same session as the conditioning procedure, there are typically strong short-term, within-session habituation effects in both autonomic (e.g., Öhman et al., 2000) and brain imaging (e.g., Raichle, 1997) measures; these effects will favor the condition that is presented first if the focus, as is the case in conditioning experiments, is on enhanced responding. Second, if the two conditions are given at different sessions, similar problems will arise because of long-term, between-session habituation. Third, there may be specific, potentially asymmetric carryover effects between conditions, depending on the order of presentation. If the contingent procedure is given before the noncontingent one, carryover conditioning effects from the first sessions will enhance responding to the noncontingent CS, thus resulting in an underestimation of conditioning effects. This problem, by the way, is not alleviated by terminating the conditioning session by an extinction series. Extinction does not break, but merely inhibits, the CS–US bond (e.g., Bouton, 2005; Milad, Rauch, Pitman, & Quirk, 2006). The intactness of the CS–US association is demonstrated, for example, by noncontingent US presentation after extinction, which reinstates the CR to the CS (Rescorla & Heth, 1975), again resulting in underestimation of conditioning effects. Similar effects will also occur when the control session precedes the conditioning session. This is because noncontingent presentation of the CS and the US will impede subsequent conditioning effects of contingent CS–US presentations as a result of latent inhibition (e.g., Lubow, 1973), US habituation (e.g., Rescorla, 1974), and learned irrelevance (Baker, 1976).

From the perspective of brain imaging, the differential conditioning design appears a more attractive option than the single-cue conditioning procedure, because it is based on within-subject contrasts (between the CS+ and the CS–) to assess conditioned changes in brain activity with stringent controls of presentation orders. However, animal studies—which are often taken as point of departures for human brain imaging experiments—more often use single-cue than differential conditioning paradigms to study brain mechanisms of conditioning, under the reasonable assumption that it has simpler brain correlates than differential conditioning has. For example, differential conditioning necessarily involves more extensive sensory analysis than single-cue conditioning, requiring more processing work in the sensory areas of the CS. Furthermore, it not only involves excitatory conditioning to the CS+, but also is likely to result in inhibitory conditioning to CS– (which becomes a "safety signal"), and therefore these two processes are confounded in a CS+ versus CS– contrast. This is highlighted in the results from a meta-analysis comparing fear conditioning in individuals diagnosed with anxiety disorder and nonanxious controls. Lissek and colleagues (2005) reported overall stronger conditioning effect in patients than in controls, and this effect was significantly larger in single cue than in differential conditioning paradigms. Indeed, examining only studies using the latter paradigm, the difference between groups was not significant. This is consistent with the hypothesis that anxiety disorder is associated with enhanced excitatory fear conditioning and difficulties in inhibiting responses to safety signals. Similarly (and interestingly), Lonsdorf and colleagues (in press) reported stronger fear-conditioned startle potentiation to the CS+ in carriers of at least one short allele than in carriers of two long alleles in the serotonin transporter gene promoter polymorphism, but no differences between these genetically defined groups in differential responding to the CS+ and to the CS–.

Some research questions are formulated in terms of single-cue rather than differential conditioning. For example, conditioning models of posttraumatic stress disorder (PTSD) posit that traumatic events may function as overwhelmingly intense USs: They support the conditioning of fear to a host of situational stimuli at a single instance, giving them the power to elicit emotionally painful flashbacks and episodes of strong anxiety when later encountered. This is clearly a case of (multiple, simultaneous) single-cue conditioning, lacking any CS– that may serve as a safety signal. Thus the very process one wants to study may be misrepresented if it is modeled by means of differential conditioning procedures. In spite of its obvious advantages, therefore, one must keep in mind that differential conditioning is not an undisputed answer to all design problems in human brain imaging research on fear conditioning.

In closing this section, I should point out that in some instances the design problems may be less acute when the focus is on brain activations rather than on behavioral responses. Behavioral responses are unidimensional in the sense that confounding effects from other processes (e.g., unconditioned effects of the CS, habituation, sensitization, generalization) than associative conditioning processes interact to influence a single index (e.g., SCRs, heart rate changes, eyeblink responses). However, brain effects of conditioning have a spatial dimension; that is, sensory effects of the CS and the US often occur at loci (e.g., sensory cortices) that are distinct from the presumed locus for associative effects (e.g., in the amygdala).

AMYGDALA ACTIVATIONS IN HUMAN FEAR CONDITIONING

Brain Imaging and Single-Cue Fear Conditioning

Perhaps because of the interpretational complications, only a few brain imaging studies have investigated brain correlates of single-cue conditioning in humans. In a pioneering attempt, Hugdahl and colleagues (1995) exposed participants to a single-cue conditioning paradigm with a tone CS and an electric shock US while they were positioned in a positron emission tomography (PET) scanner. To assess conditioning, images derived from CS-alone trials after a CS–US acquisition series were contrasted to CS-alone trials preceding conditioning. As previously discussed, such a contrast incorporates within-session habituation as a confounding factor, which is likely to underestimate conditioning effects. Accordingly, Hugdahl and colleagues did not obtain any amygdala activations, but they did see conditioning-related changes in several cortical areas.

Knight, Smith, Cheng, Stein, and Helmstetter (2004) used fMRI and a single-cue conditioning procedure to compare one group of participants subjected to a conditioning paradigm, in which a 15-sec light CS was followed by an electric shock US, with a control group in which the CS and the US were randomly related. Larger SCRs in the contingent than in the noncontingent group verified that the conditioning procedure was effective at the autonomic level. However, both groups showed significant but quantitatively similar bilateral amygdala activations to the CS (as assessed by cross-correlations to a modeled waveform of hemodynamic change) early in training; thus this study failed to support conditioned changes in amygdala activity. In contrast, between-group differences emerged in left hippocampus activation as a function of training, because subjects in the conditioning group maintained their response level, whereas it decreased in the control group. In an earlier study using a similar design, Knight, Smith, Stein, and Helmstetter (1999) also failed to show amygdala differences between groups exposed to single-cue conditioning and nonpaired control treatments, but they did report reliable conditioning changes for the anterior cingulate cortex (ACC) and the primary visual cortex.

Using PET to compare single-cue conditioning with nonpaired presentation of the CS and the US between two sessions on different days in the same participants, Bremner and colleagues (2005) reported that both women diagnosed with PTSD and healthy controls showed larger activations in the left amygdala during conditioning than during nonpaired presentation of the CS and the US. In addition, the conditioning-related changes in the left amygdala were larger in the patients with PTSD than in the healthy controls. Because the order always involved conditioning before control sessions, these conditioning data are hard to evaluate, because between-session habituation must be balanced against transfer of conditioning effects. However, interpretation of the larger left amygdala response in patients than in healthy participants is not affected by this confound.

The results of the studies reviewed here are less than convincing. In spite of the consistent finding in the animal literature (e.g., Davis, 2000; Fanselow & Poulos, 2005; LeDoux, 1996) that the amygdala is critical for single-cue conditioning in rodents, there appears to be no unequivocal demonstration of amygdala activations that can be attributed to single-cue conditioning in the limited human literature.

Brain Imaging and Differential Fear Conditioning

There are better data to support a role of the amygdala in human differential conditioning. LaBar, Gatenby, Gore, LeDoux, and Phelps (1998) used fMRI of three coronal slices centered on the amygdala to examine fear conditioning in a mixed CS+, CS– design. They reported data from 10 participants who were exposed to a differential conditioning procedure: A blue light was presented for 10 sec, followed by a mild electric shock US, and a green light (colors were counterbalanced across subjects) was presented for the same duration but was never followed by the US. Reliable SCR conditioning in 5 participants who were brought in later for a second conditioning session showed that the conditioning procedure was effective for producing differential conditioning. fMRI results demonstrated reliable larger activations primarily of the right amygdala (the periamygdaloid cortex; Talaraich coordinates –14, –4, –19) to the CS+ than the CS– during the first half of acquisition. However, this effect habituated during the second half of acquisition, to reappear as a more centrally placed amygdala activation (–17, –4, –11) early in extinction, but again to habituate on later trials. Additional areas related to conditioning included the rostral and caudal ACC, the former early and the latter late in training.

Büchel, Morris, Dolan, and Friston (1998) also used a differential conditioning design in an event-related fMRI study that included a familiarization phase (52 stimuli) and a conditioning phase (104 stimuli). The former phase involved repeated 3-sec presentations of four different neutral faces. The latter (conditioning) phase involved the same four faces, two of which served as CS+ in a 50% reinforcement schedule with a loud tone (~100 dB), and two served as CS– without any accompanying tones. That is to say, there were 26 presentations of each CS–; 26 presentations (13 of each) of the CS+ followed by the US at CS offset; and 26 presentations (13 of each) of the CS+ not followed by the US. CS+ presentations occurred in random order and were randomly intermixed with CS– presentations. The purpose of this partial reinforcement schedule was to allow assessment of SCRs and fMRI-assessed hemodynamic responses to the CS+ uncontaminated by US presentations (i.e., on the 50% of the CS+ trials that did not include the US). The CS+ versus CS– contrasts during acquisition failed to reveal any amygdala activation, but there were bilateral activations of the ACC and the anterior insula (AI). However, when Büchel and colleagues tested for an interaction between CS type (CS+ vs. CS–) and trial blocks similar to what was reported by LaBar and colleagues (1995), a significant effect was found bilaterally for the amygdala; this could be attributed to initially larger amygdala activations to the CS+ (left, –24, 3, –24; right, 27, –3, –24), but this effect disappeared across trial blocks. A very similar interaction was found for SCRs. Almost identical SCR and amygdala results, as well as activations in the ACC and anterior putamen, were reported in a second study, which used a trace rather than a delay conditioning procedure (Büchel, Dolan, Armony, & Friston, 1999).

Birbaumer and colleagues (2005) also reported a CS type × trials interaction for the right amygdala in a differential conditioning paradigm that used neutral faces (with or without mustache, counterbalanced) as CS+ and CS–, and a painful pressure as the US, in a control group of a study examining fear conditioning in psychopathy (the group with psychopathy, by the way, failed to show any evidence of fear conditioning). A similar interaction was reported for the ventromedial orbitofrontal cortex, and there were main effects of stimulus type for several structures: the ACC (rostral and caudal), posterior cingulate, and bilateral AI.

Moses and colleagues (2007) used a 306-channel magnetoencephalography (MEG) array, allowing precise timing of neural events, to estimate a dipole current source interpreted as reflecting amygdala activity. Participants were exposed to a simple differential conditioning paradigm with different visual patterns presented for 1500 msec as the CS+ and the CS–, and 100-msec binaural white noise as the US. The results showed larger and more frequent waveforms within 600 msec of CS+ than of CS– onsets, as well as late activity immediately prior to US onset and to US offset on nonreinforced CS+ trials. These effects, furthermore, were larger in response to CS+ during acquisition than during habituation and extinction. Mean peak amplitudes occurred about 300 msec after CS onset and tended to be earlier in the right than in the left amygdala. These data suggest that there were early conditioned changes in amygdala neural activity, as well as activity related to the US.

All these differential conditioning studies concur in demonstrating systematic changes in the amygdala during Pavlovian training: There is an early peak in amygdala activation that disappears with training and that may return when the contingencies are changed during extinction (Knight, Smith, et al., 2004; LaBar et al., 1998). An ingenious study by Gläscher and Büchel (2005) shed interesting light on these consistent findings by applying a formal learning theory approach to brain imaging of fear conditioning. As noted earlier in this chapter, one of the most important discoveries in modern Pavlovian conditioning research is that animals primarily learn from surprising USs—that is, when US prediction fails. The more surprising the US, the more effective it is in promoting change in the learned association between the CS and the US. At a given trial, conditioned responding is determined by the sum of two factors: an expectancy factor based on prior training, and a change factor reflecting the surprisingness of the US at the preceding trial. The latter factor is modulated by a learning parameter, which, if it is high, produces large learning changes on this trial; if it is low, little learning occurs. Gläscher and Büchel reasoned that in the latter case (i.e., a low learning parameter), learning integrates training over a considerable time period to support stable responding that is only marginally changed by events on an individual trial. If the learning parameter is high, on the other hand, changes in associative strength can be considerable from one trial to the next, which implies rapid change in order to adjust to immediate challenges. Gläscher and Büchel arranged a stimulus series composed of two CSs (a face and a house) and a US (mild pain) in which the contingencies were slowly varied so that when the US probability was high for one CS it was low for the other, and vice versa. Importantly, they also presented one series with a low (i.e., long-term integration) learning parameter and another series in which it was high. Contrasting low- against high-learning-parameter series, they reported reliable amygdala activations (as well as activation in the nucleus accumbens, ventral putamen, and hippocampus). These structures, then, reflect slow long-term changes in associative strength in CS–US association. The reverse contrast, looking for areas with a short time constant, showed strong activation of areas in the ventral visual stream (such as the fusiform facial area and the parahippocampus place area) and the orbitofrontal cortex, which suggests rapid changes in the tuning of perception in accordance with changing expectancies. It is interesting to note that Morris and Dolan (2004), in a different paradigm, reported findings consistent with those reported by Gläscher and Büchel: The amygdala resisted reversals of the CS+ and the CS−, whereas the orbitofrontal cortex rapidly adjusted to the reversal.

On the basis of their findings, Gläscher and Büchel (2005) argued that the role of the amygdala in fear conditioning is to monitor contingency changes for biologically salient stimuli. Because typical fear conditioning experiments only involve contingency changes at the junction between phases (CS-alone habituation to acquisition; acquisition to extinction), the change point is when the amygdala is most active, later to habituate when the contingency remains stable during the remaining acquisition or extinction series. In the Gläscher and Büchel experiment, on the other hand, the strength of the contingency was more or less continuously changing, which was taken to require continuous monitoring by the amygdala.

Fear Conditioning in Patients with Lesions in the Amygdala

From this review, it appears that the data quite consistently support the amygdala's involvement in differential fear conditioning, which is particularly evident early in conditioning training. However, rather than demonstrating a causal link between the amygdala and human fear conditioning, these data in effect are correlational. Thus they need to be supplemented by neuropsychological studies on patients with selective damage to the amygdala, in order to demonstrate a necessary role for the amygdala in fear conditioning. Bechara and colleagues (1995) reported an interesting double dissociation in a case study that included three patients—one with bilateral and uniquely specific damage to the amygdala because of Urbach–Wiethe disease, another with bilateral damage to the hippocampus that spared the amygdala, and the third with large temporal lesions that included both the amygdala and the hippocampus. The patients did not differ from a control group in SCRs to the loud noise used as a US, but whereas the patient with hippocampus damage showed differential SCR conditioning to both auditory and visual stimuli, the patients with amygdala damage failed to show any SCR evidence of conditioning. However, in stark contrast, the amygdala-lesioned patient, but not the hippocampus-lesioned patient, could report the CS–US contingency after the experiment. Thus the amygdala-lesioned patient learned the CS–US contingency at the cognitive level, but failed to show any evidence of emotional learning as assessed by SCRs, whereas the hippocampus-lesioned patient showed exactly the opposite pattern. Finally, the patient whose lesions included both the amygdala and the hippocampus showed neither SCR conditioning nor declarative knowledge of the CS–US contingency.

LaBar, LeDoux, Spencer, and Phelps (1995) examined about 20 patients treated by unilateral neurosurgical removal of parts of the anterior medial temporal lobe, including most of the amygdala, in order to relieve treatment-resistant epileptic seizures. The patients did not differ from a control group in unconditioned SCRs to the noise US, but whereas the control participants showed highly reliable differential SCR conditioning to a CS+ and a CS– that differed in pitch during an acquisition series, the patients (regardless of the side of the surgery) failed to show any evidence of differential conditioning, primarily because of small responses to the CS+. Similar results were reported from a more complex differential conditioning procedure in which colored lights and tones jointly defined the contingency between the CS+ and the US. The subjects were explicitly instructed to attend to the CS and "to try to detect a pattern to the stimuli, which the experimenter would ask them to report periodically throughout the session" (LaBar et al., 1995, p. 6848). Consequently, a large majority of the subjects (including about 80% of the patients) were able to report the correct contingency after each phase of the experiment. Nevertheless, the patients showed no evidence of SCR conditioning.

The results reported by LaBar and colleagues (1995) were constructively replicated by Weike and colleagues (2005), who used startle potentiation as their primary measure of conditioning. Weike and colleagues examined 30 patients subjected to standardized amygdalahippocampectomy as treatment for epilepsy (18 in the left and 12 in the right temporal lobe). The CSs were two pictures of male faces with a neutral emotional expression, one of which was followed by a brief electric shock US. Startle blinks (electromyographically measured from the left orbicularis oculi muscle) were assessed to probes (50-msec, 95-dB white noise with abrupt onset and offset) presented during some of the CS+ and the CS−, as well as alone in the intertrial intervals, and SCRs were continuously recorded. Controls showed clear evidence of conditioned startle potentiation by displaying larger responses to probes presented during the CSs than during the interstimulus interval, and larger startles to probes presented during the CS+ than the CS−, regardless of whether they were able to report the correct CS–US contingency or not. Patients as a group, on the other hand, showed no evidence of conditioned startle potentiation, regardless of which side was lesioned. However, similar to controls, who showed SCR conditioning only among aware subjects (cf. Hamm & Vaitl, 1996), the few patients (30%) who were classified as aware also showed reliable SCR conditioning. In contrast to the explicit instructions used by LaBar and colleagues, Weike and colleagues did not mention anything about the contingency in their instructions, which may account for the discrepancy in the proportion of aware subjects in the two patient samples. Another factor might have been that the lesions were larger in Weike and colleagues' patients than in LaBar and colleagues' patients, perhaps involving more of the hippocampus and thus impairing recall of the contingency. Nevertheless, among aware subjects in the two studies, reliable SCR conditioning was reported by Weike and colleagues, but not by LaBar and colleagues.

Essentially similar data were reported by Peper, Karcher, Wohlfarth, Reinshagen, and LeDoux (2001). They used the visual half-field technique to stimulate only one hemisphere at a time, to improve the odds of observing laterality effects, depending on which side of the medial temporal lobe had been subjected to surgery in their epileptic patients. In addition, they tested for conditioned SCR effects with backward-masked CSs, thus assuring that subjects were not aware of which CS they were exposed to. However, they observed lateralized conditioning effects only in control participants, who showed differential SCR conditioning to faces showing negative (CS+) and positive (CS−) emotions, when they were presented in the left (right-hemisphere) but not in the right (left-hemisphere) visual field (cf. Johnsen & Hugdahl, 1993). Patients showed no SCR conditioning effects, regardless of which field was stimulated or which side had been operated on.

To sum up, with one exception—SCR conditioning in a small group of amygdalahippocampectomy patients, who were aware of the CS–US contingency (Weike et al., 2005)—no evidence of fear conditioning has been reported for amygdala-lesioned patients (Bechara et al., 1995; LaBar et al., 1995; Peper et al., 2001; Weike et al., 2005).

DIRECT, OBSERVATIONAL, AND INSTRUCTED FEAR CONDITIONING

Pavlovian conditioning is one of several and potentially similar ways of imbuing a stimulus with predictive power in relation to a US. Indeed, both humans and monkeys can pick up a contingency between a CS and a US, and can acquire CRs, merely from watching another individual being exposed to a fear conditioning procedure (e.g., Cook & Mineka, 1989, 1990; Hygge & Öhman, 1978; Olsson & Phelps, 2004), thus learning about danger without risking to be hurt themselves. Furthermore, Pavlov (1927) described language as a "second signaling system" and argued that linguistically mediated information may turn a stimulus into a signal for other events. Accordingly, verbal instruction that a CS may be followed by a US is sufficient to induce conditioned-like SCRs (e.g., Cook & Harris, 1937; Hugdahl & Öhman, 1977) or startle potentiation to the CS (e.g., Grillon, Ameli, Woods, Merikangas, & Davis, 1991). Olsson and Phelps (2004) demonstrated SCRs of similar magnitude to stimuli that were inducted through direct, observational, and instructed conditioning. However, whereas direct and observationally conditioned responses remained significant even when backward masking blocked conscious perception of the CS, this procedure obliterated responses induced through instructions, suggesting that the instructed responses reflected a cognitive rather than basic affective level of learning (see Öhman & Mineka, 2001).

Olsson, Nearing, and Phelps (2007) delineated a neural basis for the similarity between direct and observational conditioning by demonstrating overlapping bilateral amygdala activations when participants observed a model being exposed to a CS-shock contingency and subsequently when they themselves were exposed to the CS, but without any shocks. Activations of the ACC and the AI were also reported. To examine brain correlates of instructed conditioning, Phelps and colleagues (2001) told their participants that they might feel between one and three electric shocks when exposed to one CS (e.g., a blue square) but not to another (e.g., a yellow square) CS. Like in Olsson and colleagues, the participants never received a shock. The results showed enhanced SCRs and left-amygdala activation to the threat cue, as compared to the safety cue. There was also activation of the left AI and, for a majority of the participants, of the ACC. SCRs correlated with the amygdala and AI responses. Interpreting these studies within a neural framework, Olsson and Phelps (2007) suggested that the basic subcortical fear network (e.g., LeDoux, 2000), which accounts for direct fear conditioning through plasticity in the lateral amygdala, also accounts for observational learning. However, the social analysis that is required for this type of learning necessitates interaction with cortical networks for mentalizing (medial prefrontal cortex) and empathetic emotion (ACC, AI). For instructed conditioning, given its symbolic, linguistic nature, they posited that the CS–US association, at least initially, is only represented in distributed, left-lateralized cortical networks and depends on the hippocampus for acquisition, with no necessary amygdala plasticity involved. However, to express the fear (e.g., in SCRs), similar to direct and observational conditioning, the cortical network is assumed to access the central amygdala, perhaps via the AI.

EXPRESSING LEARNED FEAR: SKIN CONDUCTANCE AND THE ORIENTING RESPONSE

Any new stimulus will evoke a pattern of autonomic changes that include SCRs, heart rate decelerations, and finger pulse volume responses, all of which can be conceptualized as components of the orienting response (OR) (see, e.g., Öhman, 1983; Öhman et al., 2000). As described in seminal work by Sokolov (1963), the motor and autonomic components of the OR are integrated parts of a centrally coordinated response, the purpose of which is to establish contact with the stimulus in order to facilitate its central processing. Indeed, it is easy to see the functionality of eliciting an OR to a novel stimulus in the prevailing context, thus commanding attentional resources to a closer analysis of its nature and possible consequences (Öhman, 1979).

As the organism learns that the CS actually has consequences (namely, is followed by the US), the OR to the CS is enhanced and then gradually habituates, to be replaced by preparatory responses in anticipation of the US as the CS–US contingency is learned (Öhman, 1979, 1983; Sokolov, 1963). Thus there is a dynamically changing pattern of responses to the CS–US complex that unfolds as a function of training. Parts of it, such as the OR, originate in unconditioned responses to the CS, and other parts (e.g., cardiovascular responses) reflect adaptive adjustments in preparation for the US (Lang et al., 1997; Öhman et al., 2000). This means that the autonomic responses often used for CR measurements are components of homeostatically controlled response patterns that provide metabolic support for whatever actions are called for, given the constraints imposed by the situation (Obrist, 1981). Thus there is no simple autonomic measure that is exclusively dedicated to tracking the conditioning process. SCRs, for example, which are often used as peripheral fear indices in brain imaging studies, are actually more closely tied to the OR and to attentional processes than to emotion (e.g., Öhman, 1979). Because the OR is part of conditioning and responds to the significance of the stimulus, the SCR indexes aspects of the conditioning process, but it can be readily dissociated from other indices of conditioned fear, such as startle potentiation (e.g., Hamm & Vaitl, 1996; Weike et al., 2005).

Knight, Helmstetter, and coworkers have analyzed the relationship between SCRs and activity in the amygdala and related structures during fear conditioning. Cheng, Knight, Smith, Stein, and Helmstetter (2003) reported a larger correlation of amygdala activity with a reference function based on SCRs than with functions based on stimulus and stimulus-convolved waveforms in a single-cue conditioning group than in an unpaired control group. They concluded that amygdala activity appeared more closely related to efferent autonomic functions than to perceptual processing of the CSs. This conclusion was further supported by Cheng, Knight, Smith, and Helmstetter (2006), who categorized CS+ and CS– trials in a differential conditioning paradigm into those that were associated with an SCR and those that did not elicit an SCR. Little amygdala activity was seen to any of the CS– categories, but among the CS+ categories, reliably more amygdala activation occurred to a CS+ accompanied by an SCR than to a CS+ without an SCR, again suggesting a link between amygdala activity and the SCR. Thus the CS+ category that did not elicit an SCR appeared insufficient to activate the amygdala.

Finally, Knight, Nguyen, and Bandettini (2005) inserted novel stimuli (tone sweeps, whistles, bursts of complex sounds) of varying durations (2–10 sec) into a differential conditioning series with tones (700 and 1300 Hz) as CS+ and CS–, and a white noise (500 msec, 100 dB) as the US. Reliable differential conditioning was demonstrated by larger SCRs to the CS+ than to the CS–, but the responses to the CS+ did not differ from SCRs to novel stimuli (which also were larger than the responses to the CS–). SCRs in general were associated with activity in several cortical (ACC, middle frontal gyrus, superior temporal gyrus, insula, inferior parietal lobule), subcortical (thalamus, caudate, putamen) and cerebellum structures (see also Critchley, Mathias, & Dolan, 2002). Areas specifically related to conditioned SCRs were located by contrasting SCRs elicited by the CS+ with all other types of SCRs. These structures included the right amygdala, right insula, right cerebellum, and left middle frontal and precentral gyri. Again, the amygdala activation was considerably stronger during conditioned SCRs than to the CS+ presentation, suggesting a closer link between the amygdala and expression of conditioned SCRs than between the amygdala and processing of the fear stimulus.

The dissociation between SCRs to novel stimuli and conditioned SCRs in terms of the suggested brain circuitry reported by Knight and colleagues (2005) conforms to a classic distinction between ORs to nonsignal and signal stimuli in the OR literature (Graham, 1979; Öhman, 1979; Öhman et al., 2000; Sokolov, 1963). The former ORs have been interpreted as bottom-up processes related to a mismatch between a stimulus and activated memorial information (e.g., Öhman, 1979), and the latter as top-down processes related to a match between a stimulus and memorial information. However, as I have argued elsewhere (Öhman, 1979), both these routes to OR activation have the joint effect of bringing the stimulus into a resource-limited focal attention channel.

EXTINCTION OF CONDITIONED FEAR

Extinction and Recovery of Fear Responses

Pavlovian CRs wane if the CS is repeatedly presented in the absence of the US. This phenomenon (and procedure) is referred to as "extinction." Extinction does not reflect the mere breaking of the bond between the CS and the US, but rather inhibitory processes that result in the suppression of the CR (Bouton, 2005; Davis & Myers, 2002).

Empirical results warrant a strong conclusion with regard to differences between the acquisition and extinction of fear CRs: The latter is more context-dependent than the former (e.g., Bouton, 2005). A fear-conditioned CR to a cue is typically elicited by that cue even if the context is changed (e.g., if an animal is exposed to the CS in a different cage). However, if a CR is conditioned in a particular context (let's call it A), and then is extinguished in a different context (B), the CR disappears. But if the experimental animal is brought back to context A and exposed to the CS, it shows a much stronger CR than a control animal extinguished in context A. This is referred to as "renewal" of the CR (see reviews by Bouton, 2005; Myers & Davis, 2007). It is as if the extinction in context B, rather than teaching the animal that the CS is no longer followed by the US, adds a contextual constraint to the CS–US contingency: It is not valid in this new situation (B). Indeed, renewal is observed also if, after extinction in context B, the CS is introduced in a completely new context (C), or even if the new context is presented after extinction in the original conditioning context (A) (see Bouton, 2005, for a review). Furthermore, an extinguished CR may be reinstated in a particular context by US-alone presentations in this context (Rescorla & Heth, 1975). Finally, as demonstrated by Pavlov (1927), spontaneous recovery of an extinguished CR can occur, merely as a consequence of the passage of time.

Renewal and Reinstatement of Conditioned SCRs

Renewal after extinction has been demonstrated in human Pavlovian conditioning. Milad, Orr, Pitman, and Rauch (2005) presented their participants with pictures of two different rooms on a computer screen. Lamps embedded in the room could be turned on and off and served as CSs, one of which was followed by shock (CS+) and the other was not (CS–). Reliable SCR conditioning in one room context, and extinction in the other context, were demonstrated in one experimental session. On the following day, participants were tested for recall of extinction in the extinction context from the previous day, and extinction remained complete. However, when the context was changed back to that of conditioning from the previous day, there was rather complete renewal, with significantly larger responses to the CS+ than to the CS–. Data indicating a similar renewal of SCR conditioning were reported by Vansteenwegen and colleagues (2005), who manipulated context by testing participants in an illuminated or a dark room. Compared to a control group having the same context throughout the experimental session, the group that switched context from conditioning to extinction showed significant renewal when switched back to the conditioning context.

LaBar and Phelps (2005) reported reinstatement of conditioned fear after extinction in humans by demonstrating context-dependent recovery of extinguished SCRs after US-alone presentations in both single-cue and differential conditioning paradigms. The effect of the US-alone presentations was mediated by the context, because US presentations had no effect when presented in a different context from that of acquisition and extinction. Consistent with this context dependence, LaBar and Phelps reported that patients with amnesia caused by damage to the hippocampus did not show reinstatement.

Brain Imaging Studies of Extinction

Animal studies suggest at least two nonexclusive routes to extinction of conditioned fear: one related to processes within the amygdala (e.g., Falls, Miserendino, & Davis, 1992; Hobin, Goosens, & Maren, 2003; see review by Walker & Davis, 2002), and the other to inhibitory influences on the amygdala, primarily from the prefrontal cortex (e.g., Morgan, Romanski, & LeDoux, 1993; Quirk & Beer, 2006; Sortres-Bayon, Cain, & LeDoux, 2006).

LaBar and colleagues (1998) reported that right amygdala activation, which had habituated from an early peak during differential conditioning, reappeared when the stimulus schedule was changed in extinction, again to disappear as extinction proceeded. Similarly, Knight, Smith, and colleagues (2004) reported right amygdala activation to the CS early in extinction in a single-cue conditioning paradigm. Moreover, based on data from aversive conditioning to an unpleasant odor, Gottfried and Dolan (2004) suggested that the diminishing amygdala activity they observed during both acquisition and extinction might be specifically located in the medial amygdala region. This diminished amygdala response could reflect the CS's loss of prediction accuracy in relation to the US as extinction proceeds (Gläscher & Büchel, 2005).

In contrast to this evanescent amygdala activation to a CS+ during extinction, Gottfried and Dolan (2004) located regions in the lateral amygdala and the orbitofrontal cortex that were more strongly and persistently active during extinction than during acquisition. These areas were interpreted as constituting an orbitofrontal–lateral amygdala network in the brain that regulates the expression of CRs during extinction.

Using a shock US, Phelps, Delgado, Nearing, and LeDoux (2004) reported a reversal of the CS+ > CS– pattern for amygdala activity observed during acquisition when the US was omitted in an extinction session that immediately followed acquisition. This reversal could be specifically attributed to decreased responses to the CS+ during extinction. However, no amygdala activations were observed in a second extinction series the following day. Phelps and colleagues also reported several distinct activations in the medial prefrontal cortex (mPFC) in their experiment. One was located in the ventral, subgenual anterior cingulate region (ventromedial prefrontal cortex, or vmPFC), and it was larger to the CS− than to the CS+. More successful behavior (SCR) extinction in the session immediately following acquisition was associated with more negative CS+ versus CS− differences in the vmPFC early in the second extinction session; this was interpreted as consistent with animal findings suggesting that the vmPFC plays a role in the retention of extinction (e.g., Quirk & Gehlert, 2003).

To address the presumed hallmark of extinction, its context dependence, Kalisch and colleagues (2006) used a design with context shifts between differential conditioning training and extinction presented together during one session. During a second day there were repeated shifts between context, each shift to the extinction context being heralded by a reinstating US presentation. Their results showed that correlated activations in vmPFC and the hippocampus were elicited by the CS+, but only in the extinction context. Further evidence was obtained by Milad and colleagues (2007), who examined recall of extinction from one day to the next. One of two CS+s was immediately extinguished in a different context from that of acquisition. Recall of extinction was tested the following day, by comparing responding to an extinguished and a nonextinguished CS+ in the extinction context. Recall of extinction was confirmed by smaller SCRs to the extinguished than to the nonextinguished CS+s. Similar fMRI contrasts revealed larger bilateral activations of the hippocampus and the vmPFC to the extinguished than to the nonextinguished CS+s. These regions were both positively related to recall of extinction as assessed by SCRs. Furthermore, connectivity analyses showed that the hippocampus and the vmPFC were significantly correlated with each other, and that the vmPFC was related to amygdala activation. Thus, consistent with animal data (e.g., Quirk & Beer, 2006), these results suggest that recall of extinction may involve hippocampal influences on the vmPFC in a context-dependent manner, and then the vmPFC, in turn, may inhibit the amygdala from expressing the CR.

AWARENESS OF THE CS–US CONTINGENCY

A Controversial Issue

Although the coupling of a CS to a fear CR is a prototypical instance of an implicit (i.e., nonconscious) memory (e.g., Squire & Knowlton, 2000), a CS–US contingency is also typically consciously perceived and gets stored as a declarative memory available to conscious awareness. Thus human participants can reflect and report on what happened in a fear conditioning experiment. Given the simplicity of most conditioning paradigms, a large majority of participants are able to describe the relationship between the CSs and the US. The simple fact that CS–US contingencies can get stored in both implicit and explicit memory systems has fueled a long-standing debate on the role of conscious cognition in human conditioning (for reviews, see Dawson & Schell, 1985; Lovibond & Shanks, 2002; Öhman, 1983; Öhman et al., 2000). The central issue in this debate concerns how fear conditioning should be understood. Is it a single unitary process, or does it reflect interactions between implicit and explicit cognitive processes? Proponents of single-process models may take a behavioral or a cognitive position. In the former case, fear conditioning is attributed to a basic, automatic, and implicit process of fear conditioning that is manifested as conditioned behavior, and awareness of the CS–US contingency is viewed merely as an epiphenomenon to this process. Alternatively, the basic process is viewed as cognitive in nature, with a critical role for awareness in the acquisition and expression of all CRs (including in animals; e.g., Lovibond, 2004). These single-process views stand against a levels-of-learning approach, which recognizes that a Pavlovian conditioning contingency engages both basic automatic and more sophisticated cognitive processes, resulting in implicit and explicit memories, respectively. The cognitive level is one of relational learning (simply picking out which environmental events go together in the prevailing context), and the other level concerns affectively tuned associative learning driven by the motivational relevance of the US, which is independent of awareness (e.g., Öhman et al., 2000: Öhman & Mineka, 2001).

In a comparative perspective, Pavlovian conditioning can be demonstrated in organisms with primitive nervous systems. Indeed, a good deal of what we know on the molecular basis of Pavlovian conditioning derives from studies of the simple sea snail genus *Aplysia* (Kandel, 2001). Furthermore, mammalian (including human; Hamm et al., 2003) fear conditioning can be achieved by subcortical circuitry in the absence of the relevant sensory cortex (e.g., Fanselow & Poulos, 2005; LeDoux, 2000). Thus a sophisticated cognitive apparatus incorporating conscious awareness is obviously not a general requirement for Pavlovian conditioning. In terms of evolution, a system for producing awareness of the CS–US contingency is a late addition to the neural architecture of fear conditioning, probably related to the emergence of human language. Nevertheless, quite a strong literature suggests that human fear conditioning is closely tied to correct reports of the CS–US contingency. For example, conditioning is typically obtained only in participants classified as aware of the CS–US contingency, and conditioned responding emerges synchronously with the conscious detection of this contingency (Dawson & Schell, 1985; Öhman, 1983). However, this correlation between conditioned behavior and verbal reports about the conditioning contingency does not by itself reveal any causal relationships between the two types of observations; one could be driven by the other, but more importantly, they may reflect more or less related (and potentially interacting) neural mechanisms.

Needless to say, this is an area of fear conditioning in which human brain imaging research has a great potential to contribute important knowledge. Animal studies have contributed decisively by delineating the basic circuitry of fear conditioning, but human research is needed to locate the circuitry whose operation results in awareness of a CS–US contingency. Obviously, this issue interfaces with one of the central challenges of contemporary cognitive science: coming to grips with the nature of consciousness.

Measuring Awareness of the CS–US Contingency

A primary challenge for research on contingency awareness in fear conditioning is to measure awareness validly and reliably, without undue interference with the conditioning procedure. Postexperimental reports do not interfere with conditioning, and simple, short recognition questionnaires assessing contingency awareness with good reliability are available (Dawson & Reardon, 1973). There are also more complex postexperimental questionnaires that assess participants' knowledge of the conditioning procedure and provide quantitative indices of awareness (Carter, Hofstötter, Tsuchiya, & Koch, 2003; Clark & Squire, 1999). However, the validity of postexperimental reports may be compromised by difficulties in recalling important aspects of the conditioning procedure after the experiment. Thus participants may be aware of the CS–US contingency during acquisition, yet may fail to remember it when exposed to the postexperimental questionnaire. These difficulties may be compounded if the conditioning session is terminated by an extinction series. For these reasons, some authors (e.g., Lovibond & Shanks, 2002) prefer procedures for concurrent measurement of awareness in which the participants continuously indicate their expectancy of the US during the experiment (e.g., by manipulating a joystick). However, such a procedure requires motor responses that may interfere with recordings of conditioning (e.g., during fMRI). Furthermore, if participants are engaged in a guessing game in which the actual US presentations provide immediate feedback on the correctness of their guesses, the motivation to perform correctly may override the (for ethical reasons) typically modest fear motivation provided by the US. At a minimum, this may prompt participants to look more closely for structure in the stimulus sequence than they would have done without the task (Wiens, Katkin, & Öhman, 2003). But it may also change the nature of the task, and as a consequence, brain systems may be recruited that have little to do with Pavlovian fear conditioning per se.

Choosing a Behavioral Index of Conditioning

The overwhelming majority of studies examining the role of awareness in human conditioning have relied on SCRs as the behavioral indices of conditioning (e.g., Dawson & Schell, 1985; Lovibond & Shanks, 2002). This may be an unfortunate choice, because SCRs appear uniquely sensitive to cognitive influences. In an important study, Hamm and Vaitl (1996) exposed participants to pictures as the CS+ and CS– in a differential conditioning paradigm in which the US for different groups was aversive (shock) or nonaversive (the imperative stimulus for a reaction time [RT] task). The measures included startle reflexes to probes presented during or in between the visual stimuli, SCRs, and heart rate responses, as well as a postexperimental questionnaire assessing the participants' awareness of the CS–US relationship. The data showed that startle magnitudes to probes presented during the CS+ were clearly larger than to those presented during the CS– or in the intertrial intervals, but only when the shock served as the US. Under these conditions, there was no relationship between conditioning as assessed by startle potentiation and the participants' ability to report the CS–US contingency verbally. With the nonaversive RT task as the US, on the other hand, no startle enhancement to the CS+ was observed. In contrast, reliable differential SCR conditioning was demonstrated regardless of the US condition, but only in participants who correctly reported the CS–US contingency. Heart rate responses were in between: Participants showing conditioned heart rate accelerations also showed conditioned startle potentiation, whereas those showing conditioned heart rate decelerations did not show any enhanced startle to probes presented during the CS. Thus it appears from these data that startle potentiation and heart rate acceleration index the conditioning of a genuine fear response, which is independent of awareness and similar to the response pattern displayed by fearful participants looking at pictures of their feared object (Globisch, Hamm, Esteves, & Öhman, 1999). Conditioned SCRs and heart rate decelerations, on the other hand, seem related to cognitive learning of the CS–US relationship in the absence of fear involvement.

Subsequent research from Hamm's laboratory has consistently showed a lack of any relationship between aversively conditioned startle potentiation and awareness of the CS–US contingency in differential conditioning paradigms; this contrasts with the consistent findings in the same experiments of SCR conditioning only among participants aware of the CS–US contingency (Weike, Schupp, & Hamm, 2007; Weike et al., 2005). It bear emphasis that this set of findings cannot be attributed to lack of validity of the postexperimental questionnaire, because it made a difference for SCR but not for startle data.

Jovanovic and colleagues (2006), in a more complex design that included examination of inhibitory (or safety signal) conditioning, reported reliable startle potentiation to a CS+ (compared to probes presented during the intertrial interval) both in participants who were aware and in those who were unaware of the contingency, thus providing an independent replication of the findings reported from Hamm's laboratory. Interestingly, awareness appeared to play a role in responding to inhibitory stimuli (CS– and a safety signal), with less responding only among participants aware of the unlikelihood of the US.

Masking the CS–US Contingency

Because the structure of a typical Pavlovian conditioning experiment is so simple, most participants pick up the contingency and show evidence of conditioning within a few trials. Therefore, there are few unaware subjects and few trials to examine for unaware conditioning preceding awareness. To deal with this problem, the conditioning procedure can be made more complex— for instance, by involving many or complex CSs (e.g., Bechara et al., 1995), or by introducing tasks to mask the contingency in order to retard conditioning. Such masking tasks, however, must be designed to occupy the participants without interfering with attention to the CSs and the US. For example, Dawson (1970) introduced a masking procedure that was presented to the subjects as a memory task, where they were asked to report the order in which four different pictures were presented after each trial. The CS+ and the CS− were the last-presented pictures in different stimulus sequences, and the shock that followed the CS+ was explained as a means of manipulating the participants' level of activation. Using this task, Dawson showed that only aware subjects (through their own eventual detection of the contingency, or through instructions) showed evidence of differential SCR conditioning. Importantly, by combining this task with intertrial reports, Dawson and Biferno (1973) showed that differential SCR responding emerged at the trial in which the subjects were able to first verbalize the contingency. Furthermore, Biferno and Dawson (1977) showed that the subjects had to understand both that the CS+ was followed by the US, and that the CS− was not, in order for differential SCRs to emerge (cf. Jovanovic et al., 2006).

Working memory tasks have also been used as a means to delay or prevent awareness of the CS–US contingency in fear conditioning experiments. For example, Carter and colleagues (2003) exposed participants to auditory CSs and shock USs while they performed a working memory task in which numbers were presented at a rate of about 1 per second. Participants were instructed to press a key when a particular digit occurred (0-back), when the digit matched the preceding number (1-back), or when it matched the digit before the previous one (2-back). Carter and colleagues reported that increasing the working memory load interfered with SCR conditioning, but less so in a single-cue conditioning paradigm than in differential delay and trace conditioning paradigms. Similar working memory tasks were use by Gläscher and Büchel (2005) and by Tabbert, Stark, Kirsch, and Vaitl (2006).

Gläscher and Büchel (2005) performed two experiments in their study that used formal learning theory to differentiate between brain substrates of changes in fear conditioning reflecting short and long time constants in adjusting to changes in the CS–US contingency. Both experiments used a face and a house as CSs, and as described earlier in this chapter (p. 127), their relationship to the pain US was systematically manipulated across time so that the two stimuli changed positions as CS+ and CS− according to a systematic schedule. However, whereas the first experiment used an implicit conditioning procedure by engaging participants in a 1-back working memory task, the second experiment used a design in which the participants were explicitly instructed about the CS–US contingencies. According to postexperimental interviews, none of the participants performing the working memory task had noted the changing roles of the face and house as CS+ and CS–. In spite of their unawareness, the participants showed reliably larger SCRs to faces when the face–pain contingency was strong than when it was weak, as well as reliable left-sided activation of the amygdala. In contrast, no differential SCRs and amygdala activations were observed for houses. Gläscher and Büchel speculated that faces, as biologically more significant stimuli than houses (cf. Öhman & Mineka, 2001), facilitated the acquisition of the contingency, particularly when the experimental conditions prevented awareness of the CS–US contingency. Accordingly, in the second experiment—which included explicit instructions of the contingency, and a task involving predicting US occurrence—both faces and houses produced reliable differential responses in SCRs and in the amygdala. Even though their primary purpose was not to address the role of awareness in conditioning, Gläscher and Büchel provided the first evidence supporting the conjecture (Öhman & Mineka, 2001) that biologically relevant stimuli may be more successful in engaging nonaware conditioning of the amygdala. Whereas the participants of their first experiment remained unaware of the stimulus contingencies, they nonetheless showed differential conditioning of the amygdala for facial but not for house CSs. In the second experiment, however, in which participants understood the contingencies, they activated the amygdala not only to facial stimuli but also to the houses.

Tabbert and colleagues (2006) used a 2-back version of a visual working memory task to manipulate awareness in a differential delay conditioning paradigm with visual shapes as CS+ and CS– and a shock US. About half of the participants were instructed about the CS–US contingency, whereas the contingency was not mentioned for the remaining participants, and the effectiveness of this manipulation was confirmed by a postexperimental questionnaire. The aware group showed clear SCR evidence of differential conditioning, but the nonaware groups failed to show any differential SCRs to the CS+ and the CS–. The brain imaging data showed the opposite results: larger amygdala, orbitofrontal, and occipital responses to the CS+ than to the CS– in the nonaware group, but no evidence of differential brain responses for the aware group. Thus there was a double dissociation effect, with awareness going together with SCR conditioning, and nonawareness with evidence of amygdala conditioning.

Such a double dissociation is broadly consistent with the levels-of-learning approach my colleagues and I have proposed (Öhman et al., 2000; Öhman & Mineka, 2001), which posits that the SCR primarily tracks a cognitive level of relational learning (unless the CS is biologically relevant), and is less sensitive to the more basic level of fear mediated by the amygdala, which is independent of awareness. This also fits the consistent data generated by Hamm and coworkers (Hamm & Vaitl, 1996; Weike et al., 2005, 2007) showing that conditioned startle potentiation (presumably closely tied to the amygdala; e.g., Davis, 2000) is independent of awareness, whereas SCR conditioning is only observed among aware subjects. The surprising feature of the findings reported by Tabbert and colleagues (2006), therefore, is not the SCR findings or the evidence of nonaware conditioning of the amygdala (as well as occipital and orbitofrontal cortex), but the complete lack of evidence of conditioning-related brain changes among aware participants. This prompted Tabbert and colleagues to perform an exploratory search with a less stringent threshold, looking for clusters that responded more to the CS+ than to the CS– among aware participants. They found clusters in the parietal (left supramarginal gyrus) and frontal (medial superior, ACC, and middle cingulate) cortex, as well as in the left inferior temporal lobe. Broadly speaking, these are areas that are related to emotional processes and to cognitive control of emotion. Thus Tabbert and colleagues suggested that the instructions given to the aware participants may have enabled them to inhibit the amygdala in order to protect the working memory performance from the distracting CSs. This argument can be boosted by examples in the literature demonstrating inverse relationships between activation of prefrontal structures and the amygdala (e.g., Carlsson et al., 2004; Cunningham et al., 2004; Hariri, Mattay, Tessitore, Fera, & Weinberger, 2003; Ochsner, Bunge, Gross, & Gabrieli, 2002).

Masking the CS

One way of preventing participants from detecting the CS–US contingency is to present the CS below the recognition threshold, under the assumption that subthreshold stimuli nevertheless can affect behavior. We (Esteves, Parra, Dimberg, & Öhman, 1994) masked briefly presented (for 30 msec) angry and happy faces by a neutral face in a differential conditioning procedure in which groups of subjects had the shock US follow a masked angry face, whereas other groups had the US follow the masked happy face. Control groups received the CSs and the US in unpaired, random order. In a subsequent extinction series, all subjects received unmasked presentations of the angry and happy faces. Differential responses during extinction were obtained only in subjects conditioned to angry faces, regardless of whether the CS+ had been followed by a short (30-msec), effective interval or a long (300-msec), ineffective interval between the CS and the masking pictures. Neither subjects conditioned to (masked or nonmasked) happy faces, nor those who had a random relationship between CSs and USs, showed any evidence of differential responding during the nonmasked extinction trials. Similarly, we (Öhman & Soares, 1998) exposed subjects to masked pictures of snakes and spiders, or masked pictures of flowers and mushrooms, in a differential paradigm in which one of the pictures was followed by a shock US. Subjects exposed to masked snakes and spiders, but not those exposed to masked flowers and mushrooms, showed reliably larger responses to the CS+ than to the CS– in a subsequent nonmasked extinction series. These data led us (Öhman & Mineka, 2001) to propose that biologically fear-relevant stimuli (snakes, spiders, angry faces) have privileged access to engaging the brain's fear system when serving as CSs for aversive USs.

In an ingenious variant of this subliminal procedure, Knight, Nguyen and Bandettini (2003) presented tone CSs (CS+ and CS−) at threshold level to participants instructed to continuously indicate their expectancy for the US by using a cursor manipulated by a computer mouse, and to press the mouse button when they detected a tone. Each time one of the tones was detected, the tone intensity was lowered for the next trial, and when a tone went undetected, its intensity was increased; this procedure introduced variation in the detection of the CSs. On consciously detected trials, subjects indicated reliably higher shock expectancy during the CS+ than during the CS−, whereas they did not elevate their shock expectancy just before the US on nondetected trials. However, they showed significant differential SCR conditioning both on detected and nondetected trials, thus demonstrating conditioning in the absence of differential expectancies.

We (Morris, Öhman, & Dolan, 1998) demonstrated that amygdala activations induced by a conditioning contingency could be expressed to stimuli that were prevented from conscious representation by backward masking. In a prescanning differential conditioning session, participants were exposed to two neutral and two angry faces, one of the latter serving as CS+ by being immediately followed by a loud noise US. During different PET scans with the US omitted, the CS+ and the other angry face (the CS−) were repeatedly presented masked by the two neutral faces. In other scans, the orders of the targets and the masks were reversed, so that the angry faces now masked the neutral ones and thus were consciously perceived. CS+ versus CS− contrasts revealed right amygdala activation when the angry faces were masked, and left amygdala activation when they were not.

These results were followed up by Morris, Büchel, and Dolan (2001), who used event-related fMRI rather than PET to assess conditioning to masked faces. While in the scanner, participants were exposed to a series of trials that included two angry faces either masked by or masking two different neutral faces. The noise US consistently followed one of the angry faces when it was masked, and none of the other pairs of faces. The effect of this conditioning procedure was assessed by contrasting the nonmasked CS+ and CS−. This contrast revealed activations in the ventral amygdala that were stable across blocks. A dorsal amygdala activation, on the other hand, showed rapid habituation of the CS+, whereas responses to the CS+ increased over time in the left fusiform gyrus.

Critchley and colleagues (2002) manipulated awareness by backward masking, and also manipulated the level of available autonomic feedback by including a patient group suffering from pure autonomic failure (i.e., a disconnection between the autonomic and the central nervous systems). Critchley and colleagues reported a main effect of conditioning on the right amygdala that was not modulated by awareness; that is, the conditioning effect was as obvious when the angry CS+ and CS− preceded a neutral face in a masking arrangement (i.e., were unseen) as when they followed the neutral face (i.e., were clearly seen). However, the amygdala effect was modulated by autonomic feedback, because it was smaller in patients with pure autonomic failure. In contrast, bilateral insula activations interacted both with awareness and autonomic feedback, showing a larger difference between the CS+ and the CS− when presented unmasked than masked, and among healthy controls than among patients with autonomic failure. On the basis of these findings, Critchley and colleagues (p. 659) proposed that "the amygdala acts as an involuntary interface between threat and body response[,] with the insula supporting representations of the response to external threat and body states," and providing "the matrix through which the subjective representation of emotion, so-called feeling states, is expressed."

A Delay versus a Trace Conditioning Paradigm

In eyeblink conditioning, there has been a recent surge of interest in the interaction between awareness of the CS–US contingency and conditioning in a delay versus a trace paradigm (see Clark, Manns, & Squire, 2002). In a delay conditioning paradigm, there is a temporal overlap between the CS and the US, such that either the CS starts before the US with the two stimuli terminating together, or the CS terminates with the onset of the US. In contrast, in a trace conditioning paradigm, the CS starts and terminates before the US is presented after a short interval without the CS. Pavlov (1927) pioneered both these procedures, arguing that delay conditioning allows a direct cortical coupling between the CS and the US, whereas in trace conditioning the US is conditioned to a memory trace of the CS. Indeed, there is evidence from both human and animal conditioning studies that in addition to the cerebellar network that mediates delay eyeblink conditioning, trace eyeblink conditioning depends on an intact hippocampus as well as on prefrontal areas, whereas delay conditioning does not (Clark et al., 2002; Fanselow & Poulos, 2005).

Inspired by this literature, Knight, Nguyen, and Bandettini (2006) incorporated delay versus trace conditioning in a second experiment using the procedure that previously provided good evidence for unaware SCR conditioning in the absence of expectancies (Knight et al., 2003). They reported differential US expectancies on perceived, but not on nonperceived, CS+ and CS− trials with both delay and trace paradigms. However, in contrast to the replicated differential SCR responses to nonperceived trials with a differential delay paradigm, no such differential responding was evident on nonperceived trace conditioning trials, thus demonstrating that contingency awareness was necessary for trace but not for delay conditioning. This conclusion was supported by Weike and colleagues (2007), who replicated their own previous findings (Hamm & Vaitl, 1996; Weike et al., 2005) that conditioned startle potentiation was independent of awareness in a differential delay fear conditioning paradigm. In contrast, however, when a trace paradigm was used, conditioned startle potentiation was observed only among aware participants.

There are few brain imaging data substantiating the animal research that has demonstrated hippocampal–prefrontal involvement in differential trace but not in differential delay conditioning (Fanselow & Poulos, 2005). How-ever, Büchel and colleagues (1998, 1999) published two closely similar studies (albeit with different CS modalities), one with a differential delay paradigm and the other with a differential trace paradigm. Both experiments resulted in stimulus type × trial interactions for the bilateral amygdala, due to large dif-ferential responses to the CS+ and CS– early in training that habituated across trials, as well as main effects in the CS+ versus CS– contrast for ACC and AI. In addition, however, the trace procedure resulted in an expected main effect for the dorsolateral prefrontal cortex, and an interaction similar to the one for the amygdala for the hippocampus. Thus this between-study comparison suggested not only a joint network for differential delay and differential trace conditioning, but a prefrontal–hippocampal network for the differential trace condition.

Knight, Cheng, Smith, Stein and Helmstetter (2004) reported an experi-ment with three distinct 10-sec visual CSs to achieve a within-subject compar-ison among a CS–, a differential delay CS+, and a trace CS+ that had the same duration as the delay CS+ but a 10-sec empty interval before the electric shock US. Joint activations in the delay and trace (including CS-elicited activations, and activations in the trace interval before the US) were observed in the ACC, medial thalamus, and supramarginal gyrus, but no activations were obtained for the amygdala. The trace interval preceding the US was uniquely associ-ated with bilateral frontal (middle frontal gyrus, frontal operculum) and right inferior parietal lobule activations. A transient hippocampal activation was observed early in training to all CSs, but it habituated quickly. In addition, participants who timed their US expectancy very accurately showed larger hippocampal activity during the trace CS than did participants who showed less well-timed US expectancy.

To sum up, awareness appears not to be necessary for fear conditioning when a differential delay paradigm is used, but to be essential if the para-digm is one of trace conditioning. Furthermore, the few human data appear to be consistent with the animal literature in supporting a role for frontal–hippocampal activity in trace but not in delay conditioning.

Final Comments on Awareness and Fear Conditioning

The data reviewed in this section may appear inconsistent and sometimes con-fusing. Nevertheless, if we take the amygdala as the core structure, the data do quite consistently suggest that awareness is not a necessary condition for fear conditioning. This conclusion is bolstered by the behavioral data that are most closely tied to the amygdala, those on startle potentiation, which quite consistently show fear conditioning effects (with delay paradigms) in the absence of CS–US awareness (Jovanovic et al., 2006; Weike et al., 2005, 2007). Similarly, several brain imaging studies show amygdala activations attributable to fear conditioning under conditions in which CS–US aware-ness can be reasonably excluded. Thus both Gläscher and Büchel (2005) and Tabbert and colleagues (2006) showed conditioning of the amygdala in participants who were unaware of the CS–US contingency because they were involved in a working memory task. Furthermore, Critchley and colleagues (2002) and Morris and colleagues (2001) demonstrated conditioned amygdala activations with masked faces as the CS+ category, and we (Morris et al., 1998) showed expression of previously conditioned amygdala changes with the same procedure. It appears, therefore, that all the studies that have tested amygdala activations in the absence of contingency awareness have demonstrated conditioned amygdala changes. Unfortunately, there appear as yet to be no amygdala or hippocampus data germane to the differential effect of delay versus trace conditioning procedures demonstrated with conditioned startle potentiation (Weike et al., 2005, 2007).

Against this background, the inconsistency in the literature primarily concerns conditioning in participants who are aware of the CS–US contingency and the results for the most frequently used autonomic indices, SCRs. To start with what is reasonably clear, participants that can be classified as aware of the CS–US contingency invariably show SCR conditioning (Carter et al., 2003; Esteves et al., 1994; Gläscher & Büchel, 2005; Hamm & Vaitl, 1996; Morris et al., 1998; Öhman & Soares, 1998; Tabbert et al., 2006; Weike et al., 2005, 2007; see review by Lovibond & Shanks, 2002). Similarly, in addition to studies that reported conditioned amygdala activations without assessment of awareness (e.g., Büchel et al., 1998, 1999) those manipulating or assessing brain activations and awareness (with one exception—Tabbert et al., 2006) showed conditioning-related changes in the amygdala in aware participants (Critchley et al., 2002; Gläscher & Büchel, 2005; LaBar et al., 1998; Morris et al., 1998). However, in spite of the previous consensus (Dawson & Schell, 1985; Lovibond & Shanks, 2002; Öhman, 1983), there are by now quite a number of studies demonstrating SCR conditioning among nonaware participants (Esteves et al., 1994; Gläscher & Büchel, 2005; Knight et al., 2003, 2006; Morris et al., 1998, 2001; Öhman & Soares, 1998). Except for the studies by Knight and colleagues (2003, 2006), these studies used biologically significant stimuli such as faces (Esteves et al., 1994; Gläscher & Büchel, 2005; Morris et al., 1998, 2001) or threatening animals (Öhman & Soares, 1998), which we (Öhman & Mineka, 2001) have proposed to be an important factor facilitating conditioning of the basic fear circuitry of the brain.

From this analysis, it appears that we are left with two anomalies: one instance of a failure of the amygdala to reflect conditioning in aware participants (Tabbert et al., 2006), and one instance of nonaware SCR conditioning with biologically arbitrary CSs (Knight et al., 2003, 2006).

A greater failure, perhaps, is the lack of any consistent findings suggesting a cerebral marker for aware conditioning. Critchley and colleagues (2002) gave such a role to the AI because it was activated only to unmasked stimuli, and its activation was enhanced in participants with intact connections between the brain and the autonomic nervous system (compared to patients with pure autonomic failure). Other studies have implicated the left (as opposed to the right) amygdala (Morris et al., 1998), or frontal areas such as the middle frontal gyrus (Carter, O'Doherty, Seymour, Koch, & Dolan, 2006; Knight, Cheng, et al., 2004; Tabbert et al., 2006).

CONCLUDING COMMENTS

There is little doubt from the data reviewed in this chapter that the amygdala, consistent with animal data (e.g., Kim & Jung, 2006), is an important or even critical structure for human fear conditioning. The strongest data come from the consistent demonstration that patients with damage to the amygdala fail to show fear conditioning. However, there are also relatively consistent findings that the amygdala is activated when a new CS–US contingency is presented, and that this activity wanes with repeated application of the contingency (e.g., Birbaumer et al., 2005; Büchel et al., 1998, 1999; Gottfried & Dolan, 2004; LaBar et al., 1998; Milad et al., 2006; Morris et al., 2001). There is even a hint that this pattern may be specific to the dorsomedial parts of the amygdala, where a ventrolaterally located activation is more sustained (Gottfried & Dolan, 2004; Morris et al., 2001). These data, however, pertain exclusively to differential conditioning paradigms. With a single-cue paradigm, there is no unequivocal demonstration of amygdala involvement in conditioning, primarily perhaps because of interpretational hazards when this type of paradigm is used in a brain imaging setting with human participants.

Another limitation of this literature is that the behavioral index of conditioning almost exclusively has been the SCR, which is a somewhat unspecific indicator of fear. Rather, it is responsive to stimuli that are relevant to the organism in a general sense, whether they are of an emotional or a cognitive nature (Öhman, 1979; Öhman et al., 2000). Thus, because effective fear stimuli are invariably relevant, they reliably elicit SCRs, but many other kinds of stimuli that are not related to fear also elicit SCRs. Indeed, this is a characteristic that the SCR may share with the amygdala, if the primary task of the latter is to monitor the environment for significant stimuli related to both avoidance and approach motivation (e.g., sexual stimuli; Hamann, Herman, Nolan, & Wallen, 2004). However, if the focus is on fear, such as in fear conditioning, SCR is not the ideal peripheral measure. Fear-potentiated startle may be a better choice, and phasic heart rate changes may provide more specific information distinguishing between defense and attention processes (Graham, 1979; Öhman et al., 2000; Öhman & Wiens, 2003).

The last few years have seen a burgeoning literature on extinction of conditioned fear (e.g., Milad et al., 2006; Myers & Davis, 2007; Sortres-Bayon et al., 2006), which derives part of its excitement from the prospect of illuminating the treatment of fear and anxiety disorders (e.g., Ressler et al., 2004), and part from its relationship to emotional regulation more generally (e.g., Quirk & Beer, 2006). The human data so far suggest differential roles for the amygdala (e.g., Gottfried & Dolan, 2004; LaBar et al., 1998), the vmPFC (e.g., Phelps et al., 2004), and the hippocampus (Kalisch et al., 2006) in different aspects of extinction.

However, like most of the brain imaging research on fear conditioning, the work on extinction has focused on examining whether similar structures are involved in humans as in other animals during the conditioning and extinction of fear. This is, of course, highly legitimate as a first step, but it carries the risk of promoting a confirmatory bias that may not be optimal as a more long-range strategy. What may be preferable is a movement from research focusing on demonstrations that human brains are similar to the brains of other animals, to more programmatic efforts directed at elucidating the interaction between systems that reflect a common mammalian heritage and systems that are more uniquely human. Extinction seems to be a promising area in this regard, because human research may provide knowledge beyond what can be obtained with animal subjects. In particular, it can interface with emotion research posing questions (e.g., about the emotional regulation of learned fear) that preferentially can be addressed in human participants.

Even more promising is the uniquely human work that has been performed on the role of contingency awareness in Pavlovian fear conditioning. So far we have learned that the amygdala can be engaged by conditioning protocols that exclude awareness, but we know little about the brain networks that promote awareness, or about the interaction between such networks and the basic fear network centered on the amygdala. This is a problem area concerned with a central problem in current cognitive neuroscience—that of conscious awareness, which might profitably be addressed in the context of what we know about the neural mechanisms of fear conditioning.

WHAT I THINK

If the focus is on understanding fear and fear learning, amygdala is clearly the brain structure of interest. Strong evidence supports its role as the central node in the fear network of the mammalian brain, which generates fear by integrating the activities of an assembly of cortical and subcortical structures. There is a body of human data supporting LeDoux's proposal of a direct route to the amygdala not involving the cortex (see Öhman, Carlsson, Lundqvist, & Ingvar, 2007, for review). This direct access to the amygdala, promoting defensive action on a minimum of sensory information, fits an evolutionary perspective because it results in fast, automatic activation of the fear network. Nonetheless, in spite of this emerging knowledge there are still many unresolved questions to ponder about the amygdala and fear learning. For example, why is it that amygdala activity shows a consistent and dramatic decline during reinforced Pavlovian training?

ACKNOWLEDGMENTS

Part of this chapter was written while I was a Fellow at the Center for Advanced Study in the Behavioral Sciences, Stanford, California. I was also supported by a Leading Investigator Award from the Swedish Research Council, and by the U.S. National Institute of Mental Health as an investigator at the Interdisciplinary Behavioral Science Center for the Study of Emotion and Attention at the University of Florida. I wish to express my gratitude to and Armita Golkar and Andreas Olsson for helpful comments.

REFERENCES

Baker, A. G. (1976). Learned irrelevance and learned helplessness: Rats learn that stimuli, reinforcers, and responses are uncorrelated. *Journal of Experimental Psychology: Animal Behavior Processes, 2*, 130–141.

Bechara, A., Tranel, D., Damasio, H., Adolphs, R., Rockland, C., & Damasio, A. R. (1995). Double dissociation of conditioning and declarative knowledge relative to the amygdala and hippocampus in humans. *Science, 269*, 1115–1118.

Biferno, M. A., & Dawson, M. E. (1977). The onset of contingency awareness and electrodermal classical conditioning: An analysis of temporal relationships during acquisition and extinction. *Psychophysiology, 14*, 164–171.

Birbaumer, N., Veit, R., Lotze, M., Eerb, M., Hermann, C., Grodd, W., et al. (2005). Deficient fear conditioning in psychopathy: A functional magnetic resonance imaging study. *Archives of General Psychiatry, 62*, 799–805.

Blanchard, D. C., & Blanchard, R. J. (1988). Ethoexperimental approaches to the biology of emotion. *Annual Review of Psychology, 39*, 43–68.

Bolles, R. C. (1970). Species-specific defense reactions and avoidance learning. *Psychological Review, 77*, 32–48.

Bouton, M. (2005). Behavior systems and the contextual control of anxiety, fear, and panic. In L. F. Barrett, P. M. Niedenthal, & P. Winkielman (Eds.), *Emotion and consciousness* (pp. 205–227). New York: Guilford Press.

Bremner, J. D., Vermetten, E., Schmahl, C., Vaccarino, V., Vythilingam, M., Afzal, N., et al. (2005). Positron emission tomographic imaging of neutral correlates of a fear acquisition and extinction paradigm in women with childhood sexual-abuse-related post-traumatic stress disorder. *Psychological Medicine, 35*, 791–806.

Büchel, C., Dolan, R. J., Armony, J. L., & Friston, K. J. (1999). Amygdala–hippocampal involvement in human aversive trace conditioning revealed through event-related functional magnetic resonance imaging. *Journal of Neuroscience, 19*, 10869–10876.

Büchel, C., Morris, J., Dolan, R. J., & Friston, K. J. (1998). Brain systems mediating aversive conditioning: An event-related fMRI study. *Neuron, 20*, 947–957.

Carlsson, K., Petersson, K. M., Lundqvist, D., Karlsson, A., Ingvar, M., & Öhman, A. (2004) Fear and the amygdala: Manipulation of awareness generates differential cerebral responses to phobic and fear-relevant (but non-feared) stimuli. *Emotion, 4*, 340–353.

Carter, R. M., Hofstötter, C., Tsuchiya, N., & Koch, C. (2003). Working memory and fear conditioning. *Proceedings of the National Academy of Sciences USA, 100*, 1399–1404.

Carter, R. M., O'Doherty, J. P., Seymour, B., Koch, C., & Dolan, R. J. (2006). Contingency awareness in human aversive conditioning involves the middle frontal gyrus. *NeuroImage, 29*, 1007–1012.

Cheng, D. T., Knight, D. C., Smith, C. N., & Helmstetter, F. J. (2006). Human amygdala activity during the expression of fear responses. *Behavioral Neuroscience, 120*, 1187–1195.

Cheng, D. T., Knight, D. C., Smith, C. N., Stein, E. A., & Helmstetter, F. J. (2003). Functional MRI of human amygdala activity during Pavlovian fear conditioning:

Stimulus processing versus response expression. *Behavioral Neuroscience, 117,* 3–10.

Clark, R. E., Manns, J. R., & Squire, L. R. (2002). Classical conditioning, awareness, and brain systems. *Trends in Cognitive Sciences, 6,* 524–531.

Clark, R. E., & Squire, L. R. (1999). Human eyeblink classical conditioning: Effects of manipulating awareness of the stimulus contingencies. *Psychological Science, 10,* 14–18.

Cook, M., & Mineka, S. (1989). Observational conditioning of fear to fear-relevant versus fear-irrelevant stimuli in rhesus monkey. *Journal of Abnormal Psychology, 98,* 448–459.

Cook, M., & Mineka, S. (1990). Selective associations in the observational conditioning of fear in rhesus monkeys. *Journal of Experimental Psychology: Animal Behavior Processes, 16,* 372–389.

Cook, S. W., & Harris, R. E. (1937) The verbal conditioning of the galvanic skin reflex. *Journal of Experimental Psychology, 21,* 202–210.

Critchley, H. D., Mathias, C. J., & Dolan, R. J. (2002). Fear conditioning in humans: The influence of awareness and autonomic arousal on functional neuroanatomy. *Neuron, 33,* 653–663.

Cunningham, W. A., Johnson, M. K., Raye, C. L., Gatenby, J. C., Gore, J. C., & Banaji, M. R. (2004). Separable neural components in the processing of black and white faces. *Psychological Science, 15,* 806–813.

Davis, M. (2000). The role of the amygdala in conditioned and unconditioned fear and anxiety. In J. P. Aggleton (Ed.), *The amygdala: A functional analysis* (2nd ed., pp. 213–288). Oxford, UK: Oxford University Press.

Davis, M., & Myers, K. (2002). The role of glutamate and gamma-aminobutyric acid in fear extinction: Clinical implications for exposure therapy. *Biological Psychiatry, 52,* 998–1007.

Dawson, M. E. (1970). Cognition and conditioning: Effect of masking the CS-UCS contingency on human GSR classical conditioning. *Journal of Experimental Psychology, 85,* 389–396.

Dawson, M. E., & Biferno, M. A. (1973). Concurrent measurement of awareness and electrodermal classical conditioning. *Journal of Experimental Psychology, 101,* 55–62.

Dawson, M. E., & Reardon, P. (1973). Construct validity of recall and recognition post-conditioning measures of awareness. *Journal of Experimental Psychology, 98,* 308–315.

Dawson, M. E., & Schell, A. M. (1985). Information processing and human autonomic classical conditioning. *Advances in Psychophysiology, 1,* 89–165.

Domjan, M. (2005). Pavlovian conditioning: A functional perspective. *Annual Review of Psychology, 56,* 179–206.

Esteves, F., Parra, C., Dimberg, U., & Öhman, A. (1994). Nonconscious associative learning: Pavlovian conditioning of skin conductance responses to masked fear-relevant facial stimuli. *Psychophysiology, 31,* 375–385.

Falls, W. A., Miserendino, M. J. D., & Davis, M. (1992). Extinction of fear-potentiated startle: Blockaded by infusion of an NMDA antagonist into the amygdala. *Journal of Neuroscience, 12,* 854–863.

Fanselow, M. S. (1994). Neural organization of the defensive behavior system responsible for fear. *Psychonomic Bulletin and Review, 1,* 429–438.

Fanselow, M. S., & Poulos, A. M. (2005). The neuroscience of mammalian associative learning. *Annual Review of Psychology, 56,* 207–234.

Gläscher, J., & Büchel, C. (2005). Formal learning theory dissociates brain regions with different temporal integration. *Neuron, 47*, 295–306.

Globisch, J., Hamm, A. O., Esteves, F., & Öhman, A. (1999). Fear appears fast: Temporal course of startle reflex potentiation in animal fearful subjects. *Psychophysiology, 36*, 66–75.

Gottfried, J. A., & Dolan, R. J. (2004). Human orbitofrontal cortex mediates extinction learning while accessing conditioned representations of value. *Nature Neuroscience, 7*, 1145–1153.

Graham, F. K. (1979). Distinguishing among orienting, defense, and startle reflexes. In H. D. Kimmel, E. H. van Olst, & J. F. Orlebeke (Eds.), *The orienting reflex in humans* (pp. 137–167). Hillsdale, NJ: Erlbaum.

Grillon, C., Ameli, R., Woods, S. W., Merikangas, K., & Davis, M. (1991). Measuring the time course of anticipatory anxiety using the fear-potentiated startle. *Psychophysiology, 30*, 340–346.

Hamann, S., Herman, R. A., Nolan, C. L., & Wallen, K. (2004). Men and women differ in amygdala response to visual sexual stimuli. *Nature Neuroscience, 7*, 411–416.

Hamm, A. O., & Vaitl, D. (1996). Affective learning: Awareness and aversion. *Psychophysiology, 33*, 698–710.

Hamm, A. O., Weike, A. I., Schupp, H. T., Treig, T., Dressel, A., & Kessler, C. (2003). Affective blindsight: Intact fear conditioning to a visual cue in a cortically blind patient. *Brain, 126*, 267–275.

Hariri, A. R., Mattay, V. S., Tessitore, A., Fera, F., & Weinberger, D. R. (2003). Neocortical modulation of the amygdala response to fearful stimuli. *Biological Psychiatry, 53*, 494–501.

Hobin, J. A., Goosens, K. A., & Maren, S. (2003). Context-dependent neuronal activity in the lateral amygdala represents fear memories after extinction. *Journal of Neuroscience, 23*, 8410–8416.

Hollis, K. (1997). Contemporary research on Pavlovian conditioning: A "new" functional analysis. *American Psychologist, 52*, 956–965.

Hugdahl, K., Berardi, A., Thompson, W. L., Kosslyn, S. M., Macy, R., Baker, D. P., et al. (1995). Brain mechanisms in human classical conditioning: A PET blood flow study. *NeuroReport, 6*, 1723–1728.

Hugdahl, K., & Öhman, A. (1980). Skin conductance conditioning to potentially phobic stimuli as a function of interstimulus interval and delay versus trace paradigm. *Psychophysiology, 17*, 348–355.

Hygge, S., & Öhman, A. (1978). Modeling processes in the acquisition of fears: Vicarious electrodermal conditioning to fear-relevant stimuli. *Journal of Personality and Social Psychology, 36*, 271–279.

Johnsen, B. H., & Hugdahl, K. (1993). Right hemisphere representation of autonomic conditioning to facial emotional expressions. *Psychophysiology, 30*, 274–278.

Jovanovic, T., Norrholm, S. D., Keyes, M., Fiallos, A., Jovanovic, S., Myers, K., et al. (2006). Contingency awareness and fear inhibition in a human fear-potentiated startle paradigm. *Behavioral Neuroscience, 120*, 995–1004.

Kalisch, R., Korenfeld, E., Stephan, K. E., Weiskopf, N., Seymour, B., & Dolan, R. J. (2006). Context-dependent human extinction memory is mediated by ventromedial prefrontal and hippocampal networks. *Journal of Neuroscience, 26*, 9503–9511.

Kamin, L. (1969). Predictability, surprise, attention, and conditioning. In B. A. Campbell & R. M. Church (Eds.), *Punishment and aversive behavior* (pp. 279–296). New York: Appleton-Century-Crofts.

Kandel, E. R. (2001). Neuroscience—the molecular biology of memory storage: A dialogue between genes and synapses. *Science, 294,* 1030–1038.

Kim, J. J., & Jung, M. W. (2006). Neural circuits and mechanisms involved in Pavlovian fear conditioning: A critical review. *Neuroscience and Biobehavioral Reviews, 30,* 188–202.

Knight, D. C., Cheng, D. T., Smith, C. N., Stein, E. A., & Helmstetter, F. J. (2004). Neural substrates mediating human delay and trace fear conditioning. *Journal of Neuroscience, 24,* 218–228.

Knight, D. C., Nguyen, H. T., & Bandettini, P. A. (2003). Expression of conditioned fear with and without awareness. *Proceedings of the National Academy of Sciences USA, 100,* 15280–15283.

Knight, D. C., Nguyen, H. T., & Bandettini, P. A. (2005). The role of the human amygdala in the production of conditioned fear responses. *NeuroImage, 26,* 1193–1200.

Knight, D. C., Nguyen, H. T., & Bandettini, P. A. (2006). The role of awareness in delay and trace fear conditioning in humans. *Cognitive, Affective, and Behavioral Neuroscience, 6,* 157–162.

Knight, D. C., Smith, C., Cheng, D. T., Stein, E. A., & Helmstetter, F. J. (2004). Amygdala and hippocampal activity during acquisition and extinction of human fear conditioning. *Cognitive, Affective, and Behavioral Neuroscience, 4,* 317–325.

Knight, D. C., Smith, C. N., Stein, E. A., & Helmstetter, F. J. (1999). Functional MRI of human Pavlovian fear conditioning: Pattern of activation as a function of learning. *NeuroReport, 10,* 3665–3670.

LaBar, K. S., Gatenby, J. C., Gore, J. C., LeDoux, J. E., & Phelps, E. A. (1998). Human amygdala activation during conditioned fear acquisition and extinction: A mixed-trial fMRI study. *Neuron, 20,* 937–945.

LaBar, K. S., LeDoux, J. E., Spencer, D. D., & Phelps, E. A. (1995). Impaired fear conditioning following unilateral temporal lobectomy in humans. *Journal of Neuroscience, 15,* 6846–6855.

LaBar, K. S., & Phelps, E. A. (2005). Reinstatement of conditioned fear in humans is context dependent and impaired in amnesia. *Behavioral Neuroscience, 119,* 677–686.

Lang, P. J., Bradley, M. M., & Cuthbert, B. N. (1997). Motivated attention: Affect, activation, and action. In P. J. Lang, R. F. Simons, & M. T. Balaban (Eds.), *Attention and orienting: Sensory and motivational processes* (pp. 97–136). Hillsdale, NJ: Erlbaum.

LeDoux, J. E. (1996). *The emotional brain.* New York: Simon & Schuster.

LeDoux, J. E. (2000). Emotion circuits in the brain. *Annual Review of Neuroscience, 23,* 155–184.

Lissek, S., Powers, A. S., McClure, E. B., Phelps, E. A., Woldehawariat, G., Grillon, C., et al. (2005). Classical fear conditioning in the anxiety disorders: A meta-analysis. *Behaviour Research and Therapy, 43,* 1391–1424.

Lonsdorf, T. B., Weike, A. I., Nikamo, P., Schalling, M., Hamm, A. O., & Öhman, A. (in press). Genetic gating of human fear learning and extinction: Implications for gene-environment interaction in anxiety disorder. *Psychological Science.*

Lovibond, P. F. (2004). Cognitive processes in extinction. *Learning and Memory, 11,* 495–500.

Lovibond, P. F., & Shanks, D. R. (2002). The role of awareness in Pavlovian conditioning: Empirical evidence and theoretical implications. *Journal of Experimental Psychology: Animal Behavior Processes, 28,* 3–31.

Lubow, R. E. (1973). Latent inhibition. *Psychological Bulletin, 79,* 398–407.

Milad, M. R., Orr, S. P., Pitman, R. K., & Rauch, S. L. (2005). Context modulation of memory for fear extinction in humans. *Psychophysiology, 42,* 456–464.

Milad, M. R., Rauch, S. L., Pitman, R., & Quirk, G. J. (2006). Fear extinction in rats: Implications for human brain imaging and anxiety disorders. *Biological Psychology, 73,* 61–71.

Milad, M. R., Wright, C. I., Orr, S. P., Pitman, R. K., Quirk, G. J., & Rauch, S. P. (2007). Recall of fear extinction in human activates the ventromedial prefrontal cortex and hippocampus in concert. *Biological Psychiatry, 62,* 446–454.

Morgan, M. A., Romanski, L. M., & LeDoux, J. E. (1993). Extinction of emotional learning: Contribution of the medial prefrontal cortex. *Neuroscience Letters, 163,* 109–113.

Morris, J. S., Büchel, C., & Dolan, R. J. (2001). Parallel neural responses in amygdala subregions and sensory cortex during implicit fear conditioning. *NeuroImage, 13,* 1044–1052.

Morris, J. S., & Dolan, R. J. (2004). Dissociable amygdala and orbitofrontal responses during reversal fear conditioning. *NeuroImage, 22,* 372–380.

Morris, J. S., Öhman, A., & Dolan, R. J. (1998). Conscious and unconscious emotional learning in the human amygdala. *Nature, 393,* 467–470.

Moses, S. N., Houck, J. M., Martin, T., Hanlon, F. M., Ryan, J. D., Thoma, R. J., et al. (2007). Dynamic neural activity recorded from human amygdala during fear conditioning using magnetoencephalography. *Brain Research Bulletin, 7,* 452–460.

Myers, K. M., & Davis, M. (2007). Mechanisms of fear extinction. *Molecular Psychiatry, 12,* 120–150.

Obrist, P. A. (1981). *Cardiovascular psychophysiology: A perspective.* New York: Plenum Press.

Ochsner, K. N., Bunge, S. A., Gross, J. J., & Gabrieli, J. D. E. (2002). Rethinking feelings: An fMRI study of the cognitive regulation of emotion. *Journal of Cognitive Neuroscience, 14,* 1215–1229.

Öhman, A. (1979). The orienting response, attention, and learning: An information processing perspective. In H. D. Kimmel, E. H. van Olst, & J. F. Orlebeke (Eds.), *The orienting reflex in humans* (pp. 443–472). Hillsdale, NJ: Erlbaum.

Öhman, A. (1983). The orienting response during Pavlovian conditioning. In D. Siddle (Ed.), *Orienting and habituation: Perspectives in human research* (pp. 315–369). Chichester, UK: Wiley.

Öhman, A., Carlsson, K., Lundqvist, D., & Ingvar, M. (2007). On the unconscious subcortical origin of human fear. *Physiology and Behavior, 92,* 180–185.

Öhman, A., Dimberg, U., & Öst, L.-G. (1985). Animal and social phobias: Biological constraints on learned fear responses. In S. Reiss & R. R. Bootzin (Eds.), *Theoretical issues in behavior therapy* (pp. 123–178). New York: Academic Press.

Öhman, A., Hamm, A., & Hugdahl, K. (2000). Cognition and the autonomic nervous system: Orienting, anticipation, and conditioning. In J. T. Cacioppo, L. G. Tassinary, & G. G. Berntson (Eds.), *Handbook of psychophysiology* (pp. 522–575). New York: Cambridge University Press.

Öhman, A., & Mineka, S. (2001). Fears, phobias, and preparedness: Toward an evolved module of fear and fear learning. *Psychological Review, 108,* 483–522.

Öhman, A., & Soares, J. J. F. (1998). Emotional conditioning to masked stimuli: Expectancies for aversive outcomes following nonrecognized fear-relevant stimuli. *Journal of Experimental Psychology: General, 127,* 69–82.

Öhman, A., & Wiens, S. (2003). On the automaticity of autonomic responses in emotion: An evolutionary perspective. In R. J. Davidson, K. R. Scherer, & H. H. Goldsmith (Eds.), *Handbook of affective sciences* (pp. 256–275). New York: Oxford University Press.

Olsson, A., Ebert, J. P., Banaji, M. R., & Phelps, E. A. (2005). The role of social groups in the persistence of learned fear. *Science, 309,* 785–787.

Olsson, A., Nearing, K. I., & Phelps, E. A. (2007). Learning fears by observing others: The neural systems of social fear transmission. *Social Cognitive and Affective Neuroscience, 2,* 3–11.

Olsson, A., & Phelps, E. A. (2004). Learned fear of "unseen" faces after Pavlovian, observational, and instructed fear. *Psychological Science, 15,* 822–828.

Olsson, A., & Phelps, E. A. (2007). Social learning of fear. *Nature Neuroscience, 10,* 1095–1102.

Pavlov, I. P. (1927). *Conditioned reflexes.* Oxford, UK: Oxford University Press.

Peper, M., Karcher, S., Wohlfarth, R., Reinshagen, G., & LeDoux, J. E. (2001). Aversive learning in patients with unilateral lesions of the amygdala and hippocampus. *Biological Psychology, 58,* 1–23.

Phelps, E. A., Delgado, M. R., Nearing, K. I., & LeDoux, J. E. (2004). Extinction learning in humans: Role of the amygdala and vmPFC. *Neuron, 43,* 897–905.

Phelps, E. A., O'Connor, K. J., Gatenby, J. C., Gore, J. C., Grillon, C., & Davis, M. (2001). Activation of the left amygdala to a cognitive representation of fear. *Nature Neuroscience, 4,* 437–441.

Prokasy, W. F. (1977). First interval skin conductance responses: Conditioned or orienting responses? *Psychophysiology, 14,* 360–367.

Quirk, G. J., & Beer, J. S. (2006). Prefrontal involvement in the regulation of emotion: Convergence of rata and human studies. *Current Opinion in Neurobiology, 16,* 723–727.

Quirk, G. J., & Gehlert, D. R. (2003). Inhibition of the amygdala: Key to pathological states. *Annals of the New York Academy of Science, 985,* 263–272.

Raichle, M. E. (1997). Automaticity: From reflective to reflexive information processing in the human brain. In M. Ito, Y. Miyashita, & E. T. Rolls (Eds.), *Cognition, computation and consciousness* (pp. 137–150). Oxford, UK: Oxford University Press.

Rescorla, R. A. (1967). Pavlovian conditioning and its proper control procedures. *Psychological Review, 74,* 71–80.

Rescorla, R. A. (1968). Probability of shock in presence and absence of CS in fear conditioning. *Journal of Comparative and Physiological Psychology, 66,* 1–5.

Rescorla, R. A. (1974). Effect of US habituation following conditioning. *Journal of Comparative and Physiological Psychology, 82,* 137–143.

Rescorla, R. A. (1988). Pavlovian conditioning: It's not what you think it is. *American Psychologist, 43,* 151–160.

Rescorla, R. A., & Heth, C. D. (1975). Reinstatement of fear to an extinguished conditioned stimulus. *Journal of Experimental Psychology: Animal Behavior Processes, 104*, 88–96.

Rescorla, R. A., & Wagner, A. R. (1972). A theory of Pavlovian conditioning: Variations in the effectiveness of reinforcement and nonreinforcement. In A. H. Black & W. F. Prokasy (Eds.), *Classical conditioning II: Current research and theory* (pp. 64–99). New York: Appleton-Century-Crofts.

Ressler, K. J., Rothbaum, B. O., Tannenbaum, L., Anderson, P., Zimand, E., Hodges, L., et al. (2004). Cognitive enhancers as adjuncts to psychotherapy: Use of D-cycloserine in phobics to facilitate extinction of fear. *Archives of General Psychiatry, 61*, 1136–1144.

Seligman, M. E. P. (1970). On the generality of the laws of learning. *Psychological Review, 77*, 406–418.

Seligman, M. E. P. (1971). Phobias and preparedness. *Behavior Therapy, 2*, 307–320.

Sokolov, E. N. (1963). *Perception and the conditioned reflex*. Oxford, UK: Pergamon Press.

Sortres-Bayon, F., Cain, C. K., & LeDoux, J. E. (2006). Brain mechanisms of fear extinction: Historical perspectives on the contribution of prefrontal cortex. *Biological Psychiatry, 60*, 329–336.

Squire, L. R., & Knowlton, B. S. (2000). The medial temporal lobe, the hippocampus, and the memory systems of the brain. In M. S. Gazzaniga (Ed.), *The new cognitive neuroscience* (pp. 765–779). Cambridge, MA: MIT Press.

Tabbert, K., Stark, R., Kirsch, P., & Vaitl, D. (2006). Dissociation of neural responses and skin conductance reactions during fear conditioning with and without awareness of stimulus contingencies. *NeuroImage, 32*, 761–770.

Vansteenwegen, D., Hermans, D., Vervliet, B., Francken, G., Beckers, T., Baeyens, F., et al. (2005). Return of fear in a human differential conditioning paradigm caused by a return to the original acquisition context. *Behaviour Research and Therapy, 43*, 323–336.

Walker, D. L., & Davis, M. (2002). The role of amygdala glutamate receptors in fear learning, fear-potentiated startle, and extinction. *Pharmacology, Biochemistry and Behavior, 71*, 379–392.

Weike, A. I., Hamm, A. O., Schupp, H. T., Runge, U., Schroeder, H. W., & Kessler, C. (2005). Fear conditioning following unilateral temporal lobectomy: Dissociation of conditioned startle potentiation and autonomic learning. *Journal of Neuroscience, 25*, 11117–11124.

Weike, A. I., Schupp, H. T., & Hamm, A. O. (2007). Fear acquisition requires awareness in trace but not in delay conditioning. *Psychophysiology, 44*, 170–180.

Wiens, S., Katkin, E. S., & Öhman, A. (2003). Effects of trial order and differential conditioning on acquisition of differential shock expectancy and skin conductance conditioning to masked stimuli. *Psychophysiology, 40*, 989–997.

CHAPTER 7

Methodological Approaches to Studying the Human Amygdala

Kevin S. LaBar and Lauren H. Warren

This chapter focuses on the multiple methods that have been used to elucidate the structure and function of the human amygdala. Progress in understanding the amygdala has been hindered by the difficulties in scientifically probing this small subcortical region buried deep within the medial temporal lobe. Since the mid-1990s, there has been a resurgent interest in the neurobiology of emotion, motivation, and social cognition; this interest can be considered an "affective revolution" in psychology and neuroscience. The amygdala has emerged at the crossroads of these endeavors, in part due to improved neuroscientific techniques and experimental paradigms that, for the first time, have permitted cogent assessments of its role in human behavior. However, each of the standard methods is fraught with technical, data-analytic, and interpretational challenges, some of which are exacerbated for the amygdala relative to other brain areas. We first present a brief historical overview of research on the human amygdala, and then critique modern approaches to its study. As will be evident, converging evidence across methodologies is essential for advancing knowledge about this fascinating almond-shaped area of the forebrain.

HISTORY

The Amygdala Concept

There remains considerable debate in the field regarding what the amygdala is, including its structural and functional boundaries. Historically, the term "amygdala" has referred to a group of roughly a dozen nuclei in the ventromedial temporal lobe (see Figure 7.1), originally identified and described by Burdach (1819–1822). The idea that the amygdala was a unified structural entity remained relatively uncontested until recently, when Swanson and Petrovich (1998) argued that the amygdala is better described as four functional units. More specifically, they provide ontological evidence that there are distinct functional subunits of the traditional amygdala: accessory olfactory, main olfactory, autonomic, and frontotemporal cortical. Moreover, they argue against the concept of the amygdala as either a structural or functional unit; their argument is primarily based on evidence from rat studies indicating disparate functions of amygdalar nuclei, such as the role of the central nucleus in controlling motor and autonomic function, and the lateral and basolateral nuclei's modulation of cognitive processes in the temporal and frontal lobes. Whether these functional divisions map onto the human amygdala remains

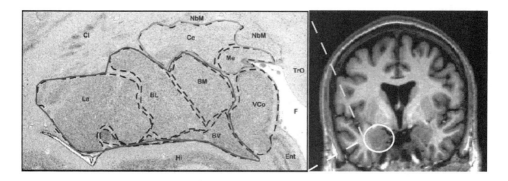

FIGURE 7.1. Anatomy of the human amygdala. *Left:* Cytoarchitecture in a coronal section obtained from postmortem tissue cut through the middle of the amygdala reveals the location of several of its subnuclei, including the basolateral nucleus (BL), basomedial nucleus (BM), basoventral nucleus (BV), central nucleus (Ce), lateral nucleus (La), medial nucleus (Me), and ventral cortical nucleus (VCo). Surrounding structures include the claustrum (Cl), entorhinal cortex (Ent), endorhinal sulcus (F), hippocampus (Hi), nucleus basalis of Meynert (NbM), optic tract (TrO), and lateral ventricle (V). The basolateral group is outlined in dark gray, and the centromedial group is outlined in light gray. From Amunts et al. (2005). Copyright 2005 by Springer Science and Business Media. Reprinted by permission. *Right:* An *in vivo* coronal section obtained from a T1-weighted structural MRI scan at approximately the same level as in the left panel. Note the lack of resolution of subnuclei in the image. From LaBar and Phelps (2005). Copyright 2005 by the American Psychological Association. Reprinted by permission.

unknown. In contrast, Aggleton and Saunders (2000) argue that although there is considerable heterogeneity in the projections of each amygdala nucleus, the disparate nuclei contain multiple intraconnections that do in fact support the notion of a coherent whole. To complicate the amygdala concept further, the term "extended amygdala" was introduced to refer to a scattered set of nuclei in the basal forebrain and ventral striatum that appear to constitute a rostral extension of the central and medial nuclei (De Olmos & Heimer, 1999). Although the structural boundaries of the amygdala remain debatable, it is well accepted that the amygdala (1) receives input from many cortical and subcortical structures; (2) serves an important role in integrating and evaluating interoceptive and exteroceptive sensory stimuli, and thus in permitting an individual to ascribe emotional meaning to events; (3) coordinates adaptive behavioral responses to emotion elicitors; and (4) modulates cognitive processing in other brain regions. The amygdala is the most densely interconnected region of the primate forebrain (Young, Flude, Hellawell, & Ellis, 1994), so its scope of influence must be wide-ranging. Further understanding of its functional and structural subdivisions is critical to guide future experimental questions and targeted hypotheses, particularly as probes of subnuclei become tractable.

Intracranial Stimulation

In the 1940s and 1950s, studies of patients with intractable epilepsy and severe behavioral disturbances provided the first *in vivo* look at the human amygdala. The earliest electrical stimulation studies were conducted by Walter Penfield and his colleagues, to assess electrocortical responses and seizure activity in patients with medial temporal lobe epilepsy. Stimulation studies and observations of patients during endogenous seizures indicated a role for the amygdala in visual hallucinations, emotional experiences, feelings of *déjà vu*, and memory recall (e.g., Feindel & Penfield, 1952; Penfield, 1958). Penfield noted that when medial temporal regions were stimulated, patients experienced vivid memories that often had strong emotional content or personal relevance. Moreover, in his discussion of phenomena preceding temporal lobe seizures, many patients reported auras or were observed to engage in automatisms that preceded their typical attacks. Chapman and colleagues (1954) noticed that during presurgical evaluation of medial temporal lobe epilepsy, four out of five patients reported sudden-onset fear and anxiety related to stimulation. Changes in heart rate and blood pressure were also observed, providing early human evidence regarding the amygdala's role in engaging autonomic effectors during emotional states.

In the 1970s and 1980s, investigations by Eric Halgren, Pierre Gloor, and colleagues extended and improved upon the initial studies of Penfield and others by employing more precise methodology and by providing details of the experiential phenomena elicited during stimulation and seizure activity (for reviews, see Gloor, 1992; Halgren, 1992). These researchers were more careful to distinguish effects arising from the amygdala relative to other medial temporal lobe structures, and noted when widespread afterdischarges accompanied the electrical activity. They found that sensations elicited by electrical activity in the amygdala almost always had emotional content, with fear being the most common emotion reported. A particularly striking example of fear elicitation is provided in the following anecdote:

> A 19-year-old woman had seizures that started with a feeling of intense fear followed by loss of consciousness and automatism in which she acted as if she were in the grips of the most intense terror. She let out a terrifying scream and her facial expression and bodily gestures were those of someone having a horrifying experience. She was able to recall her fear, but had no recollection of acting it out in the later part of her seizures. (Gloor, Olivier, Quesney, Andermann, & Horowitz, 1982, p. 132)

Although the memories elicited were vivid, they almost always had a dream-like quality, and it was sometimes difficult to determine whether the events were real or reconstructed interpretations of experiences arising from the electrical activity. For example, one patient reported the following:

> It was one of those feelings, a feeling of being someplace very far away. . . . It recalls to mind the day in the country with Tracy and brother Jamie. It was very spooky, but it was so far away. It was out by the sea and high up on a cliff, a feeling as if I were going to fall. It was a scary feeling. We are there, a world within that world, all of us were there. It is so real, yet so artificial. (quoted in Gloor et al., 1982, p. 135)

However, the researchers also found that repeated stimulation of the same site did not elicit identical emotions, memories, or hallucinations within or across patients. Thus, although such observations provided a fascinating and unique opportunity to characterize the phenomenology associated with amygdala stimulation in individual epileptic patients, the functional organization of this structure was nonetheless difficult to discern from these explorations.

Amygdalotomy as Psychosurgery

Rat and macaque studies have shown that the anterior cortical nucleus and periamygloid cortex receive direct projections from the main and accessory olfactory bulbs (Aggleton, 2000). An early set of studies (Chitanondh, 1966) provided evidence of the role of the human amygdala in olfactory processing. Stereotaxic amygdalotomy was performed on seven patients, all with olfactory hallucinations or other behavioral dysfunction. In this surgical series, the amygdala was located via ventriculography of the temporal horn of the lateral ventricle. All patients showed short-term improvement in olfactory symptoms. Despite its early promise as a treatment for intractable seizures, olfactory hallucinations, and hyperaggression, additional studies lacked appropriate control and adequate sample sizes to permit interpretation (e.g., Narabayashi & Uno, 1966). Similarly, although the use of stereotaxic amygdalotomy for medically intractable psychiatric problems such as hyperaggression has had promising results (Kim, Lee, & Choi, 2002), these studies are hampered by inadequate controls, and long-term follow-up studies are sparse and report inconsistent results. Moreover, although the advent of magnetic resonance imaging (MRI) has enhanced the spatial accuracy of amygdalotomy, the need for surgical intervention has decreased as additional medications and alternative treatments have been developed.

Critique of Early Findings

Although these early studies provided important clues about the role of the amygdala in various perceptual, cognitive, and emotional processes, some limitations are noteworthy. First, most descriptions of experiential phenomena were vague and lacked standardized probes or tests of emotional function. Second, the role of adjacent cortical structures should be considered, as surgical approaches often included the periamygdaloid cortex and hippocampus, and intracranial stimulation and seizure activity were often accompanied by afterdischarges that spread widely in the temporal lobe (Gloor, Halgren, and their colleagues attempted to clarify this issue in their analyses). Third, because these reports were limited primarily to patients with preexisting clinical conditions such as epilepsy or psychosis, the generalizability of the findings to the healthy brain is uncertain.

This literature is also notable for heterogeneity in patient selection, lesion or seizure focus locations, and techniques used. For instance, the duration and intensity of intracranial electrical stimulation or surgical approach varied across treatment sites (see also Parrent & Lozano, 2000). Stereotaxic surgery was also somewhat limited by the localization in individual patients, given the inherent variation in brain anatomy, particularly for a structure as small as the amygdala. Before the application of MRI to lesion assessment in the 1980s, there was only crude verification of the location and extent of the lesions/recording sites, and there was little standardization in terms of clinical evaluation and long-term follow-up. Furthermore, the fiber tracts that connect frontal and temporal cortices lie just lateral to the amygdala proper, and their section probably contributed to some of the behavioral effects (for a discussion of this issue in monkeys, see Meunier, Bachevalier, Murray, Malkova, & Mishkin, 1999). Finally, one must always interpret the results within the emotional context of the experimental setting. For example, Halgren, Walter, Cherlow, and Crandall (1978) noted that personality could influence the kinds of emotions elicited by brain stimulation, with individuals who were most fearful of the intracranial recording procedure being the most likely to experience fear in response to stimulation. In other words, fear may have been more readily elicited in some individuals in the experimental setting. These methodological issues are important to consider in interpreting these early results, particularly with respect to the coupling of function and brain structure in clinical–pathological correlations. Despite these concerns, there are good reasons why MRI-guided stereotaxic surgery and invasive procedures can contribute to research progress concerning the amygdala, and depth electrode monitoring in epileptic patients remains the primary way to probe its electrical activity directly.

MODERN TECHNIQUES

Electrophysiology

Intracranial Recording in Presurgical Epileptic Patients

Today, clinical assessment of seizure focus activity in patients with medically refractory temporal lobe epilepsy often includes depth electrode recording from the amygdala, although anterior temporal lobe resections are now less frequent because of the improved efficacy of anticonvulsant medications. Recordings are usually done bilaterally, with valuable information obtained from the hemisphere that is contralateral to the seizure focus (although in the case of some seizures, the activity spreads to the other hemisphere, which can exhibit additional sclerosis). A recent study (Naccache et al., 2005) obtained local field potential recordings in the amygdala during presurgical evaluation for neurosurgery in patients with seizure epileptogenesis located away from the amygdala. Data from single-photon emission computed tomography (SPECT) and electroencephalography (EEG) confirmed the structural integrity of the amygdalae in these patients. Results indicated that subliminally presented emotional words activated the amygdala prior to supraliminal processing. Another study has provided precise information regarding the temporal processing of emotional information, indicating that fear is initially processed in the amygdala prior to disgust and then spreads to cortical regions (Krolak-Salmon, Hénaff, Vighetto, Bertrand, & Mauguière, 2004). Thus intracranial recording remains a useful methodology that provides information regarding the temporal engagement of the amygdala during emotional processing. Imaging studies have also generated hypotheses that require more specific spatiotemporal resolution, and depth electrode studies can answer some of these questions, albeit in small, select patient populations.

Scalp EEG

In healthy participants, scalp recordings of the ongoing EEG and its demarcation into event-locked time averages (event-related potentials, or ERPs) are promising for identifying how emotion influences different oscillatory frequency bands in the EEG signal and for detailing the temporal profile of emotional effects on a time scale of tens of milliseconds. However, electrical signals emanating from the amygdala do not propagate readily, if at all, to the scalp. The small size and deep location of the amygdala, combined with the lack of an orderly laminar arrangement of its pyramidal neurons (which results in a relatively closed-field electrical configuration), does not permit the spatial integration and volume conduction necessary to observe electrical signals at the scalp. Moreover, emotional effects on ERPs tend to be quite broad both spatially and temporally, making spatial localization and source modeling difficult. For instance, encoding emotional relative to neutral words induces a broadly distributed positive shift in ERP activity over a long latency window, from about 450 to 1000 msec (Dillon, Cooper, Grent-'t-Jong, Woldorff, & LaBar, 2006). However, experimental manipulations that emphasize processing of a given ERP component can yield more specific findings, and downstream effects of emotion (and presumably amygdala activity) on cognition can be observed from ERPs elicited from the cortex. As an example, studies of covert attention have shown how facial expressions alter spatial orienting to subsequent targets, including enhancements of early ERP components linked to visual cortex processing (e.g., Fichtenholtz, Hopfinger, Graham, Detwiler, & LaBar, 2007; Pourtois, Grandjean, Sander, & Vuilleumier, 2004). Nonetheless, such indirect effects restrict interpretation in any attempt to combine scalp EEG and functional neuroimaging measures of emotion, given their differential sensitivity in detecting amygdala function.

Lesion Studies

Although amygdalotomy as psychosurgery is rarely performed today to treat psychiatric disorders, observations of patients with organic lesions to the amygdala provide key insights into the necessity of this brain region for socioemotional and motivational functions. The major disadvantage of this method in humans is that it is not possible to control the size, location, or extent of a lesion. An exception is the use of *en bloc* resection to treat medically refractory epilepsy, in which the surgeon uses a similar approach to excise the amygdala, hippocampus, and surrounding structures unilaterally (Spencer, Spencer, Mattson, Williamson, & Novelly, 1984). However, adjacent structures are always included in the resection to prevent recurrence of epilepsy, and there remains individual variability in the extent of cortex removed. Because of the distribution of blood supply to this region, and the nature of the syndromes that target the medial temporal lobe, it is extremely rare to observe amygdala damage in isolation (see Figure 7.2).

We remark here on a few additional limitations of neuropsychological studies of emotion and amygdala dysfunction. First, premorbid emotional/motivational status and personality characteristics are rarely quantified other than by retrospective reports from a patient or caregiver. Thus it is difficult

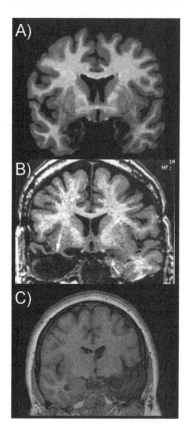

FIGURE 7.2. Human amygdala pathology associated with various disease processes in individual patients. (A) A case of Urbach–Wiethe syndrome, in which the bilateral amygdala was targeted relatively selectively, with some damage to the entorhinal cortex. From Adolphs, Tranel, and Buchanan (2005). Copyright 2005 by the Nature Publishing Group. Reprinted by permission. (B) A case of right anteromedial temporal lobe resection performed to treat medically refractory epilepsy, with selective gliosis in the left amygdala. From Phelps et al. (1998). Copyright 1998 by the Taylor & Francis Group. Reprinted by permission. (C) A case of herpes simplex encephalitis that produced widespread damage to the left temporal lobe. From Graham, Devinsky, and LaBar (2006). Copyright 2006 by Elsevier. Reprinted by permission.

to know the extent to which the onset of acquired brain damage promoted behavioral changes relative to the patient's existing baseline. Second, changes in socioemotional behavior and motivation may be secondary to lifestyle changes necessitated by the insult or disease process, rather than a direct consequence of brain damage. For instance, patients may become depressed after strokes because of their functional limitations; in this case, the depression is not directly associated with stroke-related damage to specific brain regions per se. Third, due to the extensive reciprocal interconnections of limbic forebrain structures, damage to one area, such as the amygdala, may affect the functioning of other network components, such as the anterior cingulate or orbitofrontal cortex (this phenomenon is called "diaschisis"; see Markowitsch et al., 1994). Fourth, because disease processes may be congenital or progressive, there may be long-term reorganization of brain function, and patients may compensate by using alternate strategies to solve experimental tasks. For example, amygdala-lesioned patients may use featural displacements as a perceptual heuristic to make judgments of facial affect, rather than processing the face in a holistic manner (Graham, Devinsky, & LaBar, 2006, 2007). Finally, it is difficult to determine emotional influences on select stages of information processing in patients with preexisting damage (e.g., to distinguish the effects of amygdala damage on the encoding vs. retrieval stages of emotional memory processing). These caveats notwithstanding, patients who have sustained amygdala damage have provided researchers with a wealth of valuable information. We limit our discussion here to a few neurological syndromes, although we recognize that the amygdala is implicated broadly in many neuropsychiatric disorders.

Klüver–Bucy Syndrome

The Klüver–Bucy syndrome was popularized following the publications by Klüver and Bucy (1937, 1939) that demonstrated a taming effect and inappropriate emotional reactions to stimuli in monkeys with bilateral temporal lobe lesions. The monkeys engaged in socially and motivationally inappropriate behaviors, such as hyperorality and hypersexuality, and they appeared to lack the ability to evaluate the significance of stimuli by sight alone (this lack was called "psychic blindness" by Klüver and Bucy, but today it may be considered a type of "motivational visual agnosia"). The Klüver–Bucy syndrome is rarely seen in humans, particularly in its full profile, but when it is, it generally follows amygdala damage combined with additional damage to the frontal lobes or hypothalamus. Although rare, features of Klüver–Bucy syndrome can be observed consequent to multiple etiologies, including subdural hematoma (Yoneoka et al., 2004), herpes simplex encephalitis (Bakchine, Chain, & Lhermitte, 1989; Marlowe, Mancall, & Thomas, 1975), left anterior temporal resection (Ghika-Schmid, Assal, De Tribolet, & Regli, 1995), right temporal resection (Bates & Sturman, 1995), and early Pick's disease (Cummings & Duchen, 1981). Klüver–Bucy syndrome demonstrates a difficulty with drawing strong conclusions from studies of brain-damaged patients: There is considerable variability in patient characteristics, etiology, and premorbid genetic and environmental influences that cannot be controlled. That being said, any similarities that result among patients despite these characterological differences may indicate robust findings. In these patients, the brain area that was consistently implicated was the amygdala, although the additional brain damage necessary to observe such effects implicates a broader disconnection syndrome.

Urbach–Wiethe Syndrome (Lipoid Proteinosis)

Urbach–Wiethe syndrome is a rare, autosomal recessive, multisystemic disease linked to chromosome 1q21. It is caused by mutations in the extracellular matrix protein 1 gene, and is characterized by hardening of the skin, mucosa, and viscera; hyaline deposition; and occasionally calcifications of medial temporal lobe structures (Hamada et al., 2002). In very few cases, calcifications are limited to the amygdala proper or to the amygdala plus periamygdaloid cortex. Despite an early paper detailing rage attacks and neurologic involvement in the disorder (Newton, Rosenberg, Lampert, & O'Brien, 1971), Urbach–Wiethe syndrome and its potential contribution to the study of the amygdala had remained overlooked until Tranel and Hyman's (1990) original report of patient S. M., who sustained calcifications largely restricted to the amygdala bilaterally. Subsequent studies of S. M. and similar patients have sparked interest in studying emotional functions, in much the same way that descriptions of amnesic patient H. M. bolstered memory research in the mid-20th century. For instance, Adolphs, Tranel, Damasio, and Damasio (1994) reported that patient S. M. was unable to identify facial expressions of fear, despite being able to name and identify other facial expressions. This seminal study, in conjunction with a contemporaneous report of two other patients (Markowitsch et al., 1994), provided evidence that the amygdala is essential for the evaluation of threat signals and emotional memory—themes in affective neuroscience research that have been extensively elaborated ever since.

Epilepsy

Patients who have undergone selective unilateral amygdalohippocampectomy or resection of the anteromedial temporal lobe for intractable epilepsy constitute the vast majority of patients in modern lesion studies. Although such patients provide a relatively homogeneous sample (compared to, say, those with Klüver–Bucy syndrome), the epilepsy and subsequent surgical procedure have a unilateral focus, which often yields only subtle behavioral deficits. Phelps and colleagues (1998) described an epileptic patient (S. P.) who received a unilateral right anteromedial temporal lobe resection, and who had additional gliosis that was circumscribed to the left amygdala. This patient, like patient S. M., has provided important insights into the effects of bilateral amygdala damage on emotional functions without significant comorbid impairments in other cognitive domains. S. P. exhibits deficits on tests of facial expression processing (Adolphs & Tranel, 1999; Graham et al., 2007), fear conditioning (Phelps et al., 1998), arousal-mediated memory consolidation (Phelps et al., 1998), and emotional modulation of the attentional blink paradigm (Anderson & Phelps, 2001), although her other socioemotional functions are relatively well preserved (see Anderson & Phelps, 1998, 2000; Graham et al., 2006; Phelps, Cannistraci, & Cunningham, 2003; Phelps, LaBar, & Spencer, 1997; Phelps et al., 1998).

Inducing Temporary Brain Inactivation by Transcranial Magnetic Stimulation

Given the inherent limitations in studying patients with organic brain damage, researchers have moved to inducing temporary inactivation of structures in the healthy human brain via transcranial magnetic stimulation (TMS). A major advantage of this approach is that it can be used to validate findings from patient populations about the role of specific brain regions in cognitive and emotional functioning. TMS can be applied at specific time points relative to an ongoing task to isolate a given information-processing stage, and the research subjects can serve as their own unstimulated controls. TMS has also been applied to prefrontal regions as a potential treatment for depression (e.g., George, Wassermann, & Post, 1996). Notable in these treatment studies of depressed patients is evidence that amygdalar functioning is affected, albeit indirectly. Specifically, some studies that have assessed changes in regional cerebral blood flow after repetitive TMS in the left prefrontal cortex describe changes in the left amygdala (Speer et al., 2000). However, a primary limitation of TMS is that the surface coils used to generate the magnetization pulses do not have sufficient penetration to reach the subcortical location of the amygdala. As surface coil technology improves to target deeper structures, it may be possible to temporarily inactivate the healthy amygdala with TMS, but due to the small size of this structure, it is unlikely to be selectively implicated. Because this methodology is still in its infancy, safety and practical concerns, such as optimal frequency and duration of stimulation, remain open issues (e.g., Machii, Cohen, Ramos-Estebanez, & Pascual-Leone, 2006).

Neuroimaging Techniques

Structural Imaging: Volumetry

Volume estimates of the amygdala by means of structural MRI have been used for over two decades to correlate changes in structure with altered emotional processing in neuropsychiatric disorders. High-resolution, T1-weighted, 3-D spoiled gradient recalled acquisition images with a resolution of 1.0–1.5 mm^3 are typically needed, with excellent contrast between gray and white matter in order to obtain accurate volumetric estimates. Quantifying interrater reliability is critical to validate the methodology used, given the difficulties in identifying amygdalar boundaries. Because volume changes provide only crude insight into function and are sensitive to both glial cell and neuronal atrophy, this method is often used in conjunction with other behavioral tests to determine correlations between volume changes and functional impairment.

Using computer-mouse-driven software programs to draw borders manually on individual brain slices is preferred over using automated segmentation protocols based on normalized brain atlases, although quantitative comparisons between these procedures are warranted. Borders that are most difficult to identify include the amygdalohippocampal transition area ventrocaudally, the amygdalostriatal transition area dorsorostrally, the terminus of the anterior amygdaloid area, and the anteromedial transition to entorhinal cortex, where the angular bundle becomes indistinct (Doty et al., 2008). Whereas differentiation of medial–lateral boundaries is facilitated in the coronal plane, assessment of the amygdalohippocampal transition area is facilitated in the axial plane with simultaneous co-planar visualization and verification (Convit et al., 1999). Landmarks such as the optic chiasm can facilitate definition of anterior borders, but should be used with caution and only after standard realignment prior to tracing. Inclusion of adjacent structures generally overestimates the volume of the amygdala in studies of lesser quality. A meta-analytic review by Brierley, Shaw, and David (2002) provides mean amygdala volume estimates (±95% confidence interval) of 1726.7 ± 35.1 mm^3 in the left hemisphere and 1691.7 ± 37.2 mm^3 in the right hemisphere of the adult brain.

Functional Imaging: Positron Emission Tomography

Initial activation studies using positron emission tomography (PET) have provided important insights into emotional functions of the amygdala, such as its role in facial expression processing (Morris et al., 1996) and emotional memory (Cahill et al., 1996; Hamann, Ely, Grafton, & Kilts, 1999). Recording concurrent physiological and verbal responses is more straightforward with this technique than with functional MRI (fMRI). However, analysis of typical PET data requires a degree of spatial smoothing that is larger than the extent of the amygdala itself, thereby recruiting brain signals from adjacent regions such as the hippocampus and entorhinal cortex. In addition, the temporal parameters of PET studies are limited by the half-life of the radioisotope injected into the participant (e.g., data are typically accumulated across 45- to 60-sec time periods with ^{15}O), as well as the limited repeatability of the experiment within subjects, due to ethical considerations concerning cumulative exposure to radioactive substances (George et al., 2000). For studies of sustained mood effects, the temporal scale of PET activity may be particularly useful (e.g., Schneider et al., 1995), but for investigations of emotional influences with shorter durations, trial blocking is required. In addition to untoward effects on cognitive functions (e.g., changing cognitive "set"), blocking trials by emotional category confounds emotional processing with anticipatory emotions and mood induction, and PET may miss transient amygdala activation that habituates over repeated trials (e.g., Breiter et al., 1996; Wright et al., 2001). Recent advances in PET technology have improved upon some of these issues, but this technique has been largely supplanted in cognitive activation studies by fMRI because of fMRI's superior spatial and temporal resolution, as well as other advantages (cost, noninvasiveness, etc.). PET nonetheless remains a powerful tool for examining emotional influences on resting-state cerebral blood flow and for pharmacological investigations, as radioisotopes can be designed that bind to specific receptor molecules to provide a unique view into the anatomical distribution of neurotransmitter systems in healthy and psychiatric populations.

Event-Related fMRI

Event-related fMRI has emerged in the last decade as a primary tool for neu-roimaging of amygdala function, although it is not without its challenges. A first challenge relates to the sensitivity of this technique to movement artifacts, which hinders the ability to study the generation of emotional expression/ prosody, startle reflexes, and individuals who can't lie still for extended peri-ods of time (which may be more problematic in some psychiatric disorders). There are also technical difficulties with setting up concurrent physiological recording in the MRI environment (e.g., heating of electrodes by the magnet, radiofrequency interference from the scanner pulses, blowout of frontal lobe signal with concurrent eye tracking and facial electromyography, attenuation of physiological signals prior to amplification in an external control room), but these issues have been largely resolved in recent years. Although the spa-tial resolution of fMRI is better than that of PET, it can be difficult to distin-guish amygdala responses from those of adjacent structures when standard 8-mm smoothing kernels are used, particularly for tasks where nearby struc-tures (such as the hippocampus and entorhinal cortex) make complementary and/or interactive contributions (e.g., Dolcos, LaBar, & Cabeza, 2004, 2005). The signal-averaging requirements of event-related fMRI can be problematic in terms of sustaining emotional processes over repeated exposures to the same stimulus, which can mask a transient amygdala response to novel stimuli and changes in emotional salience. Furthermore, the profile of the hemody-namic response function in the amygdala sometimes does not conform to a standard gamma function often used to model cortical responses, especially when depressed individuals are studied (Siegle, Steinhauer, Thase, Stenger, & Carter, 2002) or when healthy participants are asked to elaborate the emo-tional meaning of the stimulus (Schaefer et al., 2002). Therefore, extract-ing the raw percentage of signal change over points in time after stimulus onset without reference to a standard hemodynamic template often leads to improved measurements.

Perhaps the most troubling issue relates to the problem of overcoming sus-ceptibility artifact to obtain reliable hemodynamic signals from the amygdala. Because the amygdala is bounded medially by sinuses and ventrocaudolater-ally by the lateral ventricle, it is situated in a region characterized by magnetic-susceptibility-induced signal loss. As illustrated in Figure 7.3, quantitative analysis of signal-to-noise ratios (SNRs) in the vicinity of the amygdala shows that the signal losses contribute to intersubject and interhemispheric variabil-ity in amygdala activation during emotional processing (LaBar, Gitelman, Mesulam, & Parrish, 2001). These issues are more difficult to resolve at high field strengths, and are particularly critical for voxel-wise statistical analy-ses that require precise spatial registration of signal changes across subjects.

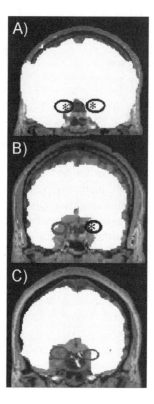

FIGURE 7.3. Quantification of fMRI signal loss in the vicinity of the amygdala for three normal adults. Computer simulations determined the minimum signal-to-noise ratios (SNRs) needed to observe reliable activation for an fMRI study that compared the processing of emotional versus neutral pictures. Location of peak amygdala activity for the *t*-test contrast (emotional > neutral) is indicated by asterisks and is overlaid onto SNR masks indicating brain regions that have sufficient sensitivity to detect a 1% signal change with α = .05 for the study. Amygdalae with sufficient SNRs are outlined in black; amygdalae located in signal voids are outlined in gray. Bilateral activity was found in an individual with no signal voids (A); unilateral activity was found in an individual with an asymmetric signal void pattern (B); and no activity was found in an individual with large signal voids (C). Results highlight the importance of considering individual differences in fMRI-related susceptibility artifacts when investigators are interpreting neuroimaging results from the human amygdala. From LaBar, Gitelman, Mesulam, and Parrish (2001). Copyright 2001 by Lippincott Williams & Wilkins. Reprinted by permission.

Specializing shimming and pulse sequences, including double-shot echoplanar and inward spiral protocols, can improve SNRs in the amygdala even at high field strengths (Posse et al., 2003; Wang, McCarthy, Song, & LaBar, 2005). Although current methods do not allow resolution of individual amygdaloid subnuclei, it is possible to segregate signals grossly into anterior–posterior, medial–lateral, and dorsal–ventral subdivisions (e.g., Anderson, Christoff, Panitz, De Rosa, & Gabrieli, 2003; Dolcos et al., 2004; Whalen et al., 1998). More detailed parsing of functional subdivisions will require high-resolution imaging techniques that also recover susceptibility artifact and are combined with analysis tools that do not rely on spatial smoothing.

Further complicating the interpretation of fMRI amygdala responses to emotional stimuli is the role of individual differences. Amygdala activity has been shown to vary across individuals according to many personality, social, and genetic factors. These include gender (Cahill, Uncapher, Kilpatrick, Alkire, & Turner, 2004; Canli, Desmond, Zhao, & Gabrieli, 2002a), age (Mather et al., 2004), extraversion (Canli, Sivers, Whitfield, Gotlib, & Gabrieli, 2002b), implicit measures of racial bias (Phelps et al., 2000), trait anxiety (Etkin et al., 2004), motivational regulatory focus (Cunningham, Raye, & Johnson, 2005), and genetic variation in serotonin receptor function (Hariri et al., 2002). Standard group-averaged analytic approaches typically neglect to account for such variables, which may reduce amygdala activity overall and contribute to the lack of replication across population samples. Other state effects also have an impact on amygdala activation, including effects of hunger (LaBar, Gitelman, Parrish, et al., 2001), state anxiety (Bishop, Duncan, & Lawrence, 2004), and mood (Wang, LaBar, & McCarthy, 2006) on the processing of visual stimuli that have emotional or motivational salience. Comprehensive characterization of personality, genomic, and demographic characteristics, as well as mood and other state variables of the participants, is becoming critical; statistical approaches that explicitly include assessment of individual differences are also urgently needed.

THE IMPORTANCE OF BEHAVIORAL ASSESSMENT AND CONCURRENT PSYCHOPHYSIOLOGY

Even with the most powerful magnets, the most selective lesions, and direct electrophysiological recordings from epileptic patients, our understanding of human amygdala function will not advance without adequate behavioral probes and psychophysiological measures. Emotion is a complex construct that consists of several underlying dimensions or categories (which vary according to different theories) and engages several stages of information processing, including evaluation, experience, and expression. Systematic characterization and experimental manipulation of these components of emotional processing are critical to infer mechanisms. Moreover, the amygdala not only is engaged during emotional processing, but also contributes to a variety of other social and motivational functions, as described throughout this book. Therefore, mere observation of amygdala signal changes during an fMRI experiment is insufficient to prove that emotion has been elicited or is contributing to task performance. Such "reverse inference" problems have been discussed with respect to other brain areas (see Poldrack & Wagner, 2004), and are especially germane when the emotional manipulation is not independently validated by concurrent psychophysiology, self-report measures, or behavioral assessments.

Although emotion research has benefited by development of standardized stimulus databases, MRI-compatible psychophysiological recording systems, and self-report batteries, efforts to link fMRI- or intracranial ERP-related amygdala activation with such data are inherently correlational in nature. As such, causality cannot be inferred, and the necessity of the structure's involvement is unknown. For this reason, obtaining converging evidence across multiple methods, including studies of patients with selective brain lesions, is of the utmost importance. A similar difficulty is that researchers must develop and rely on particular paradigms, which have been designed to be sensitive but may or may not be specific to the brain structure in question. Multiple paradigms—including fear conditioning; processing and memory for emotional auditory, olfactory, and visual stimuli; and viewing faces and other socially relevant stimuli—have been implemented to tap amygdala functioning, but also activate other brain regions due to the distributed nature of neural processing. Characterizing the amygdala's interactions with these areas and using neuroimaging observations to guide future behavioral task development would facilitate more sensitive *and* specific means to probe this enigmatic brain region.

WHAT WE THINK

Initial studies of the human amygdala pointed to its specific role in fear processing. Although some have taken the view that the amygdala is a dedicated fear module in the brain (Öhman & Mineka, 2001), the past decade has revealed an impressive diversity of emotional, motivational, and social-cognitive functions subserved by this constellation of nuclei. Moreover, its responses to specific emotional elicitors and emotion categories have been shown to change according to different experimental manipulations (e.g., Adams, Gordon, Baird, Ambady, & Kleck, 2003; Anderson et al., 2003; Schaefer et al., 2002), and patients with amygdala damage can compensate under some circumstances for their loss of fear recognition (Adolphs, Tranel, & Buchanan, 2005; Graham et al., 2006, 2007). Factors that may contribute to observing potentiated amygdala responses to fear stimuli in neuroimaging studies include (1) the scary context of the experimental setting (loud noises, dark confining chamber, etc.), which may yield a match between the stimulus presented and the context and/or a relative ease of eliciting fear in this context (see the chapter text for a similar discussion with regard to intracranial monitoring); (2) the use of blocked designs in which repeated presentations of threat signals induce potentially confounding influences of prolonged fearful states and anticipatory anxiety; and (3) the difficulty of reliably inducing highly arousing positive affect. Although there is no question that the amygdala is important for fear learning and for detecting threats in the environment, its role can also be characterized as a salience detector, whereby it monitors and signals events of most importance to the organism's state at any particular point in time (see also Sander, Grafman, & Zalla, 2003). For instance, we have observed increased amygdala activity to food stimuli when participants are in a hungry relative to a satiated state (LaBar, Gitelman, Parrish, et al., 2001); to sad images when participants are in a sad relative to a happy mood state (Wang et al., 2006); to both positively and negatively arousing pictures that are subsequently remembered, relative to those that are forgotten (Dolcos et al., 2004); and to changes in emotional salience during different phases of fear conditioning training (LaBar, Gatenby, Gore, LeDoux, & Phelps, 1998). How the amygdala combines and weights goal-directed and stimulus-driven information to determine what is important to signal from one moment to the next remains an interesting and unresolved question.

REFERENCES

Adams, R. B., Jr., Gordon, H. L., Baird, A. A., Ambady, N., & Kleck, R. E. (2003). Effects of gaze on amygdala sensitivity to anger and fear faces. *Science, 300,* 1536.

Adolphs, R., & Tranel, D. (1999). Preferences for visual stimuli following amygdala damage. *Journal of Cognitive Neuroscience, 11*(6), 610–616.

Adolphs, R., Tranel, D., & Buchanan, T. W. (2005). Amygdala damage impairs emotional memory for gist but not details of complex stimuli. *Nature Neuroscience, 8*(4), 512–518.

Adolphs, R., Tranel, D., Damasio, H., & Damasio, D. (1994). Impaired recognition of emotion in facial expressions following bilateral damage to the human amygdala. *Nature, 372,* 669–672.

Aggleton, J. P., & Saunders, R. C. (2000). The amygdala: What's happened in the last decade? In J. P. Aggleton (Ed.), *The amygdala: A functional analysis* (2nd ed., pp. 1–20). Oxford, UK: Oxford University Press.

Amunts, K., Kedo, O., Kindler, M., Pieperhoff, P., Mohlberg, H., Shah, N. J., et al. (2005). Cytoarchitectonic mapping of the human amygdala, hippocampal region and entorhinal cortex: Intersubject variability and probability maps. *Anatomy and Embryology, 210,* 343–352.

Anderson, A. K., Christoff, K., Panitz, D., De Rosa, E., & Gabrieli, J. D. (2003). Neural correlates of the automatic processing of threat facial signals. *Journal of Neuroscience, 23*(13), 5627–5633.

Anderson, A. K., & Phelps, E. A. (1998). Intact recognition of vocal expressions of fear following bilateral lesions of the human amygdala. *NeuroReport, 9*(16), 3607–3613.

Anderson, A. K., & Phelps, E. A. (2000). Expression without recognition: Contributions of the human amygdala to emotional communication. *Psychological Science, 11*(2), 106–111.

Anderson, A. K., & Phelps, E. A. (2001). Lesions of the human amygdala impair enhanced perception of emotionally salient events. *Nature, 411,* 305–309.

Bakchine, S., Chain, F., & Lhermitte, F. (1989). Herpes simplex type II encephalitis with complete Klüver–Bucy syndrome in a non-immunocompromised adult. *Journal of Neurology, Neurosurgery and Psychiatry, 52,* 290–291.

Bates, G. D. L., & Sturman, S. G. (1995). Unilateral temporal lobe damage and the partial Kluver–Bucy syndrome. *Behavioural Neurology, 8,* 103–107.

Bishop, S. J., Duncan, J., & Lawrence, A. D. (2004). State anxiety modulation of the amygdala response to unattended threat-related stimuli. *Journal of Neuroscience, 24,* 10364–10368.

Breiter, H. C., Etcoff, N. L., Whalen, P. J., Kennedy, W. A., Rauch, S. L., Buckner, R. L., et al. (1996). Response and habituation of the human amygdala during visual processing of facial expression. *Neuron, 17*(5), 875–887.

Brierley, B., Shaw, P., & David, A. S. (2002). The human amygdala: A systematic review and meta-analysis of volumetric magnetic resonance imaging. *Brain Research Reviews, 39*(1), 84–105.

Burdach, K. F. (1819–1822). *Vom Baue und Leben des Gehirns.* Leipzig.

Cahill, L., Haier, R. J., Fallon, J., Alkire, M. T., Tang, C., Keator, D., et al. (1996). Amygdala activity at encoding correlated with long-term, free recall of emotional information. *Proceedings of the National Academy of Sciences USA, 93*(15), 8016–8021.

Cahill, L., Uncapher, M., Kilpatrick, L., Alkire, M. T., & Turner, J. (2004). Sex-related hemispheric lateralization of amygdala function in emotionally influenced memory: An fMRI investigation. *Learning and Memory, 11*(3), 261–266.

Canli, T., Desmond, J. E., Zhao, Z., & Gabrieli, J. D. (2002a). Sex differences in the neural basis of emotional memories. *Proceedings of the National Academy of Sciences USA, 99*(16), 10789–10794.

Canli, T., Sivers, H., Whitfield, S. L., Gotlib, I. H., & Gabrieli, J. D. (2002b). Amygdala response to happy faces as a function of extraversion. *Science, 296,* 2191.

Chapman, W. P., Schroeder, H. R., Geyer, G., Brazier, M. A. B., Fager, C., Poppen, J. L., et al. (1954). Physiological evidence concerning importance of amygdaloid nuclear region in the integration of circulatory function and emotion in man. *Science, 120,* 949–950.

Chitanondh, H. (1966). Stereotaxic amygdalotomy in the treatment of olfactory seizures and psychiatric disorders with olfactory hallucinations. *Confinia Neurologica, 27,* 181–196.

Convit, A., McHugh, P., Wolf, O. T., de Leon, M. J., Bobinski, M., De Santi, S., et al. (1999). MRI volume of the amygdala: A reliable method allowing separation from the hippocampal formation. *Psychiatry Research, 90*(2), 113–123.

Cummings, J. L., & Duchen, L. W. (1981). Kluver–Bucy syndrome in Pick disease: Clinical and pathologic correlates. *Neurology, 31,* 1415–1422.

Cunningham, W. A., Raye, C. L., & Johnson, M. K. (2005). Neural correlates of evaluation associated with promotion and prevention regulatory focus. *Cognitive, Affective, and Behavioral Neuroscience, 5*(2), 202–211.

De Olmos, J. S., & Heimer, L. (1999). The concepts of the ventral striatopallidal system and extended amygdala. *Annals of the New York Academy of Sciences, 877,* 1–32.

Dillon, D. G., Cooper, J. J., Grent-'t-Jong, T., Woldorff, M. G., & LaBar, K. S. (2006).

Dissociation of event-related potentials indexing arousal and semantic cohesion during emotional word encoding. *Brain and Cognition, 62*(1), 43–57.

Dolcos, F., LaBar, K. S., & Cabeza, R. (2004). Interaction between the amygdala and the medial temporal lobe memory system predicts better memory for emotional events. *Neuron, 42*(5), 855–863.

Dolcos, F., LaBar, K. S., & Cabeza, R. (2005). Remembering one year later: Role of the amygdala and the medial temporal lobe memory system in retrieving emotional memories. *Proceedings of the National Academy of Sciences USA, 102*(7), 2626–2631.

Doty, T. J., Payne, M. E., Steffens, D. C., Beyer, J. L., Krishnan, K. R. R., & LaBar, K. S. (2008). Age-dependent reduction of amygdala volume in bipolar disorder. *Psychiatry Research: Neuroimaging, 163*, 84–94.

Etkin, A., Klemenhagen, K. C., Dudman, J. T., Rogan, M. T., Hen, R., Kandel, E. R., et al. (2004). Individual differences in trait anxiety predict the response of the basolateral amygdala to unconsciously processed fearful faces. *Neuron, 44*(6), 1043–1055.

Feindel, W., & Penfield, W. (1954). Localization of discharge in temporal lobe automatism. *AMA Archives of Neurology and Psychiatry, 72*, 603–630.

Fichtenholtz, H. M., Hopfinger, J. B., Graham, R., Detwiler, J. M., & LaBar, K. S. (2007). Happy and fearful emotion in cues and targets modulate event-related potential indices of gaze-directed attentional orienting. *Social Cognitive and Affective Neuroscience, 2*, 323–333.

George, M. S., Ketter, T. A., Kimbrell, T. A., Speer, A. M., Lorberbaum, J., Liberatos, C. C., et al. (2000). Neuroimaging approaches to the study of emotion. In J. C. Borod (Ed.), *The neuropsychology of emotion* (pp. 106–136). New York: Oxford University Press.

George, M. S., Wassermann, E. M., & Post, R. M. (1996). Transcranial magnetic stimulation: A neuropsychiatric tool for the 21st century. *Journal of Neuropsychiatry and Clinical Neurosciences, 8*, 373–382.

Ghika-Schmid, F., Assal, G., De Tribolet, N., & Regli, F. (1995). Klüver–Bucy syndrome after left anterior temporal resection. *Neuropsychologia, 33*, 101–113.

Gloor, P. (1992). Role of the amygdala in temporal lobe epilepsy. In J. P. Aggleton (Ed.), *The amygdala: Neurobiological aspects of emotion, memory, and mental dysfunction* (pp. 505–538). New York: Wiley-Liss.

Gloor, P., Olivier, A., Quesney, L. F., Andermann, F., & Horowitz, S. (1982). The role of the limbic system in experiential phenomena of temporal lobe epilepsy. *Annals of Neurology, 12*, 129–144.

Graham, R., Devinsky, O., & LaBar, K. S. (2006). Sequential ordering of morphed faces and facial expressions following temporal lobe damage. *Neuropsychologia, 44*(8), 1398–1405.

Graham, R., Devinsky, O., & LaBar, K. S. (2007). Quantifying deficits in the perception of fear and anger in morphed facial expressions after bilateral amygdala damage. *Neuropsychologia, 45*(1), 42–54.

Halgren, E. (1992). Emotional neurophysiology of the amygdala within the context of human cognition. In J. P. Aggleton (Ed.), *The amygdala: Neurobiological aspects of emotion, memory, and mental dysfunction* (pp. 191–228). New York: Wiley-Liss.

Halgren, E., Walter, R. D., Cherlow, D. G., & Crandall, P. H. (1978). Mental phenomena evoked by electrical stimulation of the human hippocampal formation and amygdala. *Brain, 101*(1), 83–117.

Hamada, T., McLean, W. H., Ramsay, M., Ashton, G. H., Nanda, A., Jenkins, T., et al. (2002). Lipoid proteinosis maps to 1q21 and is caused by mutations in the extracellular matrix protein 1 gene (ecm1). *Human Molecular Genetics, 11*(7), 833–840.

Hamann, S. B., Ely, T. D., Grafton, S. T., & Kilts, C. D. (1999). Amygdala activity related to enhanced memory for pleasant and aversive stimuli. *Nature Neuroscience, 2*(3), 289–293.

Hariri, A. R., Mattay, V. S., Tessitore, A., Kolachana, B., Fera, F., Goldman, D., et al. (2002). Serotonin transporter genetic variation and the response of the human amygdala. *Science, 297*, 400–403.

Kim, M. C., Lee, T. K., & Choi, C. R. (2002). Review of long-term results of stereotactic psychosurgery. *Neurologia Medico-Chirurgica (Tokyo), 42*(9), 365–371.

Klüver, H., & Bucy, P. (1937). "Psychic blindness" and other symptoms following bilateral temporal lobectomy in rhesus monkeys. *American Journal of Physiology, 119*, 352–353.

Klüver, H., & Bucy, P. (1939). Preliminary analysis of functions of the temporal lobes in monkeys. *Archives of Neurology and Psychiatry, 42*, 979–1000.

Krolak-Salmon, P., Hénaff, M., Vighetto, A., Bertrand, O., & Mauguière, F. (2004). Early amygdala reaction to fear spreading in occipital, temporal, and frontal cortex: A depth electrode ERP study in human. *Neuron, 42*, 665–676.

LaBar, K. S., Gatenby, J. C., Gore, J. C., LeDoux, J. E., & Phelps, E. A. (1998). Human amygdala activation during conditioned fear acquisition and extinction: A mixed-trial fMRI study. *Neuron, 20*(5), 937–945.

LaBar, K. S., Gitelman, D. R., Mesulam, M. M., & Parrish, T. B. (2001). Impact of signal-to-noise on functional MRI of the human amygdala. *NeuroReport, 12*, 3461–3464.

LaBar, K. S., Gitelman, D. R., Parrish, T. B., Kim, Y. H., Nobre, A. C., & Mesulam, M. M. (2001). Hunger selectively modulates corticolimbic activation to food stimuli in humans. *Behavioral Neuroscience, 115*(2), 493–500.

LaBar, K. S., & Phelps, E. A. (2005). Reinstatement of conditioned fear in humans is context dependent and impaired in amnesia. *Behavioral Neuroscience, 119*, 677–686.

Machii, K., Cohen, D., Ramos-Estebanez, C., & Pascual-Leone, A. (2006). Safety of rTMS to non-motor cortical areas in healthy participants and patients. *Clinical Neurophysiology, 117*, 455–471.

Markowitsch, H. J., Calabrese, P., Würker, M., Durwen, H. F., Kessler, J., Babinsky, R., et al. (1994). The amygdala's contribution to memory: A study on two patients with Urbach–Wiethe disease. *NeuroReport, 5*, 1349–1352.

Marlowe, W. B., Mancall, E. L., & Thomas, J. J. (1975). Complete Klüver–Bucy syndrome in man. *Cortex, 11*, 53–59.

Mather, M., Canli, T., English, T., Whitfield, S., Wais, P., Ochsner, K., et al. (2004). Amygdala responses to emotionally valenced stimuli in older and younger adults. *Psychological Science, 15*(4), 259–263.

Meunier, M., Bachevalier, J., Murray, E. A., Malkova, L., & Mishkin, M. (1999). Effects of aspiration versus neurotoxic lesions of the amygdala on emotional responses in monkeys. *European Journal of Neuroscience, 11*(12), 4403–4418.

Morris, J. S., Frith, C. D., Perrett, D. I., Rowland, D., Young, A. W., Calder, A. J., et al. (1996). A differential neural response in the human amygdala to fearful and happy facial expressions. *Nature, 383,* 812–815.

Naccache, L., Gallard, R., Adam, C., Hasboun, D., Clémenceau, S., Baulac, M., et al. (2005). A direct intracranial record of emotions evoked by subliminal words. *Proceedings of the National Academy of Sciences USA, 102,* 7713–7717.

Narabayashi, H., & Uno, M. (1966). Long range results of stereotaxic amygdalotomy for behavior disorders. *Confinia Neurologica, 27*(1), 168–171.

Newton, F. H., Rosenberg, R. N., Lampert, P. W., & O'Brien, J. S. (1971). Neurologic involvement in Urbach–Wiethe's disease (lipoid proteinosis). *Neurology, 21,* 1205–1213.

Öhman, A., & Mineka, S. (2001). Fears, phobias, and preparedness: Toward an evolved module of fear and fear learning. *Psychological Review, 108*(3), 483–522.

Parrent, A. G., & Lozano, A. M. (2000). Stereotactic surgery for temporal lobe epilepsy. *Canadian Journal of Neurological Sciences, 27*(Suppl. 1), S79–S84.

Penfield, W. (1958). Some mechanisms of consciousness discovered during electrical stimulation of the brain. *Proceedings of the National Academy of Sciences USA, 44,* 51–66.

Phelps, E. A., Cannistraci, C. J., & Cunningham, W. A. (2003). Intact performance on an indirect measure of race bias following amygdala damage. *Neuropsychologia, 41*(2), 203–208.

Phelps, E. A., LaBar, K. S., Anderson, A. K., O'Connor, K. J., Fulbright, R. K., & Spencer, D. D. (1998). Specifying the contributions of the human amygdala to emotional memory: A case study. *Neurocase, 4,* 527–540.

Phelps, E. A., LaBar, K. S., & Spencer, D. D. (1997). Memory for emotional words following unilateral temporal lobectomy. *Brain and Cognition, 35*(1), 85–109.

Phelps, E. A., O'Connor, K. J., Cunningham, W. A., Funayama, E. S., Gatenby, J. C., Gore, J. C., et al. (2000). Performance on indirect measures of race evaluation predicts amygdala activation. *Journal of Cognitive Neuroscience, 12*(5), 729–738.

Poldrack, R. A., & Wagner, A. D. (2004). What can neuroimaging tell us about the mind? *Current Directions in Psychological Science, 13*(5), 177–181.

Posse, S., Fitzgerald, D., Gao, K., Habel, U., Rosenberg, D., Moore, G. J., et al. (2003). Real-time fMRI of temporolimbic regions detects amygdala activation during single-trial self-induced sadness. *NeuroImage, 18*(3), 760–768.

Pourtois, G., Grandjean, D., Sander, D., & Vuilleumier, P. (2004). Electrophysiological correlates of rapid spatial orienting towards fearful faces. *Cerebral Cortex, 14*(6), 619–633.

Sander, D. D., Grafman, J. J., & Zalla, T. T. (2003). The human amygdala: An evolved system for relevance detection. *Reviews in the Neurosciences, 14*(4), 303–316.

Schaefer, S. M., Jackson, D. C., Davidson, R. J., Aguirre, G. K., Kimberg, D. Y., & Thompson-Schill, S. L. (2002). Modulation of amygdalar activity by the conscious regulation of negative emotion. *Journal of Cognitive Neuroscience, 14*(6), 913–921.

Schneider, F., Gur, R. E., Mozley, L. H., Smith, R. J., Mozley, P. D., Censits, D. M., et al. (1995). Mood effects on limbic blood flow correlate with emotional self-rating: A PET study with oxygen-15 labeled water. *Psychiatry Research, 61*(4), 265–283.

Siegle, G. J., Steinhauer, S. R., Thase, M. E., Stenger, V. A., & Carter, C. S. (2002). Can't shake that feeling: Event-related fMRI assessment of sustained amygdala activity in response to emotional information in depressed individuals. *Biological Psychiatry, 51*(9), 693–707.

Speer, A. M., Kimbrell, T. A., Wassermann, E. M., Repella, J. D., Willis, M. W., Herscovitch, P., et al. (2000). Opposite effects of high and low frequency rTMS on regional brain activity in depressed patients. *Biological Psychiatry, 48*, 1133–1141.

Spencer, D., Spencer, S., Mattson, R. H., Williamson, P. D., & Novelly, R. A. (1984). Access to the posterior medial temporal lobe structures in the surgical treatment of temporal lobe epilepsy. *Neurosurgery, 15*(5), 667–671.

Swanson, L. W., & Petrovich, G. D. (1998). What is the amygdala? *Trends in Neurosciences, 21*, 323–331.

Toone, B. K., Cooke, E., & Lader, M. H. (1979). The effect of temporal lobe surgery on electrodermal activity: Implications for an organic hypothesis in the aetiology of schizophrenia. *Psychological Medicine, 9*, 281–285.

Tranel, D., & Hyman, B. T. (1990). Neuropsychological correlates of bilateral amygdala damage. *Archives of Neurology, 47*(3), 349–355.

Wang, L., LaBar, K. S., & McCarthy, G. (2006). Mood alters amygdala activation to sad distractors during an attentional task. *Biological Psychiatry, 60*(10), 1139–1146.

Wang, L., McCarthy, G., Song, A. W., & LaBar, K. S. (2005). Amygdala activation to sad pictures during high-field (4 tesla) functional magnetic resonance imaging. *Emotion, 5*(1), 12–22.

Whalen, P. J., Bush, G., McNally, R. J., Wilhelm, S., McInerney, S. C., Jenike, M. A., et al. (1998). The emotional counting Stroop paradigm: A functional magnetic resonance imaging probe of the anterior cingulate affective division. *Biological Psychiatry, 44*(12), 1219–1228.

Wright, C. I., Fischer, H., Whalen, P. J., McInerney, S. C., Shin, L. M., & Rauch, S. L. (2001). Differential prefrontal cortex and amygdala habituation to repeatedly presented emotional stimuli. *NeuroReport, 12*(2), 379–383.

Yoneoka, Y., Takeda, N., Inoue, A., Ibuchi, Y., Kumagai, T., Sugai, T., et al. (2004). Human Kluver–Bucy syndrome following acute subdural hematoma. *Acta Neurochirurgica, 146*, 1267–1270.

Young, A. W., Flude, B. M., Hellawell, D. J., & Ellis, A. W. (1994). The nature of semantic priming effects in the recognition of familiar people. *British Journal of Psychology, 85*(Pt. 3), 393–411.

CHAPTER 8

The Human Amygdala and Memory

Stephan Hamann

Out of the constant stream of daily experiences, some episodes will persist in memory, whereas many others will fade into oblivion. What leads some memories to endure rather than be forgotten? Empirical research and intuition both point to emotion as one of the most potent factors that can influence the strength and subjective quality of memories. A memory system that enhances emotional memories has clear evolutionary advantages, since stimuli that trigger either negative (aversive) or positive (appetitive) emotional arousal are frequently more relevant to survival than neutral stimuli, and it would therefore be advantageous to preferentially store memories for emotional events (LeDoux, 1993; Phelps & Anderson, 1997).

The powerful ability of emotion to enhance episodic memory (memory for events) (Tulving, 2002) has long been recognized and discussed in the psychological and philosophical literatures. The psychologist William James described strong emotion, either positive or negative, as leaving "scars" on the brain—an apt and vivid metaphor for the special character and enduring nature of highly emotional episodic memories (James, 1890/1950). More recently, numerous psychological and cognitive neuroscience studies have begun to identify the cognitive and neural mechanisms involved in emotional memory encoding and retrieval (LaBar & Cabeza, 2006; Phelps, 2006).

Are there special neural mechanisms for emotional memory? There is now considerable evidence from both animal and human studies that special neural mechanisms indeed enhance and alter memories for emotionally arousing events, but are not engaged for neutral events. The key brain area orchestrating these mechanisms is the amygdala, a small spherical structure composed of several different nuclei (Amaral & Price, 1984; LeDoux, 2007), located just anterior to the hippocampus within the medial temporal lobe. The amygdala has multiple important roles in emotional responses as well as effects on cognition, including the modulation of attention and visual perception (Phelps, Ling, & Carrasco, 2006; Vuilleumier, 2005). The close proximity of the amygdala and hippocampus, and the abundant neural interconnections between them, hint at their important functional interactions—particularly in the domain of declarative memory (Cahill & McGaugh, 1998; McGaugh, 2004; Phelps, 2004).

Declarative memory, encompassing memory for facts and world knowledge (semantic memory) and events (episodic memory) that can be brought voluntarily to mind from the past, depends critically on the integrity of the medial temporal lobe memory system, which includes the hippocampal region and its closely related adjacent neocortical regions (Eichenbaum, 2006; Squire & Zola-Morgan, 1991). To anticipate a major theme in this review, the amygdala enhances memory by increasing or modulating the activity of other brain systems involved in memory (Cahill & McGaugh, 1996a; McGaugh, 2004; Packard, Cahill, & McGaugh, 1994). Thus, rather than encoding and storing emotional declarative memory itself, the amygdala facilitates ongoing memory-encoding processes in other memory systems. In this way, the amygdala performs an evolutionarily adaptive role: enhancing and prioritizing memory encoding for emotionally salient events, to ensure that survival-relevant information will be available on future occasions.

A key principle that has emerged from studies of emotional memories is that, though they have important and unique characteristics not shared with nonemotional memories, they nevertheless constitute a particular category of declarative memory and thus share many similarities with ordinary, nonemotional memories, including basic encoding, storage, and retrieval processes. For example, like nonemotional memories, emotional memories benefit from enhanced attention, cognitive elaboration, and repetition (Dolan, 2002; Hamann, 2001). Although illustrations of emotional episodic memory often focus on highly arousing events (such as the September 11, 2001, terrorist attacks), it is important to note that emotion also enhances memory for considerably less arousing emotional stimuli and events (Bonnet, Bradley, Lang, & Requin, 1995; Bradley, Greenwald, Petry, & Lang, 1992). These less arousing positive and negative events, such as those encountered in everyday situations, also engage amygdala-mediated mechanisms of emotional memory enhancement, thus facilitating their study in the laboratory.

The primary focus of the current chapter is on cognitive and neural mechanisms underlying the effects of positive and negative emotion on declarative memory for stimuli and events in humans. Emotional events also give rise to implicit or nondeclarative memory representations, such as conditioned fear responses, which exist in parallel with declarative emotional memories and can interact to guide behavior (Schacter, 1992; Squire, Knowlton, & Musen, 1993); however, these are outside the scope of the current chapter (see the "What I Think" box for a brief discussion of the relationship between declarative and nondeclarative emotional memory). Although the focus is on human studies, basic principles of emotional memory derived from animal studies have been highly influential in guiding human research, and so these principles are briefly summarized. Findings from a variety of methodological approaches are examined, including functional and structural neuroimaging studies, neuropsychological studies of patients with brain lesions, and psychophysiological and pharmacological studies.

Because the vast majority of studies have examined the enhancing effects of emotion on declarative memory, this chapter concentrates on these facilitatory effects, rather than on the impairing effects of emotion on memory. However, since the impairing effects of emotion on memory can potentially shed light on mechanisms underlying memory enhancement, these effects are briefly considered. Studies examining the amygdala's role take center stage, together with the amygdala's interactions with the medial temporal lobe memory system and neocortical regions important for declarative memory encoding and retrieval, including the prefrontal cortex. Following a brief overview of key emotion-related phenomena that occur during encoding, storage, and retrieval, the results of studies linking these phenomena to the function of the amygdala are reviewed. Finally, some key theoretical questions about the nature of the amygdala's role in declarative memory are discussed, concluding with a summary and overview of future directions.

STAGES OF EMOTIONAL MEMORY: ENCODING, STORAGE, AND RETRIEVAL

Figure 8.1 illustrates the three primary stages of emotional memory processing: (1) "encoding," the cognitive and neural events that form the initial memory representation for an emotional episode; (2) "storage," the processes by which the initially encoded memory is maintained until the memory is retrieved (including dynamic processes such as consolidation, which change the memory representation into a more enduring form); and (3) "retrieval," the cognitive and neural events involved in reactivating and reconstructing aspects of the stored memory representation. At each of these stages of memory processing, the amygdala and closely interconnected brain regions play important roles.

Current theories of emotion propose a dimensional approach to emotion, in which emotional responses can be characterized according to their arousal (emotional intensity) and degree of pleasantness or unpleasantness (valence). According to this view, the majority of emotion's effects can be understood by considering these two underlying affective dimensions, rather than on the basis of specific emotional categories such as fear or anger (Bradley et al., 1992; Ekman, 1992; Russell, 2003). Considerable evidence indicates that emotional arousal, rather than valence, is the primary factor that deter-

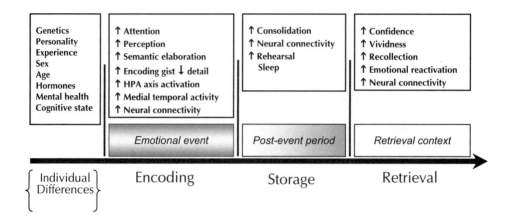

FIGURE 8.1. Stages of processing for emotional declarative memories and key associated amygdala-related factors. Illustrated are encoding, storage, and retrieval processes, which either are modulated by amygdala-mediated effects (e.g., increased attention at encoding, consolidation, enhanced vividness during retrieval), or modulate the mechanisms responsible for these effects (e.g., individual differences such as personality that affect emotional reactivity; sleep). ↑, increased; ↓, decreased; HPA, hypothalamic–pituitary–adrenal axis neurohormonal release.

mines the strength of emotional effects on declarative memory (Bradley et al., 1992; Cahill & McGaugh, 1998; Lang, Greenwald, Bradley, & Hamm, 1993; McGaugh, 2006).

To help illustrate some important phenomena associated with emotional memory across these three stages, consider this brief emotional scenario: While driving home from work, you suddenly see a neighbor's dog dart in front of your car. Reacting quickly, you narrowly miss the dog, swerving and hitting a mailbox. Though you are unhurt, your heart races. A moment later, realizing that you safely avoided the dog, you feel a wave of relief. The emotional arousal experienced during this episode is likely to trigger substantially increased encoding-related activity in the amygdala and related brain structures involved in emotional responses, setting into motion a cascade of processes both during and after the event that combine to increase the strength and subjective richness of the memory representation for the event (relative to emotionally neutral events, such as a similar but neutral scenario in which the dog remains on the sidewalk as you pass by).

Encoding

Emotional influences at encoding comprise a variety of effects, such as enhanced and focused attention; enhanced and altered perception; greater richness of elaborative, semantic processing of the stimulus attributes and meaning of the event; and enhanced activity in key memory-encoding regions, including the amygdala, the hippocampus and adjacent cortical regions, and the prefrontal cortex (Figure 8.1). When an emotionally arousing event is experienced, attention is attracted to the source of the emotional arousal, focusing enhanced attention on emotionally central aspects of the event (Armony & Dolan, 2002; Bradley, Codispoti, Cuthbert, & Lang, 2001; Easterbrook, 1959; Vuilleumier, 2005). Increased arousal also boosts attention more globally through increased alertness and physiological activation (Lang, Bradley, & Cuthbert, 1990). In the example given above, the darting dog elicits both increased attention and focused attention, which in turn will enhance declarative memory encoding through facilitation of more elaborative semantic encoding. Visual perception is also enhanced for emotionally salient stimuli through modulatory effects of the amygdala (Adolphs, 2004; Bar et al., 2006; Phelps et al., 2006). Although central elements of an emotional event are enhanced, peripheral, unrelated elements typically receive reduced attention, due to competition for limited cognitive resources. This "narrowing of attention" with increasing emotional arousal can be considered adaptive, because it focuses limited attentional resources on potentially survival-relevant emotional stimuli, ensuring that memory for the emotionally salient meaning or gist of the episode will be preferentially encoded (Adolphs, Denburg, & Tranel, 2001; Easterbrook, 1959).

At the neural level, emotional arousal triggers increased amygdala activity, which in turn modulates and enhances memory-related activity in the medial temporal lobe memory system via up-regulation of activity in the hippocampus, entorhinal cortex, and related cortical structures (McGaugh, 2004). This modulation of medial temporal lobe activity by the amygdala also increases temporally correlated activity among these structures, further enhancing memory encoding. Electrophysiological studies in animals indicate that emotional arousal increases synchrony between neuronal firing in the amygdala and hippocampus at the theta frequency, and that this effect enhances memory-related plasticity (Paré, Collins, & Pelletier, 2002). This enhanced functional connectivity is then recapitulated during the successful retrieval of emotional memories.

Highly arousing emotional events also trigger the release of adrenal stress hormones, chiefly adrenaline and cortisol, both during and after the event (Cahill, Gorski, & Le, 2003; Cahill & McGaugh, 1996b; McGaugh et al., 1993). These adrenergic and glucocorticoid hormones interact in complex ways mediated by the hypothalamic–pituitary–adrenal axis to modulate the consolidation of emotional declarative memory through amygdala-dependent mechanisms (Cahill & McGaugh, 1996b). These modulatory effects typically enhance memory, even for highly emotional stimuli such as violent films. However, it has been proposed that for some events, such as emotionally traumatic experiences that lie at the extreme upper end of the arousal continuum, the cognitive and neurohormonal responses precipitated by trauma may instead impair memory or even induce amnesia for the traumatic event. The evidence supporting these proposals remains equivocal, however, with most studies finding enhanced rather than impaired memory (LaBar & Cabeza, 2006; Rothbaum & Davis, 2003). Administration of cortisol in the absence of adrenergic activation can impair working memory and declarative memory, however, illustrating that mechanisms exist for potential memory-impairing effects of trauma (Buchanan, Tranel, & Adolphs, 2006a).

Studies of emotional memory have focused primarily on encoding, in part because of the memory modulation view, which posits a more important role for the amygdala during this stage (McGaugh, 2000). A key theoretical distinction exists between cases where memory is enhanced for an event that is intrinsically emotionally arousing, and cases where memory for a neutral stimulus is enhanced when it is experienced at the same time as an arousing event. Most studies have examined the former cases, but enhancing effects of emotional arousal have also been demonstrated for neutral events in emotional contexts, typically those that are related temporally and semantically to an emotionally arousing event (Anderson, Wais, & Gabrieli, 2006; Mather, 2007).

Storage and Consolidation

After an emotional event has ended, the nascent memory representation has not yet reached its final state. New episodic memories are hypothesized to undergo a process called "consolidation," which converts them into a more permanent form that is resistant to forgetting and interference (McGaugh, 2000). This process is thought to be gradual, taking an extended period to complete; estimates of the time required for consolidation to occur vary widely, from hours to years (McGaugh, 2004; Squire & Zola-Morgan, 1991). Emotional arousal has been hypothesized to facilitate the consolidation process through several different amygdala-mediated mechanisms. Because consolidation processes unfold gradually over time, these emotion-related effects on consolidation should not be detectable immediately after an event, but should instead evolve gradually over the postevent period. Adrenergic and glucocorticoid effects initiated during the encoding of an emotional event continue to modulate the consolidation of the memory trace after the end of the event. For example, episodic memory for the dog incident will subsequently undergo enhanced consolidation, due to stress hormones released during encoding. Growing evidence strongly suggests that consolidation of emotional memories takes place preferentially during sleep, particularly the rapid-eye-movement stage of sleep (Holland & Lewis, 2007; Wagner, Hallschmid, Rasch, & Born, 2006). In addition to these effects, cognitive processes (e.g., increased rehearsal of and rumination over the emotional event) can also reinforce and strengthen the emotional memories (LaBar & Cabeza, 2006).

Retrieval

During retrieval, retrieval cues initiate the reconstruction of the stored memory. This process involves not only retrieving stored information from the episode, but also frequently reexperiencing the originally experienced emotional responses. For example, seeing the neighbor's dog again a month later may trigger an involuntary recollection of the accident, complete with reexperiencing aspects of the emotional responses encoded during the episode. Alternatively, the same memory may be elicited through voluntary retrieval.

Emotional memory retrieval is frequently associated with a heightened feeling of vividness and confidence, relative to neutral memory retrieval. One aspect of the enhancement of episodic memory by emotion is enhanced recollection, a type of episodic memory accompanied by the retrieval of specific contextual details about the episode, rather than familiarity, where an episode is known to have been experienced previously but where the specific contextual details cannot be retrieved (Tulving, 1987; Yonelinas, 2001). Preferential effects of emotional arousal on recollection fit with studies that suggest a special role for the hippocampus in mediating recollection, and with the memory modulation view, which proposes that the hippocampus is the primary target of amgydala modulation. Although emotional arousal during encoding is typically associated with increased memory accuracy, recent theoretical interest has focused on situations where individuals can express very high confidence in emotional memories that are nonetheless objectively inaccurate (Schmolck, Buffalo, & Squire, 2000; Sharot, Delgado, & Phelps, 2004; Sharot, Martorella, Delgado, & Phelps, 2007).

Individual Differences

Emotional experiences and emotional memories associated with the same event can differ markedly among individuals as they are diffracted through the prism of individual differences in personality, genetic phenotype, prior experience, age, sex, and current mental and somatic state (see Figure 8.1) (Canli, 2007; Canli, Desmond, Zhao, & Gabrieli, 2002; Hamann, 2005a, 2005b; Hamann & Canli, 2004). For example, the emotional response and amygdala activation to the darting dog in the illustrative scenario are likely to be accentuated for an individual high in neuroticism (Canli, 2004); for a carrier of a genetic variant of the serotonin transporter gene that is linked to enhanced negative affect and increased amygdala response (Canli, 2007); or for a dog aficionado.

An intriguing example of genetic influences on emotional memory was reported in a study that examined the relation between variations in the alpha-2b-adrenergic receptor and emotional memory (de Quervain et al., 2007). Individuals with a deletion variant of the alpha-2b-adrenergic receptor showed an substantial enhancement of emotional memory for positive and negative emotional pictures (Figure 8.2), compared to individuals without the

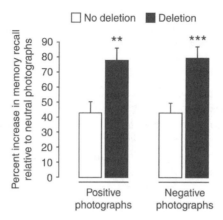

FIGURE 8.2. Genetic variation associated with enhanced emotional memory. Individuals with the deletion variant of the alpha-2b-adrenoreceptor have substantially enhanced memory for emotional photographs, of both positive and negative emotional stimuli. From de Quervain et al. (2007). Copyright 2007 by the Nature Publishing Group. Adapted by permission.

deletion variant, though emotional reactivity did not differ. In a traumatized group of Rwandan civil war survivors, this same deletion variant was linked to increased reexperiencing symptoms of posttraumatic stress disorder. This association between enhanced emotional memory effects and psychopathology is in line with theoretical views that implicate dysfunction of amygdala-dependent emotional memory mechanisms in various mood and anxiety disorders (de Quervain, 2008).

The next several sections address key findings and principles gleaned from studies of emotional memory and the role of the amygdala that have used pharmacological, neuropsychological, and neuroimaging approaches.

STRESS HORMONES AND EMOTIONAL MEMORY

Stress hormones released during and after an emotional event can strongly influence emotional memory encoding and consolidation. Initial human studies of the effects of adrenergic modulation on declarative memory were motivated by similar studies in animals, which established such basic principles as the central role of the amygdala in mediating emotional memory, the modulatory influence of the amygdala on other memory systems, the effects of stress hormones and their amygdala-dependent effects, and the importance of consolidation as a period during which the amygdala modulates memories (McGaugh, 2000, 2002). These studies in turn set the stage for later neuropsychological and neuroimaging studies.

In animals, adrenergic receptor agonists enhance memory and antagonists impair performance in emotional memory tasks, even when administered during or after encoding, thus implicating postlearning consolidation processes (McGaugh & Roozendaal, 2002). Studies in humans have largely replicated the results obtained in animal studies: Administration of beta-adrenergic antagonists blocks the memory-enhancing effects of emotional arousal, and adrenergic agonists facilitate these effects, though less consistently (McGaugh, 2004; van Stegeren, 2008; van Stegeren, Everard, Cahill, McGaugh, & Gooren, 1998). These modulatory effects are thought to be mediated by central receptors in the brain (van Stegeren, 2008), because antagonists that do not cross the blood–brain barrier (e.g., nadolol) are ineffective (see Figure 8.3). Studies that have combined functional neuroimaging during emotional memory tasks with administration of beta-adrenergic antagonists have found that amygdala activation related to the enhancing effect of emotion on memory is greatly diminished under beta-adrenergic blockade (Strange & Dolan, 2004). Behavioral stress manipulations (e.g., having subjects hold their hands in ice water) also retroactively enhance memory for material presented shortly beforehand, through endogenous release of stress hormones (Andreano & Cahill, 2006; Cahill et al., 2003).

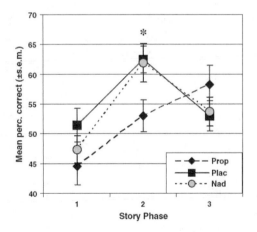

FIGURE 8.3. Central, but not peripheral, blockade of beta-adrenergic receptors impairs the enhancing effect of emotional arousal on memory. Memory results for recognition of information from three phases of an arousing illustrated story are shown for three separate drug groups. Propranolol, which reaches central beta-adrenergic receptors in the brain, blocked the boost to memory observed in the placebo group in the emotionally arousing phase 2 of the story (phases 1 and 3 are emotionally neutral). However, nadolol, a beta-adrenergic antagonist that does not cross the blood–brain barrier, did not block the emotional memory enhancement. Prop, propranolol; Plac, placebo; Nad, nadolol. From van Stegeren et al. (2008). Copyright 2008 by Elsevier. Adapted by permission.

NEUROPSYCHOLOGICAL STUDIES

Neuropsychological studies of emotional memory seek to determine the functional roles of particular brain regions by examining memory performance in patients with focal lesions. Such studies can establish whether a particular region is critical for emotional memory, but because disease processes rarely affect the amygdala selectively, extra-amygdalar damage can complicate interpretation of observed impairments. According to the memory modulation view, amygdala lesions in humans would be predicted to reduce or eliminate the enhancing effect of emotion on declarative memory, but should not impair memory for nonemotional, neutral stimuli (McGaugh, 2004). Thus the effect of amygdala lesions on memory should only be observed for emotionally salient stimuli, and rather than producing amnesia for emotional events, amygdala damage should instead cause emotional events to lose their memory boost due to emotion. To anticipate the findings of several studies, these predictions have largely been confirmed in neuropsychological studies of patients with amygdala lesions.

The amygdala also has an important role in emotional responses (Dolan, 2002; LeDoux, 1993, 2007; Phelps & LeDoux, 2005), so before concluding that amygdala lesions specifically affect emotional memory per se, it is critical to demonstrate first that any effects of amygdala lesions are not secondary to more basic impairments in emotionality. Several studies have shown that both subjective reports of valence and arousal, and physiological arousal responses (such as skin conductance responses), are not significantly impaired in patients with either unilateral or bilateral lesions to the amygdala (Adolphs & Spezio, 2006; Adolphs, Tranel, & Buchanan, 2005; Anderson & Phelps, 2002; Buchanan, Tranel, & Adolphs, 2006b; Hamann, Cahill, & Squire, 1997). Thus it appears unlikely that the effects of amygdala damage on emotional memory are generally due to attenuated emotionality. However, two recent studies have reopened this issue by reporting that trained clinicians can detect emotional abnormalities in patients with amygdala damage (Tranel, Gullickson, Koch, & Adolphs, 2006), and that subjective affective ratings of negative (but not positive) emotional stimuli are also affected (Berntson, Bechara, Damasio, Tranel, & Cacioppo, 2007). Further study of this issue is needed, particularly with respect to determining whether any deficits in emotionality may contribute to observed deficits in emotional memory.

Patients with bilateral lesions of the amygdala in general exhibit considerably stronger and more consistent emotional memory deficits than do patients with unilateral lesions, probably because of partial hemispheric redundancy of function or reorganization after unilateral lesions. Bilateral amygdala lesions have the expected effect of diminishing the enhancement of emotional memory. This effect has been shown for both negative and positive stimuli, and with a variety of stimuli, including words, sentences, pictures, faces, and films (Cahill, Babinsky, Markowitsch, & McGaugh, 1995; Hurlemann et al., 2007;

Markowitsch et al., 1994; Siebert, Markowitsch, & Bartel, 2003). Impairment in amygdala-mediated consolidation of emotional memory for emotional words has also been reported (LaBar & Phelps, 1998). Similar impairments in emotional memory enhancement have been found in neurodegenerative disorders such as Alzheimer's disease, where atrophy of the amygdala can occur together with other temporal lobe neuropathology (Hamann, Monarch, & Goldstein, 2000; Kensinger, Anderson, Growdon, & Corkin, 2004; Mori et al., 1999). Damage to the hippocampus that spares the amygdala impairs declarative memory, but does not selectively block emotional enhancement of recall or recognition (Buchanan, 2007; Buchanan, Tranel, & Adolphs, 2005, 2006b; Hamann, Cahill, McGaugh, & Squire, 1997; Hamann, Cahill, & Squire, 1997).

Emotional stimuli typically differ from neutral stimuli on other factors besides emotional arousal, including semantic characteristics, distinctiveness, and self-relevance (Bradley et al., 1992; Bradley & Lang, 1994). These stimulus factors can also contribute to enhanced memory for emotional stimuli, but these effects are independent of arousal-based effects mediated by the amygdala, as demonstrated by the preservation of these effects in patients with amygdala lesions. For example, patients with amygdala lesions after temporal lobectomy have been show to exhibit preserved enhancement of emotional memory for emotionally negative words, but not highly arousing words (Phelps, LaBar, & Spencer, 1997). Neuroimaging studies suggest that such amygdala-independent effects depend on such regions as the left inferior prefrontal cortex, which is important for mediating rich, elaborative processing (Kensinger & Corkin, 2004).

Although the amygdala has been characterized as modulating hippocampal memory function unidirectionally (McGaugh, 2004), findings from a combined neuropsychological and neuroimaging study suggest that the hippocampus also modulates amygdala activity during emotional memory encoding, implicating bidirectional amygdalohippocampal interactions (Richardson, Strange, & Dolan, 2004) (see Figure 8.4). Patients with varying degrees of temporal lobe sclerosis underwent functional magnetic resonance imaging (fMRI) as they encoded negative and neutral words. Patients with more severe hippocampal pathology had decreased activity in the left amygdala for successfully encoded emotional words, demonstrating for the first time a hippocampal modulatory influence on amygdala-mediated emotional encoding processes. The expected converse relationship showing amygdala modulation of hippocampal function was also observed, confirming the bidirectional nature of the modulation. This study illustrates the potential for combined methodological approaches to uncover complex emotional memory mechanisms.

The effects of medial temporal lobe damage on retrieval of recent and remote autobiographical memories were examined in a group of temporal lobectomy patients (Buchanan et al., 2006b). Patients with right amygdala

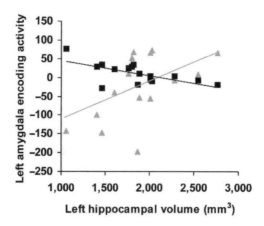

FIGURE 8.4. Codependence of the amygdala and hippocampus during the encoding of emotional words. Patients with more severe hippocampal pathology due to sclerosis had decreased activity in the left amygdala for successfully encoded emotional words. This relationship was highly specific to negative emotionality, and the corresponding converse relationship was also observed between severity of amygdala pathology and hippocampal encoding-related activity. Light triangles indicate data for emotional words (each symbol represents an individual patient); dark squares indicate corresponding data for neutral words. From Richardson, Strange, and Dolan (2004). Copyright 2004 by the Nature Publishing Group. Adapted by permission.

lesions recollected more high-intensity pleasant autobiographical memories and fewer high-intensity unpleasant memories, whereas patients with left amygdala lesions recalled fewer high-intensity positive memories and more high-intensity negative memories. These findings and those of a related study (Buchanan et al., 2005) point to complex interactions between arousal and valence in the recruitment of retrieval processes in the anteromedial temporal lobe.

NEUROIMAGING STUDIES

Neuroimaging at Encoding

Neuroimaging studies of emotional memory encoding complement neuropsychological and other approaches by identifying brain regions and regional networks in which increased activity during encoding is related to successful memory retrieval on later tests. The predictions of the memory modulation view, in which the amygdala enhances declarative memory by modulating activity in the medial temporal lobe memory system and related regions such as the prefrontal cortex (McGaugh, 2004, 2006), have been investigated in neuroimaging studies using positron emission tomography (PET) and fMRI.

In the first neuroimaging study to establish a link between amygdala activity at encoding and later emotional declarative memory, Cahill and colleagues (1996) scanned subjects with PET as they viewed highly emotionally negative or neutral films. Subjects who showed increased brain activity at encoding in the right amygdala remembered more of the emotional films on a recall test given 3 weeks later than did subjects with lower activity, and this relationship was specific to emotional stimuli. A later study (Hamann, Ely, Grafton, & Kilts, 1999) (see Figure 8.5) replicated and extended this study with positive and negative picture stimuli, showing in a PET study that bilateral amygdala activity assessed during encoding of these stimuli was highly correlated with the subsequent emotional enhancement of recognition memory for these stimuli assessed 1 month later. Consistent with the memory modulation view, hippocampal activity was correlated with amygdala activity. Activity in the ventral striatum, a region implicated in reward, was highly correlated with memory for positive (but not for negative) emotional stimuli; these results were consistent with findings of a later study (Adcock, Thangavel, Whitfield-Gabrieli, Knutson, & Gabrieli, 2006) that reward-related activity in the ventral striatum can enhance declarative memory for positive emotional stimuli.

Later studies have used event-related fMRI methods, which permit investigation of neural responses to individual items. Canli, Zhao, Brewer, Gabri-

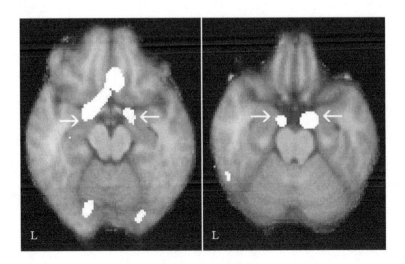

FIGURE 8.5. Amygdala activity at encoding predicts subsequent memory. Bilateral amygdala activation (arrows) predicts enhancement of memory on a subsequent recognition test, for both emotionally positive (left panel) and emotionally negative (right panel) picture stimuli. The contiguous white regions indicate where greater activity during encoding predicts subsequent emotional memory enhancement. L, left hemisphere; the left hemisphere is on the left side of each image. From Hamann, Ely, Grafton, and Kilts (1999). Copyright 1999 by the Nature Publishing Group. Adapted by permission.

eli, and Cahill (2000) used event-related fMRI to examine the encoding of
negative and neutral pictures, and found that left amygdala activity predicted
emotional memory enhancement for negative pictures—but only for highly
arousing pictures, suggesting that a minimum threshold of arousal may exist
below which amygdala activation does not modulate memory. Consistent with
this, Kensinger and Corkin (2004) showed that the memory advantage for low-
arousal emotional words was linked to activity in the hippocampus and prefrontal cortex, but not in the amygdala—results reflecting enhanced semantic
elaboration and related processes that also enhance memory for nonemotional
stimuli. Like many studies of emotional memory encoding, this study used the
so-called "subsequent memory" paradigm to contrast activity at encoding for
items that were subsequently remembered versus items that were forgotten.
In this paradigm, regions whose encoding activity predicts subsequent emotional memory are inferred to play a preferential role in emotional-memory-
encoding mechanisms. Individual differences can also influence neural correlates of emotional encoding. For example (Figure 8.6), a sex difference in
hemispheric lateralization of emotional memory encoding has been found, in

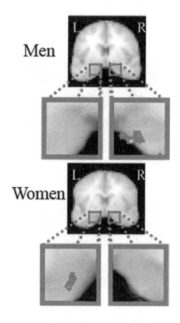

FIGURE 8.6. Hemispheric sex difference in amygdala activation during encoding
is correlated with emotional memory enhancement for negative emotionally arousing pictures. Amygdala activation during encoding predicts later emotional memory
enhancement in both men and women, but this activation is observed in the right
amygdala for men and in the left amygdala in women. From Canli, Desmond, Zhao,
and Gabrieli (2002). Copyright 2002 by the National Academy of Sciences, U.S.A.
Adapted by permission.

which men show right-lateralized amygdala activity that predicts later emotional memory, whereas women have corresponding left-lateralized amygdala activity (Canli et al., 2002). Although the psychological correlates of this sex difference are unclear, the authors suggested that it may be related to aspects of superior emotional memory ability reported for women.

Further support for the memory modulation view was reported in a study that used the subsequent memory paradigm to examine the relation between encoding activity and later cued recall for positive, negative, and neutral pictures (Dolcos, LaBar, & Cabeza, 2004). In addition to finding amygdala and medial temporal lobe activity during encoding that predicted subsequent successful emotional memory, success-related activity in the amygdala and entorhinal cortex was significantly intercorrelated for emotional (but not neutral) items, strongly supporting the view that the amygdala enhances declarative memory through increased modulatory connections with the medial temporal lobe memory system, as well as with the prefrontal cortex (Greenberg et al., 2005; LaBar & Cabeza, 2006; Richardson et al., 2004).

Neuroimaging at Retrieval

Retrieval of emotional memories has received less attention in neuroimaging studies to date, in part because of the emphasis in the memory modulation view on encoding and consolidation processes (McGaugh, 2004). Retrieval studies have examined both the retrieval of emotional events and memory retrieval of emotional contexts associated with neutral stimuli. Many of the same brain structures that are involved during emotional memory encoding are also active during retrieval, but their role during retrieval appears to be associated more with enhancing the subjective experience of remembering and retrieval of affective characteristics present during encoding than with enhancing accurate retrieval.

Dolcos, LaBar, and Cabeza (2005) used fMRI to examine recognition of emotional pictures that had been studied a year prior to scanning. Successful recognition of positive and negative emotional pictures elicited greater activation of the amygdala, hippocampus, and other medial temporal regions, particularly the entorhinal cortex; moreover, the activations in the amygdala and hippocampus were specific to recognition that was accompanied by recollection of contextual details. As predicted by the memory modulation view, the interaction between these regions also strongly predicted retrieval success for emotional items, as indexed, for example, by correlations between retrieval-success-related activations in the amygdala and entorhinal cortex (Figure 8.7).

Sharot and colleagues (2004) also examined brain activation during recognition of emotional and neutral pictures with fMRI, finding different neural correlates related to recollection for emotional versus neutral pictures (Figure 8.8). Amygdala activity during retrieval, but not activation of medial temporal lobe structures such as the parahippocampal cortex, was related

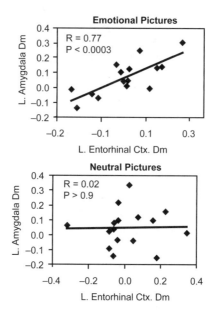

FIGURE 8.7. Stronger correlation for emotional than for neutral stimuli between activity in the left amygdala and left entorhinal cortex during encoding, which accurately predicts subsequent retrieval success. The increased coupling between activity in the amygdala and medial temporal lobe regions involved in declarative memory during successful encoding of emotional events supports the view that the amygdala influences memory encoding by modulating medial temporal lobe activity. Dm, difference in encoding activity for items subsequently remembered versus forgotten; L, left; Ctx., cortex. From Dolcos, LaBar, and Cabeza (2004). Copyright 2004 by Elsevier. Adapted by permission.

to recollection for emotional pictures; for neutral pictures, the opposite pattern was observed. Importantly, because accuracy did not differ between emotional and neutral items, the correlation between amygdala activation and recollection suggested that for emotional events the amygdala contributes to the subjective sense of recollection, but not to an increase in memory accuracy. This is consistent with behavioral dissociations between influences of emotion on memory confidence versus accuracy (Schacter & Slotnick, 2004; Schmolck et al., 2000).

In a study of autobiographical memory, Greenberg and colleagues (2005) used fMRI together with functional connectivity analyses to examine patterns of connectivity during retrieval of emotional autobiographical memories. Extending similar previous findings by Dolcos and colleagues (2005), this study found that the amygdala's interactions with medial temporal lobe memory regions and the prefrontal cortex were enhanced during emotional retrieval, indicating that dynamic interaction between the amygdala and related retrieval networks occurs during retrieval of both laboratory-induced and real-world autobiographical memories (Cabeza & St. Jacques, 2007).

Neuroimaging studies of retrieval of neutral stimuli encoded in emotional contexts have also reported amygdala activation and enhanced amygdala connectivity. Maratos, Dolan, Morris, Henson, and Rugg (2001) examined retrieval during recognition of neutral words that had been studied in either emotionally negative, positive, or neutral contexts. Whereas activation in the temporal pole was related to the attempt to retrieve emotional contexts, the

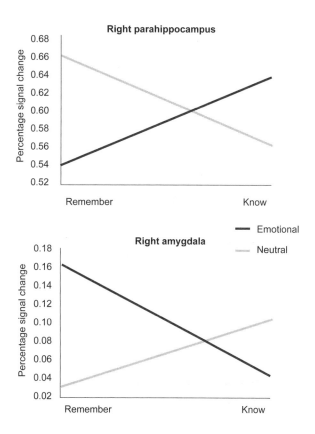

FIGURE 8.8. Amygdala activity at retrieval indexes subjective recollection. Increased right amygdala activity during a recognition test for picture stimuli correlates positively with increased subjective sense of recollection for emotional (but not neutral) pictures. In contrast, posterior parahippocampal activity correlates positively with recollection for neutral (but not emotional) stimuli. Remember indicates that the subject endorses test item as previously experienced, with concurrent retrieval of accompanying contextual details; Know indicates that the subject endorses test item as previously experienced, but with no ability to recollect the context of the item's occurrence. From Sharot, Delgado, and Phelps (2004). Copyright 2004 by the Nature Publishing Group. Adapted by permission.

amygdala was active during the successful retrieval of emotional contexts, suggesting a neural dissociation between retrieval mode and retrieval success. Smith, Stephan, Rugg, and Dolan (2006) also used fMRI to examine retrieval of emotional contexts. Successful retrieval of emotional context information was associated with enhanced bidirectional amygdalohippocampal connectivity, in line with similar interactions identified by Richardson and colleagues (2004) at encoding. Somerville, Wig, Whalen, and Kelley (2006) reported in an fMRI retrieval study that faces that had been studied with positive or negative personal affective descriptions (e.g., "John volunteers at charities") elicited activation of the amygdala even for faces for which subjects failed to remember the affective descriptions; these findings suggested that retrieval of amygdala-mediated affective information may occur without awareness.

In summary, during retrieval, regions involved in successful emotional memory encoding become reactivated and more highly functionally interconnected. Though elucidation of the full implications of these regional activations and interactions must await further study, findings to date point to an important role for the amygdala and amygdala-dependent connectivity in generating the subjective recollective experience of remembering emotional events and retrieving affective information experienced during encoding.

EMOTIONAL AROUSAL AND EMOTIONAL MEMORY

Throughout this chapter, emotional arousal has consistently figured as the primary factor driving emotional memory mechanisms. However, emotional arousal is a multidimensional construct that has subjective, physiological, and neural aspects, which are often only moderately intercorrelated (Cuthbert, Bradley, & Lang, 1996; Cuthbert, Schupp, Bradley, Birbaumer, & Lang, 2000; Lang, Bradley, & Cuthbert, 1998). The potential independent influences of each aspect of arousal on emotional memory await further investigation. A related question concerns the quantitative relationship between emotional arousal and emotional memory. The evidence reviewed here points to a markedly nonlinear relation, with low levels of arousal engaging prefrontal mechanisms involved in semantic elaboration, and moderate to high levels of arousal engaging emotion-specific mechanisms coordinated by the amygdala. However, thresholds for triggering amygdala-dependent emotional memory mechanisms differ substantially across studies. Challenges for future study will include systematically characterizing the conditions under which special emotional memory mechanisms are invoked, and relating these to underlying neurobiological processes. A further question concerns the integration across time scales between the operation of different amygdala-dependent emotional memory effects. Some emotional effects, such as attentional enhancement, exert fast, immediate effects at encoding; other influences, such as stress hormones and consolidation during sleep, operate more slowly. The mechanisms by which these fast, immediate effects and slow, delayed effects may combine and interact to influence emotional memories are as yet little understood.

Although treated as a functional unit in this review, the amygdala in fact comprises several heterogeneous nuclei, each with its own characteristic functions and pattern of connectivity (Amaral & Price, 1984; LeDoux, 2007). Animal studies have identified the amygdala's basolateral nucleus as a key site of memory modulation effects; however, limitations in the spatial resolution of neuroimaging methods have precluded the reliable identification of corresponding functions of amygdala nuclei in humans, though a few fMRI studies have attempted less fine-grained attributions—for example, between dorsal and ventral parts of the amygdala (Mackiewicz, Sarinopoulos, Cleven, & Nitschke, 2006; Whalen et al., 1998). Development of improved neuroimaging techniques for dissecting the separate functions of amygdala nuclei in humans will open a new window into the cognitive and affective functions of the amygdala.

CONCLUSION

The enhanced persistence and unique subjective characteristics of memory for emotional events can be traced to a coordinated cascade of cognitive, neural, and physiological responses that are initiated when emotional arousal triggers emotional memory mechanisms orchestrated by the amygdala. The amygdala modulates emotional memory at each of the three stages of memory processing—with particularly strong effects occurring at the encoding stage, where emotional arousal enhances attention, perception, and cognitive elaboration, which combine to form an enhanced memory representation. Active processes such as consolidation and rehearsal continue to influence and transform the memory representation after the event. During the retrieval of an emotional event, reactivation of the amygdala appears to underlie the enhanced feeling of recollection often associated with emotional memory, as well as the reexperience of emotions felt during the encoding of the original event.

The principles and neurobiological models first established in animal studies of emotional memory have been further supported and elaborated in human studies of emotional memory. Investigations of emotional declarative memory in humans via lesion, drug, and neuroimaging methods have revealed new phenomena and mechanisms that have substantially expanded our understanding of this type of memory. Neuroimaging studies have also revealed the importance of interactions among the amygdala, the medial temporal lobe memory system, and the prefrontal cortex in emotional memory. Each of the emotional memory effects reviewed here may be further modulated by individual differences in sex, genetics, personality, and other factors, and greater understanding of these individual differences may in turn shed light on neurobiological factors influencing vulnerability to mental illness (Hamann

& Canli, 2004). The challenge for future studies will be to integrate different methods and theoretical approaches to further elucidate the cognitive and
other mechanisms that mediate emotional memory, and to determine how the
amygdala works in concert with other memory systems to adaptively enhance
memory for emotionally salient events.

WHAT I THINK

What is the amygdala's role in emotional memory? Before any attempt is made
to answer this question, it may help to first unpack some of its underlying assump-
tions—for example, the notion that the amygdala plays but a single major role in
emotional memory. In fact, although this chapter has focused on the amygdala and
declarative emotional memory (conscious memory for facts and events) (Squire &
Zola-Morgan, 1991), the amygdala plays a second major role in nondeclarative
emotional memory—for example, its role in mediating classical conditioning of fear
responses (LaBar & Cabeza, 2006). Perhaps a better question might be this: Is
there a common thread or principle that can help us understand and interconnect
the amygdala's multiple emotional memory functions? And more generally, what
is the relationship between the amygdala's memory functions and its other roles in
emotion and cognition (Phelps, 2006)?

   For both declarative and nondeclarative memory, the amygdala's role can
be characterized broadly as enhancing long-term memory for emotionally arousing, biologically salient stimuli and events, both appetitive and aversive in nature
(Dolan, 2002). This memorial role can be viewed as in effect extending all of the
amygdala's adaptive functions, such as detecting and reacting to emotionally arousing stimuli, outside the window of the immediate present; it does this by facilitating
access to prior affective states, preserving salient aspects of current affective states
for future access, and planning and prospective imagining of future affective events
(Sharot, Riccardi, Raio, & Phelps, 2007). Just as memories of past emotional experiences can substantially alter an individual's current cognitive and affective state
via effects on attention, motivation, perception, decision making, and social behavior, emotional events and responses encoded in the present can in turn potentially
influence future cognitive and affective states (Adolphs, 2003; Anderson & Phelps,
2001; Davidson & Irwin, 2002).

   Although the declarative and nondeclarative emotional memory systems serve
a broadly similar adaptive function by encoding survival-relevant information, they
operate largely independently and have different operating principles. For example,
in nondeclarative classical fear conditioning, associative memory traces are stored
within the amygdala, whereas for declarative emotional memory, the amygdala
modulates the encoding of memory traces in the hippocampus and related structures that ordinarily participate in nonemotional declarative memory (McGaugh,
2000, 2002; McGaugh et al., 1993; Packard et al., 1994).

   Experiencing an emotional event gives rise to simultaneous and independent
memory changes in these two parallel emotional memory systems, with both systems
combining to affect future behavior. The evolutionarily older nondeclarative system
supports the formation of novel affective associations and initiation of rapid affective responses to emotional stimuli; yet this amygdala-based nondeclarative system

lacks the specialized structures of the hippocampus and the adjacent structures in the parahippocampal region that support representations of emotional events in declarative memory. In its modulatory role, the amygdala influences memory for emotionally arousing events in other memory systems—most notably the declarative system, but also other systems, such as skill and habit learning based in the striatum (McGaugh, Cahill, & Roozendaal, 1996; Packard et al., 1994). By modulating activity in these other memory systems rather than encoding traces within itself, the amygdala can flexibly influence multiple memory systems. This modular framework is inherently adaptive, because it allows each memory system to evolve independently of the amygdala's modulatory influence.

To return to the question posed at the outset regarding the role of the amygdala in emotional memory, it should now be evident that the amygdala plays multiple roles as it interacts with multiple memory systems, so that a complete answer must address the complex nature of the amygdala's memory functions. However, the common theme of preserving affective information to adaptively guide future responses connects these diverse roles of the amygdala in both the declarative and nondeclarative domains.

REFERENCES

Adcock, R. A., Thangavel, A., Whitfield-Gabrieli, S., Knutson, B., & Gabrieli, J. D. (2006). Reward-motivated learning: Mesolimbic activation precedes memory formation. *Neuron, 50*(3), 507–517.

Adolphs, R. (2003). Cognitive neuroscience of human social behaviour. *Nature Reviews Neuroscience, 4*(3), 165–178.

Adolphs, R. (2004). Emotional vision. *Nature Neuroscience, 7*(11), 1167–1168.

Adolphs, R., Denburg, N. L., & Tranel, D. (2001). The amygdala's role in long-term declarative memory for gist and detail. *Behavioral Neuroscience, 115*(5), 983–992.

Adolphs, R., & Spezio, M. (2006). Role of the amygdala in processing visual social stimuli. *Progress in Brain Research, 156,* 363–378.

Adolphs, R., Tranel, D., & Buchanan, T. W. (2005). Amygdala damage impairs emotional memory for gist but not details of complex stimuli. *Nature Neuroscience, 8*(4), 512–518.

Amaral, D. G., & Price, J. L. (1984). Amygdalo-cortical projections in the monkey (*Macaca fascicularis*). *Journal of Comparative Neurology, 230,* 465–496.

Anderson, A. K., & Phelps, E. A. (2001). Lesions of the human amygdala impair enhanced perception of emotionally salient events. *Nature, 411,* 305–309.

Anderson, A. K., & Phelps, E. A. (2002). Is the human amygdala critical for the subjective experience of emotion?: Evidence of intact dispositional affect in patients with amygdala lesions. *Journal of Cognitive Neuroscience, 14*(5), 709–720.

Anderson, A. K., Wais, P. E., & Gabrieli, J. D. E. (2006). Emotion enhances remembrance of neutral events past. *Proceedings of the National Academy of Sciences USA, 103*(5), 1599–1604.

Andreano, J. M., & Cahill, L. (2006). Glucocorticoid release and memory consolidation in men and women. *Psychological Science, 17*(6), 466–470.

Armony, J. L., & Dolan, R. J. (2002). Modulation of spatial attention by fear-conditioned stimuli: An event-related fMRI study. *Neuropsychologia, 40*(7), 817–826.

Bar, M., Kassam, K. S., Ghuman, A. S., Boshyan, J., Schmid, A. M., Dale, A. M., et al. (2006). Top-down facilitation of visual recognition. *Proceedings of the National Academy of Sciences USA, 103*(2), 449–454.

Berntson, G. G., Bechara, A., Damasio, H., Tranel, D., & Cacioppo, J. T. (2007). Amygdala contribution to selective dimensions of emotion. *Social Cognitive and Affective Neuroscience, 2*(2), 123–129.

Bonnet, M., Bradley, M. M., Lang, P. J., & Requin, J. (1995). Modulation of spinal reflexes: Arousal, pleasure, action. *Psychophysiology, 32*(4), 367–372.

Bradley, M. M., Codispoti, M., Cuthbert, B. N., & Lang, P. J. (2001). Emotion and motivation: I. Defensive and appetitive reactions in picture processing. *Emotion, 1*(3), 276–298.

Bradley, M. M., Greenwald, M. K., Petry, M. C., & Lang, P. J. (1992). Remembering pictures: Pleasure and arousal in memory. *Journal of Experimental Psychology: Learning, Memory, and Cognition, 18*(2), 379–390.

Bradley, M. M., & Lang, P. J. (1994). Measuring emotion: The self-assessment manikin and the semantic differential. *Journal of Behavior Therapy and Experimental Psychiatry, 25*(1), 49–59.

Buchanan, T. W. (2007). Retrieval of emotional memories. *Psychological Bulletin, 133*(5), 761–779.

Buchanan, T. W., Tranel, D., & Adolphs, R. (2005). Emotional autobiographical memories in amnesic patients with medial temporal lobe damage. *Journal of Neuroscience, 25*(12), 3151–3160.

Buchanan, T. W., Tranel, D., & Adolphs, R. (2006a). Impaired memory retrieval correlates with individual differences in cortisol response but not autonomic response. *Learning and Memory, 13*(3), 382–387.

Buchanan, T. W., Tranel, D., & Adolphs, R. (2006b). Memories for emotional autobiographical events following unilateral damage to medial temporal lobe. *Brain, 129*(Pt. 1), 115–127.

Cabeza, R., & St. Jacques, P. (2007). Functional neuroimaging of autobiographical memory. *Trends in Cognitive Sciences, 11*(5), 219–227.

Cahill, L., Babinsky, R., Markowitsch, H. J., & McGaugh, J. L. (1995). The amygdala and emotional memory. *Nature, 377*, 295–296.

Cahill, L., Gorski, L., & Le, K. (2003). Enhanced human memory consolidation with post-learning stress: Interaction with the degree of arousal at encoding. *Learning and Memory, 10*(4), 270–274.

Cahill, L., Haier, R. J., Fallon, J., Alkire, M. T., Tang, C., Keator, D., et al. (1996). Amygdala activity at encoding correlated with long-term, free recall of emotional information. *Proceedings of the National Academy of Sciences USA, 93*(15), 8016–8021.

Cahill, L., & McGaugh, J. L. (1996a). Modulation of memory storage. *Current Opinion in Neurobiology, 6*(2), 237–242.

Cahill, L., & McGaugh, J. L. (1996b). The neurobiology of memory for emotional events: Adrenergic activation and the amygdala. *Proceedings of the Western Pharmacology Society, 39*, 81–84.

Cahill, L., & McGaugh, J. L. (1998). Mechanisms of emotional arousal and lasting declarative memory. *Trends in Neurosciences, 21*(7), 294–299.

Canli, T. (2004). Functional brain mapping of extraversion and neuroticism: Learning from individual differences in emotion processing. *Journal of Personality, 72*(6), 1105–1132.

Canli, T. (2007). The emergence of genomic psychology: Insights from genomic analyses might allow psychologists to understand, predict and modify human behaviour. *EMBO Special Report No. 8,* S30–S34.

Canli, T., Desmond, J. E., Zhao, Z., & Gabrieli, J. D. (2002). Sex differences in the neural basis of emotional memories. *Proceedings of the National Academy of Sciences USA, 99*(16), 10789–10794.

Canli, T., Zhao, Z., Brewer, J., Gabrieli, J. D., & Cahill, L. (2000). Event-related activation in the human amygdala associates with later memory for individual emotional experience. *Journal of Neuroscience, 20,* RC99.

Cuthbert, B. N., Bradley, M. M., & Lang, P. J. (1996). Probing picture perception: Activation and emotion. *Psychophysiology, 33*(2), 103–111.

Cuthbert, B. N., Schupp, H. T., Bradley, M. M., Birbaumer, N., & Lang, P. J. (2000). Brain potentials in affective picture processing: Covariation with autonomic arousal and affective report. *Biological Psychology, 52*(2), 95–111.

Davidson, R. J., & Irwin, W. (2002). The functional neuroanatomy of emotion and affective style. In J. T. Cacioppo, G. G. Berntson, R. Adolphs, C. S. Carter, R. J. Davidson, M. K. McClintock, et al. (Eds.), *Foundations in social neuroscience* (pp. 473–486). Cambridge, MA: MIT Press.

de Quervain, D. J. (2008). Glucocorticoid-induced reduction of traumatic memories: Implications for the treatment of PTSD. *Progress in Brain Research, 167,* 239–247.

de Quervain, D. J., Kolassa, I. T., Ertl, V., Onyut, P. L., Neuner, F., Elbert, T., et al. (2007). A deletion variant of the alpha2b-adrenoceptor is related to emotional memory in Europeans and Africans. *Nature Neuroscience, 10*(9), 1137–1139.

Dolan, R. J. (2002). Emotion, cognition, and behavior. *Science, 298,* 1191–1194.

Dolcos, F., LaBar, K. S., & Cabeza, R. (2004). Interaction between the amygdala and the medial temporal lobe memory system predicts better memory for emotional events. *Neuron, 42*(5), 855–863.

Dolcos, F., LaBar, K. S., & Cabeza, R. (2005). Remembering one year later: Role of the amygdala and the medial temporal lobe memory system in retrieving emotional memories. *Proceedings of the National Academy of Sciences USA, 102*(7), 2626–2631.

Easterbrook, J. A. (1959). The effect of emotion on cue utilization and the organization of behavior. *Psychological Review, 66*(3), 183–201.

Eichenbaum, H. (2006). Remembering: Functional organization of the declarative memory system. *Current Biology, 16*(16), R643–645.

Ekman, P. (1992). Are there basic emotions? *Psychological Review, 99*(3), 550–553.

Greenberg, D. L., Rice, H. J., Cooper, J. J., Cabeza, R., Rubin, D. C., & Labar, K. S. (2005). Co-activation of the amygdala, hippocampus and inferior frontal gyrus during autobiographical memory retrieval. *Neuropsychologia, 43*(5), 659–674.

Hamann, S. (2001). Cognitive and neural mechanisms of emotional memory. *Trends in Cognitive Sciences, 5*(9), 394–400.

Hamann, S. (2005a). Blue genes: Wiring the brain for depression. *Nature Neuroscience, 8*(6), 701–703.

Hamann, S. (2005b). Sex differences in the responses of the human amygdala. *Neuroscientist, 11*(4), 288–293.

Hamann, S., & Canli, T. (2004). Individual differences in emotion processing. *Current Opinion in Neurobiology, 14*(2), 233–238.

Hamann, S. B., Cahill, L., McGaugh, J. L., & Squire, L. R. (1997). Intact enhancement of declarative memory for emotional material in amnesia. *Learning and Memory, 4*(3), 301–309.

Hamann, S. B., Cahill, L., & Squire, L. R. (1997). Emotional perception and memory in amnesia. *Neuropsychology, 11*(1), 104–113.

Hamann, S. B., Ely, T. D., Grafton, S. T., & Kilts, C. D. (1999). Amygdala activity related to enhanced memory for pleasant and aversive stimuli. *Nature Neuroscience, 2*(3), 289–293.

Hamann, S. B., Monarch, E. S., & Goldstein, F. C. (2000). Memory enhancement for emotional stimuli is impaired in early Alzheimer's disease. *Neuropsychology, 14*(1), 82–92.

Holland, P., & Lewis, P. A. (2007). Emotional memory: Selective enhancement by sleep. *Current Biology, 17*(5), R179–R181.

Hurlemann, R., Wagner, M., Hawellek, B., Reich, H., Pieperhoff, P., Amunts, K., et al. (2007). Amygdala control of emotion-induced forgetting and remembering: Evidence from Urbach–Wiethe disease. *Neuropsychologia, 45*(5), 877–884.

James, W. (1950). *The principles of psychology.* New York: Dover. (Original work published 1890)

Kensinger, E. A., Anderson, A., Growdon, J. H., & Corkin, S. (2004). Effects of Alzheimer disease on memory for verbal emotional information. *Neuropsychologia, 42*(6), 791–800.

Kensinger, E. A., & Corkin, S. (2004). Two routes to emotional memory: Distinct neural processes for valence and arousal. *Proceedings of the National Academy of Sciences USA, 101*(9), 3310–3315.

LaBar, K. S., & Cabeza, R. (2006). Cognitive neuroscience of emotional memory. *Nature Reviews Neuroscience, 7*(1), 54–64.

LaBar, K. S., & Phelps, E. A. (1998). Arousal-mediated memory consolidation: Role of the medial temporal lobe in humans. *Psychological Science, 9*, 527–540.

Lang, P. J., Bradley, M. M., & Cuthbert, B. N. (1990). Emotion, attention, and the startle reflex. *Psychological Review, 97*(3), 377–395.

Lang, P. J., Bradley, M. M., & Cuthbert, B. N. (1998). Emotion and motivation: Measuring affective perception. *Journal of Clinical Neurophysiology, 15*(5), 397–408.

Lang, P. J., Greenwald, M. K., Bradley, M. M., & Hamm, A. O. (1993). Looking at pictures: Affective, facial, visceral, and behavioral reactions. *Psychophysiology, 30*(3), 261–273.

LeDoux, J. E. (1993). Emotional memory systems in the brain. *Behavioural Brain Research, 58*(1–2), 69–79.

LeDoux, J. E. (2007). The amygdala. *Current Biology, 17*(20), R868–R874.

Mackiewicz, K. L., Sarinopoulos, I., Cleven, K. L., & Nitschke, J. B. (2006). The effect of anticipation and the specificity of sex differences for amygdala and hippocampus function in emotional memory. *Proceedings of the National Academy of Sciences USA, 103*(38), 14200–14205.

Maratos, E. J., Dolan, R. J., Morris, J. S., Henson, R. N., & Rugg, M. D. (2001).

Neural activity associated with episodic memory for emotional context. *Neuropsychologia, 39*(9), 910–920.

Markowitsch, H. J., Calabrese, P., Würker, M., Durwen, H. F., Kessler, J., Babinsky, R., et al. (1994). The amygdala's contribution to memory: A study on two patients with Urbach–Wiethe disease. *NeuroReport, 5*, 1349–1352.

Mather, M. (2007). Emotional arousal and memory binding: An object-based framework. *Perspectives on Psychological Science, 2*(1), 33–52.

McGaugh, J. L. (2000). Memory: A century of consolidation. *Science, 287*, 248–251.

McGaugh, J. L. (2002). Memory consolidation and the amygdala: A systems perspective. *Trends in Neurosciences, 25*(9), 456.

McGaugh, J. L. (2004). The amygdala modulates the consolidation of memories of emotionally arousing experiences. *Annual Review of Neuroscience, 27*, 1–28.

McGaugh, J. L. (2006). Make mild moments memorable: Add a little arousal. *Trends in Cognitive Sciences, 10*(8), 345–347.

McGaugh, J. L., Cahill, L., & Roozendaal, B. (1996). Involvement of the amygdala in memory storage: Interaction with other brain systems. *Proceedings of the National Academy of Sciences USA, 93*(24), 13508–13514.

McGaugh, J. L., Introini-Collison, I. B., Cahill, L. F., Castellano, C., Dalmaz, C., Parent, M. B., et al. (1993). Neuromodulatory systems and memory storage: Role of the amygdala. *Behavioural Brain Research, 58*(1–2), 81–90.

McGaugh, J. L., & Roozendaal, B. (2002). Role of adrenal stress hormones in forming lasting memories in the brain. *Current Opinion in Neurobiology, 12*, 205–210.

Mori, E., Ikeda, M., Hirono, N., Kitagaki, H., Imamura, T., & Shimomura, T. (1999). Amygdalar volume and emotional memory in Alzheimer's disease. *American Journal of Psychiatry, 156*(2), 216–222.

Packard, M. G., Cahill, L., & McGaugh, J. L. (1994). Amygdala modulation of hippocampal-dependent and caudate nucleus-dependent memory processes. *Proceedings of the National Academy of Sciences USA, 91*(18), 8477–8481.

Paré, D., Collins, D. R., & Pelletier, J. G. (2002). Amygdala oscillations and the consolidation of emotional memories. *Trends in Cognitive Sciences, 6*(7), 306–314.

Phelps, E. A. (2004). Human emotion and memory: Interactions of the amygdala and hippocampal complex. *Current Opinion in Neurobiology, 14*(2), 198–202.

Phelps, E. A. (2006). Emotion and cognition: Insights from studies of the human amygdala. *Annual Review of Psychology, 57*, 27–53.

Phelps, E. A., & Anderson, A. K. (1997). Emotional memory: What does the amygdala do? *Current Biology, 7*(5), R311–R314.

Phelps, E. A., LaBar, K. S., & Spencer, D. D. (1997). Memory for emotional words following unilateral temporal lobectomy. *Brain and Cognition, 35*(1), 85–109.

Phelps, E. A., & LeDoux, J. E. (2005). Contributions of the amygdala to emotion processing: From animal models to human behavior. *Neuron, 48*(2), 175–187.

Phelps, E. A., Ling, S., & Carrasco, M. (2006). Emotion facilitates perception and potentiates the perceptual benefits of attention. *Psychological Science, 17*(4), 292–299.

Richardson, M. P., Strange, B. A., & Dolan, R. J. (2004). Encoding of emotional memories depends on amygdala and hippocampus and their interactions. *Nature Neuroscience, 7*(3), 278–285.

Rothbaum, B. O., & Davis, M. (2003). Applying learning principles to the treatment of post-trauma reactions. *Annals of the New York Academy of Sciences, 1008*(1), 112–121.

Russell, J. A. (2003). Core affect and the psychological construction of emotion. *Psychological Review, 110*(1), 145–172.

Schacter, D. L. (1992). Understanding implicit memory: A cognitive neuroscience approach. *American Psychologist, 47*(4), 559–569.

Schacter, D. L., & Slotnick, S. D. (2004). The cognitive neuroscience of memory distortion. *Neuron, 44*(1), 149–160.

Schmolck, H., Buffalo, E. A., & Squire, L. R. (2000). Memory distortions develop over time: Recollections of the O. J. Simpson trial verdict after 15 and 32 months. *Psychological Science, 11*(1), 39–45.

Sharot, T., Delgado, M. R., & Phelps, E. A. (2004). How emotion enhances the feeling of remembering. *Nature Neuroscience, 7*(12), 1376–1380.

Sharot, T., Martorella, E. A., Delgado, M. R., & Phelps, E. A. (2007). How personal experience modulates the neural circuitry of memories of September 11. *Proceedings of the National Academy of Sciences USA, 104*(1), 389–394.

Sharot, T., Riccardi, A. M., Raio, C. M., & Phelps, E. A. (2007). Neural mechanisms mediating optimism bias. *Nature, 450*, 102-105.

Siebert, M., Markowitsch, H. J., & Bartel, P. (2003). Amygdala, affect and cognition: Evidence from 10 patients with Urbach–Wiethe disease. *Brain, 126*(Pt. 12), 2627–2637.

Smith, A. P., Stephan, K. E., Rugg, M. D., & Dolan, R. J. (2006). Task and content modulate amygdala–hippocampal connectivity in emotional retrieval. *Neuron, 49*(4), 631–638.

Somerville, L. H., Wig, G. S., Whalen, P. J., & Kelley, W. M. (2006). Dissociable medial temporal lobe contributions to social memory. *Journal of Cognitive Neuroscience, 18*(8), 1253–1265.

Squire, L. R., Knowlton, B., & Musen, G. (1993). The structure and organization of memory. *Annual Review of Psychology, 44*, 453–495.

Squire, L. R., & Zola-Morgan, S. (1991). The medial temporal lobe memory system. *Science, 253*, 1380–1386.

Strange, B. A., & Dolan, R. J. (2004). Beta-adrenergic modulation of emotional memory-evoked human amygdala and hippocampal responses. *Proceedings of the National Academy of Sciences USA, 101*(31), 11454–11458.

Tranel, D., Gullickson, G., Koch, M., & Adolphs, R. (2006). Altered experience of emotion following bilateral amygdala damage. *Cognitive Neuropsychiatry, 11*(3), 219–232.

Tulving, E. (1987). Multiple memory systems and consciousness. *Human Neurobiology, 6*(2), 67–80.

Tulving, E. (2002). Episodic memory: From mind to brain. *Annual Review of Psychology, 53*, 1–25.

van Stegeren, A. H. (2008). The role of the noradrenergic system in emotional memory. *Acta Psychologica, 127*(3), 532–541.

van Stegeren, A. H., Everaerd, W., Cahill, L., McGaugh, J. L., & Gooren, L. J. (1998). Memory for emotional events: Differential effects of centrally versus peripherally acting beta-blocking agents. *Psychopharmacology (Berlin), 138*(3–4), 305–310.

Vuilleumier, P. (2005). How brains beware: Neural mechanisms of emotional attention. *Trends in Cognitive Sciences, 9*(12), 585–594.

Wagner, U., Hallschmid, M., Rasch, B., & Born, J. (2006). Brief sleep after learning keeps emotional memories alive for years. *Biological Psychiatry, 60*(7), 788–790.

Whalen, P. J., Rauch, S. L., Etcoff, N. L., McInerney, S. C., Lee, M. B., & Jenike, M. A. (1998). Masked presentations of emotional facial expressions modulate amygdala activity without explicit knowledge. *Journal of Neuroscience, 18*(1), 411–418.

Yonelinas, A. P. (2001). Components of episodic memory: The contribution of recollection and familiarity. *Philosophical Transactions of the Royal Society of London, Series B, 356,* 1363–1374.

CHAPTER 9

The Human Amygdala
and the Control of Fear

Elizabeth A. Phelps

Research on the amygdala has highlighted its role in the acquisition, expression, and recognition of fear. Although the function of the amygdala extends beyond fear processing, our detailed understanding of its importance in fear, particularly Pavlovian fear conditioning, has formed the basis for the exploration of its broader role in emotion and social behavior (Phelps, 2006). Recently, many studies of fear processing and the human amygdala have shifted from understanding fear acquisition to examining the control of fear. The ability to control and modify emotional responses, especially fear, is critical for both adaptive behavior and the treatment of psychopathology. In this chapter, I review research on the role of the amygdala in the control of fear, starting with a brief introduction to the neural mechanisms identified in animal models and extending to investigations in humans.

Several techniques and approaches can be used to control fear. In general, these techniques highlight the amygdala's interaction with other neural structures, with the consequence being a diminished amygdala response in the presence of previously fear-eliciting events. Although the term "emotion regulation" has typically been used to describe the use of cognitive strategies to control emotion (Ochsner & Gross, 2005), in a broader sense all of these techniques are employed to regulate emotion—with some being applied via conscious effort, and others being more passive, automatic, or reflexive. To date, four primary techniques have been investigated as a means to control fear. Two of these techniques (extinction and cognitive regulation strategies) have been studied extensively in humans, whereas the other techniques (active coping and the blockade of reconsolidation) have, so far, primarily been investigated with animal models.

EXTINCTION

In Pavlovian fear conditioning, a neutral event, the conditioned stimulus (CS), comes to elicit fear by virtue of its pairing with an aversive event, the unconditioned stimulus (US). After a few pairings, the presentation of the previously neutral CS alone results in a range of fear responses indicating the acquisition of a conditioned response (CR). This fear learning is rapid, robust, and generally long-lasting. However, the expression of conditioned fear can be diminished or eliminated through extinction. During extinction, the CS is presented alone (unreinforced) for a number of trials; the organism eventually learns that the CS no longer predicts the US, and the CR is diminished. Even though extinction training can eliminate the expression of conditioned fear, there is abundant evidence that extinction does not erase or undo the fear learning. After extinction, conditioned fear can return in a range of circumstances, including the simple passage of time (spontaneous recovery), exposure to the US (reinstatement), or exposure to the CS in a novel context (renewal) (for a review, see Bouton, 2002). This recovery of fear indicates that extinction training results in new learning to inhibit the expression of conditioned fear, rather than eliminating the underlying representation of conditioned fear.

Investigations of the neural mechanisms underlying extinction have highlighted the interaction of three neural structures: the amygdala, the ventromedial prefrontal cortex (vmPFC), and the hippocampus. All these structures play an important role in extinction learning and expression, with their differential involvement unfolding over time and contexts.

In order to fully understand the complex role of each of these regions in fear extinction, it is necessary to briefly review the organization of the amygdala. As noted in earlier chapters of this volume (see LeDoux & Schiller, Chapter 2, and Myers et al., Chapter 3), the amygdala is composed of a number of substructures, each with unique roles. The lateral nucleus (LA) receives the CS and US sensory input and is proposed to be the site of plasticity for the CS–US association during fear acquisition. The LA projects directly to the central nucleus (CE), which outputs to various regions controlling specific fear CRs. The LA also projects to the CE indirectly through intermediate connections within the amygdala. Specifically, the LA projects to the basal nucleus (B) and the intercalated cells (ITC), all of which project to the CE. In addition, the B has direct projections to the ITC, providing another pathway to modify CE responses.

Within the LA, there are some populations of cells that show diminished CS-related responses with extinction training, and other cell populations in which activity is elevated throughout extinction (Repa et al., 2001). These extinction-resistant cells are consistent with behavioral data suggesting that extinction does not erase the fear memory, as evidenced by the recovery of conditioned fear following extinction. However, the diminished CS-related response of some LA cell populations suggests possible modifications of responses within the LA during extinction training, although these CS-related responses may return with renewal (Hobin, Goosens, & Maren, 2003). Because the amygdala is needed to express fear CRs, most work on the role of the amygdala in extinction has used pharmacological manipulations rather than lesions. Davis and colleagues (see Myers & Davis, 2007, for a review, and Myers et al., Chapter 3, this volume) have shown that blockade of N-methyl-D-aspartate (NMDA) receptors in the amygdala disrupts extinction, and that facilitation of NMDA receptor function with D-cycloserine (DCS) enhances extinction training. The enhancement of the effectiveness of extinction with DCS occurs both when the drug is administered prior to extinction and in the time window immediately following extinction, with less effectiveness as time since training increases up to a few hours, after which there is no benefit (Ledgerwood, Richardson, & Cranney, 2003). These results suggest that DCS may play a role in the acquisition and early consolidation of extinction-related changes within the amygdala, and they highlight a role for plasticity within the amygdala in the acquisition of extinction learning.

In an elegant series of studies that I do not review in detail here, Davis and colleagues (see Davis, Myers, Chhatwal, & Ressler, 2006) have extended the use of DCS, administered systemically in humans, to facilitate the effectiveness of exposure therapy in the treatment of phobias. For example, by administering DCS prior to each exposure therapy session, they were able to reduce the number of sessions needed for clinically significant results (Ressler et al., 2004). These initial findings have led to the exploration of DCS as a time-limited cognitive enhancer to increase the effectiveness of other therapeutic approaches. This groundbreaking work provides a powerful example of how research on the mechanisms of controlling fear conducted in the laboratory can be applied directly to the treatment of fear-related disorders.

Although the amygdala plays a role in the acquisition and early consolidation of extinction learning, the maintenance of extinction learning requires its interaction with the vmPFC. Interest in the role of the vmPFC in extinction emerged when it was shown that damage to this region left the expression of conditioned fear unaltered, but impaired extinction training over days (Morgan & LeDoux, 1995). Quirk, Russo, Barron, and Lebron (2000) demonstrated that damage to the infralimbic cortex (IL), a subregion of the vmPFC, did not impair the short-term (i.e., same-day) expression of extinction learning; rather, it led to little retention of extinction training on subsequent days, thus highlighting a role of the IL in the recall of extinction. Consistent with these lesion studies, electrophysiological recording of IL neurons showed potentiation to a CS specifically during the recall of extinction (Milad & Quirk, 2002).

There are reciprocal connections between the amygdala and vmPFC. These connections may facilitate the consolidation of the extinction memories within the vmPFC, and may also play a critical role in the vmPFC's inhibition of amygdala responses during the recall of extinction (see Quirk, Garcia, & González-Lima, 2006, and Sotres-Bayon, Cain, & LeDoux, 2006, for reviews). One primary means by which it is suggested the vmPFC inhibits the amygdala during the recall of extinction is through connections between the IL region within the vmPFC and the ITC within the amygdala. The ITC are inhibitory neurons that connect the B, the LA, and the CE. It is proposed that during the recall of extinction, CS-related responses in the vmPFC (the IL subregion) lead to the excitation of ITC, which in turn inhibit the communication between the LA (where fear memories are stored) and the CE (the output for the fear response) (Quirk et al., 2000). Consistent with this model, stimulation of the IL region of the vmPFC resulted in decreased excitability of neurons in the CE and the expression of conditioned fear (Quirk, Likhtik, Pelletier, & Paré, 2003; Milad, Vidal-Gonzalez, & Quirk, 2004). When communication between the LA and CE is inhibited, the storage of the fear memory is intact, but the expression of fear is inhibited. It has also been suggested that projections from the vmPFC to the LA subregion of the amygdala may play a role in the inhibition of fear during extinction (Rosenkranz, Moore, & Grace, 2003).

In animal models of fear extinction, the other brain structure that plays an important role is the hippocampus. In both the acquisition and extinction of conditioned fear, the hippocampus has been shown to be involved in the modulation of fear expression by context (Fanselow, 2000; Ji & Maren, 2007). Behavioral research on extinction has shown that context plays an important role in the expression of extinction learning (see Bouton, 2002, for a review). For instance, in contextual renewal, an extinguished CR may return when the extinguished CS is presented in a novel context. In contextual reinstatement, presentations of the US alone may lead to the return of a CR to an extinguished CS, but only when the US is presented in the same context. Evidence from animal models suggests that the hippocampus mediates the return of previously extinguished fear in both renewal (Corcoran & Maren, 2001) and contextual reinstatement (Wilson, Brooks, & Bouton, 1995). The hippocampus projects to both the amygdala and the vmPFC. It is suggested that one function of hippocampal projections to the vmPFC is to modify the vmPFC's inhibition of the amygdala during the recall of extinction learning so that it is only expressed in the appropriate context. Specifically, it is suggested that the hippocampus may inhibit extinction-related responses in the vmPFC to the CS, which leads to the failure to inhibit the expression of a previously extinguished CR in situations where the context signals that the previous extinction learning may not be relevant (see Ji & Maren, 2007, for a review). The hippocampal projections to the amygdala have also been suggested to play a role in the contextual modulation of fear extinction (see Sotres-Bayon et al., 2006, for a review). By working in concert, the amygdala, vmPFC, and hippocampus mediate the initial acquisition, recall, and contextually appropriate expression of extinction learning.

Our ability to study the details of the neural circuitry mediating extinction in humans is necessarily limited by technical and ethical constraints when studying the human brain. However, there are functional magnetic resonance imaging (fMRI), lesion, and anatomical data to support the model of extinction outlined above. Using fMRI, recent studies have provided initial support for the roles of the amygdala, vmPFC, and hippocampus in the extinction of conditioned fear (Gottfried & Dolan, 2004; Kalisch et al., 2006; Knight, Smith, Cheng, Stein, & Helmstetter, 2004; Phelps, Delgado, Nearing, & LeDoux, 2004). Initial reports of extinction of conditioned fear in humans suggested that the amygdala shows an increased response during early extinction when the CS–US stimulus contingency is first altered (Gottfried & Dolan, 2004; Knight et al., 2004; LaBar, Gatenby, Gore, LeDoux, & Phelps, 1998), followed by a decrease in amygdala activation as extinction progresses (Phelps et al., 2004). In a study examining the initial learning and the retention of extinction after 24 hours, amygdala activation was observed to a CS that predicted shock during fear acquisition. As extinction progressed, activation to the CS diminished, both during initial extinction learning and at the recall of extinction. However, only during initial learning did this decrease in amygdala activation correlate with the physiological expression of extinction. In other words, those participants who showed a greater decrease in their CR during the initial learning of extinction also showed a greater decrease in amygdala activation to the CS. This correlation was not observed after a 24-hour delay. These results support a role for the amygdala in the learning of extinction.

fMRI studies of extinction in humans generally report activation of the vmPFC during all stages of fear conditioning, including acquisition (Gottfried & Dolan, 2004; Phelps et al., 2004). During acquisition, this activation is characterized as a decrease, relative to the resting baseline, in the blood-oxygenation-level-dependent (BOLD) signal. As extinction progresses, BOLD responses in the vmPFC increase, consistent with the pattern observed in electrophysiological studies in nonhuman animals (Milad & Quirk, 2002). In the study mentioned above examining the retention of extinction (Phelps et al., 2004), activation of the vmPFC was observed in a region of the subgenual anterior cingulate that is suggested to be analogous to the IL region of the vmPFC investigated in animal models of extinction (Kim, Somerville, Johnstone, Alexander, & Whalen, 2003). Although responses in this region were observed during the acquisition, initial learning, and retention of extinction, it was only during the recall of extinction that these responses correlated with the expression of the CR. Specifically, those subjects who showed greater retention of extinction learning after a 24-hour delay also showed a greater BOLD response in the vmPFC (see also Milad et al., 2007, for a similar finding). Furthermore only at retention test was there a correlation between responses in the vmPFC and the amygdala, such that increased vmPFC activation correlated with decreased amygdala activation during extinction recall. These results are consistent with a role for the vmPFC in inhibiting the amygdala during the recall of extinction. Further supporting this role for the vmPFC in the retention of extinction is a study examining anatomical differences that predict extinction success (Milad et al., 2005). Across subjects, the cortical thickness of a region of the vmPFC similar to that observed in fMRI investigations (Milad et al., 2007; Phelps et al., 2004) predicted the success of extinction recall after a delay.

Finally, studies in humans examining the contextual modulation of the expression of extinction have reported evidence for the involvement of the hippocampus. With fMRI, the modulation of context can be challenging, because the consistency of the scanner environment makes the investigation of the renewal and contextual reinstatement procedures used in animal models difficult. However, several studies have demonstrated activation of the hippocampus during extinction (Kalisch et al., 2006; Knight et al., 2004; Milad et al., 2007), and a few of these have explicitly manipulated context via changes in the background screen on which a visual CS is presented. A study designed to examine the retention of extinction in which the background context differed during acquisition and extinction found a correlation between activation of the hippocampus and the recall of extinction after a delay, along with a correlation between the vmPFC and hippocampus (Milad et al., 2007). A second fMRI study manipulated the context of the background screen during learning so that extinction of the CS was associated with one background context, but not with the other. During the retention of extinction, there was a correlated CS-related response between the vmPFC and the hippocampus only when the CS was presented in the extinction context. These results are consistent with a role for the hippocampus in mediating the contextual dependence of the expression of extinction via its influence on the vmPFC. In an effort to explicitly link studies in nonhuman animals examining the contextual modulation of extinction to humans, a lesion study explored the role of the hippocampus in contextual reinstatement (LaBar & Phelps, 2005). Similar to findings obtained in rats (Wilson et al., 1995), damage to the hippocampus in humans impaired the contextual reinstatement of the CR following extinction. When these data are combined with the brain imaging results, there is strong evidence that the human hippocampus plays an important role in the contextual mediation of the expression of extinction.

Although extinction is only one means by which we humans can control fear, it has a long history of demonstrated clinical relevance, in addition to practical relevance in our everyday experiences of confronting our fears. The convergence of findings from studies with animal models and humans provides assurance that the details of the neural circuitry investigated in animal models of extinction are relevant and important to understanding the control of fear in humans.

COGNITIVE REGULATION STRATEGIES

In contrast to extinction, the use of cognitive strategies to control fear has been studied exclusively in humans. In everyday life, we regularly use our thoughts to alter our emotions. Whether we are choosing to reinterpret the significance of an event or deciding to focus attention on the less fearful aspects of a situation, we tune our cognition in the service of generating more adaptive emotional and social reactions. Although many different cognitive strategies can be used to control fear, the use of these techniques generally requires the active engagement of the participants in an effort to alter their emotional responses through changing their thoughts. These cognitive strategies can be taught and practiced, as demonstrated in cognitive therapy techniques, and they may also become habitual and easier to enact over time, as exemplified by the individual who has learned to see the "glass as half full" when approaching tough situations.

Research outlining the neural systems mediating the cognitive regulation of fear has only recently emerged. These studies have examined a range of cognitive regulation strategies. Two of the earliest studies on this topic demonstrated how a cognitive strategy can both increase (Phelps et al., 2001) and decrease (Ochsner, Bunge, Gross, & Gabrieli, 2002) the expression of fear or negative affect, along with a corresponding increase or decrease in activation of the amygdala. A study examining how thoughts can generate fear examined instructed fear, in which participants were verbally instructed that they might receive a shock paired with one stimulus (threatening), but not with another (safe). In this paradigm, a shock was never delivered, but simply anticipating a potential shock with the threat stimulus led to increased arousal and increased activation of the left amygdala (Phelps et al., 2001). In addition, it was shown that damage to the left, but not right, amygdala resulted to an impaired expression of instructed fear (Funayama, Grillon, Davis, & Phelps, 2001)—perhaps because the potential threat was communicated symbolically through language, which typically has a left-hemisphere representation. This laterality of instructed fear is in contrast to fear conditioning, in which lesions of either the right or left amygdala will result in impaired fear expression (LaBar, LeDoux, Spencer, & Phelps, 1995). Unlike fear conditioning, it is unlikely that the symbolic, cognitive representation generated in instructed fear relies on the amygdala for the formation or storage of the fear representation; nevertheless, the amygdala plays a critical role in the expression of this cognitive means of fear learning. These findings suggest that even though humans have developed complex cognitive and social means for acquiring and representing fear, they take advantage of phylogenetically shared mechanisms for fear expression (see Olsson & Phelps, 2007).

The majority of studies on the cognitive regulation of fear or negative affect have examined means to diminish fear and have relied almost exclusively on fMRI to investigate the underlying neural circuitry. Although a few cognitive techniques have been investigated to diminish fear, most studies examine strategies that emphasize reinterpreting the emotional significance of the event (see Ochsner & Gross, 2008, for a review). For example, Ochsner and colleagues (2002) used a reappraisal strategy, in which participants were presented with negative emotional scenes and asked to reinterpret the events depicted in the scene to reduce their negative affective response. When using this strategy, a participant might imagine when a scene depicts a bloody wound that it is fake, or that the wound is less painful than it appears. Reappraisal has been shown to be effective at reducing negative affect in research using both self-report and physiological measures of emotion (Ochsner & Gross, 2008). An examination of the patterns of brain activation in the initial study revealed that the reappraisal of negative scenes, as opposed to just attending to them, resulted in increased activation of both dorsolateral PFC (dlPFC) and ventrolateral PFC (vlPFC) regions along with dorsal anterior cingulate, and in decreased activation of a region of the orbitofrontal cortex and the amygdala (Ochsner et al., 2002). It was proposed that underlying the reappraisal of negative affect, the engagement of the dlPFC may be linked to executive control processes required in the online manipulation of the interpretation of scenes, and the decrease of amygdala activation may reflect the cognitive control of subcortical mechanisms linked to the representation of negative emotional value (Ochsner et al., 2002).

Since this initial report (see also Beauregard, Lévesque, & Bourgouin, 2001), a number of studies have examined the reinterpretation of negative affect. These studies consistently report decreased amygdala activation, increased activation of the dlPFC and/or vlPFC, along with some involvement of medial PFC (mPFC) regions. However, across studies the precise location and/or laterality of these PFC regions varies, perhaps due to subtle difference in the stimuli or strategy used (see Ochsner & Gross, 2008, for a review). In spite of these differences, a general model of the cognitive regulation of fear or negative affect has emerged. In this model, the dlPFC (e.g., Delgado, Nearing, LeDoux, & Phelps, 2008; Ochsner et al., 2002) is involved in the effortful manipulation or interpretation of the stimulus, and the vlPFC may play a role in the selection of emotion interpretation (e.g., Wager, Davidson, Hughes, Lindquist, & Ochsner, 2008). The changes observed in the amygdala result from the top-down modulation of the emotional meaning of the stimulus. One important aspect of this model is that the dlPFC does not project directly to the amygdala (Barbas, 2000; McDonald, Mascagni, & Guo, 1996). Instead, its influence on the amygdala is likely to be mediated by ventral PFC and medial PFC regions that have stronger connections with the amygdala (Urry et al., 2006). Although this model of emotion regulation is somewhat speculative, given the inconsistency of precise PFC regions observed across studies (see Ochsner & Gross, 2008) and the dependence on a single neuroscience technique, it provides a preliminary neural framework for further efforts to understand the cognitive regulation of fear.

A critical aspect of the studies of cognitive regulation of fear is that the amygdala response is decreased as a result of inhibition from the PFC. Much as in extinction, it is suggested that this PFC inhibition is critical to the control of fear. In an effort to directly compare the role of the PFC in the inhibition of the amygdala across extinction and cognitive regulation, the Delgado and colleagues (2008) study examined the regulation of conditioned fear. In this study, the CSs were colored squares. When instructed to regulate, participants used a strategy in which they generated an image of a soothing nature scene containing the color of the square. In contrast to attend trials, using this cognitive strategy resulted in a decrease in the CR. This decrease in fear was accompanied by increased activation of the dlPFC, decreased activation of the amygdala, and increased activation of a region of the vmPFC overlapping with that observed in a similar study on fear extinction (Delgado et al., 2008; Phelps et al., 2004). In a direct comparison with data from the extinction study, similar patterns of activation were observed in the amygdala and vmPFC when fear was diminished through either extinction or cognitive regulation, although only the regulation study reported increased activation of the dlPFC, consistent with a role for this region in the online manipulation or reinterpretation of the meaning of the CS. When responses across these regions were compared, it was found that responses in the vmPFC were correlated with those observed in both the dlPFC and the amygdala. These results suggest a model by which the dlPFC inhibition of the amygdala during cognitive regulation is mediated through the same vmPFC region thought to mediate the inhibition of fear with extinction. It is possible that, much as the generation of fear through cognitive means relies on the amygdala for expression, the inhibition of fear through cognitive means relies on a phylogenetically shared vmPFC–amygdala circuitry. Although most cognitive regulation techniques are unique to humans, by linking components of the neural circuitry of extinction with regulation, we gain some insight into additional potential details of the neural mechanisms underlying the cognitive control of fear.

ACTIVE COPING AND RECONSOLIDATION

The final two techniques that can be used to control fear have yet to be investigated extensively in humans. For this reason, I only briefly review them here. "Active coping" is a general term that refers to taking an instrumental action to diminish exposure to a fear-eliciting stimulus. In everyday life, choosing to engage in an action to reduce exposure to fearful events is a common coping mechanism, perhaps our most common. In light of this, and of the extensive literature examining instrumental actions to approach rewarding events (Rangel, Camerer, & Montague, 2008), the lack of human research on this means of regulating emotion is somewhat surprising.

A study exploring the role of the amygdala in mediating the active coping of fear using an animal model examined the escape-from-fear (EFF) paradigm. In the EFF paradigm, the rat first undergoes fear conditioning. In a second stage, the rat is given the option to take an action to terminate the CS, thus reducing exposure to the fear-eliciting event. In this paradigm, the termination of the CS becomes a conditioned reinforcer for the instrumental action. An investigation by Amorapanth, LeDoux, and Nader (2000) found that diminishing fear through active coping relies on a circuitry within the amygdala that can be dissociated from the expression of conditioned fear. As outlined earlier, the physiological expression of conditioned fear is proposed to depend on a circuitry of amygdala subnuclei by which the LA, which is necessary for the formation of the CS–US association, projects to the CE, which outputs to a number of regions mediating the physiological expression of conditioned fear. By placing lesions in the different amygdala subnuclei, Amorapanth and colleagues found that although damage to the LA impaired both the physiological expression and active coping of fear, damage to the CE only disrupted the physiological expression of fear. Rats with lesions confined to the CE were able to learn an action to terminate the CS, even though they failed to show the typical expression of conditioned fear. In contrast, damage to the B resulted in the opposite pattern of results—that is, failure to learn an action to terminate the CS, but normal expression of the CR. It is suggested that B may not be the site of storage for active coping representations in the EFF paradigm, but rather that B projects to the striatum, which is known to have a broader role in motor control and reinforcement of action. In short, the pathway for active coping is hypothesized to involve the LA, which projects to the B, which in turn projects to the striatum to convey the reinforcing nature of the instrumental action (see LeDoux & Gorman, 2001).

The final technique currently under investigation as a means to control fear is the blockade of reconsolidation. The classic view of memory suggests that immediately after learning there is a period of time during which the memory is fragile and labile, but that after sufficient time has passed, the memory is more or less permanent. During this consolidation period, it is possible to disrupt the formation of the memory; once this time window has passed, the memory may be modified or inhibited, but not eliminated. Recently, however, there has been renewed interest in an alternative view of memory suggesting that every time a memory is retrieved, the underlying memory trace is once again labile and fragile—requiring another consolidation period, called "reconsolidation." This reconsolidation period allows another opportunity to disrupt the memory. Given that fear memories can at times be maladaptive, resulting in fear or anxiety disorders, the possibility of disrupting a previously acquired fear memory by blocking reconsolidation may have important clinical implications.

This renewed interest in reconsolidation and its role in the control of fear emerged from a study by Nader, Schafe, and LeDoux (2000), in which they demonstrated that conditioned fear can be eliminated by blocking reconsolidation. In this study, rats were conditioned to fear a tone (the CS), and the fear memory was consolidated for 1–14 days. After consolidation, some of the rats were presented with an unreinforced presentation of the CS. This CS reminder served to reactivate the fear memory trace. This reactivation was followed immediately by an injection of either anisomycin, a protein synthesis inhibitor, or a saline solution into the amygdala. Protein synthesis is required for the formation of a memory trace, and blocking protein synthesis has been previously shown to block the consolidation of fear memories. Even though the time window of consolidation had passed, the rats that received anisomycin following reactivation failed to show evidence of conditioned fear. The rats that received either a saline injection following reactivation of the CS or anisomycin without reactivation showed normal conditioned fear. These results suggest that fear memories undergo reconsolidation every time they are retrieved, and that this reconsolidation process can be disrupted, essentially eliminating the previously learned fear.

Since this initial report, several studies have explored the nature of the blockade of reconsolidation, examining issues such as its relation to initial consolidation and its underlying mechanisms (see Alberini, 2005, and Dudai, 2006, for reviews). However, research on the blockade of the reconsolidation of fear memories has only slowly been extended to humans, for a few reasons. A primary reason initially was that the blockade of reconsolidation required the administration of protein synthesis inhibitors, which is not viable in humans. However, it has recently been demonstrated that propranolol, a beta-adrenergic antagonist safe to administer to humans, may block reconsolidation by indirectly influencing protein synthesis in the amygdala (Debiec & LeDoux, 2004). Although the discovery that propranolol can be used to block reconsolidation provides an avenue for examining this process in humans, preliminary results are only now emerging (Brunet et al., 2008). It is still unclear how effective and specific this approach will be in controlling fear in humans (Brunet et al., 2008).

CONCLUSIONS

Although research on the human amygdala and the control of fear has used a limited range of neuroscience methods, by linking this research with animal models, we can begin to develop an overarching model for at least two of these approaches—extinction and emotion regulation (see Figure 9.1). As outlined earlier, research in humans suggests that the basic mechanisms of extinction are preserved across species. For this reason, our model of extinction in humans is the same as that suggested by research in other species. However, humans have developed unique cognitive capabilities for the control of fear. These cognitive techniques may in part influence the amygdala and the expression of fear through neural mechanisms overlapping with those of extinction. However, these shared mechanisms are driven or engaged not by the passive experience of exposure, but in a top-down, effortful manner via regions of the PFC that may differ more substantially across species, such as the dlPFC.

Future research on the human amygdala and the control of fear will expand this working model to include additional approaches, such as active coping and the blockade of reconsolidation, and ideally will utilize a broader range of human neuroscience methods. By developing a more complete understanding of the circuitry mediating the control of fear in humans and its impact on the amygdala, we can gain insight into when and how different techniques

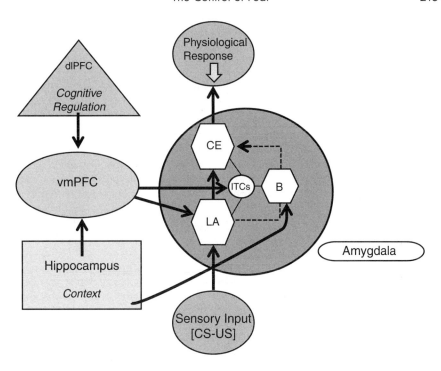

FIGURE 9.1. Working model for the control of conditioned fear in humans through extinction and cognitive regulation. The control of fear in humans requires a network of brain regions. Within the amygdala, the lateral nucleus (LA) receives sensory input and is the site of CS–US plasticity. The LA projects to the central nucleus (CE), which outputs to a number of brain regions responsible for the expression of conditioned fear. During the recall of extinction, the ventromedial prefrontal cortex (vmPFC) inhibits the expression of conditioned fear through excitation of the intercalated cells (ITC), which inhibit communication from the LA to the CE, this reducing the expression of conditioned fear. In addition, the vmPFC projects to the LA, which may also play a role in the inhibition of fear with extinction. The hippocampus mediates the contextual expression of extinction via projections to the vmPFC. Moreover, hippocampal projections to the basal nucleus (B), which in turn modulates the CE, may play a role in modulating the expression of extinction by context. The dorsolateral PFC (dlPFC) is involved in cognitive regulation of conditioned fear, influencing the expression of conditioned fear by projections to the vmPFC, which inhibits the amygdala.

might be most effective and how their combination could be most beneficial, as we attempt to apply this research to the treatment of clinical disorders.

WHAT I THINK

My answer to the question "What does the amygdala do?" is inspired by the work of some colleagues on the nature of emotion, combined with my research and that of others on the role of the amygdala. "Emotion" is a broad concept that encompasses a range of processes and components, only some of which involve the amygdala. However, in theorizing about the function of emotion, Nico Frijda, Klaus Scherer, and others have suggested that emotion is a "relevance detector." Emotions inform us of what is important and what matters as we navigate a complex world. In my view, the amygdala is a relevance detector for the brain and cognition. This does not mean that the amygdala is necessary for the generation of emotion broadly. In fact, the amygdala may play a minimal role in the subjective experience of emotion, and it underlies only some physiological expressions of emotion. Rather, the amygdala detects when there is something in the environment that is potentially important, and, through its extensive connectivity, modulates other neural systems to be especially attuned to this information. If one looks at a connectivity map of the brain, the amygdala looks something like Grand Central Station. It gets signals from throughout the brain and sends signals throughout the brain. This places the amygdala in a prime position to incorporate information concerning the emotional significance of events we encounter, in order to ensure that our cognitive functions, such as perception, attention, memory, and decisions, are modified to give priority to these events. Of course, the amygdala also plays a role in learning what is relevant. This is best known in fear conditioning, but the amygdala is involved in learning appetitive values as well. Determining the precise contribution of the amygdala and other regions, such as the striatum, in coding appetitive and aversive learning is an important future challenge; however, the amygdala, in conjunction with other learning and memory systems, is important for the flexible assessment of what is relevant in a changing and uncertain world. In short, the amygdala helps us learn what is relevant, detects when there is something relevant in the environment, and tunes our cognitive and social processes to give priority to these relevant events.

REFERENCES

Alberini, C. M. (2005). Mechanisms of memory stabilization: Are consolidation and reconsolidation similar or distinct processes? *Trends in Neurosciences, 28*, 51–56.

Amorapanth, P., LeDoux, J. E., & Nader, K. (2000). Different lateral amygdala outputs mediate reactions and actions elicited by a fear-arousing stimulus. *Nature Neuroscience, 3*, 74–79.

Barbas, H. (2000). Connections underlying the synthesis of cognition, memory, and emotion in primate prefrontal cortices. *Brain Research Bulletin, 52*, 319–330.

Beauregard, M., Lévesque, J., & Bourgouin, P. (2001). Neural correlates of conscious self-regulation of emotion. *Journal of Neuroscience, 21*, RC165.

Bouton, M. E. (2002). Context, ambiguity, and unlearning: Sources of relapse after behavioral extinction. *Biological Psychiatry, 52*, 976–986.

Brunet, A., Orr, S. P., Tremblay, J., Robertson, K., Nader, K., & Pitman, R. K. (2008). Effect of post-retrieval propranolol on psychophysiologic responding during subsequent script-driven traumatic imagery in post-traumatic stress disorder. *Journal of Psychiatric Research, 46*, 503–506.

Corcoran, K. A., & Maren, S. (2001). Hippocampal inactivation disrupts contextual retrieval of fear memory after extinction. *Journal of Neuroscience, 21*, 1720–1726.

Davis, M., Myers, K. M., Chhatwal, J., & Ressler, K. J. (2006). Pharmacological treatments that facilitate extinction of fear: Relevance to psychotherapy. *NeuroRx, 3*, 82–96.

Debiec, J., & LeDoux, J. E. (2004). Disruption of reconsolidation but not consolidation of auditory fear conditioning by noradrenergic blockade in the amygdala. *Neuroscience, 129*, 267–272.

Delgado, M. R., Nearing, K. I., LeDoux, J. E., & Phelps, E. A. (2008). Neural circuitry underlying the regulation of conditioned fear and its relation to extinction. *Neuron, 59*, 829–838.

Dudai, Y. (2006). Reconsolidation: The advantage of being refocused. *Current Opinion in Neurobiology, 16*, 174–178.

Fanselow, M. S. (2000). Contextual fear, gestalt memories, and the hippocampus. *Behavioral Brain Research, 110*, 73–81.

Funayama, E. S., Grillon, C., Davis, M., & Phelps, E. A. (2001). A double dissociation in the affective modulation of startle in humans: Effects of unilateral temporal lobectomy. *Journal of Cognitive Neuroscience, 13*, 721–729.

Gottfried, J. A., & Dolan, R. J. (2004). Human orbitofrontal cortex mediates extinction learning while accessing conditioned representations of value. *Nature Neuroscience, 7*, 1144–1152.

Hobin, J. A., Goosens, K. A., & Maren, S. (2003). Context-dependent neuronal activity in the lateral amygdala represents fear memories after extinction. *Journal of Neuroscience, 23*, 8410–8416.

Ji, J., & Maren, S. (2007). Hippocampal involvement in contextual modulation of fear extinction. *Hippocampus, 17*, 749–758.

Kalisch, R., Korenfeld, E., Stephan, K. E., Weiskopf, N., Seymour, B., & Dolan, R. J. (2006). Context-dependent human extinction memory is mediated by a ventromedial prefrontal and hippocampal network. *Journal of Neuroscience, 26*, 9503–9511.

Kim, H., Somerville, L. H., Johnstone, T., Alexander, A. L., & Whalen, P. J. (2003). Inverse amygdala and medial prefrontal cortex responses to surprised faces. *NeuroReport, 14*, 2317–2322.

Knight, D. C., Smith, C. N., Cheng, D. T., Stein, E. A., & Helmstetter, F. J. (2004). Amygdala and hippocampal activity during acquisition and extinction of human fear conditioning. *Cognitive, Affective, and Behavioral Neuroscience, 4*, 317–325.

LaBar, K. S., Gatenby, J. C., Gore, J. C., LeDoux, J. E., & Phelps, E. A. (1998). Human amygdala activation during conditioned fear acquisition and extinction: A mixed-trial fMRI study. *Neuron, 20*, 937–945.

LaBar, K. S., LeDoux, J. E., Spencer, D. D., & Phelps, E. A. (1995). Impaired fear conditioning following unilateral temporal lobectomy in humans. *Journal of Neuroscience, 15,* 6846–6855.

LaBar, K. S., & Phelps, E. A. (2005). Reinstatement of conditioned fear in humans is context-dependent and impaired in amnesia. *Behavioral Neuroscience, 119,* 677–686.

LeDoux, J. E., & Gorman, J. M. (2001). A call to action: Overcoming anxiety through active coping. *American Journal of Psychiatry, 158,* 1953–1955.

Ledgerwood, L., Richardson, R., & Cranney, J. (2003). Effects of D-cycloserine on extinction of conditioned freezing. *Behavioral Neuroscience, 117,* 341–349.

McDonald, A. J., Mascagni, F., & Guo, L. (1996). Projections of the medial and lateral prefrontal cortices to the amygdala: A *Phaseolus vulgaris* leucoagglutinin study in the rat. *Neuroscience, 71,* 55–75.

Milad, M. R., Quinn, B. T., Pitman, R. K., Orr, S. P., Fischl, B., & Rauch, S. L. (2005). Thickness of ventromedial prefrontal cortex in humans is correlated with extinction memory. *Proceedings of the National Academy of Sciences USA, 102,* 10706–10711.

Milad, M. R., & Quirk, G. J. (2002). Neurons in medial prefrontal cortex signal memory for fear extinction. *Nature, 420,* 70–74.

Milad, M. R., Vidal-González, I., & Quirk, G. J. (2004). Electrical stimulation of medial prefrontal cortex reduces conditioned fear in a temporally specific manner. *Behavioral Neuroscience, 118,* 389–394.

Milad, M. R., Wright, C. I., Orr, S. P., Pitman, R. K., Quirk, G. J., & Rauch, S. L. (2007). Recall of fear extinction in humans activates the ventromedial prefrontal cortex and hippocampus in concert. *Biological Psychiatry, 62,* 446–454.

Morgan, M. A., & LeDoux, J. E. (1995). Differential contribution of dorsal and ventral medial prefrontal cortex to the acquisition and extinction of conditioned fear in rats. *Behavioral Neuroscience, 109,* 681–688.

Myers, K. M., & Davis, M. (2007). Mechanisms of fear extinction. *Molecular Psychiatry, 12,* 120–150.

Nader, K., Schafe, G. E., & LeDoux, J. E. (2000). Fear memories require protein synthesis in the amygdala for reconsolidation after retrieval. *Nature, 406,* 722–726.

Ochsner, K. N., Bunge, S. A., Gross, J. J., & Gabrieli, J. D. (2002). Rethinking feelings: An FMRI study of the cognitive regulation of emotion. *Journal of Cognitive Neuroscience, 14,* 1215–1229.

Ochsner, K. N., & Gross, J. J. (2005). The cognitive control of emotion. *Trends in Cognitive Sciences, 9,* 243–249.

Ochsner, K. N., & Gross, J. J. (2008). Cognitive emotion regulation: Insights from social, cognitive and affective neuroscience. *Current Directions in Psychological Science, 17,* 153–158.

Olsson, A., & Phelps, E. A. (2007). Social learning of fear. *Nature Neuroscience, 10,* 1095–1102.

Phelps, E. A. (2006). Emotion and cognition: Insights from studies of the human amygdala. *Annual Review of Psychology, 57,* 27–53.

Phelps, E. A., Delgado, M. R., Nearing, K. I., & LeDoux, J. E. (2004). Extinction learning in humans: Role of the amygdala and vmPFC. *Neuron, 43,* 897–905.

Phelps, E. A., O'Connor, K. J., Gatenby, J. C., Gore, J. C., Grillon, C., & Davis, M. (2001). Activation of the left amygdala to a cognitive representation of fear. *Nature Neuroscience, 4,* 437–441.

Quirk, G. J., Garcia, R., & González-Lima, F. (2006). Prefrontal mechanisms in extinction of conditioned fear. *Biological Psychiatry, 60*, 337–343.

Quirk, G. J., Likhtik, E., Pelletier, J. G., & Paré, D. (2003). Stimulation of medial prefrontal cortex decreases the responsiveness of central amygdala output neurons. *Journal of Neuroscience, 23*, 8800–8807.

Quirk, G. J., Russo, G. K., Barron, J. L., & Lebron, K. (2000). The role of ventromedial prefrontal cortex in the recovery of extinguished fear. *Journal of Neuroscience, 20*, 6225–6231.

Rangel, A., Camerer, C., & Montague, P. R. (2008). A framework for studying the neurobiology of value-based decision making. *Nature Reviews Neuroscience, 9*, 545–556.

Repa, J. C., Muller, J., Apergis, J., Desrochers, T. M., Zhou, Y., & LeDoux, J. E. (2001). Two different lateral amygdala cell populations contribute to the initiation and storage of memory. *Nature Neuroscience, 4*, 724–731.

Ressler, K. J., Rothbaum, B. O., Tannenbaum, L., Anderson, P., Graap, K., Zimand, E., et al. (2004). Cognitive enhancers as adjuncts to psychotherapy: Use of D-cycloserine in phobic individuals to facilitate extinction of fear. *Archives of General Psychiatry, 61*, 1136–1144.

Rosenkranz, J. A., Moore, H., & Grace, A. A. (2003). The prefrontal cortex regulates lateral amygdala neuronal plasticity and responses to previously conditioned stimuli. *Journal of Neuroscience, 23*, 11054–11064.

Sotres-Bayon, F., Cain, C. K., & LeDoux, J. E. (2006). Brain mechanisms of fear extinction: Historical perspectives on the contribution of prefrontal cortex. *Biological Psychiatry, 60*, 329–336.

Urry, H. L., van Reekum, C. M., Johnstone, T., Kalin, N. H., Thurow, M. E., Schaefer, H. S., et al. (2006). Amygdala and ventromedial prefrontal cortex are inversely coupled during regulation of negative affect and predict the diurnal pattern of cortisol secretion among older adults. *Journal of Neuroscience, 26*, 4415–4425.

Wager, T. D., Davidson, M. L., Hughes, B. L., Lindquist, M. A., & Ochsner, K. N. (2008). Prefrontal–subcortical pathways mediating successful emotion regulation. *Neuron, 59*, 1037–1050.

Wilson, A., Brooks, D. C., & Bouton, M. E. (1995). The role of the rat hippocampal system in several effects of context in extinction. *Behavioral Neuroscience, 109*, 828–836.

CHAPTER 10

The Role of the Human Amygdala in Perception and Attention

Patrik Vuilleumier

The amygdala is one of the brain regions most extensively scrutinized and most frequently invoked for its critical involvement in emotion processing. This central role holds across different theoretical frameworks in neuroscience and psychology, and reflects the fact that amygdala functions encompass several essential aspects of emotions. Not only is it associated with the ability to detect and retain the motivational value of environmental events, but it is crucial for orchestrating a wide range of physiological reactions that allow the organism to adjust to these events. Thus the amygdala not only receives and integrates various inputs from external and internal sources, but also projects to many output systems that can then modulate autonomic, motor, memory, cognitive, and perceptual processes. Even though theorists still disagree on the best defining features of emotions, this faculty of appraising and responding to important events is generally considered the hallmark of emotional processing (Scherer & Peper, 2001), and the amygdala combines these distinct facets within a unique, small, but highly intricate brain structure.

Among its various influences on other brain systems, the amygdala is particularly well positioned to exert modulations on cortical pathways involved in perception and attention, which may in turn produce a range of downstream effects on cognitive and memory functions. The present chapter focuses on recent evidence from neuroimaging and neuropsychology studies in humans that have begun to unveil the neural mechanisms underlying such interactions between attention and emotion in the amygdala. Attention is in itself a vital

and complex cognitive function, with a key role in the regulation of awareness and goal-directed behavior. Due to limitations in processing resources,
the brain has to discern relevant information in the environment and therefore needs selection mechanisms, such as attention, in order to encode the
more pertinent information in preference to concomitant events of less interest
(Kastner & Ungerleider, 2000). As a consequence, unattended information
in a scene usually fails to be fully processed and does not enter awareness.
However, emotion appears to have a similar and complementary role in controlling the allocation of processing resources for perception and awareness.
Compelling evidence has accrued to indicate that specific mechanisms may act
to facilitate attention toward emotionally significant stimuli—an ability with
obvious evolutionary advantages (Öhman, 1986)—and that neural circuits
underlying these effects are intimately linked to amygdala function (Vuilleumier, 2005). Hence attention and emotion do not constitute entirely separate systems; rather, both contribute to regulate the access of sensory inputs
to conscious awareness, though via partly distinct neural mechanisms. This in
turn suggests that emotion processing not only may serve to imbue experience
with affective values and "feelings," but may directly shape the content of perception itself. This is obviously an important function for promoting adaptive
behavior and survival in typical conditions, although it may also contribute
to some pathological situations where distribution of attention and hence perceptual contents in awareness could be altered by abnormal emotional processing, such as in anxiety or phobia. This chapter provides a general overview
of this reciprocal interplay between attention and emotion, and in particular
describes our current knowledge of the underlying neural circuits.

ENHANCED PERCEPTUAL PROCESSING
FOR EMOTIONAL INFORMATION

In keeping with our common subjective experience that emotionally charged
events make stronger impressions, brain imaging studies in humans have consistently demonstrated increased neural responses to a great variety of emotional stimuli, relative to comparable but neutral stimuli. This research has
used a variety of experimental paradigms and techniques, including functional magnetic resonance imaging (fMRI), positron emission tomography
(PET), electroencephalography (EEG), and magnetoencephalography (MEG).
The amygdala is thought to be critically involved in such increases and may
exert its influences through both direct and indirect mechanisms, as described
in more detail below.

In the visual domain, an emotional "boosting" of neural responses to
emotional stimuli has been observed in early visual areas, including primary
visual cortex in the occipital lobe (Lang et al., 1998; Pessoa, McKenna, Gutierrez, & Ungerleider, 2002; Vuilleumier, Armony, Driver, & Dolan, 2001),
as well as in higher-level regions associated with object and face recogni-

tion (Morris et al., 1998; Sabatinelli, Bradley, Fitzsimmons, & Lang, 2005). For instance, scenes with emotional content produce greater activation in the lateral occipital cortex than neutral scenes do (Lane, Chua, & Dolan, 1999), whereas faces with emotional expressions (such as fear) produce selective increases in the fusiform face area (FFA) (Vuilleumier et al., 2001), and emotional body expressions activate both the fusiform and extrastriate body areas (FBA and EBA) (Peelen, Atkinson, Andersson, & Vuilleumier, 2007). Likewise, in the auditory domain, vocal and nonvocal sounds with emotional significance (such as prosody, animal cries, or gunshots) may evoke significantly higher neural responses in auditory cortical areas than similar but more mundane sounds do (Fecteau, Belin, Joanette, & Armony, 2007; Grandjean et al., 2005; Sander, Grandjean, & Scherer, 2005). These findings suggest a selective modulation by emotion of cortical areas that are specifically involved in processing the stimulus category (see Plate 10.1 in color insert).

Stimulus-specific modulation has recently been demonstrated in a study using a multivoxel pattern analysis of fMRI data (Peelen et al., 2007). In this study, participants viewed short movies with either faces or bodies expressing various emotional expressions (e.g., neutral or fearful, angry, happy, etc.). Face and body stimuli elicited overlapping activation in fusiform cortex, in accord with previous reports on the FFA and FBA (Peelen & Downing, 2005), but a voxel-by-voxel analysis demonstrated a significant correlation between emotion-related activation and category-related activation, for each individual voxel within the fusiform cortex, in each individual participant. In other words, the amount of emotional modulation by body expressions was correlated with the magnitude of body selectivity in fusiform (and also in the occipital EBA), whereas there was no relation with the magnitude of responses to faces. Conversely, emotional modulation of fusiform cortex by facial expressions was correlated with the degree of response selectivity to faces, but not with the degree of responses to bodies (all relative to a third visual category of tools). These results indicate that emotional modulations induced by face or body expressions are exerted on distinct voxels that have different preferences for faces or bodies, respectively, supporting a stimulus-specific enhancement rather than more general boosting of visual processing. Nonetheless, some effects due to increased vigilance or alertness may also arise in different brain areas or in different situations.

Increased responses in visual (Armony & Dolan, 2002; Tabbert, Stark, Kirsch, & Vaitl, 2005) or auditory (Büchel, Morris, Dolan, & Friston, 1998) cortical areas are also obtained for previously neutral stimuli after these have acquired a particular emotional value, such as through aversive Pavlovian conditioning. This suggests that these effects are not simply due to intrinsic sensory features of the stimuli, but directly relate to their emotional significance—which may result from previous experience and learning. These findings are consistent with a role of the amygdala in driving these responses, since the amygdala is known to represent a key neural substrate underlying affective conditioning (Phelps & LeDoux, 2005). Thus several studies have found that when a face is repeatedly paired with unpleasant sounds, it will produce greater activation in face-sensitive regions of the visual cortex when it is subsequently presented without the sound than the same face without such preexposure will (Armony & Dolan, 2002; Glascher & Büchel, 2005), and that such increases in visual areas are usually accompanied by concomitant activation in the amygdala. Similar conditioning effects arising in parallel in visual areas and amygdala have been found with abstract, nonfacial stimuli, such as geometric shapes (Tabbert et al., 2005).

In several studies showing increased activation of visual cortical areas to emotional relative to neutral stimuli such as faces, bodies, or scenes, the magnitude of these increases was significantly correlated with amygdala responses (Morris et al., 1998; Peelen et al., 2007; Sabatinelli et al., 2005). That is, the greater the amygdala's sensitivity to the emotional meaning of a visual stimulus, the greater the responses of visual areas to this stimulus. Furthermore, studies comparing different stimulus categories in individuals with different types of phobias have shown parallel increases in visual cortices and amygdala for the relevant fear cues (e.g., pictures of snakes), which do not arise for the same stimulus category in individuals without phobias (Sabatinelli et al., 2005). These findings support the view that the amygdala may be functionally implicated in these emotional effects on stimulus-processing areas, although such correlation alone does not demonstrate a true directional or causal role.

Research examining electrophysiological responses to emotional stimuli with EEG or MEG has brought similar results, indicating that perceptual processes are modulated by emotion at several cortical stages. Most remarkably, event-related potentials (ERPs) show that early components associated with sensory processing (within 100–200 msec after stimulus onset) are enhanced in response to emotional cues (for a review, see Olofsson, Nordin, Sequeira, & Polich, 2008), such as facial expressions or fear-conditioned stimuli (Dolan, Heinze, Hurlemann, & Hinrichs, 2006; Eimer & Holmes, 2002; Pourtois, Schwartz, Seghier, Lazeyras, & Vuilleumier, 2005; Schupp, Junghofer, Weike, & Hamm, 2003, 2004). These emotional effects in ERPs include increases in the amplitude of exogenous visual components such as P1 or N1, which are generated in early extrastriate cortex and are known to index general attentional factors (Hopfinger, Woldorff, Fletcher, & Mangun, 2001). Emotional increases can also affect subsequent, more specific components such as N170 (Pizzagalli et al., 2002) or posterior negative waveforms (Kissler, Herbert, Peyk, & Junghofer, 2007; Schupp et al., 2003), which are associated with face or object recognition processes in higher-level visual regions, respectively. In some cases, emotional effects have been observed for the earliest visual cortical responses recorded in EEG (C1 component), thought to reflect neuronal activity in striate cortex (Pourtois, Grandjean, Sander, & Vuilleumier, 2004; Stolarova, Keil, & Moratti, 2006). Altogether, these effects are suggestive of enhanced processing within early perceptual pathways. In addition, emotional stimuli produce distinctive electrophysiological responses at longer latencies after stimulus onset (i.e., 300–400 msec), characterized by modulations of the classic P3 component (Carretie, Iglesias, Garcia, & Ballesteros, 1997; Lang, Nelson, & Collins, 1990; Schupp et al., 2003) or sustained late positive potentials (Cuthbert, Schupp, Bradley, Birbaumer, & Lang, 2000; Krolak-Salmon, Fischer, Vighetto, & Mauguiere, 2001), which may be related to more elaborate affective and cognitive evaluations of these stimuli, subsequent autonomic arousal, and/or memory formation (Olofsson et al., 2008). Source localization analyses suggest that these late ERP components reflect the activity of a widespread cortical network including prefrontal, cingulate, and parietal regions (Carretie, Martin-Loeches, Hinojosa, & Mercado, 2001), although a recent study combining EEG with fMRI in the same participants found that the amplitude of late positive potentials was also correlated with blood-oxygen-level-dependent (BOLD) responses in occipitotemporal cortex (Sabatinelli, Lang, Keil, & Bradley, 2007).

Because emotional influences on perception and attention have long been perceived as vital for efficient detection of potential dangers (Öhman, 1986), the vast majority of imaging and electrophysiology studies investigating these effects have generally focused on threat-related cues (such as fearful or angry faces, as well as unpleasant or aversively conditioned scenes). This also reflects the traditional view that the amygdala plays a well-established role in fear processing and may be responsible for these influences. However, a similar enhancement of cortical responses has now consistently been observed in both visual and auditory areas for other types of emotional stimuli, including positive visual scenes, erotica, or joyful voices (Fecteau et al., 2007; Sabatinelli et al., 2005; Wiethoff et al., 2008). These positive emotional stimuli also activate the amygdala, in accord with the view that the latter may not respond to fear cues only, but also more generally to arousing, ambiguous, or self-relevant information (Anderson, Christoff, Stappen, et al., 2003; Baxter & Murray, 2002; Sander, Grafman, & Zalla, 2003). Nevertheless, it still remains to be determined what critical affective dimensions are driving human amygdala responses, and whether different types of emotional cues (e.g., fear, anger, disgust, joy) produce similar influences on perceptual and attentional processes, inasmuch as they produce similar responses in the amygdala. Although the amygdala may be activated in response to, and may modulate, sensory processing of both positive and arousing stimuli, some studies have found greater effects for fearful than for happy faces that cannot be simply explained by differences in arousal (Morris et al., 1998; Surguladze et al., 2003).

Taken together, data from functional imaging and electrophysiology therefore converge to show that emotion signals may boost perceptual processing in early sensory cortices, and may do so for different sensory modalities or stimulus categories. Such boosting may consist of stimulus-specific and nonspecific increases in processing, leading to a more robust representation of the affectively relevant event or more general effects on vigilance and responsiveness to other accompanying stimuli. Both specific and nonspecific effects may serve to enhance cortical analysis and/or plasticity in response to emotional information.

BEHAVIORAL CONSEQUENCES
OF EMOTIONAL INFLUENCES ON PERCEPTION

In keeping with neuroimaging evidence of enhanced neural responses to emotional information, a large number of behavioral results indicate that perception is facilitated and attention is prioritized for emotionally significant stimuli as compared with neutral ones. Classic examples come from visual search studies, where the detection of a visual target among distractors is typically quicker when the target is emotional as opposed to neutral. Although this has often been shown with negative or threat-related stimuli, such as angry faces, snakes, or spiders (Eastwood, Smilek, & Merikle, 2001; Fox, 2002; Öhman, Flykt, & Esteves, 2001), similar effects have also occasionally been reported with positive or appetitive stimuli (Lucas & Vuilleumier, 2008; Williams, Moss, Bradshaw, & Mattingley, 2005). Conversely, emotional distractors may slow target detection during search or other selective attention tasks (Fenske & Eastwood, 2003; Horstmann, Scharlau, & Ansorge, 2006). However, a greater efficiency of search for emotional targets does not imply that emotional stimuli are processed without attention or "pop out" like targets defined by salient feature differences (e.g., color), as was sometimes inferred from early studies (Hansen & Hansen, 1988). Instead, attention appears to be preferentially drawn toward and speeded up for emotionally distinctive information, reflecting biases in the allocation of attention rather than a bypass or shortcut to conscious perception. Thus the detection time slopes are typically shallower when targets are emotional rather than neutral, but do not remain flat, regardless of the number of items in the search display (Figure 10.1).

These findings show that attentional priority tends to be given to emotional stimuli in cluttered visual scenes in which concurrent objects compete for processing resources. Such effects suggest in turn that emotional information may be extracted prior to selective attention and used to guide attention to the location of relevant stimuli. Accordingly, the advantage for emotional targets is abolished when search is performed with a restricted aperture revealing items one by one as a function of each successive fixation (Smilek, Frischen, Reynolds, Gerritsen, & Eastwood, 2007); this demonstrates that the facilitation of detection times depends on some coarse perceptual analysis prior to attentive fixation, but is not due to quicker identification or response selection after the stimulus has been fixated.

Nevertheless, it remains somewhat uncertain whether the critical dimensions responsible for attracting attention are directly related to processing of the emotional meaning per se or of associated perceptual characteristics of the stimuli (Horstmann, Borgstedt, & Heumann, 2006; Huang, Baddeley, & Young, 2008). The degree of attentional capture by emotional stimuli does not necessarily correspond to the strength of affective evaluations for the same stimuli, even when measured by other implicit tests such as affective priming (Purkis & Lipp, 2007). However, a role for emotional processes is supported by the findings that attentional biases are often exaggerated in people with

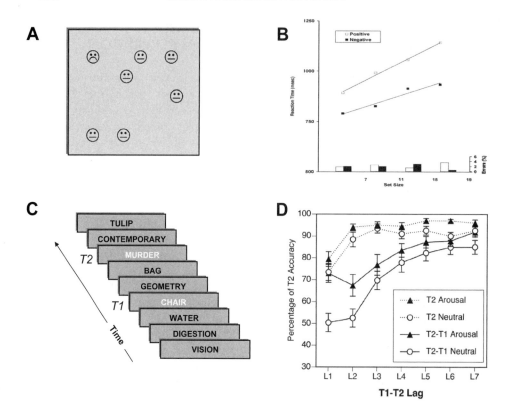

FIGURE 10.1. Emotional facilitation of attentional tasks. (A) Visual search requiring detection of a target face with either negative or positive expression among distractor faces with neutral expression. (B) Detection becomes slower with increasing number of distractors, but consistently quicker for negative than for positive faces. A and B are from Eastwood, Smilek, and Merikle (2001). Copyright 2001 by the Psychonomic Society. Reprinted by permission. (C) Attentional blink paradigm requiring detection of target words cued by green print in a rapid visual stream. (D) Detection is impaired when a second target (T2) follows a first target (T1) after a short interval, but with fewer misses when T2 is emotionally arousing rather than neutral. This advantage is observed only when attentional resources are taxed by task demands (reporting both T1 and T2), but does not reflect better perceptual discrimination of arousing compared to neutral words when there is no competition for attention (reporting T2 alone).

high anxiety or specific phobia. Thus attention is directed faster to pictures of snakes than spiders in persons with snake phobia, but vice versa in persons with spider phobia (Öhman et al., 2001). Specific physiological responses may also accompany faster detection of emotional targets during visual search (Flykt, 2005). But even though this suggests that emotion may drive attention, it is also possible that these effects reflect a greater sensitivity or tuning of perceptual systems to critical sensory features, or that different processes operate in parallel.

A role for emotion meaning in inducing attentional biases is also supported by behavioral studies using words with emotional or nonemotional content, which have shown that emotional words are better detected than neutral words when presented in rapid succession (Anderson, 2005; Anderson & Phelps, 2001) or when masked (Gaillard et al., 2006). These findings imply that written words may receive sufficient semantic processing under conditions where attentional resources are limited by the current task demands (Naccache et al., 2005), and that they may enjoy a lower threshold for gaining access to awareness as a function of their meaning. In particular, this phenomenon has been well established by studies of the "attentional blink" (Anderson, 2005; Huang et al., 2008; Keil & Ihssen, 2004). Whereas visual search highlights competition for processing resources between concurrent stimuli distributed in space, the attentional blink reveals a similar limitation for processing stimuli that appear in close temporal proximity. Thus the detection of a target word in a rapid serial visual presentation (with different items appearing serially at fixation) is impaired when it occurs shortly after another target (as if attention capacity transiently "blinked"). However, this impairment may be reduced when the second target is emotional rather than neutral (Anderson, 2005; Keil & Ihssen, 2004). Conversely, the attentional blink for a second (neutral) target may increase when the first is emotional, suggesting that the emotional meaning of words tends to either grab or divert attention in situations where resources cannot be equally deployed to every successive stimulus. Moreover, this advantage for emotional words is specifically observed in conditions requiring dual-target detection (Figure 10.1), where processing resources are taxed, but not in conditions with single targets where no competition occurs (Anderson, 2005); again, this suggests that emotional processes act on capacity-limited stages controlling access to awareness, rather than on stimulus recognition per se. These affective influences on attentional blink seem to reflect primarily the arousal value of words, rather than their valence or verbal distinctiveness (Anderson, 2005; Keil & Ihssen, 2004), although a few studies have reported greater effects on attentional blink with fearful faces or threatening pictures than with positive stimuli in people who show high anxiety or phobias (Fox, Russo, & Georgiou, 2005; Trippe, Hewig, Heydel, Hecht, & Miltner, 2007). Likewise, suppression of perception by binocular manipulations, such as rivalry (Alpers & Gerdes, 2007) or continuous flash suppression (in which stimuli presented to one eye are rendered invisible by dynamic "noise" presented to the other eye; see Yang, Zald, & Blake, 2007), show that fearful faces emerge into awareness more frequently and more quickly than neutral or happy faces do. These effects can also be obtained by fear conditioning with previously neutral stimuli (Alpers, Ruhleder, Walz, Muhlberger, & Pauli, 2005; Smith, Most, Newsome, & Zald, 2006).

Interestingly, modulation of detection performance for emotional relative to neutral words in attentional blink conditions may occur only when semantic processing of the stimuli is required, not when a purely perceptual or phonological task is required instead (Huang et al., 2008). This suggests that emotional significance is not automatically extracted in these conditions, but depends on the level of semantic analysis. A role for task-related factors in allowing the activation of semantic representations or associations may be particularly important for emotional influences from words; however, this may be less obvious for visual cues in faces or pictures of objects in which semantic and emotion information tends to be extracted effortlessly even when task-relevant (Boucart, Humphreys, & Lorenceau, 1995; Ganel & Goshen-Gottstein, 2004). Moreover, emotional Stroop effects indicate that sometimes word meaning can produce involuntary effects on attention even when semantic processing is not required (Williams, Mathews, & MacLeod, 1996)—just as facial expressions can also slow down face color judgments (van Honk, Tuiten, de Haan, van den Hout, & Stam, 2001).

Critically, affective influences on target detection in the attentional blink have been found to depend on amygdala functions, consistent with the idea that the latter may be responsible for enhanced perceptual processing in sensory cortical areas. A pioneer study by Anderson and Phelps (2001) showed that unlike healthy people, who demonstrate a robust reduction of the attentional blink for verbal stimuli with aversive content as compared with neutral stimuli, patients with left or bilateral damage to the amygdala showed no benefits for such negative stimulus events. In spite of this, all patients still understood normally the affective meaning of negative words. These results point to a direct causal role of the amygdala for affective influences on perception and attention, beyond its well-established involvement in the affective modulation of learning and memory. Moreover, the impact of left but not right amygdala lesions on the detection of emotionally salient words is consistent with imaging studies showing a predominant activation of the left amygdala in response to verbal material (Hamann & Mao, 2002; but see Isenberg et al., 1999; Kensinger & Schacter, 2006). In addition, a critical influence of the arousal value of words (Anderson, 2005; Keil & Ihssen, 2004) or faces (Brosch, Sander, & Scherer, 2007; Lucas & Vuilleumier, 2008; Williams, Moss, et al., 2005) on attentional biases induced by emotional cues accords with evidence from neuroimaging that the amygdala may primarily represent arousal (or relevance) of sensory events, rather than their valence (Anderson, Christoff, Stappen, et al., 2003; Lewis, Critchley, Rotshtein, & Dolan, 2007).

Taken together, behavioral and imaging data converge to indicate that perceptual processing is enhanced for emotionally significant information, and that such enhancement is related to intact amygdala activity: It allows the neural representation of potentially relevant or threatening events to be strengthened under conditions of limited attention, and thus prioritized for their access to awareness. This enhancement of perceptual processing is analogous to that produced in sensory cortical areas by attentional signals, which are thought to reflect top-down influences from frontal and parietal areas (Kastner & Ungerleider, 2000; Vuilleumier & Driver, 2007) and to mediate similar changes in awareness due to selective attention (e.g., Beck, Rees, Frith, & Lavie, 2001). For emotional stimuli, however, such enhancement appears to be critically dependent on the amygdala, rather than the frontoparietal cortex, as described in further detail below.

NEURAL PATHWAYS FOR THE AMYGDALA'S DIRECT AND INDIRECT INFLUENCES ON SENSORY PROCESSING

Direct access of the amygdala to sensory cortical areas is made possible by dense feedback connections that project from amygdala nuclei to widespread regions in the cortex, including all stages along the perceptual pathways (Amaral, Behniea, & Kelly, 2003). Tracing studies in the macaque monkey have shown that such projections to visual cortices have a precise topographical organization (Figure 10.2) with a rostral-to-caudal gradient, such that more rostral regions of the amygdala project to higher-level areas in more rostral parts of the ventral temporal stream (e.g., area TE), whereas more caudal regions of the amygdala project to earlier, more caudal visual areas (e.g., area V1). These connections are not strictly reciprocal, because cortical projections from the amygdala are more divergent than cortical projections to the amygdala. In the visual system, the main cortical inputs are provided by rostral areas such as TE and terminate predominantly in the lateral nucleus, while the amygdala projections originate primarily in the basal nucleus and target all areas from V1 to TE, in a relatively distributed and punctuated manner, but with area TE receiving additional return projections from the lateral and accessory basal nucleus (Amaral et al., 2003; Freese & Amaral, 2005). Interestingly, in the macaque monkey, the most dense projections were found in the ventral bank of the superior temporal sulcus (STS), corresponding to regions known to contain neurons with selective responses to faces (Baylis, Rolls, & Leonard, 1987). In addition, at the microscopic level, amygdala projections terminate exclusively in the superficial layers (border of I–II) of area V1, and in both the superficial (I–II) and deep layers (V–VI) of area TE (Freese & Amaral, 2005), consistent with an excitatory feedback input that primarily influences pyramidal neurons in these cortices (Freese & Amaral, 2006). Thus, as the basal nucleus is highly interconnected with other amygdala nuclei and receives inputs from the lateral nucleus (Stefanacci et al., 1992), these circuits may be ideally suited to provide a modulatory feedback signal enhancing the cortical processing of visual stimuli that activate the amygdala (Figure 10.2). Moreover, although in primates the most abundant inputs to the amygdala are received from the visual system, a similar pattern of afferent and efferent projections has been observed for the auditory and somatosensory modalities. For example, amygdala connections to areas TC and TA of the auditory cortex primarily originate in the basal nucleus, with a rostrocaudal topography of neurons within the basal nucleus, and additional projections from the accessory basal and lateral nuclei to the more rostral auditory cortex (Yukie, 2002).

Similar feedback connections are likely to exist in the human brain, and may underlie the enhanced responses to emotional stimuli observed in behavioral and neuroimaging studies. Recent MRI studies using diffusion tensor imaging have identified topographically organized fibers in the white matter between occipital cortex and anterior medial temporal lobe, named the inferior longitudinal fasciculus, which may contain such back-projections from the amygdala to early visual areas and/or fast transfer of visual signals to anterior temporal structures (Catani, Jones, Donato, & ffytche, 2003). More direct evidence for a modulatory influence of the amygdala on cortical responses in humans is provided by imaging studies showing that amygdala lesions cause abnormal functional activation in distant connected sites (Vuil-

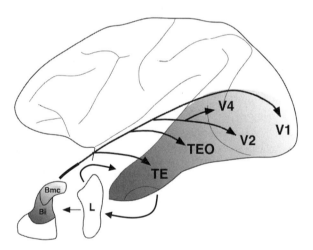

FIGURE 10.2. Feedback projections from amygdala to visual cortex. Results from tracing studies in the macaque show topographically organized connections with denser projections to rostral than to caudal visual areas. Whereas the lateral nucleus (L) receives and projects mainly to higher-level areas (such as TE), the basal nucleus shows a progressive gradient, such that its dorsal part (magnocellular; Bmc) projects predominantly to earlier areas (such as V1) and its more ventral part (intermediate; Bi) projects predominantly to later areas (such as TEO and TE). From Freese and Amaral (2005). Copyright 2005 by Wiley. Reprinted by permission.

leumier, Richardson, Armony, Driver, & Dolan, 2004). Patients with medial temporal lobe sclerosis have been examined by fMRI while they viewed faces with fearful or neutral expressions, in order to compare neural responses in fusiform cortex for those patients who had damage to both the amygdala and hippocampus, relative to those who had damage to the hippocampus alone, in addition to healthy controls. In this study (Vuilleumier et al., 2004), participants were presented with pairs of faces or houses that were the same or different, either vertically or horizontally aligned (Plate 10.2 in color insert). In different blocks, participants had to focus on the vertical pair while ignoring the horizontal pair, or vice versa, and then judged whether the pictures in each pair (houses or faces) were the same or different. Faces were either both fearful or both neutral. Healthy controls and patients with hippocampus damage only showed increased activation in visual cortex, and particularly fusiform gyrus, to the fearful faces as compared to the neutral faces, indicating that these areas were activated by fearful expressions beyond the activation produced by neutral faces. Moreover, this increase was observed regardless of whether the participants focused their attention on the face pair or the house pair (replicating earlier findings in healthy individuals; see Vuilleumier et al., 2001). However, such an increase was not observed in the patients with amygdala plus hippocampus damage (Plate 10.2). Furthermore, correlation analyses could show that the loss in such modulation was parametrically related to the degree of sclerosis in the amygdala ipsilateral to the visual areas tested. In other words, left amygdala damage abolished the increased activation to fearful faces in the left fusiform gyrus, but right amygdala damage abolished increased activation in the right fusiform.

These findings imply that although each amygdala may project diffusely to widespread regions along the ventral visual stream, these projections are predominantly acting within the same hemisphere (ipsilaterally), in keeping with anatomical data from tracing studies in monkeys (Amaral et al., 2003; Freese & Amaral, 2005). These fMRI results thus clearly demonstrate that the amygdala plays a direct causal role in the enhanced cortical processing of emotional stimuli. By contrast, regardless of lesions in amygdala and/or hippocampus, the fusiform cortex was still modulated by attention in all patients, as shown by normal increases in activity when conditions where faces were task-relevant versus irrelevant were compared. This is consistent with the notion that such attentional effects are mediated by top-down influences from frontal and parietal cortical systems (Kastner & Ungerleider, 2000; Vuilleumier & Driver, 2007), which were intact in all patients.

Abnormal activation in several visual and temporal areas was also reported in another fMRI study of face recognition in patients with medial temporal lobe epilepsy (Benuzzi et al., 2004), with more severe deficits in cases with right lesions and disease onset in early life. These patients also had difficulties in recognizing fearful expressions in faces, suggesting that some long-lasting changes may also arise in visual cortices subsequent to amygdala dysfunction (Grelotti, Gauthier, & Schultz, 2002). Likewise, recent ERP results have pointed to functional anomalies in visual responses to emotional faces in patients with amygdala lesions (Rotshtein et al., 2006), with a reduction of differential responses to fearful versus neutral expressions affecting both the early P1 component (~100–150 msec after stimulus onset) and the later components (arising at ~500 msec). In this ERP study, the severity of amygdala pathology determined the magnitude of both these effects, consistent with a causal role for the amygdala. These results suggest two distinct phases during which the amygdala may influence the processing of emotional faces. More recent data applying causal connectivity analysis to visual ERPS have also shown increased coupling between visual and parietal areas during exposure to emotional pictures, relative to neutral pictures; this was interpreted as evidence for reentrant signals from attentional systems to lower-level sensory areas (Keil et al., in press).

Another pathway by which the amygdala may modulate perception and attention involves indirect influences on cortical areas through cholinergic projections. Cholinergic nuclei in the basal forebrain receive dense inputs from the amygdala, particularly the central nucleus, which may thereby play a major role in attentional orienting and vigilance (Holland & Gallagher, 1999; Holland, Han, & Gallagher, 2000). The basal forebrain nuclei in turn project to many regions in frontal, parietal, and sensory cortices where cholinergic signals generally act to enhance the processing of stimulus information in attention-demanding contexts, by amplifying and sustaining neuronal responses (Sarter, Hasselmo, Bruno, & Givens, 2005). Such effects may contribute to the modulation of perception by emotional processing in the amygdala, as well as to top-down influences by executive control systems in frontal or parietal cortex. In animals, electrical stimulation of the amygdala may increase cortical arousal via its influences on the activity of cholinergic neurons of the nucleus basalis (Dringenberg, Saber, & Cahill, 2001; Kapp, Supple, & Whalen, 1994).

In humans, these cholinergic influences have been investigated by fMRI in combination with procholinergic drugs, such as the cholinesterase inhibitor physostigmine (Bentley, Vuilleumier, Thiel, Driver, & Dolan, 2003), during a visual task with neutral and fearful faces similar to that previously used in healthy subjects (Vuilleumier et al., 2001) and patients with medial temporal sclerosis (Vuilleumier et al., 2004). In this task, again, faces and houses were presented in vertical or horizontal pairs, while participants focused their attention on one pair of stimuli but ignored the other pair, and faces could be both fearful or both neutral (see Plate 10.2 in color insert). On the one hand, physostigmine (relative to placebo) was found to enhance visual responses to emotional faces in fusiform cortex (and dorsolateral prefrontal cortex)—but only when attention was directed to the faces, not when attention was directed to houses and faces were ignored instead (Bentley et al., 2003). On the other hand, physostigmine also increased responses to fearful faces in the lateral orbitofrontal and anterior cingulate cortex, whereas it decreased responses in intraparietal cortex, but specifically when attention was directed away from faces (Plate 10.3 in color insert). The latter changes in activation paralleled changes in behavioral performance, with slower response times to houses when unattended faces were fearful versus neutral; these results suggested an inter-ference due to emotional distractors that was enhanced under physostigmine, and mediated by modulations of attentional control systems in intraparietal and orbitofrontal cortex. The amygdala itself was modulated by neither phys-ostigmine nor attention (Bentley et al., 2003). Taken together, these findings indicate that acetylcholine is not directly responsible for the usual enhanced activation to emotional stimuli in sensory areas (Morris et al., 1998; Sabatinelli et al., 2005; Vuilleumier et al., 2001), but that it can modulate frontoparietal areas to promote the allocation of attention to emotional information.

Lastly, interactions between attention and emotion processing may also implicate projections from the amygdala to the orbitofrontal and cingulate cortices, together with their reciprocal connections with other prefrontal areas (Cavada, Compañy, Tejedor, Cruz-Rizzolo, & Reinoso-Suarez, 2000), through which emotional limbic circuits may affect ongoing cognitive pro-cesses mediated by dorsal and lateral prefrontal areas, or vice versa (Dol-cos & McCarthy, 2006; Yamasaki, LaBar, & McCarthy, 2002). In addition, orbitofrontal and ventromedial prefrontal cortex may also regulate emotional processing through their inputs to the basal nucleus of the amygdala, and thus in turn indirectly affect its output and feedback to various brain regions. However, the exact dynamics and functional roles of these different circuits still remain to be determined.

COMPLEMENTARITY AND INDEPENDENCE OF EMOTIONAL REGULATION AND ATTENTION

The existence of neural circuits enabling direct modulatory feedback from the amygdala on sensory pathways suggests that emotional influences may affect cortical activity in parallel to influences exerted on the same areas by other top-down signals, particularly those due to voluntary attention under the control of frontal and parietal networks (Vuilleumier, 2005). Thus top-down enhancement of sensory inputs may be determined by additive influences from different sources, including both emotional and attentional processes, which can then converge on common neural sites or pathways in order to regulate perceptual analysis and access to awareness. Partly separate and parallel influ-ences of emotion on perception should be useful, in order to ensure that threat or affectively relevant information can be monitored even when it is outside the current focus of attention and unexpected by the current goal settings, so as to allow the brain to reorient processing resources and plan adaptive responses. Indeed, since selective attention gates the access to awareness and goal-directed behavior, it would potentially be highly deleterious if any signifi-cant event was always ignored whenever attention was focused elsewhere and already occupied by less significant information.

A number of imaging studies have provided evidence supporting these parallel influences of emotion and attention on perception. For instance, in research using fMRI in experimental conditions where attention and emotion factors were manipulated separately, it was found that the response to faces in visual cortex (Bentley et al., 2003; Vuilleumier et al., 2001) or to voices in auditory cortex (Grandjean et al., 2005) could be modulated by each factor independently. In a study similar to the one described above (Vuilleumier et al., 2004; see Plate 10.2 in color insert), healthy participants were presented with brief displays of two faces and two houses, and had to judge one pair of stimuli at precued locations (same–different matching task); brain responses to fearful expressions could be compared when the faces appeared at either the cued (task-relevant) or uncued (irrelevant) locations—that is, inside or outside the focus of attention. In this study (Vuilleumier et al., 2001), face-sensitive regions in fusiform cortex showed increased activation when attention was directed to faces versus houses (as expected); more importantly, fusiform activity was also greater for fearful than for neutral faces, both when faces were task-relevant and when they were ignored (with houses now task-relevant). In other words, fear expression could boost fusiform activity, in a manner both parallel and additive to the modulation of the same region by spatial attention. A similar fMRI paradigm with emotional voices heard on the attended or unattended side revealed similar results (Grandjean et al., 2005). In the latter study, participants performed a dichotic listening task with two voices, one in the left ear and one in the right ear. Voices could be either neutral or angry. As illustrated in Plate 10.4 (in color insert), results showed that voice-selective regions in superior temporal gyrus were modulated by voluntary attention (with greater responses when participants were focusing on the contralateral than on the ipsilateral ear), regardless of voice prosody; in addition, however, the same regions were modulated by emotional prosody (with greater responses to angry than neutral voices), regardless of the side of the angry voices (i.e., in the attended or unattended ear). These fMRI data demonstrate that face or voice processing may be modulated by emotional cues, over and above the concomitant influence of endogenously driven attention, and that such emotional responses may still persist when attention is diverted and cortical processing is reduced for the emotionally relevant stimulus.

Additive effects of emotion and attention on early perceptual responses to emotional stimuli were also observed in ERP studies manipulating these two factors systematically (Keil, Moratti, Sabatinelli, Bradley, & Lang, 2005; Schupp, Flaisch, Stockburger, & Junghofer, 2006; Schupp et al., 2007). For instance, Keil and colleagues (2005) presented pairs of emotional and neutral pictures, one in each visual hemifield, while participants directed attention to one side only (right or left). Amplitude of ERPs was increased and latencies were reduced for emotional relative to neutral pictures, regardless of their location, but also for all attended relative to unattended pictures, regardless of their emotional content. Such findings again suggest that visual processing along the occipitotemporal pathways may be regulated by both affective and attentional processes.

Nevertheless, this independent neural circuitry for attentional and emotional control of perception does not necessarily imply that both factors do not interact in some conditions and/or some brain areas. Whereas emotional processing can modulate attention, attention is in turn likely to influence emotional responses, even though each type of processing may be largely activated independently of the other (Compton, 2003; Okon-Singer, Tzelgov, & Henik, 2007). For instance, directing attention away from faces may reduce amygdala responses in tasks where attentional load is particularly high (Erthal et al., 2005; Pessoa et al., 2002; Pessoa, Padmala, & Morland, 2005; Silvert et al., 2007), and thus possibly also reduce the impact of emotion on perceptual processing. In many cases, however, some emotional responses may still occur without explicit attention to the stimuli or even without awareness (Anderson, Christoff, Panitz, De Rosa, & Gabrieli, 2003; Critchley, Mathias, & Dolan, 2002; Jiang & He, 2006; Pasley, Mayes, & Schultz, 2004; Whalen et al., 1998; Williams, McGlone, Abbott, & Mattingley, 2005; Williams, Morris, McGlone, Abbott, & Mattingley, 2004). Such responding is perhaps driven by elementary sensory features that are sufficient to activate the amygdala despite incomplete processing in the cortex, such as low spatial frequency (Alorda, Serrano-Pedraza, Campos-Bueno, Sierra-Vazquez, & Montoya, 2007; Carretie, Hinojosa, Lopez-Martin, & Tapia, 2007; Vuilleumier, Armony, Driver, & Dolan, 2003) and/or simple "diagnostic" cues (Whalen et al., 2004; Yang et al., 2007)). Critically, ERP recordings suggest that some emotional effects may affect early perceptual processes (~100–120 msec after stimulus onset) prior to the modulation by voluntary attention (~170–300 msec after stimulus onset) (Holmes, Vuilleumier, & Eimer, 2003; Schupp et al., 2007), and that dynamic interactions between emotion and attention may vary, depending on the perceptual stages at which they arise.

Furthermore, the effectiveness of emotional processing and its attenuation by attentional control or goal settings may also depend on individual factors, such as anxiety (Bishop, Duncan, & Lawrence, 2004) or harm avoidance (Most, Chun, Johnson, & Kiehl, 2006), consistent with behavioral findings that some personality traits may determine attentional biases to emotional information (Bradley, Mogg, & Millar, 2000; Fox et al., 2005; Öhman et al., 2001; Trippe et al., 2007). These task-related or personality-related influences may act on emotional pathways through projections from prefrontal and orbitofrontal areas on the basal nucleus of the amygdala, by gating the relay of inputs within the feedback loop to sensory cortices (Freese & Amaral, 2005). In our own studies, however, attentional load or anxiety factors were found to correlate with activity in anterior cingulate and prefrontal areas, but without significant effects on amygdala responses (Vuilleumier, Armony, & Schwartz, unpublished data).

Most importantly, the independence of attentional and emotional influences on perception is further supported by neuropsychological evidence that emotional biases may still arise in patients in whom attentional mechanisms are selectively impaired after brain damage. These patients may present with a syndrome of spatial hemineglect, characterized by failures in orienting attention to left space subsequent to frontal or parietal lesions in the right hemisphere (Driver, Vuilleumier, & Husain, 2004; Vuilleumier, 2004). Therefore, such patients typically remain unaware of stimuli or events arising on their left (contralesional) side, especially when presented with another competing stimulus on the right (intact/ipsilesional) side or with multielement search display. However, this loss in awareness has been found to be less severe for emotional stimuli, such as faces with angry or happy expressions as compared with neutral faces (Fox, 2002; Lucas & Vuilleumier, 2008; Vuilleumier & Schwartz, 2001b); bodies with emotional gestures as compared with neutral bodies (Tamietto, Geminiani, Genero, & de Gelder, 2007); or pictures of spiders as compared with pictures of flowers (Vuilleumier & Schwartz, 2001a). Likewise, these patients often fail to perceive left-sided information when presented with auditory stimuli in both ears simultaneously, but their deficit is less for voices with emotional prosody than for voices with neutral prosody (Grandjean, Sander, Lucas, Scherer, & Vuilleumier, 2008). Altogether, these results accord with the findings from healthy subjects that emotional stimuli tend to attract attention effectively under conditions of competition with neutral stimuli (Anderson, 2005; Eastwood, Smilek, & Merikle, 2003; Fox et al., 2000). However, such emotional effects also produce additive influences over and above the abnormal spatial biases associated with hemineglect, but by no means indicate that emotional stimuli are processed "without attention" or somehow "escape" the effects of inattention to the left space (see Plate 10.5 in color insert). Furthermore, a systematic analysis of brain lesions in patients with hemineglect reveals that those with the largest "benefits" in detection rates for emotional relative to neutral stimuli have lesions centered on lateral frontal and parietal regions, whereas those with weaker emotional biases have more frequent lesions in basal ganglia and orbitofrontal regions; these results for orbitofrontal lesions have been obtained for both emotional faces (Lucas & Vuilleumier, 2008) and emotional voices (Grandjean et al., 2008) (see Plate 10.5 in color insert). These neuropsychological data add to the evidence that emotional influences on perception are not mediated by frontoparietal networks controlling spatial attention (Vuilleumier et al., 2002); they further suggest that orbitofrontal regions may be involved in these interactions between emotion and attention.

REFLEXIVE ORIENTING OF SPATIAL ATTENTION INDUCED BY EMOTIONAL CUES

Once attention has been drawn to and engaged by emotional stimuli, it may also dwell longer at this location and influence the processing of subsequent events. Such orienting effects have been demonstrated in numerous studies using variants of the "dot probe task," initially developed by Posner and subsequently adapted for use with emotional stimuli (Bradley et al., 2000; Fox,

Russo, Bowles, & Dutton, 2001; Mathews, May, Mogg, & Eysenck, 1990). In this classic paradigm, a target (e.g., a dot) must be detected or discriminated as rapidly as possible after a brief cue in which an emotional stimulus (e.g., a face or word) is presented either at the same location (valid) or at a different location (invalid). Typical results show faster responses when the target appears at the location previously occupied by an emotional cue, as compared to when the target follows a neutral cue and the emotional stimulus is presented at another, invalid location. Emotional cueing may also increase contrast sensitivity for the subsequent target, suggesting a modulation of early visual processing (Phelps, Ling, & Carrasco, 2006). These effects are essentially exogenous and reflexive, since they occur despite the fact that the cue is not predictive of the target location (i.e., valid and invalid trials are equally probable). They may arise with both negative and positive cues (Brosch et al., 2007), and operate even across sensory modalities (i.e., for visual targets following auditory cues; Brosch, Grandjean, Sander, & Scherer, 2008), suggesting a supramodal effect on spatial attention. Likewise, emotional distractors may cause transient shifts in covert attention that can then bias eye movements toward their location, even when people are explicitly instructed to avoid looking at these items (Nummenmaa, Hyona, & Calvo, 2006).

Neuroimaging results show that such spatial orienting induced by peripheral emotional stimuli is associated with an activation of the classic frontoparietal networks controlling attention (Armony & Dolan, 2002; Pourtois, Schwartz, Seghier, Lazeyras, & Vuilleumier, 2006). A recent fMRI study (Pourtois et al., 2006) compared brain responses to a simple visual target (a straight line) when it appeared at the same location as a fearful face or at a different location (after a brief interval), and could dissociate responses to these targets from responses to the cues alone (faces without a subsequent target). Results showed a selective activation in the intraparietal sulcus (IPS) for targets following a valid (same location) rather than an invalid (different location) fearful face; conversely, there was an activation of the orbitofrontal cortex for targets following an invalid rather than a valid fearful face. Moreover, increased IPS activation arose on valid trials with ipsilateral targets, but contrasted with a decreased activation on invalid trials, suggesting that the IPS was unresponsive to targets appearing in the ipsilateral hemifield after an invalid fearful face in the contralateral hemifield. These data demonstrate a reduced processing of ipsilateral targets due to the initial focusing of attention on the contralateral side after an invalid fearful cue. By contrast, the IPS was strongly activated by targets in the ipsilateral hemifield when these were preceded by a valid fearful face at the same location (Plate 10.6 in color insert). In other words, attentional processing mediated by the IPS may be restricted to contralateral targets following a fearful face on that same side, but more bilaterally recruited by targets on either side in other conditions—a pattern that corresponds to the prolonged attentional disengagement from emotional stimuli observed behaviorally in similar tasks (Fox et al., 2001). In addition, this fMRI study showed an increased activation of occipital cortex for the visual targets following a valid fearful face, consistent with enhanced visual processing induced by reflexive orienting of attention toward the emotionally cued location (Hopfinger et al., 2001).

In keeping with these fMRI findings, ERP recordings during the same paradigm (Pourtois et al., 2004; Pourtois, Thut, Grave de Peralta, Michel, & Vuilleumier, 2005) revealed a higher amplitude of visual potentials (i.e., the P1 component) evoked by targets when the latter followed a fearful face (valid) rather than a neutral face (invalid). As the P1 is known to be generated in extrastriate occipital cortex and modulated by spatial attention (Hopfinger, Buonocore, & Mangun, 2000), these data further demonstrate that emotional cues may bias attention to their location and enhance perceptual processing of subsequent stimuli (Phelps et al., 2006). A detailed spatiotemporal analysis of these ERPs also revealed that the enhancement of P1 was preceded by a modulation of parietal activity, which correlated with the magnitude of P1 increases (Pourtois, Thut, et al., 2005), suggesting that this earlier parietal activity was possibly responsible for generating top-down influences on visual cortex after the presentation of the emotional cue (Keil et al., in press).

Taken together, these results point to a distinctive cascade of neural events induced by an emotional stimulus, which will influence the allocation of attention and thus enhance perception for this stimulus and others at the same location. Not only may emotional processing in the amygdala act directly on sensory cortices to boost the neural representation of such stimulus and thus promote its access to awareness; this may then also influence frontoparietal mechanisms responsible for orienting and shifting attention in space, so that subsequent information arising at the same location as emotional cues will also benefit from enhanced processing resources.

CONCLUSION

Research in recent years has provided us with a remarkable amount of new knowledge concerning the neural mechanisms by which perception and attention may be influenced by emotional processing. Compelling evidence supports a key role for the amygdala in some of these influences. However, this role involves a dynamic interplay between the amygdala and many other brain regions—including not only sensory cortices but also parietal and prefrontal areas, as well as neuromodulatory pathways such as the cholinergic system, and perhaps even subnuclei within the amygdala itself.

An emerging model of functional interactions between emotion and attention is illustrated in Figure 10.3. An initial response of the amygdala based on partial stimulus information may induce direct feedback from the lateral and basal nuclei on sensory cortices, which could be responsible for the initial boosting of the neural representation of emotional stimuli, and thus promote their selection by attention and privileged access to awareness among competing stimuli. These effects may correspond to the early emotional responses

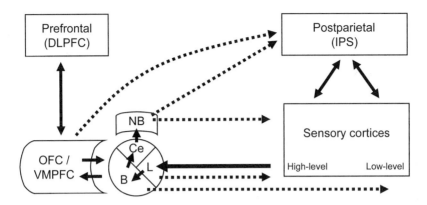

FIGURE 10.3. Schematic diagram of reciprocal pathways between emotional and attentional control. Feedback from lateral (L) and basal (B) nuclei from amygdala can amplify neural representations of emotionally relevant information at different stages along sensory cortical areas. Amygdala output via the central nucleus (Ce) can also activate cholinergic projections from nucleus basalis (NB) in forebrain to posterior parietal (IPS) as well as frontal and sensory cortical regions, which may promote alerting reactions and shifts of attention. Projections to other systems in brainstem (noradrenergic) are not shown here. Top-down interactions between parietal cortex and sensory areas may then focus attentional resources on the location of emotional events. The gain of these feedback loops may be modulated by influences from orbito-frontal cortex (OFC), as well as indirectly by interconnections with anterior cingulate cortex (ACC) and dorsolateral prefrontal cortex (DLPFC).

recorded by ERPs (~120–150 msec after stimulus onset) (Eimer & Holmes, 2002; Kawasaki et al., 2001), prior or in parallel to top-down influences of voluntary attention (occurring at about 170–200 msec) (Holmes et al., 2003; Hopfinger et al., 2001), such that both types of modulation might act simultaneously on the same cortical sites (Grandjean et al., 2005; Vuilleumier et al., 2001). Although emotional influences arise without voluntary control and outside awareness, they may be amplified or attenuated by current goals or internal emotional states via gating mechanisms in the basal nucleus of the amygdala, possibly mediated by inputs from orbitofrontal cortex. Because amygdala nuclei project differentially to successive stages along sensory pathways (Freese & Amaral, 2005), these contextual factors may also determine whether feedback is primarily exerted on lower- or higher-level areas (e.g., V1 or fusiform). In addition, amygdala outputs may activate other brain systems directly implicated in attentional control, including subcortical cholinergic nuclei and medial prefrontal regions (Bentley et al., 2003; Sarter et al., 2005), potentially contributing to shift attention away from its current focus and reorient it to more relevant information. The engagement of attention by emotional stimuli may in turn bias the activity of intraparietal cortex in favor of their location (Pourtois, Thut, et al., 2005; Pourtois et al., 2006), perhaps through direct coupling with extrastriate cortex (Keil et al., 2007) or via connections between parietal and orbitofrontal cortex (Cavada et al., 2000). This may then lead to a subsequent improvement in perceptual sensitivity for information presented at the same location in space (Phelps et al., 2006; Pourtois et al., 2004), even across different sensory modalities (Brosch et al., 2008). Some potentiation between attention and emotion may also arise in certain pathways (e.g., V1), such that emotional signals may amplify the effect of attention or vice versa (Phelps et al., 2006; Vuilleumier, Armony, Driver, & Dolan, 2001). Concurrently, the activity of orbitofrontal and cingulate regions may be increased when emotional cues must be ignored or interfere with current task goals (Bentley et al., 2003; Pourtois, Thut, et al., 2005; Pourtois et al., 2006; Vuilleumier et al., 2001), consistent with strong projections from these regions to both amygdala and lateral prefrontal cortex (Dolcos & McCarthy, 2006; Yamasaki et al., 2002). Such activations in frontal and parietal areas underlying executive and attentional adjustment to emotional signals may be reflected by the later components of ERPs (~250–400 msec after stimulus onset), which are more sensitive to current task demands (Carretie et al., 2001; Olofsson et al., 2008; Schupp et al., 2007). Altogether, these dynamic interactions among distributed brain regions implement a powerful machinery by which emotion can control perception and behavior. Furthermore, besides transient effects on attentional functioning, emotional modulations may produce long-lasting changes in perceptual pathways that enhance memory (Talmi, Schimmack, Paterson, & Moscovitch, 2007) and increase functional tuning of cortical systems (Weinberger, 2004).

In sum, these data demonstrate that emotional processing not only serves to appraise the value of sensory events and generate internal feelings, but may directly regulate perception and its content. These mechanisms complement other "traditional" attentional systems that are known to select and organize sensory inputs based on spatial or object-based dimensions (Kastner & Ungerleider, 2000), and as such constitute specialized neural systems for "emotional attention" (Vuilleumier, 2005). Although common wisdom has long recognized that emotion may alter sensation as well as reason, the recent insights from cognitive and affective neurosciences have now clearly shown that this notion is not just a metaphor.

WHAT I THINK

Interactions between emotion and attention in the amygdala are reciprocal. Hence it is necessary to distinguish between questions on how emotional processes may influence attentional operations (as described in this chapter) and questions on how attentional processes modulate emotional responses (in the amygdala or connected regions). Nevertheless, such reciprocity also raises questions on the interdependence of these bidirectional effects: For example, to what extent may attentional control of emotion affect the emotional impact on attention (or vice versa)? This has given rise to several controversies, but is still unresolved.

I believe that an important feature of emotional influences on perception and attention is that their functioning is essentially reflexive and automatic, in the sense that their elicitation and action do not rely on voluntary intention or conscious monitoring. However, this does not imply that these effects are impermeable to contextual or attentional factors. Cognitive psychology often assumes that automatic processes should be purely stimulus-driven and goal-independent, but neurophysiology teaches us that many reflexive processes can be modulated by higher-level factors. (Even primitive reflexes in the spinal cord can be controlled, as shown, for instance, by our ability to voluntarily inhibit urination depending on current priorities, or by cognitive effects on expression of some motor reflexes.) In fact, the classic Stroop interference during color naming with words illustrates that some "automaticity" may arise without intentionality (despite harmful consequences for performance), whereas subliminal priming demonstrates that abstract semantic information is extracted from words without conscious awareness—although such effects do not require a special or unique route for word reading. Rather, these phenomena may simply reflect the fact that the brain is wired in such a way that it is somehow prepared to process and organize sensory information along specialized "highways," perhaps related to some default mode or particular selectivity among neuronal populations. Different highways may be more or less amenable to control by task-related factors.

Furthermore, in the domain of emotion processing and amygdala activity, the influences of attention are usually considered unitary and univocal. However, I believe that such influences are likely to be more complex and composite than is commonly assumed. Several pathways exist by which attention may influence processing of emotional stimuli, including different sources in frontal or parietal networks, and different sites in sensory cortices or in the amygdala itself. Using fMRI to dissociate "automatic" responses and top-down influences in the human amygdala may be limited by the slow temporal sensitivity of BOLD signals and their macroscopic resolution, pooling neural activity over several phases of neuronal activity and different cell populations. Moreover, neurophysiological data suggest that sensory-driven and top-down effects are likely to arise in different amygdala nuclei—a factor that is usually neglected in fMRI studies, but may partly account for conflicting results. Finally, although most research has focused on whether changes in attentional settings may reduce amygdala responses to emotional information, it is plausible that such changes could also affect baseline activity and responses to neutral stimuli, in relation to variations in motivation, relevance, or ambiguity. Therefore, much remains to be done to disentangle the multiple reciprocal links between emotion and attention, as each of these two terms encompasses a wide collection of distinct neural processes.

REFERENCES

Alorda, C., Serrano-Pedraza, I., Campos-Bueno, J. J., Sierra-Vazquez, V., & Montoya, P. (2007). Low spatial frequency filtering modulates early brain processing of affective complex pictures. *Neuropsychologia, 45*(14), 3223–3233.

Alpers, G. W., & Gerdes, A. B. (2007). Here is looking at you: Emotional faces predominate in binocular rivalry. *Emotion, 7*(3), 495–506.

Alpers, G. W., Ruhleder, M., Walz, N., Muhlberger, A., & Pauli, P. (2005). Binocular rivalry between emotional and neutral stimuli: A validation using fear conditioning and EEG. *International Journal of Psychophysiology, 57*(1), 25–32.

Amaral, D. G., Behniea, H., & Kelly, J. L. (2003). Topographic organization of projections from the amygdala to the visual cortex in the macaque monkey. *Neuroscience, 118*(4), 1099–1120.

Anderson, A. K. (2005). Affective influences on the attentional dynamics supporting awareness. *Journal of Experimental Psychology: General, 134*(2), 258–281.

Anderson, A. K., Christoff, K., Panitz, D., De Rosa, E., & Gabrieli, J. D. (2003). Neural correlates of the automatic processing of threat facial signals. *Journal of Neuroscience, 23*(13), 5627–5633.

Anderson, A. K., Christoff, K., Stappen, I., Panitz, D., Ghahremani, D. G., Glover, G., et al. (2003). Dissociated neural representations of intensity and valence in human olfaction. *Nature Neuroscience, 6*(2), 196–202.

Anderson, A. K., & Phelps, E. A. (2001). Lesions of the human amygdala impair enhanced perception of emotionally salient events. *Nature, 411*, 305–309.

Armony, J. L., & Dolan, R. J. (2002). Modulation of spatial attention by fear-conditioned stimuli: An event-related fMRI study. *Neuropsychologia, 40*, 817–826.

Baxter, M. G., & Murray, E. A. (2002). The amygdala and reward. *Nature Reviews Neuroscience, 3*(7), 563–573.

Baylis, G. C., Rolls, E. T., & Leonard, C. M. (1987). Functional subdivisions of the temporal lobe neocortex. *Journal of Neuroscience, 7*(2), 330–342.

Beck, D. M., Rees, G., Frith, C. D., & Lavie, N. (2001). Neural correlates of change detection and change blindness. *Nature Neuroscience, 4*(6), 645–650.

Bentley, P., Vuilleumier, P., Thiel, C. M., Driver, J., & Dolan, R. J. (2003). Cholinergic enhancement modulates neural correlates of selective attention and emotional processing. *NeuroImage, 20*(1), 58–70.

Benuzzi, F., Meletti, S., Zamboni, G., Calandra-Buonaura, G., Serafini, M., Lui, F., et al. (2004). Impaired fear processing in right mesial temporal sclerosis: A fMRI study. *Brain Research Bulletin, 63*(4), 269–281.

Bishop, S. J., Duncan, J., & Lawrence, A. D. (2004). State anxiety modulation of the amygdala response to unattended threat-related stimuli. *Journal of Neuroscience, 24*, 10364–10368.

Boucart, M., Humphreys, G. W., & Lorenceau, J. (1995). Automatic access to object identity: Attention to global information, not to particular physical dimensions, is important. *Journal of Experimental Psychology: Human Perception and Performance, 21*(3), 584–601.

Bradley, B. P., Mogg, K., & Millar, N. H. (2000). Covert and overt orienting of attention to emotional faces in anxiety. *Cognition and Emotion, 14*(6), 789–808.

Brosch, T., Grandjean, D., Sander, D., & Scherer, K. R. (2008). Behold the voice of wrath: Cross-modal modulation of visual attention by anger prosody. *Cognition, 106*(3), 1497–1503.

Brosch, T., Sander, D., & Scherer, K. R. (2007). That baby caught my eye ... : Attention capture by infant faces. *Emotion, 7*(3), 685–689.

Büchel, C., Morris, J., Dolan, R. J., & Friston, K. J. (1998). Brain systems mediating aversive conditioning: An event-related fMRI study. *Neuron, 20*(5), 947–957.

Carretie, L., Hinojosa, J. A., Lopez-Martin, S., & Tapia, M. (2007). An electrophysiological study on the interaction between emotional content and spatial frequency of visual stimuli. *Neuropsychologia, 45*(6), 1187–1195.

Carretie, L., Iglesias, J., Garcia, T., & Ballesteros, M. (1997). N300, P300 and the emotional processing of visual stimuli. *Electroencephalography and Clinical Neurophysiology, 103*(2), 298–303.

Carretie, L., Martin-Loeches, M., Hinojosa, J. A., & Mercado, F. (2001). Emotion and attention interaction studied through event-related potentials. *Journal of Cognitive Neuroscience, 13*(8), 1109–1128.

Catani, M., Jones, D. K., Donato, R., & ffytche, D. H. (2003). Occipito-temporal connections in the human brain. *Brain, 126*(Pt. 9), 2093–2107.

Cavada, C., Compañy, T., Tejedor, J., Cruz-Rizzolo, R. J., & Reinoso-Suarez, F. (2000). The anatomical connections of the macaque monkey orbitofrontal cortex. A review. *Cerebral Cortex, 10*(3), 220–242.

Compton, R. J. (2003). The interface between emotion and attention: A review of evidence from psychology and neuroscience. *Behavioral and Cognitive Neuroscience Reviews, 2*(2), 115–129.

Critchley, H. D., Mathias, C. J., & Dolan, R. J. (2002). Fear conditioning in humans: The influence of awareness and autonomic arousal on functional neuroanatomy. *Neuron, 33*(4), 653–663.

Cuthbert, B. N., Schupp, H. T., Bradley, M. M., Birbaumer, N., & Lang, P. J. (2000). Brain potentials in affective picture processing: Covariation with autonomic arousal and affective report. *Biological Psychology, 52*(2), 95–111.

Dolan, R. J., Heinze, H. J., Hurlemann, R., & Hinrichs, H. (2006). Magnetoencephalography (MEG) determined temporal modulation of visual and auditory sensory processing in the context of classical conditioning to faces. *NeuroImage, 32*(2), 778–789.

Dolcos, F., & McCarthy, G. (2006). Brain systems mediating cognitive interference by emotional distraction. *Journal of Neuroscience, 26*(7), 2072–2079.

Dringenberg, H. C., Saber, A. J., & Cahill, L. (2001). Enhanced frontal cortex activation in rats by convergent amygdaloid and noxious sensory signals. *NeuroReport, 12*(11), 2395–2398.

Driver, J., Vuilleumier, P., & Husain, M. (2004). Spatial neglect and extinction. In M. Gazzaniga (Ed.), *The new cognitive neurosciences* (3rd ed., pp. 589–606). Cambridge, MA: MIT Press.

Eastwood, J. D., Smilek, D., & Merikle, P. M. (2001). Differential attentional guidance by unattended faces expressing positive and negative emotion. *Perception and Psychophysics, 63*(6), 1004–1013.

Eastwood, J. D., Smilek, D., & Merikle, P. M. (2003). Negative facial expression captures attention and disrupts performance. *Perception and Psychophysics, 65*(3), 352–358.

Eimer, M., & Holmes, A. (2002). An ERP study on the time course of emotional face processing. *NeuroReport, 13*, 427–431.

Erthal, F. S., de Oliveira, L., Mocaiber, I., Pereira, M. G., Machado-Pinheiro, W., Volchan, E., et al. (2005). Load-dependent modulation of affective picture processing. *Cognitive, Affective, and Behavioral Neuroscience, 5*(4), 388–395.

Fecteau, S., Belin, P., Joanette, Y., & Armony, J. L. (2007). Amygdala responses to nonlinguistic emotional vocalizations. *NeuroImage, 36*(2), 480–487.

Fenske, M. J., & Eastwood, J. D. (2003). Modulation of focused attention by faces expressing emotion: Evidence from flanker tasks. *Emotion, 3*(4), 327–343.

Flykt, A. (2005). Visual search with biological threat stimuli: Accuracy, reaction times, and heart rate changes. *Emotion, 5*(3), 349–353.

Fox, E. (2002). Processing of emotional facial expressions: The role of anxiety and awareness. *Cognitive, Affective, and Behavioral Neuroscience, 2*(1), 52–63.

Fox, E., Lester, V., Russo, R., Bowles, R. J., Pichler, A., & Dutton, K. (2000). Facial expressions of emotion: Are angry faces detected more efficiently? *Cognition and Emotion, 14*, 61–92.

Fox, E., Russo, R., Bowles, R. J., & Dutton, K. (2001). Do threatening stimuli draw or hold visual attention in subclinical anxiety? *Journal of Experimental Psychology: General, 130*(4), 681–700.

Fox, E., Russo, R., & Georgiou, G. A. (2005). Anxiety modulates the degree of attentive resources required to process emotional faces. *Cognitive, Affective, and Behavioral Neuroscience, 5*(4), 396–404.

Freese, J. L., & Amaral, D. G. (2005). The organization of projections from the amygdala to visual cortical areas TE and V1 in the macaque monkey. *Journal of Comparative Neurology, 486*(4), 295–317.

Freese, J. L., & Amaral, D. G. (2006). Synaptic organization of projections from the amygdala to visual cortical areas TE and V1 in the macaque monkey. *Journal of Comparative Neurology, 496*(5), 655–667.

Gaillard, R., Del Cul, A., Naccache, L., Vinckier, F., Cohen, L., & Dehaene, S. (2006). Nonconscious semantic processing of emotional words modulates conscious access. *Proceedings of the National Academy of Sciences USA, 103*(19), 7524–7529.

Ganel, T., & Goshen-Gottstein, Y. (2004). Effects of familiarity on the perceptual integrality of the identity and expression of faces: The parallel-route hypothesis revisited. *Journal of Experimental Psychology: Human Perception and Performance, 30*(3), 583–597.

Glascher, J., & Büchel, C. (2005). Formal learning theory dissociates brain regions with different temporal integration. *Neuron, 47*(2), 295–306.

Grandjean, D., Sander, D., Lucas, N., Scherer, K. R., & Vuilleumier, P. (2008). Effects of emotional prosody on auditory extinction for voices in patients with spatial neglect. *Neuropsychologia, 46*(2), 487–496.

Grandjean, D., Sander, D., Pourtois, G., Schwartz, S., Seghier, M. L., Scherer, K. R., et al. (2005). The voices of wrath: Brain responses to angry prosody in meaningless speech. *Nature Neuroscience, 8*(2), 145–146.

Grelotti, D. J., Gauthier, I., & Schultz, R. T. (2002). Social interest and the development of cortical face specialization: What autism teaches us about face processing. *Developmental Psychobiology, 40*(3), 213–225.

Hamann, S., & Mao, H. (2002). Positive and negative emotional verbal stimuli elicit activity in the left amygdala. *NeuroReport, 13*(1), 15–19.

Hansen, C. H., & Hansen, R. D. (1988). Finding the face in the crowd: an anger superiority effect. *Journal of Personality and Social Psychology, 54*(6), 917–924.

Holland, P. C., & Gallagher, M. (1999). Amygdala circuitry in attentional and representational processes. *Trends in Cognitive Sciences, 3*(2), 65–73.

Holland, P. C., Han, J. S., & Gallagher, M. (2000). Lesions of the amygdala central nucleus alter performance on a selective attention task. *Journal of Neuroscience, 20*(17), 6701–6706.

Holmes, A., Vuilleumier, P., & Eimer, M. (2003). The processing of emotional facial expression is gated by spatial attention: Evidence from event-related brain potentials. *Brain Research: Cognitive Brain Research, 16*(2), 174–184.

Hopfinger, J. B., Buonocore, M. H., & Mangun, G. R. (2000). The neural mechanisms of top-down attentional control. *Nature Neuroscience, 3*, 284–291.

Hopfinger, J. B., Woldorff, M. G., Fletcher, E. M., & Mangun, G. R. (2001). Dissociating top-down attentional control from selective perception and action. *Neuropsychologia, 39*(12), 1277–1291.

Horstmann, G., Borgstedt, K., & Heumann, M. (2006). Flanker effects with faces may depend on perceptual as well as emotional differences. *Emotion, 6*(1), 28–39.

Horstmann, G., Scharlau, I., & Ansorge, U. (2006). More efficient rejection of happy than of angry face distractors in visual search. *Psychonomic Bulletin and Review, 13*(6), 1067–1073.

Huang, Y. M., Baddeley, A., & Young, A. W. (2008). Attentional capture by emotional stimuli is modulated by semantic processing. *Journal of Experimental Psychology: Human Perception and Performance, 34*(2), 328–339.

Isenberg, N., Silbersweig, D., Engelien, A., Emmerich, S., Malavade, K., Beattie, B., et al. (1999). Linguistic threat activates the human amygdala. *Proceedings of the National Academy of Sciences USA, 96*(18), 10456–10459.

Jiang, Y., & He, S. (2006). Cortical responses to invisible faces: Dissociating subsystems for facial-information processing. *Current Biology, 16*, 2023–2029.

Kapp, B. S., Supple, W. F., Jr., & Whalen, P. J. (1994). Effects of electrical stimulation of the amygdaloid central nucleus on neocortical arousal in the rabbit. *Behavioral Neuroscience, 108*(1), 81–93.

Kastner, S., & Ungerleider, L. G. (2000). Mechanisms of visual attention in the human cortex. *Annual Review of Neuroscience, 23*, 315–341.

Kawasaki, H., Kaufman, O., Damasio, H., Damasio, A. R., Granner, M., Bakken, H., et al. (2001). Single-neuron responses to emotional visual stimuli recorded in human ventral prefrontal cortex. *Nature Neuroscience, 4*(1), 15–16.

Keil, A., & Ihssen, N. (2004). Identification facilitation for emotionally arousing verbs during the attentional blink. *Emotion, 4*(1), 23–35.

Keil, A., Moratti, S., Sabatinelli, D., Bradley, M. M., & Lang, P. J. (2005). Additive effects of emotional content and spatial selective attention on electrocortical facilitation. *Cerebral Cortex, 15*(8), 1187–1197.

Keil, A., Sabatinelli, D., Ding, M., Lang, P. J., Ihssen, N., & Heim, S. (in press). Re-entrant projections modulate visual cortex in affective perception: Evidence from Granger causality analysis. *Human Brain Mapping.*

Kensinger, E. A., & Schacter, D. L. (2006). Processing emotional pictures and words: Effects of valence and arousal. *Cognitive, Affective, and Behavioral Neuroscience, 6*(2), 110–126.

Kissler, J., Herbert, C., Peyk, P., & Junghofer, M. (2007). Buzzwords: Early cortical responses to emotional words during reading. *Psychological Science, 18*(6), 475–480.

Krolak-Salmon, P., Fischer, C., Vighetto, A., & Mauguiere, F. (2001). Processing of facial emotional expression: Spatio-temporal data as assessed by scalp event-related potentials. *European Journal of Neuroscience, 13*(5), 987–994.

Lane, R. D., Chua, P. M., & Dolan, R. J. (1999). Common effects of emotional valence, arousal and attention on neural activation during visual processing of pictures. *Neuropsychologia, 37*(9), 989–997.

Lang, P. J., Bradley, M. M., Fitzsimmons, J. R., Cuthbert, B. N., Scott, J. D., Moulder, B., et al. (1998). Emotional arousal and activation of the visual cortex: An fMRI analysis. *Psychophysiology, 35*(2), 199–210.

Lang, S. F., Nelson, C. A., & Collins, P. F. (1990). Event-related potentials to emotional and neutral stimuli. *Journal of Clinical Experimental Neuropsychology, 12*(6), 946–958.

Lewis, P. A., Critchley, H. D., Rotshtein, P., & Dolan, R. J. (2007). Neural correlates of processing valence and arousal in affective words. *Cerebral Cortex, 17*(3), 742–748.

Lucas, N., & Vuilleumier, P. (2008). Effects of emotional and non-emotional cues on visual search in neglect patients: Evidence for distinct sources of attentional guidance. *Neuropsychologia, 46*(5), 1401–1414.

Mathews, A., May, J., Mogg, K., & Eysenck, M. (1990). Attentional bias in anxiety: Selective search or defective filtering? *Journal of Abnormal Psychology, 99*(2), 166–173.

Morris, J. S., Friston, K. J., Büchel, C., Frith, C. D., Young, A. W., Calder, A. J., et al. (1998). A neuromodulatory role for the human amygdala in processing emotional facial expressions. *Brain, 121*(Pt. 1), 47–57.

Most, S. B., Chun, M. M., Johnson, M. R., & Kiehl, K. A. (2006). Attentional modulation of the amygdala varies with personality. *NeuroImage, 31*(2), 934–944.

Naccache, L., Gaillard, R., Adam, C., Hasboun, D., Clemenceau, S., Baulac, M., et al. (2005). A direct intracranial record of emotions evoked by subliminal words. *Proceedings of the National Academy of Sciences USA, 102*, 7713–7717.

Nummenmaa, L., Hyona, J., & Calvo, M. G. (2006). Eye movement assessment of selective attentional capture by emotional pictures. *Emotion, 6*(2), 257–268.

Öhman, A. (1986). Face the beast and fear the face: Animal and social fears as prototypes for evolutionary analyses of emotion. *Psychophysiology, 23*(2), 123–145.

Öhman, A., Flykt, A., & Esteves, F. (2001). Emotion drives attention: Detecting the snake in the grass. *Journal of Experimental Psychology: General, 130*(3), 466–478.

Okon-Singer, H., Tzelgov, J., & Henik, A. (2007). Distinguishing between automaticity and attention in the processing of emotionally significant stimuli. *Emotion, 7*(1), 147–157.

Olofsson, J. K., Nordin, S., Sequeira, H., & Polich, J. (2008). Affective picture processing: An integrative review of ERP findings. *Biological Psychology, 77*(3), 247–265.

Pasley, B. N., Mayes, L. C., & Schultz, R. T. (2004). Subcortical discrimination of unperceived objects during binocular rivalry. *Neuron, 42*(1), 163–172.

Peelen, M. V., Atkinson, A. P., Andersson, F., & Vuilleumier, P. (2007). Emotional modulation of body-selective visual areas. *Social Cognitive and Affective Neuroscience, 2*, 274–283.

Peelen, M. V., & Downing, P. E. (2005). Selectivity for the human body in the fusiform gyrus. *Journal of Neurophysiology, 93*(1), 603–608.

Pessoa, L., McKenna, M., Gutierrez, E., & Ungerleider, L. G. (2002). Neural processing of emotional faces requires attention. *Proceedings of the National Academy of Sciences USA, 99*(17), 11458–11463.

Pessoa, L., Padmala, S., & Morland, T. (2005). Fate of unattended fearful faces in the amygdala is determined by both attentional resources and cognitive modulation. *NeuroImage, 28*(1), 249–255.

Phelps, E. A., & LeDoux, J. E. (2005). Contributions of the amygdala to emotion processing: From animal models to human behavior. *Neuron, 48*(2), 175–187.

Phelps, E. A., Ling, S., & Carrasco, M. (2006). Emotion facilitates perception and potentiates the perceptual benefits of attention. *Psychological Science, 17*(4), 292–299.

Pizzagalli, D. A., Lehmann, D., Hendrick, A. M., Regard, M., Pascual-Marqui, R.

D., & Davidson, R. J. (2002). Affective judgments of faces modulate early activity (approximately 160 ms) within the fusiform gyri. *NeuroImage, 16*(3, Pt. 1), 663–677.

Pourtois, G., Grandjean, D., Sander, D., & Vuilleumier, P. (2004). Electrophysiological correlates of rapid spatial orienting towards fearful faces. *Cerebral Cortex, 14*(6), 619–633.

Pourtois, G., Schwartz, S., Seghier, M. L., Lazeyras, F., & Vuilleumier, P. (2005). Portraits or people?: Distinct representations of face identity in the human visual cortex. *Journal of Cognitive Neuroscience, 17*(7), 1043–1057.

Pourtois, G., Schwartz, S., Seghier, M. L., Lazeyras, F., & Vuilleumier, P. (2006). Neural systems for orienting attention to the location of threat signals: An event-related fMRI study. *NeuroImage, 31*(2), 920–933.

Pourtois, G., Thut, G., Grave de Peralta, R., Michel, C., & Vuilleumier, P. (2005). Two electrophysiological stages of spatial orienting towards fearful faces: Early temporo-parietal activation preceding gain control in extrastriate visual cortex. *NeuroImage, 26*(1), 149–163.

Purkis, H. M., & Lipp, O. V. (2007). Automatic attention does not equal automatic fear: Preferential attention without implicit valence. *Emotion, 7*(2), 314–323.

Rotshtein, P., Richardson, M., Winston, J., Kiebel, S., Vuilleumier, P., Eimer, M., et al. (2006). *Early brain responses to fearful faces are modulated by amygdala lesion.* Paper presented at the meeting of the Human Brain Mapping Organization, Florence, Italy.

Sabatinelli, D., Bradley, M. M., Fitzsimmons, J. R., & Lang, P. J. (2005). Parallel amygdala and inferotemporal activation reflect emotional intensity and fear relevance. *NeuroImage, 24*(4), 1265–1270.

Sabatinelli, D., Lang, P. J., Keil, A., & Bradley, M. M. (2007). Emotional perception: Correlation of functional MRI and event-related potentials. *Cerebral Cortex, 17*(5), 1085–1091.

Sander, D., Grafman, J., & Zalla, T. (2003). The human amygdala: An evolved system for relevance detection. *Review of Neuroscience, 14*(4), 303–316.

Sander, D., Grandjean, D., & Scherer, K. R. (2005). A systems approach to appraisal mechanisms in emotion. *Neural Networks, 18*(4), 317–352.

Sarter, M., Hasselmo, M. E., Bruno, J. P., & Givens, B. (2005). Unraveling the attentional functions of cortical cholinergic inputs: Interactions between signal-driven and cognitive modulation of signal detection. *Brain Research: Brain Research Reviews, 48*(1), 98–111.

Scherer, K. R., & Peper, M. (2001). Psychological theories of emotion and neuropsychological research. In G. Gainotti (Ed.), *Emotional behavior and its disorders* (pp. 17–48). Amsterdam: Elsevier.

Schupp, H. T., Flaisch, T., Stockburger, J., & Junghofer, M. (2006). Emotion and attention: Event-related brain potential studies. *Progress in Brain Research, 156,* 31–51.

Schupp, H. T., Junghofer, M., Weike, A. I., & Hamm, A. O. (2003). Emotional facilitation of sensory processing in the visual cortex. *Psychological Science, 14*(1), 7–13.

Schupp, H. T., Junghofer, M., Weike, A. I., & Hamm, A. O. (2004). The selective processing of briefly presented affective pictures: An ERP analysis. *Psychophysiology, 41*(3), 441–449.

Schupp, H. T., Stockburger, J., Codispoti, M., Junghofer, M., Weike, A. I., & Hamm,

A. O. (2007). Selective visual attention to emotion. *Journal of Neuroscience*, 27(5), 1082–1089.

Silvert, L., Lepsien, J., Fragopanagos, N., Goolsby, B., Kiss, M., Taylor, J. G., et al. (2007). Influence of attentional demands on the processing of emotional facial expressions in the amygdala. *NeuroImage*, 38(2), 357–366.

Smith, S. D., Most, S. B., Newsome, L. A., & Zald, D. H. (2006). An emotion-induced attentional blink elicited by aversively conditioned stimuli. *Emotion*, 6(3), 523–527.

Stefanacci, L., Farb, C. R., Pitkänen, A., Go, G., LeDoux, J. E., & Amaral, D. G. (1992). Projections from the lateral nucleus to the basal nucleus of the amygdala: A light and electron microscopic PHA-L study in the rat. *Journal of Comparative Neurology*, 323(4), 586–601.

Stolarova, M., Keil, A., & Moratti, S. (2006). Modulation of the C1 visual event-related component by conditioned stimuli: Evidence for sensory plasticity in early affective perception. *Cerebral Cortex*, 16(6), 876–887.

Surguladze, S. A., Brammer, M. J., Young, A. W., Andrew, C., Travis, M. J., Williams, S. C., et al. (2003). A preferential increase in the extrastriate response to signals of danger. *NeuroImage*, 19(4), 1317–1328.

Tabbert, K., Stark, R., Kirsch, P., & Vaitl, D. (2005). Hemodynamic responses of the amygdala, the orbitofrontal cortex and the visual cortex during a fear conditioning paradigm. *International Journal of Psychophysiology*, 57(1), 15–23.

Talmi, D., Schimmack, U., Paterson, T., & Moscovitch, M. (2007). The role of attention and relatedness in emotionally enhanced memory. *Emotion*, 7(1), 89–102.

Tamietto, M., Geminiani, G., Genero, R., & de Gelder, B. (2007). Seeing fearful body language overcomes attentional deficits in patients with neglect. *Journal of Cognitive Neuroscience*, 19(3), 445–454.

Trippe, R. H., Hewig, J., Heydel, C., Hecht, H., & Miltner, W. H. (2007). Attentional blink to emotional and threatening pictures in spider phobics: Electrophysiology and behavior. *Brain Research*, 1148, 149–160.

van Honk, J., Tuiten, A., de Haan, E., van den Hout, M., & Stam, H. (2001). Attentional biases for angry faces: Relationships to trait anger and anxiety. *Cognition and Emotion*, 15(3), 279–297.

Vuilleumier, P. (2004). Héminégligence spatiale et extinction visuelle. In A. Safran & T. Landis & A. Vighetto (Eds.), *Traité de neuro-opthalmologie clinique* (pp. 140–145). Paris: Masson.

Vuilleumier, P. (2005). How brains beware: Neural mechanisms of emotional attention. *Trends in Cognitive Science*, 9(12), 585–594.

Vuilleumier, P., Armony, J. L., Clarke, K., Husain, M., Driver, J., & Dolan, R. J. (2002). Neural response to emotional faces with and without awareness: Event-related fMRI in a parietal patient with visual extinction and spatial neglect. *Neuropsychologia*, 40(12), 2156–2166.

Vuilleumier, P., Armony, J. L., Driver, J., & Dolan, R. J. (2001). Effects of attention and emotion on face processing in the human brain: An event-related fMRI study. *Neuron*, 30(3), 829–841.

Vuilleumier, P., Armony, J. L., Driver, J., & Dolan, R. J. (2003). Distinct spatial frequency sensitivities for processing faces and emotional expressions. *Nature Neuroscience*, 6(6), 624–631.

Vuilleumier, P., & Driver, J. (2007). Modulation of visual processing by attention and emotion: Windows on causal interactions between human brain regions. *Philosophical Transactions of the Royal Society of London, Series B, 362,* 837–855.

Vuilleumier, P., Richardson, M. P., Armony, J. L., Driver, J., & Dolan, R. J. (2004). Distant influences of amygdala lesion on visual cortical activation during emotional face processing. *Nature Neuroscience, 7*(11), 1271–1278.

Vuilleumier, P., & Schwartz, S. (2001a). Beware and be aware: Capture of spatial attention by fear-related stimuli in neglect. *NeuroReport, 12*(6), 1119–1122.

Vuilleumier, P., & Schwartz, S. (2001b). Emotional facial expressions capture attention. *Neurology, 56*(2), 153–158.

Weinberger, N. M. (2004). Specific long-term memory traces in primary auditory cortex. *Nature Reviews Neuroscience, 5*(4), 279–290.

Whalen, P. J., Kagan, J., Cook, R. G., Davis, F. C., Kim, H., Polis, S., et al. (2004). Human amygdala responsivity to masked fearful eye whites. *Science, 306,* 2061.

Whalen, P. J., Rauch, S. L., Etcoff, N. L., McInerney, S. C., Lee, M. B., & Jenike, M. A. (1998). Masked presentations of emotional facial expressions modulate amygdala activity without explicit knowledge. *Journal of Neuroscience, 18*(1), 411–418.

Wiethoff, S., Wildgruber, D., Kreifelts, B., Becker, H., Herbert, C., Grodd, W., et al. (2008). Cerebral processing of emotional prosody: Influence of acoustic parameters and arousal. *NeuroImage, 39*(2), 885–893.

Williams, J. M., Mathews, A., & MacLeod, C. (1996). The emotional Stroop task and psychopathology. *Psychological Bulletin, 120*(1), 3–24.

Williams, M. A., McGlone, F., Abbott, D. F., & Mattingley, J. B. (2005). Differential amygdala responses to happy and fearful facial expressions depend on selective attention. *NeuroImage, 24*(2), 417–425.

Williams, M. A., Morris, A. P., McGlone, F., Abbott, D. F., & Mattingley, J. B. (2004). Amygdala responses to fearful and happy facial expressions under conditions of binocular suppression. *Journal of Neuroscience, 24*(12), 2898–2904.

Williams, M. A., Moss, S. A., Bradshaw, J. L., & Mattingley, J. B. (2005). Look at me, I'm smiling: Visual search for threatening and nonthreatening facial expressions. *Visual Cognition, 12*(1), 29–50.

Yamasaki, H., LaBar, K. S., & McCarthy, G. (2002). Dissociable prefrontal brain systems for attention and emotion. *Proceedings of the National Academy of Sciences USA, 99*(17), 11447–11451.

Yang, E., Zald, D. H., & Blake, R. (2007). Fearful expressions gain preferential access to awareness during continuous flash suppression. *Emotion, 7*(4), 882–886.

Yukie, M. (2002). Connections between the amygdala and auditory cortical areas in the macaque monkey. *Neuroscience Research, 42*(3), 219–229.

CHAPTER 11

Individual Differences
in Human Amygdala Function

Turhan Canli

Advances in noninvasive brain imaging methodologies have inspired researchers to investigate the neural basis of ever more complex human behaviors. Although a great deal of research effort continues to be devoted to basic perceptual and cognitive processes, such as vision, there is a rapidly accelerating trend toward publication of studies related to emotion, traits, and social behavior. Plate 11.1 (in color insert) illustrates this trend, which compares the publication rates (indexed at 1 for the period between 1990 and 1994) for several topic areas using functional magnetic resonance imaging (fMRI). For example, the publication rate for fMRI studies of vision and other basic processes has increased linearly between 1990 and 2004, and has dropped slightly since. In contrast, the publication rate for fMRI studies of such complex processes as emotion, traits, or social behavior has grown exponentially. The fastest-growing topic area is fMRI research on individual differences; this is astounding, considering that earlier studies in cognitive neuroscience regarded any form of between-subject variance simply as statistical noise (Plomin & Kosslyn, 2001).

The recent interest in individual differences contrasts with a more traditional approach in cognitive neuroscience, which seeks to identify brain regions that show consistent activation across studies and across individuals. This traditional approach was critical in the first decade of cognitive neuroscience, when one of the principal goals in the emerging field was to demonstrate the reliability of fMRI and other noninvasive imaging techniques. In that spirit, a consortium of investigators conducted an fMRI study using a spatial working memory task (Casey et al., 1998) to demonstrate the reliability of their findings with different scanners across four institutions. Another example is the display of data, which intended to highlight consistency in neural activation. For example, the authors of one fMRI study illustrated the consistency of hippocampal activation associated with memory encoding and retrieval by showing activation data from each of six scanned individuals (Gabrieli, Brewer, Desmond, & Glover, 1997).

Very quickly, however, investigators began to appreciate the power of individual differences in predicting behavior. In a follow-up to the Gabrieli and colleagues (1997) study, the same group showed that individual differences in hippocampal activation predicted how well individual participants performed in a subsequent memory task (Brewer, Zhao, Desmond, Glover, & Gabrieli, 1998). With the emergence of affective neuroscience, the interest in individual differences began to blossom, as more studies turned to the neural basis of emotion and emotion-related traits.

EMOTION

Individuals can differ greatly in their response to identical emotional stimuli. In one early study of individual differences in emotional experience (Canli, Desmond, Zhao, Glover, & Gabrieli, 1998), we used fMRI to measure lateralized brain responses to negative and positive images. From Davidson's (1995) work, we expected left-lateralized activation to positive (relative to negative) pictures, and right-lateralized activation to negative (relative to positive) pictures. Indeed, we confirmed this laterality pattern in a group of participants who, although they experienced the negative and positive pictures as different in pleasantness (valence), felt that both sets of stimuli were of comparable emotional intensity (arousal). However, half of the sample had a different emotional experience: These individuals experienced negative pictures not only as more unpleasant (more negative valence) than positive pictures, but also as more emotionally intense (higher arousal) than positive pictures. For these individuals, the laterality pattern was reversed, with greater *right*-lateralized activation to positive (relative to negative) pictures, and greater *left*-lateralized activation to negative (relative to positive) pictures. This was the first demonstration that individual differences in emotional experience can have a profound effect on observable brain activation patterns.

Given the central role of the amygdala in the animal literature (Aggleton, 1992), neuroimaging studies of emotion almost immediately focused on this structure in humans. For example, in the middle to late 1990s, three different groups focused on the question of how individual differences in amygdala activation were related to subsequent emotional memory (Cahill et al., 1996;

Canli, Zhao, Desmond, Glover, & Gabrieli, 1999; Hamann, Ely, Grafton, & Kilts, 1999). (For a detailed review of amygdala function in memory, see Hamann, Chapter 8, this volume.)

Individual differences in emotional experience, evaluation, and regulation also implicate the amygdala. For example, we conducted an event-related fMRI study in which participants provided online ratings of their emotional arousal in response to a set of images that ranged from neutral to highly unpleasant (Canli, Zhao, Brewer, Gabrieli, & Cahill, 2000). The design of the study allowed us to investigate neural activation as a function of within-subject variability, as each individual provided ratings across the set of shown stimuli. We found that activation in the left amygdala increased as ratings of subjective emotional arousal increased.

Two other studies have reported left-lateralized amygdala activation as a function of experienced emotional arousal in a rating task. We saw this pattern for both males and females in an emotional encoding study (Canli, Desmond, Zhao, & Gabrieli, 2002). Phan and colleagues (2004) saw this pattern in a study of emotional appraisal: Participants were shown negative, positive, and neutral pictures, and were asked to rate either their subjective experience of emotional arousal (valence task) or the degree to which a given stimulus was perceived to be related to one's self (association task). The authors reported significant left amygdala activation during the valence task, but no significant amygdala activation during the association task. Furthermore, activation in the left amygdala increased as individual ratings of subjective emotional intensity increased.

From these data, one should expect that ratings of individual emotional experience might be better predictors of amygdala activation than normative ratings. This question was explicitly addressed by Phan and colleagues (2003), who examined the signal obtained from the amygdala when presentation of emotional stimuli was predicted by a simple boxcar regressor that was identical for all subjects, versus a regressor that was based on each subject's rating of each stimulus. They found that the ratings regressor, but not the boxcar regressor, detected significant amygdala activation in response to emotional stimuli.

Appraisal of emotional information is particularly valuable when the information is incomplete or ambiguous, and the amygdala may play a critical role in the evaluation of ambiguous information (Whalen, 1998). For example, facial expressions of surprise may signal a positive or negative consequence. Given the role that the amygdala plays in generating a state of vigilance (Davis & Whalen, 2001), appraisal of surprised facial expressions may moderate amygdala activation. This hypothesis was tested by Kim, Somerville, Johnstone, Alexander, and Whalen (2003), who had participants rate the perceived valence of surprised facial expressions. They found that higher negative ratings of surprised faces were associated with greater amygdala activation to these faces, compared to amygdala activation to neutral expressions.

TRAITS

Individual differences in emotional experience can give us important clues about the structure of personality. Rather than reflecting random noise, stable differences across individuals in their response to emotional stimuli may reflect the underlying dispositions, biases, and behavioral response styles that we commonly identify as "traits." For example, extraverted individuals have a greater tendency to be sociable and to experience positive affect than introverted individuals do (Costa & McCrae, 1980). Neurotic individuals have a greater tendency to be anxious and to experience negative affect than less neurotic individuals do (Costa & McCrae, 1980). We have built a program of research based on these personality traits to investigate the neural basis of personality, using an individual-difference approach to studying emotional processing (Canli, 2004).

In the first study of this series (Canli et al., 2001), we scanned individuals as they passively viewed alternating blocks of negative and positive pictures. We then correlated the fMRI signal with individuals' scores for extraversion and neuroticism. We predicted (1) that extraversion would be positively correlated with activation to positive (relative to negative) pictures, and (2) that neuroticism would be positively correlated with activation to negative (relative to positive) pictures. Our analyses confirmed these predictions, but were particularly exciting with respect to the amygdala. We found that activation of the amygdala (among other regions) to positive pictures was significantly correlated with extraversion. This suggested that the amygdala would respond to positive stimuli (which at the time was not a widely held view), but that the *degree* of the response would be moderated by personality.

Our second study focused on individual differences in amygdala response to facial expressions of emotion (Canli, Sivers, Whitfield, Gotlib, & Gabrieli, 2002). Prior work had consistently reported amygdala responsiveness to fearful facial expressions (Breiter et al., 1996; Morris et al., 1996; Whalen et al., 1998), which was consistent with a substantial animal literature on the amygdala's role in fear-related processes (Davis, 2000; LeDoux, 2003). On the other hand, these same studies had yielded inconsistent conclusions about the amygdala's responsiveness to happy facial expressions. On the basis of our earlier personality study (Canli et al., 2001), we hypothesized that amygdala activation to happy facial expressions would be associated with participants' degree of extraversion. As shown in Plate 11.2 (in color insert), this prediction was borne out. These data may help explain prior inconsistencies, because extraversion was an extraneous variable that was not controlled in these earlier studies.

Other studies have illustrated how individual trait differences may modulate amygdala responsiveness to negative stimuli. For example, amygdala activation to videos depicting snakes in individuals without snake phobia was correlated with dispositional pessimism (Fischer, Tillfors, Furmark, & Fredrikson, 2001). Two PET studies reported that dispositional negative affect or depression severity was correlated with increased amygdala resting blood flow and glucose metabolism in depressed patients (Abercrombie et al., 1998; Drevets et al., 1992), and amygdala activation to negative images was also correlated with dispositional negative affect in an fMRI study of healthy individuals (Davidson & Irwin, 1999). Trait rumination was associated with greater amygdala activation in participants who viewed negative, compared to neutral, pictures (Ray et al., 2005). Interestingly, rumination was also associated with changes in amygdala activation when participants consciously regulated their emotions to feel more negative affect (producing greater amygdala activation) or to feel less negative affect (producing less amygdala activation). This second observation appears somewhat counterintuitive: Individuals who score high on trait rumination appear to be more effective in decreasing amygdala activation to negative stimuli than individuals who score low on this trait seem to be. However, the greater decrease in amygdala activation in higher-scoring ruminators is driven by a higher level of activation in the control condition, rather than by a higher level of deactivation in the experimental (i.e., emotion regulation) condition (R. D. Ray, personal communication, April 4, 2006). This caveat serves to remind us that fMRI always involves comparisons of relative differences, which may or may not be driven by the condition of experimental interest. (I return to this point in the next section.)

A construct that is loosely related to emotion regulation is regulatory focus, which is hypothesized to consist of two motivational systems: one that imbues the individual with a tendency to be sensitive to gains (promotion focus), and one that imbues the individual with a tendency to be sensitive to losses (prevention focus). Cunningham, Raye, and Johnson (2005) showed that individual differences in promotion focus were correlated with amygdala activation to positive (relative to negative) word stimuli, and that individual differences in prevention focus were correlated with amygdala activation to negative (relative to positive) word stimuli. These data reinforce the view that amygdala processing tags personally relevant emotional information, regardless of valence.

As shown in the cases of emotion regulation and regulatory focus, personality traits can modulate amygdala activation during conscious processing of emotional stimuli. However, recent work illustrates that personality traits can modulate amygdala activation during nonconscious processing as well. For example, individual differences in state anxiety were associated with amygdala activation to unattended, but not attended, threat stimuli (Bishop, Duncan, & Lawrence, 2004). Another study found a similar pattern as a function of trait (as opposed to state) anxiety. Using high-resolution fMRI, Etkin and colleagues (2004) reported that unconscious perception of (masked) fearful faces was associated with basolateral amygdala activation, and that the degree of activation was associated with individual differences in trait anxiety. On the other hand, *conscious* perception of fearful faces was associated with dorsal amygdala activation, and this activation was *independent* of individual differences in trait anxiety. The results from Bishop and colleagues (2004) and Etkin and colleagues (2004) may explain why we did not observe amygdala activation to fearful faces to be moderated by neuroticism (Canli et al., 2001), because participants had a conscious perception of these faces. Thus conscious and unconscious processing of fear may both involve the amygdala, but may engage distinct neural networks and processes.

GENOMIC IMAGING

In the previous sections, I have presented evidence from a diverse set of task paradigms and a number of independent laboratories that individual differences in amygdala function are associated with complex human behavior related to emotions and traits. What are the underlying cellular and molecular mechanisms that can explain individual differences in amygdala activation? One promising strategy lies in "genomic imaging," in which variance in neuroimaging signals (such as the fMRI blood-oxygenation-level-dependent [BOLD] response) is associated with genetic variance. In this section, I briefly highlight two genetic systems in which variance at the molecular level has been related to variance in amygdala function.

Variation in the Serotonin Transporter Gene

The first system relates to the transport of serotonin (5-hydroxytryptamine, or 5-HT) from the synaptic cleft. The serotonin transporter gene (*5-HTT*) has a common variation (polymorphism) in the transcriptional control region (5-HTTLPR), which results in either a short (s) or long (l) variant (allele). Because any individual carries two alleles of any gene (one from each parent), there are three categories of individuals: those with two short alleles (s/s), those with two long alleles (l/l), and those with one of each (s/l). Lesch and colleagues (1996) discovered that individuals carrying either one or two copies of the short allele (s/s or s/l, referred to hereafter as the "S-group") scored higher in self-reported neuroticism than did individuals who were noncarriers—that is, were homozygous for the long allele (l/l, referred to hereafter as the "L-group").

Hariri and colleagues (2002) demonstrated that amygdala activation to angry and fearful faces (relative to a visuospatial control task) was greater in the S-group than in the L-group. What was particularly impressive about this demonstration was the effect size: Whereas the association between 5-HTTLPR genotype and self-reported neuroticism accounted for 3–4% of the variance, the association between 5-HTTLPR genotype and amygdala activation accounted for 20% of the variance (Hamer, 2002). The effect size was greater because genetic function related to neurotransmitter regulation is more closely associated with neural processes than with higher-level behavioral processes (such as those measured by self-report questionnaires).

In addition to replication by the same group with a larger sample (Hariri et al., 2005), other groups have demonstrated greater amygdala activation to emotional stimuli in carriers of the 5-HTTLPR short allele than in non-carriers, as confirmed by a recent meta-analysis (Munafo, Brown, & Hariri, 2007). In aggregate, these studies have been conducted across a number of task paradigms, including face matching (Hariri et al., 2002, 2005; Pezawas et al., 2005), passive viewing of pictures (Heinz et al., 2005), and an anxiety-producing speaking task (Furmark et al., 2004).

Importantly, each of these studies compared brain activation during the emotional condition to a neutral baseline control condition, which is assumed not to generate any activation of interest itself. We (Canli, Omura, et al., 2005) explicitly tested this assumption with an experimental design that featured two baseline conditions, one consisting of neutral words and the other of a resting condition. When we compared amygdala activation to emotional words to the neutral control condition, we replicated the observation that the S-group showed greater amygdala activation than the L-group (see Plate 11.3 in color insert). We reasoned that this activation could be driven by an increase to negative words or by a decrease to neutral words. To disentangle these two possibilities, we compared activation to emotional and to neutral words separately, using the resting baseline condition. As shown in Plate 11.3, the S-group showed no significant increase in activation to negative words, but did show a significant decrease to neutral words, compared to the resting condition. Importantly, this observation was independently replicated (Heinz et al., 2007), although the interpretation of this observation continues to be a matter of debate, as reviewed elsewhere (Canli & Lesch, 2007).

How can one reconcile this observation with the fact that the presence of the short allele is associated with negative affect? One interpretation is that the S-group is characterized by tonic amygdala activation at rest (Canli & Lesch, 2007), which may be interrupted by phasic decreases in activation in response to brief presentation of stimuli. We conducted an explicit test of this interpretation by using perfusion imaging to measure absolute levels of amygdala activation at rest, as a function of 5-HTTLPR genotype (Canli et al., 2006). Using this methodology, we confirmed that the S-group is indeed characterized by elevated amygdala resting activation, compared to the L-group. This observation was again independently replicated by others (Rao et al., 2007). The debate now focuses on the question of whether elevated amygdala activation in the absence of task constraints reflects a reaction to the uncertainty of the environment of the scanner, as suggested by some (Heinz et al., 2007), or instead a tonically elevated level of activity that is independent of external stimuli, as we suggest in our tonic model of 5-HTTLPR function (Canli & Lesch, 2007).

The effects of 5-HTTLPR genotype on amygdala function are amplified by life stress experience (Canli et al., 2006). We asked participants to complete a simple questionnaire in which they noted whether they had ever experienced any of 28 different types of events (stressful experiences in social relationships, health, legal or financial problems, loss of loved ones, etc.). We found that the number of life stress experiences correlated positively with amygdala resting activation in the S-group, but *negatively* in the L-group. Furthermore, the same pattern was observed with respect to rumination: Life stress correlated positively with rumination in the S-group, but negatively in the L-group. These findings suggest that both types of individuals respond to life stress, but in opposite ways. Future work will have to address which psychological and neural processes can explain this pattern of data. For example, future work may address whether L-group individuals benefit from life stress experience to strengthen neural circuits that regulate emotions. Alternatively, it is possible that life stress in these individuals leads to "burnout" of the amygdala, which renders them emotionally unresponsive.

Variation in the Tryptophan Hydroxylase-2 Gene

The second system also relates to the serotonergic system and involves the tryptophan hydroxylase-2 gene (TPH2), which codes for the rate-limiting enzyme during serotonin synthesis in the brain. A number of TPH2 polymorphisms have been linked to psychopathology, including depression (Zill et al., 2004), bipolar disorder (Harvey, 2003), attention-deficit/hyperactivity disorder (Sheehan et al., 2005; Walitza et al., 2005), and dysfunction in behavioral inhibition (Stoltenberg et al., 2006).

Cools and colleagues (2005) examined the effects of acute tryptophan depletion (ATD), which results in a transient reduction of cerebral serotonin, on amygdala activation to fearful faces. One question of interest was whether the degree of change in amygdala responsiveness was moderated by individual differences in self-reported threat sensitivity. They found that ATD enhanced amygdala activation to fearful (vs. happy) faces, relative to a placebo condition. Furthermore, they found that the degree of amygdala enhancement by ATD was positively correlated with participants' threat sensitivity scores.

Whereas ATD represents an artificial means of studying the effect of individual differences in available serotonin on amygdala function, variation within TPH2 may provide a natural mechanism. Brown and colleagues (2005) used fMRI to provide evidence that the presence of the T allele in a single-nucleotide polymorphism (SNP; specifically, the TPH2 rs4570625 SNP) was associated with increased amygdala reactivity to angry and fearful facial expressions, compared to a visuospatial matching task. Independently of Brown and colleagues, we investigated amygdala activation to both negative and positive emotional facial expressions as a function of the same polymorphism (Canli, Congdon, Gutknecht, Constable, & Lesch, 2005). As shown in Plate 11.4 (in color insert), we observed greater amygdala activation in carriers of the *TPH2* T allele in response to fearful, happy, and sad (compared to neutral) faces, and additional analyses showed that the effect was not carried by *TPH2* modulation in amygdala processing of neutral faces. Thus this genetic variation may modulate amygdala processing of emotional stimuli, regardless of valence.

The effects of 5-HTTLPR and *TPH2* are additive when assessed with event-related potentials during viewing of emotional pictures (Herrmann et al., 2007), and also when assessed with fMRI (Canli, Congdon, Constable, & Lesch, in press): Individuals who carried genetic variants that were associated with greater emotional reactivity (relative to neutral stimuli) for both genes exhibited the greatest degree of brain activation (primarily in the putamen, but also in the amygdala at reduced threshold levels), whereas those individuals who carried neither of these variants for the two genes exhibited the lowest degree of brain activation, and those who carried one or the other gene variant exhibited intermediate levels of activation. This pattern was observed across two tasks, using word and face stimuli.

CONCLUSIONS

The prospect for understanding the neurobiological basis of individual differences in human amygdala function is bright. A number of neuroimaging paradigms have been, and continue to be, developed that capture individual differences in a number of complex behaviors, as I have illustrated in this chapter for emotion and traits. The advent of genomic imaging has now begun to identify genetic variations that are associated with these processes, and is beginning to reveal interactions with environmental factors, such as life stress experience, and among genes. Undoubtedly, these neurogenetic models will grow in complexity and richness, as molecular techniques are used to assess larger numbers of genetic and epigenetic markers (Canli, 2008).

WHAT I THINK

I think that the study of individual differences in amygdala function will become more comprehensive and integrative with respect to both higher-order and lower-order levels of analysis in the next decade.

With respect to higher-order levels of analysis, I think that the behaviors under study will become more complex. Although studies of emotional behavior and traits will continue to flourish, there will be much excitement about social processes. One catalyst is the emergent field of "neuroeconomics" (Sanfey, Loewenstein, McClure, & Cohen, 2006), in which investigators borrow task paradigms from game theory to study social interactions with well-defined parameters. The recent inauguration of journals specifically devoted to "social neuroscience" will likewise accelerate the trend toward study of social behavior. Indeed, some studies have already begun to conduct "hyperscanning" experiments, in which two individuals are scanned at the same time while interacting with each other (King-Casas et al., 2005; Montague et al., 2002; Tomlin et al., 2006).

With respect to lower-order levels of analysis, I think that genomic imaging will become the dominant imaging approach to the study of the amygdala in particular and of brain function in general. This is because the genetic characterization of individuals greatly enhances our ability to develop molecular models of neural function. Even better is that these models will be closely related to behavior, because most imaging studies will continue to use a functional imaging approach that seeks to identify neural correlates of behavior. In the process, the focus will move away from single genes' effects on brain function (for which the term "imaging genetics" may be more appropriate) (Hariri, Drabant, & Weinberger, 2006) and toward whole-genome analyses, which consider the effects of large sets of genes. This development, however, will depend critically on the advancement of novel analysis methods that are currently in development (Zapala & Schork, 2006).

The focus on genetic moderators of individual differences in amygdala function does not dismiss environmental variables. Indeed, several studies have begun to identify gene × environment (G × E) interactions that are specific to polymorphic genes in humans (Caspi et al., 2002, 2003; Eley et al., 2004; Grabe et al., 2005; Kaufman et al., 2004; Kendler, Kuhn, Vittum, Prescott, & Riley, 2005), and we were the first to show the role of G × E interactions for a specific gene (5-HTTLPR) in the brain (Canli et al., 2006). Future work will focus on the underlying molecular mechanisms of these interactions, which are very likely to involve modulation of the epigenome (Wong, Gottesman, & Petronis, 2005), as has recently been illustrated in animal studies on the effects of early maternal experience on glucocorticoid gene methylation (Weaver et al., 2004; Weaver, Meaney, & Szyf, 2006).

As our understanding of G × E interactions grows, and as we begin to associate these interactions with brain function in humans, the need for causal explanations will grow. The human data will always be correlational, because we cannot manipulate people's environments or genotypes. On the other hand, methods for genetic manipulation in animals continue to be refined, and therefore make it possible to test causal models that were derived from human correlational data. Thus I think that in the next decade, there will be an increased drive toward integration of human and animal research approaches. The results of this integration will change the field of psychology and will probably revolutionize clinical neuroscience approaches to the treatment and prevention of mental illness. I am grateful to be associated with a scientific discipline that can offer such a hopeful message for the future.

REFERENCES

Abercrombie, H. C., Schaefer, S. M., Larson, C. L., Oakes, T. R., Lindgren, K. A., Holden, J. E., et al. (1998). Metabolic rate in the right amygdala predicts negative affect in depressed patients. *NeuroReport, 9*, 3301–3307.

Aggleton, J. P. (Ed.). (1992). *The amygdala: Neurobiological aspects of emotion, memory, and mental dysfunction.* New York: Wiley-Liss.

Bishop, S. J., Duncan, J., & Lawrence, A. D. (2004). State anxiety modulation of the amygdala response to unattended threat-related stimuli. *Journal of Neuroscience, 24*, 10364–10368.

Breiter, H. C., Etcoff, N. L., Whalen, P. J., Kennedy, W. A., Rauch, S. L., Buckner, R. L., et al. (1996). Response and habituation of the human amygdala during visual processing of facial expression. *Neuron, 17*, 875–887.

Brewer, J. B., Zhao, Z., Desmond, J. E., Glover, G. H., & Gabrieli, J. D. E. (1998). Making memories: Brain activity that predicts how well visual experience is remembered. *Science, 281*, 1185–1187.

Brown, S. M., Peet, E., Manuck, S. B., Williamson, D. E., Dahl, R. E., Ferrell, R. E., et al. (2005). A regulatory variant of the human tryptophan hydroxylase-2 gene biases amygdala reactivity. *Molecular Psychiatry, 10*(9), 884–888.

Cahill, L., Haier, R. J., Fallon, J., Alkire, M. T., Tang, C., Keator, D., et al. (1996). Amygdala activity at encoding correlated with long-term, free recall of emotional information. *Proceedings of the National Academy of Sciences USA, 93,* 8016–8021.

Canli, T. (2004). Functional brain mapping of extraversion and neuroticism: Learning from individual differences in emotion processing. *Journal of Personality, 72*(6), 1105–1132.

Canli, T. (2008). Toward a neurogenetic theory of neuroticism. In D. Pfaff & M. B. Kiefer (Eds.), Molecular and biophysical mechanisms of arousal, alertness and attention. *Annals of the New York Academy of Science, 1129,* 153–174.

Canli, T., Congdon, E., Constable, R. T., & Lesch, K. P. (in press). Additive effects of serotonin transporter and tryptophan hydroxylase-2 gene variation on neural correlates of affective processing. *Biological Psychology.*

Canli, T., Congdon, E., Gutknecht, L., Constable, R. T., & Lesch, K. P. (2005). Amygdala responsiveness is modulated by tryptophan hydroxylase-2 gene variation. *Journal of Neural Transmission, 112*(11), 1479–1485.

Canli, T., Desmond, J. E., Zhao, Z., & Gabrieli, J. D. E. (2002). Sex differences in the neural basis of emotional memories. *Proceedings of the National Academy of Sciences USA, 99,* 10789–10794.

Canli, T., Desmond, J. E., Zhao, Z., Glover, G., & Gabrieli, J. D. E. (1998). Hemispheric asymmetry for emotional stimuli detected with fMRI. *NeuroReport, 9,* 3233–3239.

Canli, T., & Lesch, K. P. (2007). Long story short: The serotonin transporter in emotion regulation and social cognition. *Nature Neuroscience, 10*(9), 1103–1109.

Canli, T., Omura, K., Haas, B. W., Fallgatter, A. J., Constable, R. T., & Lesch, K. P. (2005). Beyond affect: A role for genetic variation of the serotonin transporter in neural activation during a cognitive attention task. *Proceedings of the National Academy of Sciences USA, 102,* 12224–12229.

Canli, T., Qiu, M., Omura, K., Congdon, E., Haas, B. W., Amin, Z., et al. (2006). Neural correlates of epigenesis. *Proceedings of the National Academy of Sciences USA, 103,* 16033–16038.

Canli, T., Sivers, H., Whitfield, S. L., Gotlib, I. H., & Gabrieli, J. D. E. (2002). Amygdala response to happy faces as a function of extraversion. *Science, 296,* 2191.

Canli, T., Zhao, Z., Brewer, J., Gabrieli, J. D. E., & Cahill, L. (2000). Event-related activation in the human amygdala associates with later memory for individual emotional experience. *Journal of Neuroscience, 20*(19), RC99.

Canli, T., Zhao, Z., Desmond, J. E., Glover, G., & Gabrieli, J. D. E. (1999). fMRI identifies a network of structures correlated with retention of positive and negative emotional memory. *Psychobiology, 27,* 441–452.

Canli, T., Zhao, Z., Desmond, J. E., Kang, E., Gross, J., & Gabrieli, J. D. E. (2001). An fMRI study of personality influences on brain reactivity to emotional stimuli. *Behavioral Neuroscience, 115*(1), 33–42.

Casey, B. J., Cohen, J. D., O'Craven, K., Davidson, R. J., Irwin, W., Nelson, C. A., et al. (1998). Reproducibility of fMRI results across four institutions using a spatial working memory task. *NeuroImage, 8*(3), 249–261.

Caspi, A., McClay, J., Moffitt, T. E., Mill, J., Martin, J., Craig, I. W., et al. (2002). Role of genotype in the cycle of violence in maltreated children. *Science, 297,* 851–854.

Caspi, A., Sugden, K., Moffitt, T. E., Taylor, A., Craig, I. W., Harrington, H., et al. (2003). Influence of life stress on depression: Moderation by a polymorphism in the 5-HTT gene. *Science, 301,* 386–389.

Cools, R., Calder, A. J., Lawrence, A. D., Clark, L., Bullmore, E., & Robbins, T. W. (2005). Individual differences in threat sensitivity predict serotonergic modulation of amygdala response to fearful faces. *Psychopharmacology (Berlin), 180*(4), 670–679.

Costa, P. T., Jr., & McCrae, R. R. (1980). Influence of extraversion and neuroticism on subjective well-being: Happy and unhappy people. *Journal of Personality and Social Psychology, 38,* 668–678.

Cunningham, W. A., Raye, C. L., & Johnson, M. K. (2005). Neural correlates of evaluation associated with promotion and prevention regulatory focus. *Cognitive, Affective, and Behavioral Neuroscience, 5*(2), 202–211.

Davidson, R. J. (1995). Cerebral asymmetry, emotion, and affective style. In R. J. Davidson & K. Hugdahl (Eds.), *Brain asymmetry.* Cambridge, MA: MIT Press.

Davidson, R. J., & Irwin, W. (1999). The functional neuroanatomy of emotion and affective style. *Trends in Cognitive Sciences, 3,* 11–21.

Davis, M. (2000). The role of the amygdala in conditioned and unconditioned fear and anxiety. In J. P. Aggleton (Ed.), *The amygdala: A functional analysis* (2nd ed., pp. 213–288). Oxford, UK: Oxford University Press.

Davis, M., & Whalen, P. J. (2001). The amygdala: Vigilance and emotion. *Molecular Psychiatry, 6*(1), 13–34.

Drevets, W. C., Videen, T. O., Price, J. L., Preskorn, S. H., Carmichael, S. T., & Raichle, M. E. (1992). A functional anatomical study of unipolar depression. *Journal of Neuroscience, 12,* 3628–3641.

Eley, T. C., Sugden, K., Corsico, A., Gregory, A. M., Sham, P., McGuffin, P., et al. (2004). Gene–environment interaction analysis of serotonin system markers with adolescent depression. *Molecular Psychiatry, 9*(10), 908–915.

Etkin, A., Klemenhagen, K. C., Dudman, J. T., Rogan, M. T., Hen, R., Kandel, E. R., et al. (2004). Individual differences in trait anxiety predict the response of the basolateral amygdala to unconsciously processed fearful faces. *Neuron, 44*(6), 1043–1055.

Fischer, H., Tillfors, M., Furmark, T., & Fredrikson, M. (2001). Dispositional pessimism and amygdala activity: A PET study in healthy volunteers. *NeuroReport, 12,* 1635–1638.

Furmark, T., Tillfors, M., Garpenstrand, H., Marteinsdottir, I., Langstrom, B., Oreland, L., et al. (2004). Serotonin transporter polymorphism related to amygdala excitability and symptom severity in patients with social phobia. *Neuroscience Letters, 362*(3), 189–192.

Gabrieli, J. D. E., Brewer, J. B., Desmond, J. E., & Glover, G. H. (1997). Separate neural bases of two fundamental memory processes in the human medial temporal lobe. *Science, 276,* 264–266.

Grabe, H. J., Lange, M., Wolff, B., Volzke, H., Lucht, M., Freyberger, H. J., et al. (2005). Mental and physical distress is modulated by a polymorphism in the 5-HT transporter gene interacting with social stressors and chronic disease burden. *Molecular Psychiatry, 10*(2), 220–224.

Hamann, S. B., Ely, T. D., Grafton, S. T., & Kilts, C. D. (1999). Amygdala activity related to enhanced memory for pleasant and aversive stimuli. *Nature Neuroscience, 2*, 289–293.

Hamer, D. (2002). Genetics: Rethinking behavior genetics. *Science, 298*, 71–72.

Hariri, A. R., Drabant, E. M., Munoz, K. E., Kolachana, B. S., Mattay, V. S., Egan, M. F., et al. (2005). A susceptibility gene for affective disorders and the response of the human amygdala. *Archives of General Psychiatry, 62*(2), 146–152.

Hariri, A. R., Drabant, E. M., & Weinberger, D. R. (2006). Imaging genetics: Perspectives from studies of genetically driven variation in serotonin function and corticolimbic affective processing. *Biological Psychiatry, 59*(10), 888–897.

Hariri, A. R., Mattay, V. S., Tessitore, A., Kolachana, B., Fera, F., Goldman, D., et al. (2002). Serotonin transporter genetic variation and the response of the human amygdala. *Science, 297*, 400–403.

Harvey, J. A. (2003). Role of the serotonin 5-HT(2A) receptor in learning. *Learning and Memory, 10*(5), 355–362.

Heinz, A., Braus, D. F., Smolka, M. N., Wrase, J., Puls, I., Hermann, D., et al. (2005). Amygdala–prefrontal coupling depends on a genetic variation of the serotonin transporter. *Nature Neuroscience, 8*(1), 20–21.

Heinz, A., Smolka, M. N., Braus, D. F., Wrase, J., Beck, A., Flor, H., et al. (2007). Serotonin transporter genotype (5-HTTLPR): Effects of neutral and undefined conditions on amygdala activation. *Biological Psychiatry, 61*(8), 1011–1014.

Herrmann, M. J., Huter, T., Muller, F., Muhlberger, A., Pauli, P., Reif, A., et al. (2007). Additive effects of serotonin transporter and tryptophan hydroxylase-2 gene variation on emotional processing. *Cerebral Cortex, 17*(5), 1160–1163.

Kaufman, J., Yang, B. Z., Douglas-Palumberi, H., Houshyar, S., Lipschitz, D., Krystal, J. H., et al. (2004). Social supports and serotonin transporter gene moderate depression in maltreated children. *Proceedings of the National Academy of Sciences USA, 101*, 17316–17321.

Kendler, K. S., Kuhn, J. W., Vittum, J., Prescott, C. A., & Riley, B. (2005). The interaction of stressful life events and a serotonin transporter polymorphism in the prediction of episodes of major depression: A replication. *Archives of General Psychiatry, 62*(5), 529–535.

Kim, H., Somerville, L. H., Johnstone, T., Alexander, A. L., & Whalen, P. J. (2003). Inverse amygdala and medial prefrontal cortex responses to surprised faces. *NeuroReport, 14*(18), 2317–2322.

King-Casas, B., Tomlin, D., Anen, C., Camerer, C. F., Quartz, S. R., & Montague, P. R. (2005). Getting to know you: Reputation and trust in a two-person economic exchange. *Science, 308*, 78–83.

LeDoux, J. (2003). The emotional brain, fear, and the amygdala. *Cellular and Molecular Neurobiology, 23*(4–5), 727–738.

Lesch, K. P., Bengel, D., Heils, A., Sabol, S. Z., Greenberg, B. D., Petri, S., et al. (1996). Association of anxiety-related traits with a polymorphism in the serotonin transporter gene regulatory region. *Science, 274*, 1527–1531.

Montague, P. R., Berns, G. S., Cohen, J. D., McClure, S. M., Pagnoni, G., Dhamala, M., et al. (2002). Hyperscanning: Simultaneous fMRI during linked social interactions. *NeuroImage, 16*(4), 1159–1164.

Morris, J. S., Frith, C. D., Perrett, D. I., Rowland, D., Young, A. W., Calder, A. J., et al. (1996). A differential neural response in the human amygdala to fearful and happy facial expressions. *Nature, 383*, 812–815.

Munafo, M. R., Brown, S. M., & Hariri, A. R. (2008). Serotonin transporter (5-HTTLPR) genotype and amygdala activation: A meta-analysis. *Biological Psychiatry, 63*(9), 852–857.

Pezawas, L., Meyer-Lindenberg, A., Drabant, E. M., Verchinski, B. A., Munoz, K. E., Kolachana, B. S., et al. (2005). 5-HTTLPR polymorphism impacts human cingulate–amygdala interactions: A genetic susceptibility mechanism for depression. *Nature Neuroscience, 8*(6), 828–834.

Phan, K. L., Taylor, S. F., Welsh, R. C., Decker, L. R., Noll, D. C., Nichols, T. E., et al. (2003). Activation of the medial prefrontal cortex and extended amygdala by individual ratings of emotional arousal: A fMRI study. *Biological Psychiatry, 53*(3), 211–215.

Phan, K. L., Taylor, S. F., Welsh, R. C., Ho, S. H., Britton, J. C., & Liberzon, I. (2004). Neural correlates of individual ratings of emotional salience: A trial-related fMRI study. *NeuroImage, 21*(2), 768–780.

Plomin, R., & Kosslyn, S. M. (2001). Genes, brain and cognition. *Nature Neuroscience, 4*(12), 1153–1154.

Rao, H., Gillihan, S. J., Wang, J., Korczykowski, M., Sankoorikal, G. M., Kaercher, K. A., et al. (2007). Genetic variation in serotonin transporter alters resting brain function in healthy individuals. *Biological Psychiatry, 62*(6), 600–606.

Ray, R. D., Ochsner, K. N., Cooper, J. C., Robertson, E. R., Gabrieli, J. D., & Gross, J. J. (2005). Individual differences in trait rumination and the neural systems supporting cognitive reappraisal. *Cognitive, Affective, and Behavioral Neuroscience, 5*(2), 156–168.

Sanfey, A. G., Loewenstein, G., McClure, S. M., & Cohen, J. D. (2006). Neuroeconomics: Cross-currents in research on decision-making. *Trends in Cognitive Sciences, 10*(3), 108–116.

Sheehan, K., Lowe, N., Kirley, A., Mullins, C., Fitzgerald, M., Gill, M., et al. (2005). Tryptophan hydroxylase 2 (TPH2) gene variants associated with ADHD. *Molecular Psychiatry, 10*(10), 944–949.

Stoltenberg, S. F., Glass, J. M., Chermack, S. T., Flynn, H. A., Li, S., Weston, M. E., et al. (2006). Possible association between response inhibition and a variant in the brain-expressed tryptophan hydroxylase-2 gene. *Psychiatric Genetics, 16*(1), 35–38.

Tomlin, D., Kayali, M. A., King-Casas, B., Anen, C., Camerer, C. F., Quartz, S. R., et al. (2006). Agent-specific responses in the cingulate cortex during economic exchanges. *Science, 312*, 1047–1050.

Walitza, S., Renner, T. J., Dempfle, A., Konrad, K., Wewetzer, C., Halbach, A., et al. (2005). Transmission disequilibrium of polymorphic variants in the tryptophan hydroxylase-2 gene in attention-deficit/hyperactivity disorder. *Molecular Psychiatry, 10*(12), 1126–1132.

Weaver, I. C., Cervoni, N., Champagne, F. A., D'Alessio, A. C., Sharma, S., Seckl, J. R., et al. (2004). Epigenetic programming by maternal behavior. *Nature Neuroscience, 7*(8), 847–854.

Weaver, I. C., Meaney, M. J., & Szyf, M. (2006). Maternal care effects on the hippocampal transcriptome and anxiety-mediated behaviors in the offspring that are reversible in adulthood. *Proceedings of the National Academy of Sciences USA, 103*(9), 3480–3485.

Whalen, P. J. (1998). Fear, vigilance, and ambiguity: Initial neuroimaging studies of the human amygdala. *Current Directions in Psychological Science, 7,* 177–188.

Whalen, P. J., Rauch, S. L., Etcoff, N. L., McInerney, S. C., Lee, M. B., & Jenike, M. A. (1998). Masked presentations of emotional facial expressions modulate amygdala activity without explicit knowledge. *Journal of Neuroscience, 18,* 411–418.

Wong, A. H., Gottesman, I. I., & Petronis, A. (2005). Phenotypic differences in genetically identical organisms: The epigenetic perspective. *Human Molecular Genetics, 14*(Spec. No. 1), R11–R18.

Zapala, M. A., & Schork, N. J. (2006). Multivariate regression analysis of distance matrices for testing associations between gene expression patterns and related variables. *Proceedings of the National Academy of Sciences USA, 103,* 19430–19435.

Zill, P., Baghai, T. C., Zwanzger, P., Schule, C., Eser, D., Rupprecht, R., et al. (2004). SNP and haplotype analysis of a novel tryptophan hydroxylase isoform (TPH2) gene provide evidence for association with major depression. *Molecular Psychiatry, 9*(11), 1030–1036.

CHAPTER 12

Human Amygdala Responses
to Facial Expressions of Emotion

*Paul J. Whalen, F. Caroline Davis, Jonathan A. Oler,
Hackjin Kim, M. Justin Kim, and Maital Neta*

As the first section of this volume describes, much of what we know about the amygdala has been obtained from studies of animals undergoing aversive Pavlovian conditioning. The dependent measure in these studies is most often a decrease in movement, called "freezing." This behavior is interpreted as an indication of fear, originally observed to the unconditioned stimulus (US), which after training is observed to a once neutral stimulus, or conditioned stimulus (CS). In addition to being the quintessential manifestation of a state of fear, freezing can serve another purpose—the facilitation of learning. During the freezing response, the animal arrests any ongoing movement. This allows the animal time to survey the environment and develop a plan of action. In addition, the freezing response often begins with a quick shift of the body that "aims" the sensory organs (e.g., eyes, ears) in the direction that is the animal's "best guess" at the direction that will be most instructive ("where a potentially predictive stimulus was noticed the last time a US occurred"). Nonspecific attentional responses such as these have been referred to as "associative orienting" (Gallagher & Holland, 1994; Kapp, Whalen, Supple, & Pascoe, 1992; Whalen, 1998), because they influence the eventual acquisition rate of other conditioned responses (see Kapp et al., 1992; Weisz, Harden, & Xiang, 1992). Critically, they are observed during the early stages of acquisition, as well as at any time during learning when the outcome predicted by a particular cue is not entirely clear (see Whalen, 1998).

Numerous studies have shown that the amygdala is critical to the acquisition and expression of conditioned freezing behavior (LeDoux, 1996). Thus
increased amygdala responsivity accompanies a learned state of fear. However, lesions of the amygdala also block associative orienting responses. Our
task then is to try to dissociate the role of the amygdala in this attentional
function from the fear state that conspires to overshadow its direct study.
What is needed is a CS that in and of itself does not evoke a strong fear state,
but whose reinforcement history calls for an increase in nonspecific arousal.
In addition, this CS should include a dimension of clear negativity, but should
also include a separate dimension where the nature of the predicted negativity
is unclear and will thus require associative orienting. Our work, presented in
this chapter, is based on the premise that fearful facial expressions constitute
such a multidimensional CS.

We begin by briefly reviewing the anatomy of the amygdala, highlighting
a distinction between the human dorsal and ventral amygdala, especially as it
relates to our attempts to use functional magnetic resonance imaging (fMRI)
to investigate amygdala function. The reader is referred to Freese and Amaral
(Chapter 1, this volume) for a detailed account of the anatomy of the nonhuman primate amygdala and the implications of this information for understanding human amygdala anatomy.

THE AMYGDALOID COMPLEX

The nuclei that constitute the basolateral amygdala complex (BLA; lateral,
basal, and accessory basal nuclei) are directly connected with widespread
cortical regions. The sensory neocortex and thalamus send prominent projections to the lateral nucleus, suggesting that the lateral nucleus acts as a sensory interface for the amygdala (LeDoux, Cicchetti, Xagoraris, & Romanski,
1990; Pitkänen, 2000). The lateral nucleus then projects in a medial direction to the basal nuclei within the BLA. The basal nuclei have heavy reciprocal connections with the prefrontal and parahippocampal cortices, which
allow for convergent processing of stimuli following detection by the lateral
nucleus.

The BLA projects in a dorsal direction to the central nucleus of the
amygdala (CeA; see Plate 12.1 in color insert). The CeA is the main output
structure for amygdalofugal projections to the hypothalamus, midbrain, pons,
and medulla (Davis, 2000; McDonald, 2003). Although there is very little if
any CeA input to the cerebral cortex (Pitkänen, 2000), the CeA can have
a profound indirect effect on cortical function via direct projections to all
major corticopetal neuromodulatory systems—that is, the ventral tegmental
area (dopamine), the raphe nuclei (serotonin), the nucleus basalis of Meynert
(NBM) (acetylcholine), and the locus coeruleus (norepinephrine).

Physically imposed between the BLA and the CeA are gamma-
aminobutyric acid-ergic "islands" of neurons known as the intercalated cell

masses (ICMs; Royer, Martina, & Paré, 1999). Like the BLA, the ICMs receive a direct projection from the prefrontal cortex, and this pathway can inhibit CeA and NBM activity (Quirk, Likhtik, Pelletier, & Paré, 2003). Thus, if BLA projections to CeA initiate activity that could potentially result in increased autonomic nervous system activation and concomitant increased cortical neuronal activation, the ICMs can override this call for increased arousal and vigilance, based on an additional assessment of the situation by the prefrontal cortex. An example would be a response to the detection of a snake by the BLA. An initiation of autonomic and cortical activation would be adaptive if the snake is encountered in a field. But, at a zoo, the prefrontal cortex would likely override this call for help from the BLA via the ICMs, based on knowledge of something the BLA couldn't possibly understand—Plexiglas.

One way to conceptualize this system is that the BLA and CeA function as an orienting subsystem for the rest of the brain, alerting other systems at times when it would be expedient to gather information. Stimuli detected by the BLA can evoke responses from the CeA that can affect the state of cortical processing, fundamentally changing the vigilance level of the organism. These changes can increase environmental monitoring in the service of eliciting assistance from the cortex in assessing the predictive value of a given environmental event (see Kapp et al., 1992; Whalen, 1998). Such a basic associative function fits well with the amygdaloid complex as a part of an integrative neurobiological system subserving various adaptive functions that cross the categorical boundaries of such constructs as motivation, emotion, vigilance, attention, and cognition (Gallagher & Holland, 1994; Davis & Whalen, 2001).

Using fMRI to Study the Human Amygdaloid Complex

In humans, the ventral region of the amygdaloid complex comprises the BLA, and the CeA is located within the dorsal amygdala (see Plate 12.1 in color insert). Within the BLA, the lateral nucleus is situated at the most lateral aspects of the BLA, and the basal nuclei are situated medially. The central and medial nuclei lie dorsal to the BLA (Heimer & Van Hoesen, 2006). It is important to note that this dorsal–ventral distinction is specific to the human amygdala. Comparison to the rat amygdala (for example) shows that the amygdala is rotated in a clockwise direction, so that the lateral nucleus has both a dorsal and a ventral component (see Figure 12.1).

Though fMRI activations located within the human ventral amygdala can be unequivocally localized to the BLA, activations located within the dorsal amygdala are difficult to localize to the CeA and/or medial nucleus. First, many believe that the CeA and the medial nucleus constitute the posterior and inferior extent of the so-called "extended amygdala" (Alheid, 2003; de Olmos & Heimer, 1999). To elaborate, neurons that are similar to those found in the central and medial nuclei extend in a superior and medial direction through the ventral basal forebrain, remaining below the lentiform nucleus as they

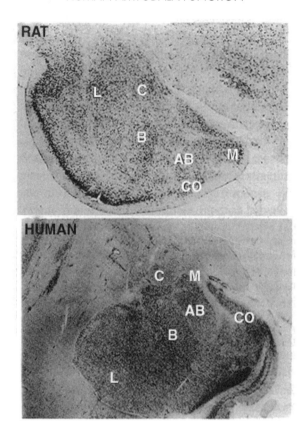

FIGURE 12.1. Comparison of the rat and human amygdala. Note that the human amygdala is rotated in a counterclockwise direction relative to that of the rat. This creates a clear dorsal–ventral distinction between the central nucleus (C), located dorsally, and the basolateral amygdala (L, B, and AB), located ventrally in the human. Note that in the rat, aspects of the lateral nucleus are quite dorsal. From Gloor (1997), who attributes the rat specimen to Dr. Barbara Jones, and the human specimen to the Yakolev Collection. Copyright 1997 by Oxford University Press. Adapted by permission.

continue toward the anterior commissure. Here a proportion of these neurons congregate to constitute the bed nucleus of the stria terminalis (BNST). These neurons then extend in an anterior direction from the BNST, finally terminating in the ventral striatum. Given the similarity of these neurons to those of the CeA and medial nucleus in terms of projection targets and cytoarchitechtonics (de Olmos & Heimer, 1999) and their location within the region of the ventral basal forebrain located just below the lentiform nucleus, these neurons are referred to as "sublenticular extended amygdala" (SLEA) neurons. Intermingled with SLEA neurons located immediately superior to the dorsal extent of the amygdala are large corticopetal cholinergic neurons making up the NBM. Projections from the CeA to these NBM neurons can directly influence their activity (Jolkkonen, Miettinen, Pikkarainen, & Pitkänen, 2002), and in turn the amount of cholinergic release at the cortex.

Though it has become a bit of a trend to label fMRI activations immediately dorsal to the amygdala (within the ventral basal forebrain) as "extended amygdala" activations, the intermingled presence of these larger corticopetal cholinergic neurons muddles this assertion. Indeed, the intermingled nature of CeA, SLEA, BNST, and NBM neurons within this region of the ventral basal forebrain is the basis for referring to this brain region as "substantia innominata" (SI), or "unnamed substance." Advances in histochemical techniques that can easily discern these cell groups have caused some neuroanatomists to declare the term "substantia innominata" obsolete (Heimer, Harlan, Alheid, Garcia, & de Olmos, 1997). But since fMRI responses in the SI region cannot be specifically localized to any one of these cell groups, human functional neuroimaging can make good use of this antiquated neuroanatomical term. Importantly, because previous data in animal subjects show that these neuronal groups probably work in concert to modulate central and peripheral vigilance levels when a predictive stimulus associated with an arousing biologically relevant outcome is encountered (Kapp, Supple, & Whalen, 1994; Whalen, Kapp, & Pascoe, 1994), discerning the unique contributions of each group need not be a central goal of fMRI. Thus the dorsal amygdala/SI activation detailed in numerous functional neuroimaging studies (Breiter et al., 1996; Kim, Somerville, Johnstone, Alexander, & Whalen, 2003; LaBar, Gatenby, Gore, LeDoux, & Phelps, 1998; Pessoa, McKenna, Gutierrez, & Ungerleider, 2002; Whalen, 1998; Whalen, Shin, McInerney, & Fischer, 2001) could reflect activity of dorsal amygdala nuclei, SLEA, BNST, and/or NBM neurons.

Spatial Resolution and the Human Amygdala

The spatial resolution of most current fMRI studies allows for only coarse spatial dissociations within the amygdaloid complex. But given that the anatomical borders of the unilateral amygdaloid complex extend approximately 15–20 mm in all directions, it is possible to demonstrate fMRI response dissociations within the amygdala in each direction: dorsal versus ventral amygdala (Kim et al., 2003, 2004; Morris, Buchel, & Dolan, 2001; Whalen, 1998; Whalen et al., 2001), medial versus lateral amygdala (Kim et al., 2003; Zald & Pardo, 2002), or anterior versus posterior amygdala (Gottfried, O'Doherty, & Dolan, 2002; Morris, deBonis, & Dolan, 2002; Wang et al., 2008). The hypotheses driving the prediction of such effects can be based on the knowledge of which subnuclei reside within these regions, as long as it is remembered that the resulting data cannot provide incontrovertible evidence of the involvement of these subnuclei, especially within the dorsal amygdala/SI region. Such claims must await higher-resolution scanning tools and techniques.

A final caveat, as far as amygdala anatomy relates to fMRI, is that signal quality across the amygdaloid complex is not uniform. The ventral amygdala (particularly the medial portion, where the basal nuclei are located) generally yields lower signal-to-noise ratios (i.e., is more difficult to image). This will be particularly important to consider when evaluating null effects reported within the amygdala. One strategy would be to have another experimental condition demonstrating activation within the ventral amygdala; this would then allow for the interpretation of a null effect observed within a separate condition (see the discussion of Plate 12.2, below, for such a condition).

USING FACIAL EXPRESSIONS
TO STUDY THE HUMAN AMYGDALA

Facial expressions mediate a critical portion of our human nonverbal communication. From the expressions of others, we can glean information about their internal emotional state, their intentions, and/or their reaction to contextual events in our immediate environment. Facial expressions of emotion have predicted important events for us in the past, and we can use these previous experiences to respond appropriately to expressions as we perceive them. In this way, facial expressions can be considered CSs. Because these CSs do not necessarily evoke strong emotional states when presented in an experimental context, they are well suited for addressing the dissociation between associative orienting and the fear state itself.

Human Amygdala Responses
to Fearful Facial Expressions

Based on animal research showing the importance of the amygdala in fear conditioning (Davis, 1992; Kapp et al., 1992; LeDoux, 2000), and studies of patients with bilateral amygdala lesions showing deficits in processing the facial expression of fear (Adolphs, Tranel, Damasio, & Damasio, 1994; Broks et al., 1998), early human neuroimaging investigations of amygdala responses to facial expressions focused on fearful expressions (Breiter et al., 1996; Morris et al., 1996; Phillips et al., 1997; Whalen et al., 1998). Subsequent studies have replicated robust amygdala activations to fearful faces (Pessoa & Ungerleider, 2004; Whalen et al., 1998, 2001). These findings have been presented as consistent with the traditional view of the amygdala—that it is dedicated to processing negative emotion or threat-related information exclusively.

However, further research has shown that the human amygdala is also responsive to other types of facial expressions, including positive expressions of emotion (Somerville, Kim, Johnstone, Alexander, & Whalen, 2004; Yang et al., 2002). These findings suggest that the amygdala may not be exclusively responsive to negative emotion or threat-related information. Indeed, studies compared to low-level fixation baselines or non-face-related control conditions, have shown that the human amygdala was responsive to happy, sad, surprised, disgusted, and even neutral faces, which have been traditionally viewed as devoid of a specific emotional state (Fitzgerald, Angstadt,

Jelsone, Nathan, & Phan, 2006; Kim et al., 2003; Somerville et al., 2004; Yang et al., 2002). Altogether, we can conclude from these studies that the human amygdala is responsive to faces in general, supporting the view that the amygdala may be involved in processing emotionally and socially salient stimuli rather than being restricted to threat-related information. One caveat when considering such data is whether amygdala activations in response to a particular expression are in any way causal to a behavioral outcome. That is, patients with bilateral lesions of the amygdala are not impaired in their processing of many of these expressions, though subjects without brain damage show amygdala activation in response to such expressions. Thus the amygdala could monitor the presence of some expressions in the environment without directly influencing behavioral responses to these expressions. Alternatively, it is possible that we simply have not yet figured out the behaviors that should be measured to document such a causal link.

Many studies assessing human amygdala responses to all expressions continue to provide evidence that the amygdala is most sensitive to fearful faces. For example, a study showing that amygdala responses to fearful, angry, disgusted, sad, neutral, and happy faces were not statistically significantly different also showed that the degree of activation and the spatial extent tended to be greatest for fearful faces (Fitzgerald et al., 2006). In addition, studies directly pitting fearful faces against other primary expressions have shown significantly greater amygdala activity to fearful faces than to angry (Whalen et al., 2001), happy (Morris et al., 1996), disgusted (Phillips et al., 1997), and surprised (Kim et al., 2003) faces. Indeed, we now discuss studies directly comparing fear with other expressions as a useful way to isolate the meaning of amygdala responses to fearful expressions, and more generally the fundamental role of the human amygdala in processing predictive stimuli of biological relevance.

USING FACIAL EXPRESSIONS TO ASSESS REGIONAL fMRI RESPONSE DIFFERENCES ACROSS THE HUMAN AMYGDALOID COMPLEX

We have noted above that it should be possible to demonstrate coarse spatial dissociations across the amygdaloid complex with fMRI. The BLA can process sensory input on the basis of learned valence representations (e.g., "That stimulus predicted a negative outcome"). Additional data show that the CeA, on the other hand, is the substrate of associative orienting responses that facilitate learning. Recall that these responses are often observed to stimuli that have uncertain predictive value (e.g., "there are at least two possible outcomes predicted by that stimulus, and I'm not sure which one applies here"). Critically, recall that in the human brain, the BLA is located within the ventral amygdala, while the CeA, NBM, BNST, and SLEA are located within the dorsal amygdala/SI region.

The Facial Expressions of Fear and Anger

Since angry and fearful faces both signal the presence of threat, activity within the BLA should increase in response to this negative predictive value (i.e., in the ventral amygdala, fear = anger). But because fearful faces signal an unknown source of the threat relative to anger, dorsal amygdala/SI output systems that can change the level of cortical processing (i.e., increase vigilance) should be more active (i.e., in the dorsal amygdala/SI, fear > anger). Figure 12.2. summarizes our predictions of how these expressions would be handled by the amygdaloid complex.

Plate 12.2 (in color insert) presents fMRI data showing that when fearful faces (i.e., uncertain negativity) were directly contrasted with angry faces (i.e., certain negativity), significant signal increases were observed only in the dorsal amygdala/SI region (Whalen et al., 2001). The lack of signal increases in the ventral amygdala was not related to signal quality issues, as we observed ventral amygdala activation to both fearful versus neutral and angry versus neutral faces in these same subjects. These data are consistent with the notion that the detection of negativity will most readily produce changes in ventral amygdala fMRI signal, whereas dorsal amygdala/SI signal changes can be

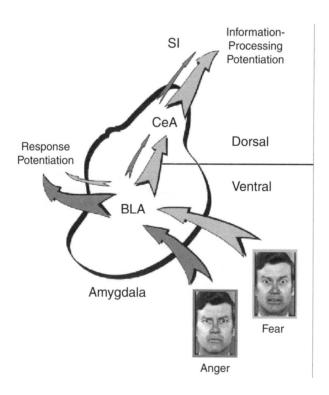

FIGURE 12.2. A proposed model of amygdala response to fearful and angry facial expressions.

related to the predictive uncertainty of the same stimulus. If signal changes within the dorsal amygdala/SI region were truly related to the ambiguity of the event that elicited the fearful expression, then a compelling demonstration would involve showing a similar signal increase in the dorsal amygdala to a facial expression that has a similar ambiguity of source, but is not necessarily negatively valenced.

The Facial Expression of Surprise

Surprised expressions provide an important comparison for fear. Though neither expression (fear nor surprise) indicates the exact nature of its eliciting event, fearful expressions do provide additional information concerning predicted negative valence. Surprise, on the other hand, can be interpreted either positively or negatively (Tomkins & McCarter, 1964). For example, a surprised expression might be observed in response to an oncoming car (negative) or an unexpected birthday party (positive). Thus surprised facial expressions can be used to reveal important individual differences in both (1) the propensity to subjectively ascribe positive or negative valence to an ambivalent stimulus and (2) the relationship between these subjective ratings and fMRI signal changes in the amygdala. We (Kim et al., 2003) predicted that when subjects were viewing surprised facial expressions, responses within the ventral amygdala should be consistent with the ascribed valence of the faces, but that activity in the dorsal amygdala/SI should increase across all subjects, regardless of positive versus negative valence interpretations. Plate 12.3A (in color insert) shows that a lateral ventral region of the amygdala tracked individual differences in valence interpretations of surprised faces. Subjects who interpreted the surprised faces negatively showed signal increases that correlated with the intensity of these ratings. Plate 12.3B shows that despite these differences of opinion related to the valence of the faces, all subjects showed a main effect for surprise manifested as strong signal increases across other regions of the amygdala, strongest within the dorsal amygdala/SI region. These data are consistent with the fact that different portions of the amygdala can work on different parts of the problem—predictive aspects of an expression that appear clear to the viewer ("That face looks negative to me"), and, simultaneously, other aspects that remain unclear ("I wonder what that person is reacting to").

That some individuals would show such a positivity bias associated with lower amygdala activity might seem a bit surprising for a brain region that functions to monitor the environment for potential threat. One might have thought that the ventral amygdala would have responded to the potential negativity of the surprised faces similarly in all subjects. Individual differences of this type suggested to us that another region of the brain might be exerting a regulatory influence over the amygdala. Based on the anatomical connections of the ventral amygdala (discussed above), we focused our search on the medial prefrontal cortex (mPFC). Accordingly, we observed two regions of the mPFC that were correlated with subjects' valence interpretations of surprised faces. Like the amygdala, a dorsal region of the mPFC (specifically, the rostral anterior cingulate cortex [ACC]; see Kim et al., 2003) displayed a positive relationship with negative valence ratings (i.e., higher activity with more negative ratings). A ventral region of the mPFC (ventral ACC; see Kim et al., 2003) showed an opposite relationship with valence ratings of surprised faces to that shown by the amygdala and dorsal mPFC (i.e., higher activity with more positive ratings). Plate 12.4A (in color insert) presents a three-dimensional representation of these regions, where activity in the ventral mPFC is inversely related to activity in the amygdala and dorsal mPFC. Plate 12.4B presents a bar graph focusing on the inverse relationship between the ventral mPFC and the amygdala, showing that subjects who interpreted these faces negatively showed high amygdala responses and low ventral mPFC responses, while the subjects who interpreted them positively showed high ventral mPFC responses and low amygdala responses. Note that this inversely correlated ventral mPFC–amygdala fMRI activity was observed during passive viewing. That is, activity measured while subjects viewed repeating surprised faces predicted the valence ratings they assigned to these faces after the scanning session. These data are consistent with the notion that these valence calculations were relatively automatic/implicit (Kim et al., 2003).

One interpretation of these data is that in response to surprised expressions, a regulatory override message from the ventral region of the mPFC is required to interpret these faces as positively valenced. Inherent in this assertion is the presumption that the amygdala has an initial default negative interpretation of surprised faces in all subjects, after which some subjects are able to regulate and respond more positively. Such a hypothesis is consistent with data showing that the amygdala is especially sensitive to eye widening (Morris et al., 2002; Whalen et al., 2004), a particularly salient feature of surprised faces.

Linking Prefrontal–Amygdala Response to Surprised Faces with the Extinction Literature

Following fear conditioning, if the tone CS is repeatedly presented in the absence of the US (i.e., now tone = no shock), the conditioned response will diminish over time—a phenomenon known as extinction. At this point, the CS is inherently ambiguous, having predicted both shock and the absence of shock in the past (see Bouton, 1994).

Of relevance to the present discussion, neurons within the ventral mPFC of the rat show robust firing to extinguished tones, but only in animals that remember the new meaning of the tone (i.e., the tone now predicts the absence of shock) (Milad & Quirk, 2002). In other words, the animals that show greater ventral mPFC activity in response to the extinguished tone do not show concomitant fear responses (i.e., freezing), suggesting they have learned that the tone is safe. If one simply assumes that not being shocked is a positive thing, then the neural circuitry supporting successful extinction training sounds much like the circuit we see in response to surprised faces (Oler,

Quirk, & Whalen, in press). That is, greater ventral mPFC activity in response to surprised faces predicts that the subjects will interpret those faces more positively. Thus, whether rats are listening to tone CSs or humans are viewing face CSs, greater ventral mPFC activity predicts that the subjects will recall the more positive hypothesis concerning the CS. Consistent with this line of reasoning, studies examining extinction training in human subjects document involvement of a similar ventral mPFC region (Phelps, Delgado, Nearing, & LeDoux, 2004). Pragmatically, these data suggest that future studies could use surprised faces as presented stimuli to engage a circuitry thought to be critical for regulating fear responses to past predictive stimuli. Failure of such regulation is thought to be at the heart of the anxiety disorders (e.g., Shin et al., 2005; Whalen et al., 2008), as well as of the negativity bias that accompanies major depression (e.g., Alloy & Abramson, 1979; Bouhuys, Geerts, & Gordijn, 1999; Fales et al., 2008; Johnstone, van Reekum, Urry, Kalin, & Davidson, 2007; Ramel et al., 2007).

Likening fearful faces to consistently reinforced CSs (those that consistently predict a negative event) and surprised facial expressions to inconsistently reinforced CSs (those that sometimes predict positive and sometimes predict negative events) allows for several interesting predictions. One prediction follows from the partial reinforcement extinction effect—that is, the fact that inconsistently reinforced events take longer to extinguish than consistently reinforced ones do (Gibbs, Latham, & Gormezano, 1978; Rescorla, 1999; Sheffield, 1949; Weinstock, 1954). If we view facial expressions as CSs, then we would predict that amygdala activity should extinguish at a faster rate in response to consistently reinforced stimuli (fearful faces) than to inconsistently reinforced stimuli (surprised faces). With these predictions in mind, we reanalyzed data from a previously published paper that presented subjects with both fearful and surprised expressions (Kim et al., 2003). Plate 12.5 (in color insert) presents these data, showing that initially robust amygdala responses to fearful faces decrease in magnitude with repeated (unreinforced) presentations. In contrast, amygdala responsivity to surprised faces is moderate in magnitude (compared to amygdala response to fearful faces), but is uniquely sustained over repeated presentations (Kim & Whalen, 2008). These data support the assertions that (1) facial expressions are usefully thought of as CSs, because of their past reinforcement history; and (2) nonreinforced presentations of these expressions in a controlled laboratory environment are tantamount to extinction trials.

MORE THAN MEETS THE FACE: OTHER THINGS WE CAN LEARN FROM FACIAL EXPRESSIONS

Some lessons we have learned from studying facial expressions offer us new ways to think about some very old psychological questions. Here we consider but a few.

Valence and Arousal

An increasing trend in human neuroimaging research involves attempting to characterize amygdala responses based on the dimensions of valence and arousal. A recent meta-analysis (Costafreda, Brammer, David, & Fu, 2008) found that although human amygdala activity is best evoked by negative emotional stimuli such as facial expressions of fear and disgust, amygdala activity is also strongly evoked by highly arousing positive emotions such as humor (as opposed to happiness, which is less likely to be associated with amygdala activity). The authors interpret these data as suggesting that emotional arousal may drive amygdala activity more than valence. We suggest that one need not choose which is the more important dimension to the amygdala. Ample data show that both valence and arousal are critical determinants of amygdala activity (e.g., Kapp et al., 1992; LeDoux, 1996). Indeed, panels A and B of Plate 12.3 (in color insert) show a within-group fMRI spatial distinction across the amygdala: One region is tracking valence, while another region tracks arousal (in this example, uncertainty of eliciting source). However, though it is often useful to employ spatial distinctions within the amygdala to characterize the role of the amygdaloid complex in processing valence and arousal, it is also worthwhile to appreciate their overlapping nature.

We re-present here the data of Bradley, Cuthbert, and Lang (1996), because we think they are particularly instructive in terms of considering the difficulty one will have disentangling valence effects from arousal effects. Figure 12.3 presents eyeblink startle magnitudes in response to negative, neutral,

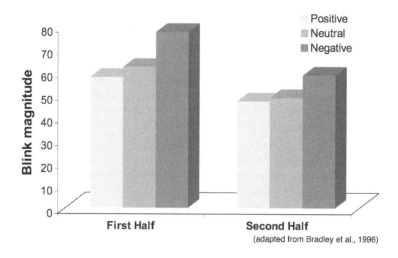

(adapted from Bradley et al., 1996)

FIGURE 12.3. A re-presentation of startle eyeblink data from Bradley et al. (1996), showing decreasing arousal responses but sustained valence effects over time. From Bradley, Cuthbert, and Lang (1996). Copyright 1996 by the Society for Psychophysiological Research. Adapted by permission.

and positive picture stimuli. Note that the data are divided by early versus late stimulus presentation trials (a very instructive strategy for examining habituation of amygdala responses, and one that has been adopted in a number of fMRI studies). The most obvious and overshadowing effect is the large decrement in response magnitude observed for all three valence conditions over time (i.e., between early and late trials). But it is critical to note that a response distinction between valence conditions is observed early and maintained late, despite the large decrease in overall response magnitude. We take these data to suggest that although the overwhelming effects of arousal may sometimes overshadow subtle valence effects, it is clear that both valence and arousal can be represented simultaneously. Indeed, psychophysiological measures of emotional responses can differentiate between responses to valence (facial electromyography—Cacioppo, Petty, Losch, & Kim, 1986; Lang, Greenwald, Bradley, & Hamm, 1993; Tassinary, Cacioppo, & Vanman, 2007) and responses to arousal (electrodermal activity—Lang et al., 1993; Lang, Bradley, & Cuthbert, 1998). Future studies will find it useful to attempt to correlate these measures with amygdala activity. Data presented in this chapter suggest that such studies are likely to find that the amygdala is influenced by *both* valence and arousal. Furthermore, depending on the experimental design in question, the amygdala may choose one over the other, and this choice may differ from study to study (see "Conclusions").

Of Dimensions and Categories

We have approached our studies of fearful facial expressions by directly comparing and contrasting them with other categorical facial expressions. Although many would conduct similar studies in the hopes of delineating a neural circuit that is unique to each expression, we have described in this chapter numerous fMRI studies comparing two categorical facial expressions, where the specific contrasts were chosen to elucidate the neural substrates of dimensional constructs that cross the categorical boundary. For example, by pitting fearful against angry expressions, we held the dimensions of arousal and valence constant (as they cross this categorical boundary) and were able to more cleanly assess the differing information value that these expressions communicate to the viewer. Thus we have utilized this dimensional approach to better understand the categories of emotion (at least as much as these relate to the processing these facial expressions).

These arguments are not specific to the amygdala. If the amygdala has shown an affinity for the facial expression of fear, then the analogous brain region for disgusted expressions would be the insular cortex. Neuroimaging as well as depth electrode recording studies show that the human insular cortex responds to disgusted faces (Krolak-Salmon et al., 2003; Phillips et al., 1997; Sambataro et al., 2006; Stark et al., 2007; Wicker et al., 2003), and that damage to the insula produces deficits in the recognition of disgust faces (Adolphs, Tranel, & Damasio, 2003; Calder, Keane, Manes, Antoun, & Young,

2000). Furthermore, insular pathology in Huntington's disorder is associated with a decreased disgust response and a similar recognition deficit of disgust (Gray, Young, Barker, Curtis, & Gibson, 1997; Sprengelmeyer et al., 1996). Although it is tempting to divide duties for the amygdala and insular cortex between fear and disgust, and to suggest that they represent unique neural substrates for their processing, other work suggests that these reciprocally connected regions will interact along dimensions such as arousal, valence, and/or attention—dimensions that cross expression categories (Anderson, Christoff, Panitz, De Rosa, & Gabrieli, 2003; Gorno-Tempini et al., 2001; Krolak-Salmon et al., 2003; Phan, Wager, Taylor, & Liberzon, 2002; Schienle et al., 2002). For example, Anderson, Christoff, Panitz, and colleagues (2003) have shown that the amygdala will track the presence of disgusted faces, but only implicitly—that is, when subjects' attention is directed away from presented faces. They suggest that the amygdala widens its focus from fear-specific to more generalized threat-specific as attention to faces moves from explicit to implicit. These data provide a nice example that these neural circuits can track a functional dimension (such as attention) across categories of emotional expressions. But in this way, they help us to understand better what the categories themselves actually represent (i.e., a collection of overlapping and nonoverlapping dimensions).

Automaticity

Numerous studies using techniques that mitigate subjective awareness (e.g., backward masking, binocular suppression) have shown robust amygdala responses to fearful facial expressions (Armony, Corbo, Clement, & Brunet, 2005; Etkin et al., 2004; Morris, Öhman, & Dolan, 1998, 1999; Rauch et al., 2000; Sheline et al., 2001; Whalen et al., 1998; Williams, Morris, McGlone, Abbott, & Mattingly, 2004). A fearful face contains an immense amount of information, though much of it is subtle (e.g., raised brows, wide eyes, slightly open mouth, etc.). It is likely that the amygdala does not compute all this information in such a short time frame. Taking a lead from the work of Joseph LeDoux suggesting that the amygdala's initial reactions are based on crude representations of CSs, we showed that presentation of fearful eye whites using backward masking is sufficient to produce amygdala reactivity (see Plate 12.6 in color insert; Whalen et al., 2004). A control condition (inverse fearful and happy "eye blacks") supported the specificity of this response for the more ecologically valid eye whites. These data suggest that the amygdala may use widened eyes as a crude proxy for the presence of fearful faces.

Plate 12.6 shows that the amygdala response to 17-msec masked presentations of fearful eye whites is convincingly localized to the ventral amygdala. Plate 12.7 (in color insert) re-presents this activation, breaking down our subjects' responses during passive viewing on the basis of their performance in the subsequent forced-choice objective detection task. First, consistent with other reports (Pessoa, Japee, Sturman, & Ungerleider, 2006; Pessoa, Japee, &

Ungerleider, 2005), roughly half of our subjects could detect fearful faces above chance levels, though subjectively they reported not seeing them (see Whalen et al., 2004, "Supplemental Materials"). The other half of our subjects could not detect fearful faces when actively searching for them, making it highly unlikely that they could have done so during the earlier passive viewing task, when they were naïve to the presence of the fearful faces. Critically, there was no difference in the magnitude of the response to masked fearful eye whites within the ventral amygdala for subjects who could detect these stimuli above chance (good detectors) versus those who could not (poor detectors) (Whalen et al., 2004, "Supplemental Materials"). Note that in the dorsal amygdala/SI region, we did see activation in good detectors that was not observed in poor detectors, consistent with other reports (Pessoa et al., 2006).

These data suggest that one portion of the amygdala may show more automated responses (i.e., the ventral amygdala), while another portion of the amygdala may be more sensitive to manipulations that affect attention or awareness (i.e., the dorsal amygdala/SI). Such an assertion could be consistent with the role of dorsal amygdala subnuclei in attentional responses (Gallagher & Holland, 1994; Kapp et al., 1992).

CONCLUSIONS

In this chapter, we have presented studies that seek to define some dimensional constructs (e.g., valence, arousal, information value, predictability) that might explain human amygdala responses to specific facial expressions of emotion (i.e., fearful, angry, and surprised). We have offered a very biased view that the amygdala will respond to these expressions on the basis of their predictive value as CSs. The fundamental role of the amygdala in modulating vigilance in the service of learning (see Whalen, 1998) means that it will track the best predictor of outcomes at any given moment. For example, it can track arousal in one instance (Anderson, Christoff, Stappen, et al., 2003; Canli, Zhao, Brewer, Gabrieli, & Cahill, 2000; Demos, Kelley, Ryan, Davis, & Whalen, in press; Garavan, Pendergrass, Ross, Stein, & Risinger, 2001; Kensinger & Schacter, 2006; Lewis, Critchley, Rothstein, & Dolan, 2007; Somerville, Wig, Whalen, & Kelley, 2006), but then valence in another (Anders, Lotze, Erb, Grodd, & Birbaumer, 2004; Kim et al., 2003, 2004; Pessoa, Padmala, & Morlan, 2005; Straube, Pohlack, Mentzel, & Miltner, 2008); as we have seen, it can also track them both simultaneously (Kim et al., 2003; Whalen et al., 1998, 2001; see also Britton et al., 2006; Williams et al., 2004; Winston, Gottfried, Kilner, & Dolan, 2005). It will track fearful faces one moment, then disgusted faces the next (Anderson, Christoff, Stappen, et al., 2003). It will track static displays of expressions in one study (Whalen et al., 2001), but ignore them in another experimental context that includes dynamic displays (LaBar, Crupain, Voyvodic, & McCarthy, 2003). Thus the amygdala will be a bit of a chameleon—eluding categorization based on responses along a single dimension, but rather tracking whatever stimulus dimension shows the most promise for learning.

Though we struggle with issues of spatial resolution in fMRI, all available data suggest that it will be necessary to effectively measure spatial differences across the human amygdaloid complex. Here we have offered initial data showing coarse spatial dissociations across the amygdala, as we await future scanning protocols that will allow for higher spatial resolutions. To date, we have offered data suggesting that more automatic amygdala responses (i.e., more immune to attentional effects) should be observed within the ventral amygdala (see Plate 12.7 in color insert; see also Whalen et al., 2004, "Supplemental Materials"). These data fit well with our studies of surprised faces showing that ventral regions of the amygdala can work on issues of valence, while other regions of the amygdala (most notably the dorsal amygdala/SI region) work on the arousal value of these faces, regardless of valence (see Plate 12.3 in color insert; see also Kim et al., 2003). The finding that the inversely correlated ventral mPFC–amygdala activity that predicted valence interpretations of surprised faces was specific to the *ventral* amygdala is consistent with the location of known prefrontal–amygdala connections in non-human primates (Ghashghaei, Hilgetag, & Barbas, 2006).

One aim of this chapter has been to show the fruitfulness of using facial expressions as experimental stimuli to study how and what the human amygdala learns. Though use of these stimuli will mean that we lack the ability to control for individual differences in reinforcement history, these differences constitute a worthy subject of study in their own right. In this way, facial expressions offer a relatively innocuous strategy with which to investigate normal variations in affective processing, as well as the promise of elucidating what role the aberrance of such processing may play in emotional disorders (Armony et al., 2005; Bouhuys et al., 1999; Fales et al., 2008; Rauch et al., 2000; Sheline et al., 2001; Shin et al., 2005; Whalen et al., 1998).

WHAT WE THINK

We have opened this chapter by pointing out the role of the amygdala in learning situations that are more emotionally subtle than fear conditioning (e.g., attention, orienting, etc.). This is because most of our lives are not spent at the extreme ends of the emotional continuum, but rather play out within the subtler, central region of this continuum. The fundamental role of the amygdala is to *facilitate* biologically relevant learning, be it subtle or extreme, on a moment-by-moment basis.

The Amygdala Is Unpredictable

The amygdala takes note of the order of events solely to determine their predictive value. This suggests that an amygdala response to a US is also about determining whether any other contingent events occurred. With this calculation, the organism will be in a better position to predict this US on the *next* trial.

During the initial acquisition of experiences suggesting contingency between two events, neuronal activation will be observed across the entire amygdaloid complex. When this contingency becomes clear, much of the activity across the amygdala will wane, as will amygdala-mediated peripheral responses (see Kapp et al., 1992; Weisz et al., 1992; Whalen, 1998). However, some regions of the amygdala will continue to represent the associative nature of these two events (Maren, 2000; Repa et al., 2001; Wilensky, Schafe, Kristensen, & LeDoux, 2006; Zimmerman, Rabinak, McLachlan, & Maren, 2007), in case this learned contingency should change. In this way, unpredictability will rule the amygdala's day (see Whalen, 1998). The recent demonstration in both mouse and human subjects that the amygdala was sensitive to unpredictability per se (i.e., inconsistently presented tones), even for these seemingly biologically irrelevant stimuli, is consistent with this assertion (Herry et al., 2007).

The Amygdala Is Subtle

The amygdala *optimizes* biologically relevant learning; it will not always determine whether learning will or will not occur. For example, rats with amygdala lesions show impaired conditioning to a 65-dB tone, but have no problem learning about the predictive value of an 85-dB tone (Weisz et al., 1992). Human patients with bilateral lesions who cannot extract predictive information from fearful faces can suddenly do so if instructed to focus on the eye region of the face (Adolphs et al., 2005). These data are highly consistent with the discussion of associative orienting presented at the beginning of this chapter. The amygdala mediates attentional orienting responses that make us better consumers of predictive information.

Consider the fact that electrical stimulation of the amygdala in patients with epilepsy causes increased scanning of the environment (Bancaud, Talairach, Morel, & Bresson, 1966). To elaborate, in reaction to electrical stimulation of the amygdala, one subject engaged in what could be termed "vacuous orienting": He oriented to a specific point in the periphery, though he knew nothing was there. Such an effect is consistent with the amygdala's known efferent connectivity with regions that can initiate spatial orienting (see Jolkkonen et al., 2002). Therefore, one way the amygdala facilitates biologically relevant learning is to orient us to look for predictive cues in the location that taught us best last—be it the corner of a cage from which a potentially predictive tone was emitted, or the upper half of a face where the eyes are located. And, apparently, the amygdala will be most useful when these predictive cues are particularly subtle. For, as far as facial features are concerned, the amygdala has been shown to be sensitive to signals in others as subtle as eye widening (Morris et al., 2002; Whalen et al., 2004) and pupil dilation (Demos et al., in press; Harrison, Singer, Rotshtein, Dolan, & Critchley, 2006). Moreover, electrical stimulation of the amygdala also produces eye widening and pupil dilation (Gloor, 1997; Kapp et al., 1992). Taken together, these data suggest that the amygdala is sensitive to the facial reactions in others that it controls in us—reactions indicating that "someone else is learning right now, and perhaps I would do well to do the same."

REFERENCES

Adolphs, R., Gosselin, F., Buchanan, T. W., Tranel, D., Schyns, P., & Damasio, A. R. (2005). A mechanism for impaired fear recognition after amygdala damage. *Nature, 433,* 68–72.

Adolphs, R., Tranel, D., & Damasio, A. R. (2003). Dissociable neural systems for recognizing emotions. *Brain and Cognition, 52*(1), 61–69.

Adolphs, R., Tranel, D., Damasio, A. R., & Damasio, H. (1994). Impaired recognition of emotion in facial expressions following bilateral damage to the human amygdala. *Nature, 372,* 669–672.

Alheid, G. F. (2003). Extended amygdala and basal forebrain. *Annals of the New York Academy of Sciences, 985*(1), 185–205.

Alloy, L. B., & Abramson, L. Y. (1979). Judgment of contingency in depressed and nondepressed students: Sadder but wiser? *Journal of Experimental Psychology: General, 108, 441–485.*

Anders, S., Lotze, M., Erb, M., Grodd, W., & Birbaumer, N. (2004). Brain activity underlying emotional valence and arousal: A response-related fMRI study. *Human Brain Mapping, 23,* 200–209.

Anderson, A. K., Christoff, K., Panitz, D., De Rosa, E., & Gabrieli, J. D. (2003). Neural correlates of the automatic processing of threat facial signals. *Journal of Neuroscience, 23*(13), 5627–5633.

Anderson, A. K., Christoff, K., Stappen, I., Panitz, D., Ghahremani, D. G., Glover, G., et al. (2003). Dissociated neural representations of intensity and valence in human olfaction. *Nature Neuroscience, 6,* 196–202.

Armony, J. L., Corbo, V., Clement, M. H., & Brunet, A. (2005). Amygdala response in patients with acute PTSD to masked and unmasked emotional facial expressions. *American Journal of Psychiatry, 162*(10), 1961–1963.

Bancaud, J., Talairach, J., Morel, P., & Bresson, M. (1966). La corne d'Ammon et le noyau amygdalien: Effets cliniques et electriques de leur stimulation chez l'homme. *Revue Neurologique (Paris), 115*(3), 329–352.

Bouhuys, A. L., Geerts, E., & Gordijn, M. C. M. (1999). Depressed patients' perceptions of facial emotions in depressed and remitted states are associated with relapse. *Journal of Nervous and Mental Disease, 187,* 595–602.

Bouton, M. E. (1994). Context, ambiguity, and classical conditioning. *Current Directions in Psychological Science, 3*(2), 49–53.

Bradley, M. M., Cuthbert, B. N., & Lang, P. J. (1996). Lateralized startle probes in the study of emotion. *Psychophysiology, 33*(2), 156–161.

Breiter, H. C., Etcoff, N. L., Whalen, P. J., Kennedy, W. A., Rauch, S. L., Buckner, R. L., et al. (1996). Response and habituation of the human amygdala during visual processing of facial expression. *Neuron, 17*(5), 875–887.

Britton, J. C., Phan, K. L., Taylor, S. F., Welsh, R. C., Berridge, K. C., & Liberzon, I. (2006). Neural correlates of social and nonsocial emotions: An fMRI study. *NeuroImage, 31,* 397–409.

Broks, P., Young, A. W., Maratos, E. J., Coffey, P. J., Calder, A. J., Isaac, C. L., et al. (1998). Face processing impairments after encephalitis: Amygdala damage and recognition of fear. *Neuropsychologia, 36*(1), 59–70.

Cacioppo, J. T., Petty, R. E., Losch, M. E., & Kim, H. S. (1986). Electromyographic activity over facial muscle regions can differentiate the valence and intensity of affective reactions. *Journal of Personality and Social Psychology, 50,* 260–268.

Calder, A. J., Keane, J., Manes, F., Antoun, N., & Young, A. W. (2000). Impaired recognition and experience of disgust following brain injury. *Nature Neuroscience, 3*(11), 1077–1078.

Canli, T., Zhao, Z., Brewer, J., Gabrieli, J. D., & Cahill, D. (2000). Event-related activation in the human amygdala associates with later memory for individual emotional experience. *Journal of Neuroscience, 20*(19), RC99.

Costafreda, S. G., Brammer, M. J., David, A. S., & Fu, C. H. (2008). Predictors of amygdala activation during the processing of emotional stimuli: A meta-analysis of 385 PET and fMRI studies. *Brain Research Reviews, 58*(1), 57–70.

Davis, M. (1992). The role of the amygdala in fear and anxiety. *Annual Review of Neuroscience, 15*, 353–375.

Davis, M., & Whalen, P. J. (2001). The amygdala: Vigilance and emotion. *Molecular Psychiatry, 6*(1), 13–34.

Demos, K. E., Kelley, W. M., Ryan, S. L., Davis, F. C., & Whalen, P. J. (in press). Human amygdala sensitivity to the pupil size of others. *Cerebral Cortex*.

de Olmos, J. S., & Heimer, L. (1999). The concepts of the ventral striatopallidal system and extended amygdala. *Annals of the New York Academy of Sciences, 877*, 1–32.

Etkin, A., Klemenhagen, K. C., Dudman, J. T., Rogan, M. T., Hen, R., Kandel, E. R., et al. (2004). Individual differences in trait anxiety predict the response of the basolateral amygdala to unconsciously processed fearful faces. *Neuron, 44*(6), 1043–1055.

Fales, C. L., Barch, D. M., Rundle, M. M., Mintun, M. A., Snyder, A. Z., Cohen, J. D., et al. (2008). Altered emotional processing in affective and cognitive-control brain circuitry in major depression. *Biological Psychiatry, 63*, 377–384.

Fitzgerald, D. A., Angstadt, M., Jelsone, L. M., Nathan, P. J., & Phan, K. L. (2006). Beyond threat: Amygdala reactivity across multiple expressions of facial affect. *NeuroImage, 30*(4), 1441–1448.

Gallagher, M., & Holland, P. C. (1994). The amygdala complex: Multiple roles in associative learning and attention. *Proceedings of the National Academy of Sciences USA, 91*, 11771–11776.

Garavan, H., Pendergrass, J. C., Ross, T. J., Stein, E. A., & Risinger, R. C. (2001). Amygdala response to both positively and negatively valenced stimuli. *NeuroReport, 12*, 2779–2783.

Ghashghaei, H. T., Hilgetag, C. C., & Barbas, H. (2006). Sequence of information processing for emotions based on the anatomic dialogue between prefrontal cortex and amygdala. *NeuroImage, 34*, 905–923.

Gibbs, C. M., Latham, S. B., & Gormezano, I. (1978). Classical conditioning of the rabbit nictitating membrane response: Effects of reinforcement schedule on response maintenance and resistance to extinction. *Animal Learning and Behavior, 6*(2), 209–215.

Gloor, P. (1997). *The temporal lobe and limbic system*. New York: Oxford University Press.

Gorno-Tempini, M. L., Pradelli, S., Serafini, M., Pagnoni, G., Baraldi, P., Porro, C., et al. (2001). Explicit and incidental facial expression processing: An fMRI study. *NeuroImage, 14*(2), 465–473.

Gottfried, J. A., O'Doherty, J., & Dolan, R. J. (2002). Appetitive and aversive olfactory learning in humans studied using event-related functional magnetic resonance imaging. *Journal of Neuroscience, 22*, 10829–10837.

Gray, J. M., Young, A. W., Barker, W. A., Curtis, A., & Gibson, D. (1997). Impaired recognition of disgust in Huntington's disease gene carriers. *Brain, 120*(11), 2029–2038.

Harrison, N. A., Singer, T., Rotshtein, P. Dolan, R. J., & Critchley, H. D. (2006). Pupillary contagion: Central mechanisms engaged in sadness processing. *Social Cognitive and Affective Neuroscience, 1,* 5–17.

Heimer, L., Harlan, R. E., Alheid, G. F., Garcia, M. M., & de Olmos, J. (1997). Substantia innominata: A notion which impedes clinical–anatomical correlations in neuropsychiatric disorders. *Neuroscience, 76*(4), 957–1006.

Heimer, L., & Van Hoesen, G. W. (2006). The limbic lobe and its output channels: Implications for emotional functions and adaptive behavior. *Neuroscience and Biobehavioral Reviews, 30*(2), 126–147.

Herry, C., Bach, D. R., Esposito, F., Di Salle, F., Perrig, W. J., Scheffler, K., et al. (2007). Processing of temporal unpredictability in human and animal amygdala. *Journal of Neuroscience, 27*(22), 5958–5966.

Johnstone, T., van Reekum, C. M., Urry, H. L., Kalin, N. H., & Davidson, R. J. (2007). Failure to regulate: Counterproductive recruitment of top-down prefrontal–subcortical circuitry in major depression. *Journal of Neuroscience, 27,* 8877–8884.

Jolkkonen, E., Miettinen, R., Pikkarainen, M., & Pitkänen, A. (2002). Projections from the amygdaloid complex to the magnocellular cholinergic basal forebrain in rat. *Neuroscience, 111*(1), 133–149.

Kapp, B. S., Supple, W. F. J., & Whalen, P. J. (1994). Effects of electrical stimulation of the amygdaloid central nucleus on neocortical arousal in the rabbit. *Behavioral Neuroscience, 108,* 81–93.

Kapp, B. S., Whalen, P. J., Supple, W. F., & Pascoe, J. P. (1992). Amygdaloid contributions to conditioned arousal and sensory information processing. In J. P. Aggleton (Ed.), *The amygdala: Neurobiological aspects of emotion, memory, and mental dysfunction* (pp. 229–254). New York: Wiley-Liss.

Kensinger, E. A., & Schacter, D. L. (2006). Processing emotional pictures and words: Effects of valence and arousal. *Cognitive, Affective, and Behavioral Neuroscience, 6,* 110–126.

Kim, H., Somerville, L. H., Johnstone, T., Alexander, A. L., & Whalen, P. J. (2003). Inverse amygdala and medial prefrontal cortex responses to surprised faces. *NeuroReport, 14*(18), 2317–2322.

Kim, H., Somerville, L. H., Johnstone, T., Polis, S., Alexander, A. L., Shin, L. M., et al. (2004). Contextual modulation of amygdala responsivity to surprised faces. *Journal of Cognitive Neuroscience, 16*(10), 1730–1745.

Kim, H., & Whalen, P. J. (2008). *A computational model of amygdala function in the detection and resolution of predictive uncertainty.* Manuscript submitted for publication.

Krolak-Salmon, P., Henaff, M. A., Isnard, J., Tallon-Baudry, C., Guenot, M., Vighetto, A., et al. (2003). An attention modulated response to disgust in human ventral anterior insula. *Annals of Neurology, 53*(4), 446–453.

LaBar, K. S., Crupain, M. J., Voyvodic, J. T., & McCarthy, G. (2003). Dynamic perception of facial affect and identity in the human brain. *Cerebral Cortex, 13*(10), 1023–1033.

LaBar, K. S., Gatenby, J. C., Gore, J. C., LeDoux, J. E., & Phelps, E. A. (1998).

Human amygdala activation during conditioned fear acquisition and extinction: A mixed-trial fMRI study. *Neuron, 20*(5), 937–945.

Lang, P. J., Bradley, M. M., & Cuthbert, B. N. (1998). Emotion, motivation, and anxiety: Brain mechanisms and psychophysiology. *Biological Psychiatry, 44*, 1248–1263.

Lang, P. J., Greenwald, M. K., Bradley, M. M., & Hamm, A. O. (1993). Looking at pictures: Affective, facial, visceral, and behavioral reactions. *Psychophysiology, 30*(3), 261–273.

LeDoux, J. E. (1996). *The emotional brain: The mysterious underpinnings of emotional life.* New York: Simon & Schuster.

LeDoux, J. E. (2000). The amygdala and emotion: A view through fear. In J. P. Aggleton (Ed.), *The amygdala: A functional analysis* (2nd ed., pp. 289–310). New York: Oxford University Press.

LeDoux, J. E., Cicchetti, P., Xagoraris, A., & Romanski, L. M. (1990). The lateral amygdaloid nucleus: Sensory interface of the amygdala in fear conditioning. *Journal of Neuroscience, 10*, 1062–1069.

Lewis, P. A., Critchley, H. D., Rotshtein, P., & Dolan, R. J. (2007). Neural correlates of processing valence and arousal in affective words. *Cerebral Cortex, 17*, 742–748.

Maren, S. (2000). Auditory fear conditioning increases CS-elicited spike firing in lateral amygdala neurons even after extensive overtraining. *European Journal of Neuroscience, 12*, 4047–4054.

Milad, M. R., & Quirk, G. J. (2002). Neurons in medial prefrontal cortex signal memory for fear extinction. *Nature, 420*, 70–74.

Morris, J. S., Buchel, C., & Dolan, R. J. (2001). Parallel neural responses in amygdala subregions and sensory cortex during implicit fear conditioning. *NeuroImage, 13*(6, Pt. 1), 1044–1052.

Morris, J. S., deBonis, M., & Dolan, R. J. (2002). Human amygdala responses to fearful eyes. *NeuroImage, 17*(1), 214–222.

Morris, J. S., Frith, C. D., Perrett, D. I., Rowland, D., Young, A. W., Calder, A. J., et al. (1996). A differential neural response in the human amygdala to fearful and happy facial expressions. *Nature, 383*, 812–814.

Morris, J. S., Öhman, A., & Dolan, R. J. (1998). Conscious and unconscious emotional learning in the human amygdala. *Nature, 393*, 467–470.

Morris, J. S., Öhman, A., & Dolan, R. J. (1999). A subcortical pathway to the right amygdala mediating "unseen" fear. *Proceedings of the National Academy of Sciences USA, 96*(4), 1680–1685.

Oler, J. A., Quirk, G. J., & Whalen, P. J. (in press). Cingulo-amygdala interactions in surprise and extinction: Interpreting associative ambiguity. In B. Vogt (Ed.), *Cingulate neurobiology and disease: Vol. 1. Infrastructure, diagnosis, and treatment.* New York: Oxford University Press.

Pessoa, L., Japee, S., Sturman, D., & Ungerleider, L. G. (2006). Target visibility and visual awareness modulate amygdala responses to fearful faces. *Cerebral Cortex, 16*(3), 366–375.

Pessoa, L., Japee, S., & Ungerleider, L. G. (2005). Visual awareness and the detection of fearful faces. *Emotion, 5*, 243–247.

Pessoa, L., McKenna, M., Gutierrez, E., & Ungerleider, L. G. (2002). Neural processing of emotional faces requires attention. *Proceedings of the National Academy of Sciences USA, 99*, 11458–11463.

Pessoa, L., Padmala, S., & Morlan, T. (2005). Fate of unattended fearful faces in the amygdala is determined by both attentional resources and cognitive modulation. *NeuroImage, 28,* 249–255.

Phan, K. L., Wager, T., Taylor, S. F., & Liberzon, I. (2002). Functional neuroanatomy of emotion: A meta-analysis of emotion activation studies in PET and fMRI. *NeuroImage, 16*(2), 331–348.

Phelps, E. A., Delgado, M. R., Nearing, K. I., & LeDoux, J. E. (2004). Extinction learning in humans: Role of the amygdala and vmPFC. *Neuron, 43*(6), 897–905.

Phillips, M. L., Young, A. W., Senior, C., Brammer, M., Andrew, C., Calder, A. J., et al. (1997). A specific neural substrate for perceiving facial expressions of disgust. *Nature, 389,* 495–498.

Pitkänen, A. (2000). Connectivity of the rat amygdaloid complex. In J. P. Aggleton (Ed.), *The amygdala: A functional analysis* (2nd ed., pp. 31–117). New York: Oxford University Press.

Quirk, G. J., Likhtik, E., Pelletier, J. G., & Paré, D. (2003). Stimulation of medial prefrontal cortex decreases the responsiveness of central amygdala output neurons. *Journal of Neuroscience, 23*(25), 8800–8807.

Ramel, W., Goldin, P. R., Eyler, L. T., Brown, G. G., Gotlib, I. H., & McQuaid, J. R. (2007). Amygdala reactivity and mood-congruent memory in individuals at risk for depressive relapse. *Biological Psychiatry, 61,* 231–239.

Rauch, S. L., Whalen, P. J., Shin, L. M., McInerney, S. C., Macklin, M. L., Lasko, N. B., et al. (2000). Exaggerated amygdala response to masked facial stimuli in posttraumatic stress disorder: A functional MRI study. *Biological Psychiatry, 47,* 769–776.

Repa, J. C., Muller, J., Apergis, J., Desrochers, T. M., Zhou, Y., & LeDoux, J. E. (2001). Two different lateral amygdala cell populations contribute to the initiation and storage of memory. *Nature Neuroscience, 4*(7), 724–731.

Rescorla, R. A. (1999). Partial reinforcement reduces the associative change produced by nonreinforcement. *Journal of Experimental Psychology: Animal Behavior Processes, 25,* 403–414.

Royer, S., Martina, M., & Paré, D. (1999). An inhibitory interface gates impulse traffic between the input and output stations of the amygdala. *Journal of Neuroscience, 19*(23), 10575–10583.

Sambataro, F., Dimalta, S., Di Giorgio, A., Taurisano, P., Blasi, G., Scarabino, T., et al. (2006). Preferential responses in amygdala and insula during presentation of facial contempt and disgust. *European Journal of Neuroscience, 24*(8), 2355–2362.

Schienle, A., Stark, R., Walter, B., Blecker, C., Ott, U., Kirsch, P., et al. (2002). The insula is not specifically involved in disgust processing: An fMRI study. *NeuroReport, 13*(16), 2023–2026.

Sheffield, V. F. (1949). Extinction as a function of partial reinforcement and distribution of practice. *Journal of Experimental Psychology, 39*(4), 511–526.

Sheline, Y. I., Barch, D. M., Donnelly, J. M., Ollinger, J. M., Snyder, A. Z., & Mintun, M. A. (2001). Increased amygdala response to masked emotional faces in depressed subjects resolves with antidepressant treatment: An fMRI study. *Biological Psychiatry, 50*(9), 651–658.

Shin, L. M., Wright, C. I., Cannistraro, P. A., Wedig, M. M., McMullin, K.,

Martis, B., et al. (2005). A functional magnetic resonance imaging study of amygdala and medial prefrontal cortex responses to overtly presented fearful faces in posttraumatic stress disorder. *Archives of General Psychiatry, 62*(3), 273–281.

Somerville, L. H., Kim, H., Johnstone, T., Alexander, A. L., & Whalen, P. J. (2004). Human amygdala responses during presentation of happy and neutral faces: Correlations with state anxiety. *Biological Psychiatry, 55*(9), 897–903.

Somerville, L. H., Wig, G. S., Whalen, P. J., & Kelley, W. M. (2006). Dissociable medial temporal lobe contributions to social memory. *Journal of Cognitive Neuroscience, 18*, 1253–1265.

Sprengelmeyer, R., Young, A. W., Calder, A. J., Karnat, A., Lange, H., Homberg, V., et al. (1996). Loss of disgust: Perception of faces and emotions in Huntington's disease. *Brain, 119*(5), 1647–1665.

Stark, R., Zimmermann, M., Kagerer, S., Schienle, A., Walter, B., Weygandt, M., et al. (2007). Hemodynamic brain correlates of disgust and fear ratings. *NeuroImage, 37*(2), 663–673.

Straube, T., Pohlack, S., Mentzel, H. J., & Miltner, W. H. (2008). Differential amygdala activation to negative and positive emotional pictures during an indirect task. *Behavioral Brain Research, 191*, 285–288.

Tassinary, L. G., Cacioppo, J. T., & Vanman, E. J. (2007). The skeletomotor system: Surface electromyography. In J. T. Cacioppo, L. G. Tassinary, & G. G. Berntson (Eds.), *Handbook of psychophysiology* (3rd ed., pp. 267–302). New York: Cambridge University Press.

Tomkins, S. S., & McCarter, R. (1964). What and where are the primary affects?: Some evidence for a theory. *Perceptual and Motor Skills, 18*, 119–158.

Wang, G. J., Tomasi, D., Backus, W., Wang, R., Telang, F., Geliebter, A., et al. (2008). Gastric distention activates satiety circuitry in the human brain. *NeuroImage, 39*, 1824–1831.

Weinstock, S. (1954). Resistance to extinction of a running response following partial reinforcement under widely spaced trials. *Journal of Comparative and Physiological Psychology, 47*(4), 318–322.

Weisz, D. J., Harden, D. G., & Xiang, Z. (1992). Effects of amygdala lesions on reflex facilitation and conditioned response acquisition during nictitating membrane response conditioning in rabbit. *Behavioral Neuroscience, 106*(2), 262–273.

Whalen, P. J. (1998). Fear, vigilance, and ambiguity: Initial neuroimaging studies of the human amygdala. *Current Directions in Psychological Science, 7*(6), 177–188.

Whalen, P. J., Johnstone, T., Somerville, L. H., Nitschke, J. B., Polis, S., Alexander, A. L., et al. (2008). A functional magnetic resonance imaging predictor of treatment response to venlafaxine in generalized anxiety disorder. *Biological Psychiatry, 63*(9), 858–863.

Whalen, P. J., Kagan, J., Cook, R. G., Davis, F. C., Kim, H., Polis, S., et al. (2004). Human amygdala responsivity to masked fearful eye whites. *Science, 306*, 2061.

Whalen, P. J., Kapp, B. S., & Pascoe, J. P. (1994). Neuronal activity within the nucleus basalis and conditioned neocortical electroencephalographic activation. *Journal of Neuroscience, 14*, 1623–1633.

Whalen, P. J., Rauch, S. L., Etcoff, N. L., McInerney, S. C., Lee, M. B., & Jenike,

M. A. (1998). Masked presentations of emotional facial expressions modulate amygdala activity without explicit knowledge. *Journal of Neuroscience, 18*(1), 411–418.

Whalen, P. J., Shin, L. M., McInerney, S. C., & Fischer, H. (2001). A functional MRI study of human amygdala responses to facial expressions of fear versus anger. *Emotion, 1*(1), 70–83.

Wicker, B., Keysers, C., Plailly, J., Royet, J.-P., Gallese, V., & Rizzolatti, G. (2003). Both of us disgusted in my insula: The common neural basis of seeing and feeling disgust. *Neuron, 40*(3), 655–664.

Wilensky, A. E., Schafe, G. E., Kristensen, M. P., & LeDoux, J. E. (2006). Rethinking the fear circuit: The central nucleus of the amygdala is required for the acquisition, consolidation, and expression of Pavlovian fear conditioning. *Journal of Neuroscience, 26*, 12387–12396.

Williams, M. A., Morris, A. P., McGlone, F., Abbott, D. F., & Mattingly, J. B. (2004). Amygdala responses to fearful and happy expressions under conditions of binocular suppression. *Journal of Neuroscience, 24*, 2898–2904.

Winston, J. S., Gottfried, J. A., Kilner, J. M., & Dolan, R. J. (2005). Integrated neural representations of odor intensity and affective valence in human amygdala. *Journal of Neuroscience, 25*, 8903–8907.

Yang, T. T., Menon, V., Eliez, S., Blasey, C., White, C. D., Reid, A. J., et al. (2002). Amygdalar activation associated with positive and negative facial expressions. *NeuroReport, 13*(14), 1737–1741.

Zald, D. H., & Pardo, J. V. (2002). The neural correlates of aversive stimulation. *NeuroImage, 16*, 746–753.

Zimmerman, J. M., Rabinak, C. A., McLachlan, I. G., & Maren, S. (2007). The central nucleus of the amygdala is essential for acquiring and expressing conditional fear after overtraining. *Learning and Memory, 14*, 634–644.

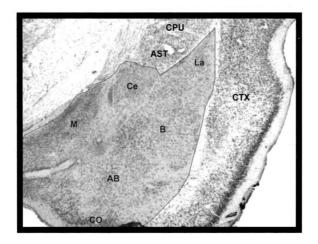

PLATE 2.1. The amygdala.

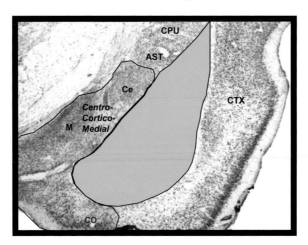

PLATE 2.2. The basolateral and centrocorticomedial divisions.

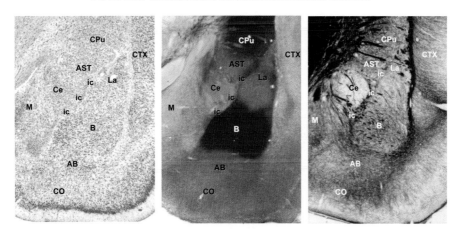

PLATE 2.3. Nuclei of the amygdala.

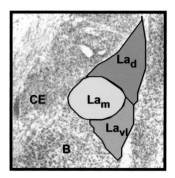

PLATE 2.4. Subareas of the lateral nucleus.

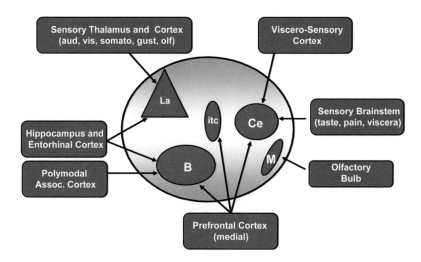

PLATE 2.5. Input connections.

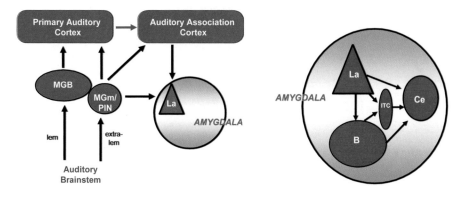

PLATE 2.6. Auditory inputs to the lateral amygdala.   **PLATE 2.7.** Intra-amygdala connections.

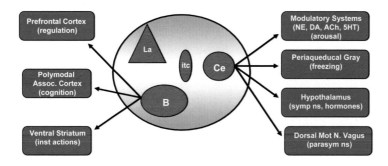

PLATE 2.8. Output connections.

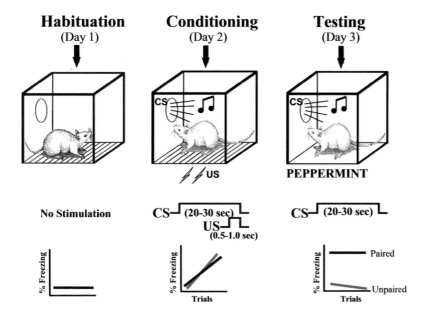

PLATE 2.9. Fear conditioning.

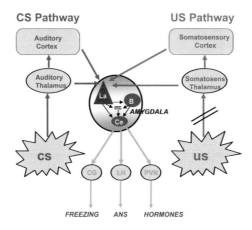

PLATE 2.10. Fear conditioning circuit.

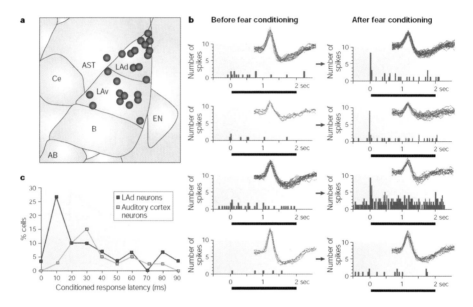

PLATE 2.11. Conditioned cellular responses.

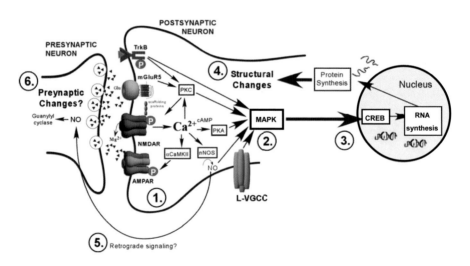

PLATE 2.12. Signal transduction pathways involved in fear conditioning in the lateral amygdala: Molecular mechanisms.

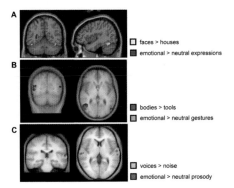

PLATE 10.1. Emotional enhancement of neural responses in fMRI. (A) Faces with a fearful relative to a neutral expression produce increased activation in fusiform cortex, overlapping with the fusiform area selectively activated by faces (FFA) as compared with houses. (B) Bodies with dynamic gestures expressing various emotions (fear, anger, happiness, or disgust) produce increased activation in lateral occipital area cortex, overlapping with the extrastriate area selectively activated by bodies (EBA) as compared with tools. (C) Voices with angry prosody produce increased activation in temporal cortex, overlapping with an area in superior temporal gyrus selectively activated by human voices (TVA) as compared with noises with similar acoustic energy.

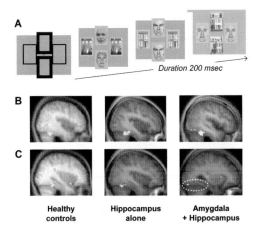

PLATE 10.2. Distant influences of the amygdala on visual cortex in humans. (A) Paradigm used to compare modulation of face processing by attention and by emotion. During fMRI, participants are instructed by visual cues to make same–different judgments for either vertical pairs (as illustrated here) or horizontal pairs of stimuli (two neutral or fearful faces, or two houses). (B) Activity in fusiform cortex is increased when faces are presented at the cued (attended) as compared to uncued (ignored) location; this attentional modulation is similar in healthy controls, patients with hippocampus sclerosis, and patients with hippocampus plus amygdala sclerosis ($n = 13$ in each group). (C) Activity in fusiform cortex is also increased when faces are fearful as compared to neutral (regardless of location), but this emotional modulation is not found in patients with amygdala sclerosis.

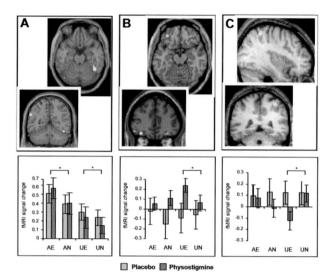

PLATE 10.3. Effect of cholinergic stimulation on emotion and attention. Two groups of participants performed the same attentional task as shown in Plate 10.2A, with neutral and fearful faces at task-relevant or task-irrelevant locations, after receiving either a procholinergic drug (physostigmine) or placebo. (A) Activity in right fusiform cortex showed additive modulation by emotion (*) and by attention, without any increase under physostigmine. (B) Physostigmine increased activity (*) in left orbito-frontal cortex when fearful faces appeared at task-irrelevant locations. (C) Physostigmine decreased activity (*) in right parietal cortex when fearful faces appeared at task-irrelevant locations. A, faces attended; U, faces unattended; F, fearful; N, neutral. From Bentley, Vuilleumier, Thiel, Driver, and Dolan (2003). Copyright 2003 by Elsevier. Reprinted by permission.

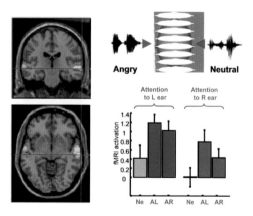

PLATE 10.4. Effects of emotional prosody and spatial attention on voice processing. Participants were presented with one voice in each ear, either neutral or angry, but had to concentrate on either the left (blue) or right (red) side in order to judge gender. Voice-sensitive regions in superior temporal gyrus showed increased activation when attention was directed to the contralateral ear (regardless of prosody) and when one voice was angry (regardless of attention), as illustrated for the right hemisphere here. Ne, neutral; A, angry; L, left; R, right.

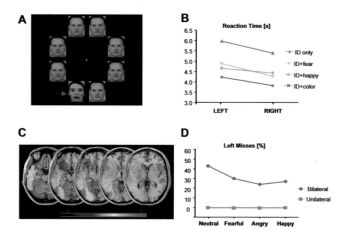

PLATE 10.5. Emotional influences on spatial attentional biases in patients with left spatial neglect. (A) Visual search requiring detection of a target face that could differ from distractors by either identity alone, identity + expression (fearful or happy), or identity + color (red hue). (B) Patients with left neglect after right-hemisphere lesion (*n* = 13) show longer reaction times for all types of targets on the left relative to the right side of the array, but a facilitation by color or expression still operates on the impaired/left as well as on the intact/right side, despite the attentional neglect bias. (C) Lesion analysis of patients with large versus small benefits from emotional expression during face search, showing more frequent damage to posterior temporoparietal areas in the former (red–orange), but to orbitofrontal regions in the latter (blue). Color scale represents chi-square values. (D) Dichotic listening task (similar to that shown in Plate 10.4) in patients with left neglect (*n* = 6). Voices in the left ear are accurately detected during unilateral presentation but often missed during bilateral presentation, but with an advantage for emotional stimuli on bilateral trial.

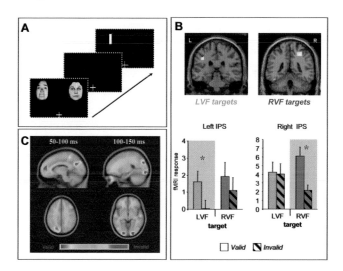

PLATE 10.6. Emotional influences on spatial orienting of attention in healthy subjects. (A) Variant of the "dot probe task" in which a target (vertical or horizontal bar) is preceded by two faces (one neutral and one emotional) and appears either on the same or the opposite side as the emotional face (valid vs. invalid trial, respectively). (B) On fMRI, valid versus invalid targets produce greater activation in intraparietal sulcus (IPS), due to relative suppression of responses to the ipsilateral visual field after an invalid emotional face; this is consistent with enhanced focusing of attention in the contralateral visual field. A and B are from Pourtois, Schwartz, Seghier, Lazeyras, and Vuilleumier (2006). Copyright 2006 by Elsevier. Reprinted by permission. (C) In EEG, parietal activity is already selectively increased for valid targets 50–100 msec after target onset (i.e., 100–300 msec after presentation of faces), and correlates with increased activation in occipital visual areas 100–150 msec after target onset that corresponds to amplification of the P1 component. From Pourtois, Thut, Grave de Peralta, Michel, and Vuilleumier (2005). Copyright 2005 by Elsevier. Reprinted by permission.

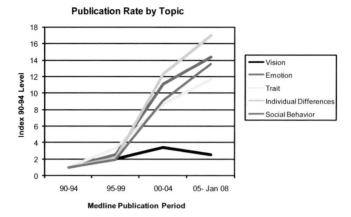

PLATE 11.1. Publication trends since 1990. Data were derived from the PubMed database (searched Jan 30, 2008). Searches were limited to human studies, using the search terms "functional magnetic resonance imaging and ___," where the blank refers to the topic area of interest. For each topic area, raw publication numbers (based on the number of citations minus review articles) were indexed at 1 for the period 1990–1994.

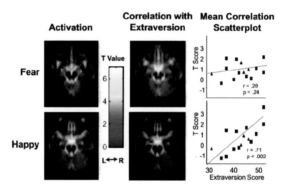

PLATE 11.2. Amygdala activation to happy faces correlates with extraversion. From Canli, Sivers, Whitfield, Gotlib, and Gabrieli (2002). Copyright 2002 by the American Association for the Advancement of Science. Reprinted by permission.

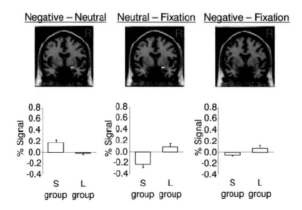

PLATE 11.3. Amygdala activation as a function of 5-HTTLPR genotype. From Canli, Omura, et al. (2005). Copyright 2005 by the National Academy of Sciences. Reprinted by permission.

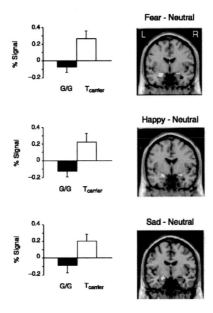

PLATE 11.4. Amygdala activation as a function of TPH2 genotype. From Canli, Congdon, Gutknecht, Constable, and Lesch (2005). Copyright 2005 by Springer Verlag Wien. Reprinted by permission.

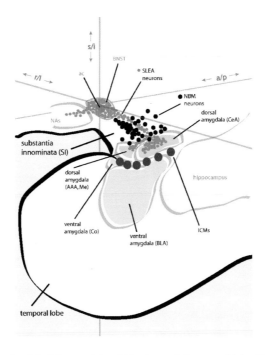

PLATE 12.1. Schematic of the left amygdala within the medial temporal lobe. NAs, nucleus accumbens (shell); ac, anterior commissure; BNST, bed nucleus of the stria terminalis; SLEA, sublenticular extended amygdala; NBM, nucleus basalis of Meynert; CeA, central nucleus of the amygdala; ICMs, intercalated cell masses; BLA, basolateral amygdala; Co, cortical nucleus; AAA, anterior amygdala area; Me, medial nucleus; r/l, right–left; s/i, superior–inferior; a/p, anterior–posterior. The chapter authors thank Lennart Heimer for his suggested changes to this figure.

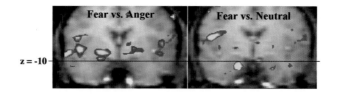

PLATE 12.2. Direct contrast of fearful and angry faces reveals signal increases within the dorsal amygdala/SI region. In the same subjects, fearful contrasted with neutral faces activated the ventral amygdala. Angry faces also activated the ventral amygdala in this study (see Whalen et al., 2001). The horizontal line on both pictures represents a dorsal–ventral dividing line of z = –10 (i.e., 10 mm below the anterior commissure). From Whalen et al. (2001). Copyright 2001 from the American Psychological Association. Reprinted by permission.

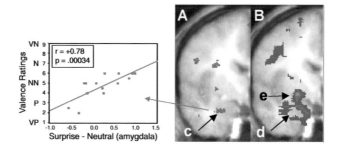

PLATE 12.3. (A) The orange voxels depict the location within the ventral amygdala where a positive correlation with ratings of surprise was observed (arrow c) from the results of Kim et al. (2003). Scatterplot to the left presents these data. The x-axis presents fMRI responses to surprised versus neutral faces, while the y-axis presents the valence scale from 1 to 9. Labels on the y-axis: VN, very negative; N, negative; NN, neither negative nor positive; P, positive; VP, very positive. (B) Voxels at this same anterior–posterior level (y = –3) showing a significant main effect for surprised versus neutral faces across all subjects. The maximally activated voxel for this main effect is located in the dorsal amygdala/SI (arrow e). Note that these voxels do not include the voxels in which we observed the significant correlation based upon individual differences (arrow d). Image B is thresholded liberally (p < .05, uncorrected), to make the points that (1) no trend toward a main effect for surprise existed in the voxels presented in A, and (2) we have signal coverage across the entirety of the amygdaloid complex.

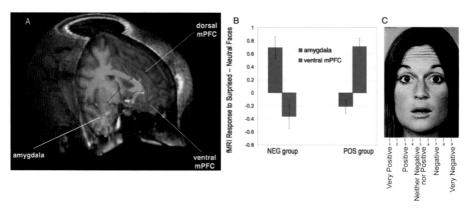

PLATE 12.4. (A) A three-dimensional depiction of the correlational results of Kim et al. (2003). Amygdala and dorsal mPFC loci that showed a positive correlation with valence ratings of surprise (colored in orange) are also positively correlated with one another (red arrow; r = +.66). The ventral mPFC locus that showed a negative correlation with valence ratings of surprise (colored in blue) is also negatively correlated with the amygdala (blue arrow; r = –.69) and the dorsal mPFC (blue arrow; r = –.62). (B) Bar graph focusing on the inverse relationship between the amygdala and ventral mPFC in subjects who interpreted the surprised faces either positively (POS) or negatively (NEG). (C) An example of the surprised faces and the valence scale used to rate them.

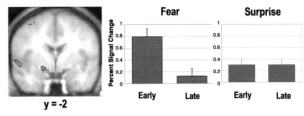

$y = -2$

PLATE 12.5. A reanalysis of data from Kim et al. (2003) where subjects viewed fearful and surprised faces in separate scans. Note the different habituation rates of activity within the right dorsal amygdala for fearful compared to surprised faces for early scans (first half of scans) versus late scans (last half of scans). From Kim and Whalen (2008).

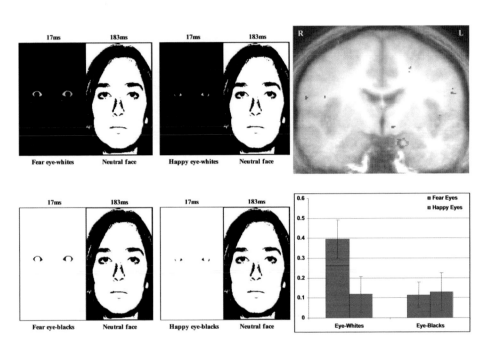

PLATE 12.6. Four stimulus conditions (fearful eye whites, happy eye whites, fearful eye blacks, and happy eye blacks) from the study by Whalen et al. (2004) showing that fearful eye whites are sufficient to activate the amygdala. The eye stimuli were presented for 17 msec and were immediately followed by neutral face line drawings presented for 183 msec, which effectively mitigated subjects' reported awareness of the presence of the eye stimuli (i.e., backward masking). Brain activation observed to the fearful eye whites but not to the other three conditions (see bar graph) located within the ventral amygdala.

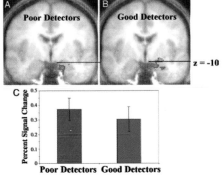

PLATE 12.7. Response to fearful versus happy masked eye whites separated as a function of detection ability. This figure breaks the activation pictured in Plate 12.6 down by subjects who were able to detect fearful eye whites above chance levels (good detectors) versus at or below chance levels (poor detectors) in a subsequent detection task. The bar graph reflects percentage of signal change in the ventral amygdala (below $z = -10$) to fearful versus happy masked eye whites; there was no significant difference in the ventral amygdala between poor and good detectors. Only good detectors showed signal changes in the dorsal amygdala/SI region (above $z = -10$).

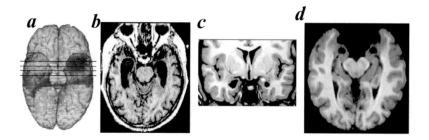

PLATE 13.1. Neuroanatomy of three different etiologies that resulted in amygdala lesions. (a) This ventral view of a brain maps the lesions of 17 subjects who had left ($n = 10$) or right ($n = 7$) neurosurgical temporal lobectomy (note that none of the lesions are bilateral, so the lesions shown in left and right temporal lobes are from different subjects). Color encodes the density of overlaps of lesions, showing maximal overlaps in the medial temporal lobe including the amygdala, but also variably extending to surrounding tissue. The horizontal black lines indicate sections that would include the entire extent of the amygdala. (b) Magnetic resonance scan of a patient with limbic encephalitis that resulted in complete bilateral amygdala lesions, as well as damage to more posterior medial temporal lobe structures. (c) The lesions of patient A. P., restricted to bilateral amygdala. (d) The lesions of patient S. M., likewise relatively restricted to bilateral amygdala. S. M.'s lesions are more extensive than A. P.'s and include some of anterior entorhinal cortex.

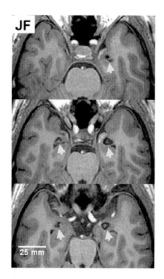

PLATE 13.2. Detailed portrayal of the lesions in patient A. P. showing focal damage restricted to parts of the amygdala on both sides (yellow arrowheads). Images are at a 1-mm isotropic voxel resolution obtained at 3T.

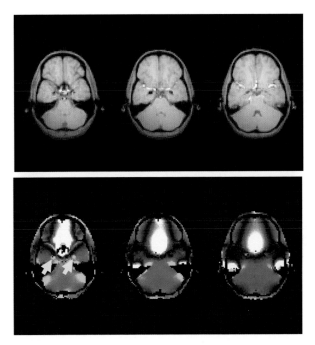

PLATE 13.3. B0 maps for patient A. P. At the top are EPI images on which the bilateral amygdala lesions are just visible as tiny black regions. The B0 maps in the bottom panel show a very small phase shift of about −30 Hz just inferior to the lesion itself (arrowheads), but this is very small compared to the field inhomogeneity due to air–tissue interfaces (e.g., in ventromedial prefrontal cortex). Scale is a full scale from −50 Hz to 50 Hz. Data are from a Siemens 3T Trio scanner.

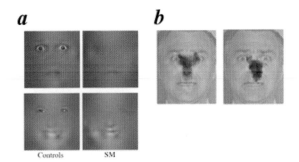

PLATE 13.4. Face processing in S. M. (a) Classification images from controls (left) and S. M. (right) for fearful faces (top row) or happy faces (bottom row). Shown are regions of faces that correlated significantly ($p < .05$, corrected) with performance accuracy. Whereas controls used the eyes and mouth, S. M. failed to make use of information from the eyes. (b) Furthermore, S. M. failed to fixate the eyes in faces. Fixation density maps are overlaid on a sample stimulus face, and encode more fixations with redder colors. From Adolphs et al. (2005). Copyright 2005 by the Nature Publishing Group. Reprinted by permission.

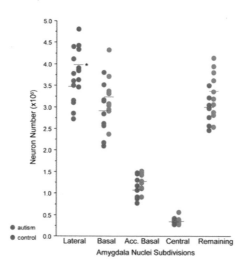

PLATE 16.1. Number of neurons in five subdivisions of the amygdala in autistic (red dots) and control (blue dots) brains. Asterisk indicates significant difference ($p = .03$) in neuron number between autistic and control lateral nuclei. From Schumann and Amaral (2006). Copyright 2006 by the Society for Neuroscience. Reprinted by permission.

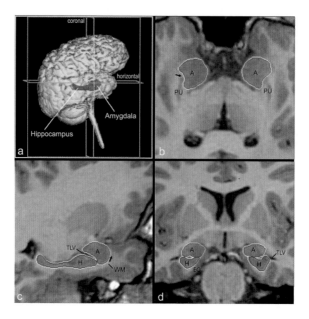

PLATE 16.2. MRI showing human amygdala (red) and adjacent hippocampus (blue). From Schumann et al. (2004). Copyright 2004 by the Society for Neuroscience. Reprinted by permission.

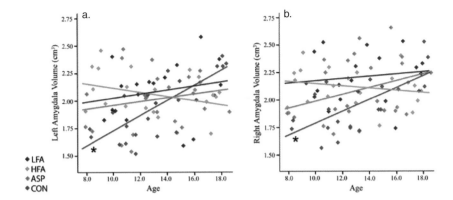

PLATE 16.3. Linear regression scatterplot for absolute amygdala volume (in cubic centimeters) by age. Typically developing subjects showed a positive correlation of age with amygdala volume for both the left (a) and right (b) amygdala (*$p < .05$). Amygdala volume in participants with autism was not correlated with age. Abbreviations: LFA, participants with low-functioning autism; HFA, participants with high-functioning autism; ASP, participants with Asperger syndrome; CON, typically developing control participants. From Schumann et al. (2004). Copyright 2004 by the Society for Neuroscience. Adapted by permission.

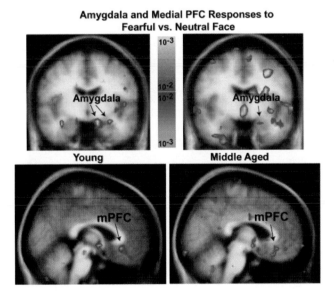

PLATE 17.1. Age-related amygdala and medial prefrontal cortex (PFC) responses to fearful faces. Top panels shows coronal T1-weighted Talairach brain images with superimposed colorized statistical maps. Greater activation to the contrast between fearful and neutral faces was present in the young (top left panel) than in the middle-aged (top right panel) subjects. Bottom panels show sagittal T1-weighted Talairach brain images with superimposed colorized statistical maps. For discussion of these, see the "What I Think" box. Young subjects (bottom left panel) had less activity (deactivations) in the medial PFC than middle-aged subjects (bottom right panel), who showed medial PFC signal increases to the same contrast.

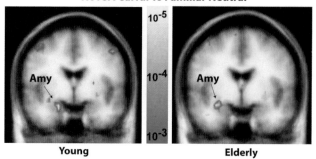

Amygdala Responses to Novel Fearful vs Familiar Neutral

Young

Elderly

PLATE 17.2. Similar amygdala responses to human faces in young and elderly subjects. Coronal Talairach T1-weighted images with superimposed colorized statistical maps demonstrating similar amygdala activation in young (*n* = 18) and elderly (*n* = 18) subjects. The activations shown are for the comparison between novel fearful faces and familiar neutral faces. From Wright, Wedig, et al. (2006). Copyright 2006 by Elsevier. Adapted by permission.

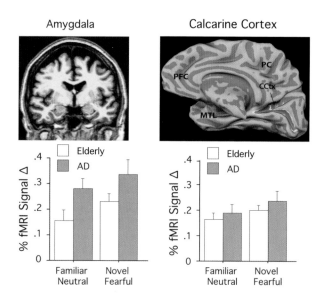

PLATE 17.3. Exaggerated amygdala responses to human faces in AD. Left upper panel shows high-resolution coronal MRI image demonstrating amygdala tracings used. for anatomically based fMRI analyses. Bar graphs show percent (%) blood-oxygen-level-dependent (BOLD) signal change for elderly controls (*n* = 12) and patients with mild AD (*n* = 12). Bar graphs below show right amygdala responses to familiar neutral and novel fearful faces versus fixation. The amygdala in the patients with AD versus the healthy elderly subjects had significantly greater responses to both face conditions. Right upper panel shows the partially inflated reconstruction of the medial cortical surface demonstrating the right calcarine cortex parcellation (CCtx, purple). This was used for anatomically based fMRI analyses. The medial prefrontal cortex (PFC), medial temporal lobe (MTL), and parietal cortex (PC) are indicated. Bar graphs below show similar responses in the calcarine cortex of the two subjects groups. From Wright, Dickerson, et al. (2007). Copyright 2007 by the Society of Biological Psychiatry. Adapted by permission.

CHAPTER 13

The Human Amygdala
in Social Function

Tony W. Buchanan, Daniel Tranel, and Ralph Adolphs

W hat is the role of the amygdala in social function? Although this question has been the topic of considerable research, many past studies have addressed this question only indirectly, in the context of research on emotion or learning. In such studies, the sights, sounds, and smells of conspecifics have been used to induce emotional states or to influence learning. These social stimuli are often the most effective in producing emotional responses. But what gives these stimuli their potency in the production of affect and influence on learning? The social environment is first encountered immediately after birth in the form of mother–infant interactions and continues to be of tremendous importance throughout an animal's lifespan. The bond formed with the mother is necessary for the survival of an organism (at least for most mammals), and this bond influences social behavior from infancy through adulthood. The primacy of the social environment in the survival of an organism makes it necessary for neural mechanisms to acclimate quickly to and learn from social situations. While many neural structures are involved in this process, the amygdala occupies a central position in both the recognition of and response to socially salient stimuli.

Perhaps an appropriate reformulation of the question at the beginning of the chapter is this: To *what* in the social environment does the amygdala respond? Some researchers have postulated that it is *ambiguity* or *relevance* to which the amygdala is sensitive (Sander, Grafman, & Zalla, 2003; Whalen, 1998). Stimuli that predict threat some of the time, as in a partial reinforcement schedule, produce greater amygdala-dependent conditioned responses than those that consistently predict threat do (Lloyd & Kling, 1991). With regard to the human social environment, Whalen (1998) has argued that the amygdala response to facial expressions of fear (and, by extension, the facial fear recognition deficit in patients with amygdala damage) is due to the inherent ambiguity expressed in the fearful face. Whereas angry faces indicate both a threat and the source of that threat, fearful faces indicate only the presence of a threat, but not its source. In this view, the amygdala response is in the service of disambiguating the threat stimulus. Taken to its logical extreme, what could be more ambiguous than our social environment? Stimuli in the social environment include family members, coworkers, potential mates, potential enemies, and many others; they constitute a multifaceted system of interactions, which are sometimes predictable, but never certain. We humans by nature attempt to explain other humans' behavior, which is often erratic and can constitute threats to our survival, or at least to our well-being. In this sense, then, activation of the amygdala while we are navigating our social environment is an index of the amygdala's role in deciphering ambiguity.

We postulate that the unpredictable nature of social interactions is what influences amygdala function (and perhaps even its structure, although this is beyond the scope of our analysis). Within this chapter, we describe work showing the specific instances in which the amygdala is implicated in the processing of inherently unpredictable social stimuli. We begin by describing some of the early work done in nonhuman primates and discussing how this work influenced subsequent work in humans. Next, we review recent work on social cognition and the amygdala, which has used functional neuroimaging and neurophysiology approaches in humans. We then turn to descriptions of some rare amygdala-damaged patients we have had an opportunity to study, and discuss these patients in terms of both their performance on social tasks and their real-life social behavior. We conclude with a proposal for an integrative model of the functions of the human amygdala in social processing.

HISTORICAL CONTEXT, FOCUSING ON ANIMAL RESEARCH

Some of the earliest writings on the role of the amygdala in behavior emphasized its social function (Brown & Schafer, 1888). Klüver and Bucy (1937), in their classic paper on the behavior of rhesus monkeys that had undergone bilateral removal of the temporal lobes (including the amygdala, hippocampus, and surrounding cortex), included descriptions of altered sexual behavior and increased tameness toward humans and conspecifics. This work was followed by many studies documenting changes in social behavior, and increased compliance with experimenters, in monkeys with bilateral damage limited primarily to the amygdala (Dicks, Myers, & Kling, 1968; Thompson, Bergland, & Towfighi, 1977; Weiskrantz, 1956). The specific results of amygdala damage in animals depended on the age of the animals at the time the damage occurred, the dominance status of the animals in their social hierarchy, and how the animals were housed (laboratory cage housing vs. a natural habitat).

In a classic study assessing the effects of amygdala damage on social behavior in the wild, Dicks and colleagues (1968) examined the effects of juvenile-onset and adult-onset lesions to the amygdala (and uncus) in rhesus monkeys. Animals that received the operation as juveniles (between 2 and 3 years of age) showed a transient social impairment, following which these animals rejoined their social group and within a month of the procedure were behaving within normal limits of social behavior. By contrast, the adult-onset cases were unable to display appropriate social signals, resulting in social ostracism. During the initial social reintroduction, both the adult- and juvenile-onset cases were described as "retarded in their ability to foresee and avoid dangerous confrontations." They did not show appropriate submissive gestures toward more dominant animals. Although the juvenile-onset animals were able to overcome these social impairments, the adult-onset cases were not so fortunate and, forced to live on their own, died within a month of the operation. On the basis of findings with animals having either early- or adult-onset amygdala damage, Thompson and colleagues (1977) suggested that damage to the amygdala did not result merely in tameness or placidity, but that these animals were "slow in conforming to the social etiquette normally associated with a subordinate status and behave in ways that prolong the hostility directed at them." This conclusion is more in tune with the idea that damage to the amygdala results in inappropriate responses to ambiguous social cues, rather than merely producing a pattern of tameness.

More recent research has assessed the effects of amygdala damage on the development of social behavior by examining the effects of neonatal amygdala damage on social interactions (Bauman, Lavenex, Mason, Capitanio, & Amaral, 2004a, 2004b). These authors have shown that the amygdala is not essential for the development of social behavior in rhesus monkeys. Damage to the amygdala does, however, alter certain aspects of social function. The primary social effect of neonatal amygdala damage—like that previously described for adult-onset lesions—is an inability to appreciate the threat value of a situation and to modify behavior accordingly. The amygdala, then, plays a modulatory role: While the development of fundamental social behavior with both the mother and peers proceeds (mostly) normally after early-onset amygdala damage, these animals are unable to regulate their social behavior later in life, especially in response to potentially fear-inducing situations. This pattern of results is analogous to that reported for the role of the amygdala in long-term declarative memory. Although the amygdala is not essential for the encoding, consolidation, and retrieval of memories, it does play a modulatory role. Specifically, the amygdala participates in the enhancement of memory for emotionally arousing material (Buchanan & Adolphs, 2004; McGaugh, Cahill, & Roozendaal, 1996). Just as normal memory performance develops in monkeys or humans with amygdala damage, social development proceeds normally for the most part. It is only in certain social situations in which differences in social behavior or emotional memory are evidenced following amygdala damage.

These findings in animals with early- and adult-onset amygdala damage are instructive, in that they relate to the patterns of deficits seen in humans with amygdala damage due to either a developmental disease process or adult-onset changes in amygdala function, as we review in more detail later in this chapter.

NEUROPHYSIOLOGY AND FUNCTIONAL IMAGING IN PRIMATES

The altered social behavior described after damage to the amygdala suggests that it is involved in processing social signals—specifically, those related to potential threat—and modifying behavior accordingly. Neurophysiology and neuroimaging studies have allowed for the assessment of the specific stimuli in the social environment that activate the amygdala.

Neurophysiological studies have shown that neurons in the primate amygdala are responsive to faces (Leonard, Rolls, Wilson, & Baylis, 1985) and other social stimuli (Brothers & Ring, 1993; Brothers, Ring, & Kling, 1990). Leonard and colleagues (1985) described neurons in the basal accessory nucleus of the amygdala in the rhesus macaque that responded selectively to human and monkey faces. Similar findings have since been reported from single-neuron activity measured from the human amygdala (Fried, MacDonald, & Wilson, 1997). These results suggest a mechanism whereby amygdala damage could result in the altered social behavior previously documented in monkeys following amygdalectomy. If neurons in the amygdala are responsive to faces, and specifically to the faces of individuals within a dominance hierarchy, then damage to these neurons may result in an inability either to recognize members of a hierarchy or to produce the proper behavioral response to those individuals. This deficit, then, may alter the social and affective behavior of an individual in the presence of animals above or below that individual in the dominance hierarchy. Interestingly, Leonard and colleagues found that face-responsive neurons in the amygdala were slower to respond to facial stimuli than were neurons in the superior temporal sulcus area (110–200 msec compared to 90–140 msec, respectively). This delayed response suggests that the amygdala is receiving preprocessed information from cortical areas sensitive to social stimuli. The amygdala may utilize this processed social information, orchestrating the proper affective response when presented with an unpredictable social situation.

Other studies have shown that the amygdala response in social situations is potentiated when the situations can be interpreted as ambiguous (Kling, Steklis, & Deutsch, 1979; Lloyd & Kling, 1991; Whalen, 1998). Kling and colleagues (1979) showed that amygdala activity in squirrel monkeys increased when animals were presented with ambiguous social behaviors by conspecifics, such as approach or genital inspection. A number of outcomes are possible in these situations, including aggression or sexual behavior. Amygdala activity was greatest in the conditions characterized by uncertainty than in any other conditions in the experiment, including situations involving overt physical aggression. Interestingly, these authors also found increased amygdala activity in a study in which squirrel monkeys were placed in a nonsocial situation in which they had previously received uncued—and therefore unpredictable—shock (Lloyd & Kling, 1991). Amygdala activity in the uncued shock chamber was greater than that recorded in a chamber in which shock had been presented reliably. These authors suggested that unpredictability, in the behavior of conspecifics as well as in the possibility of shock, was what elicited the amygdala activity.

Following from neurophysiological and neuropsychological studies, researchers have used functional neuroimaging techniques such as positron emission tomography (PET) and functional magnetic resonance imaging (fMRI) to address the role of the human amygdala in social function. The results of many of these studies are discussed at length in other chapters in this volume, but we describe a selection of those studies that have specifically addressed social functioning.

The initial finding of amygdala response to facial expression stimuli in humans came from a PET study in which subjects viewed faces expressing fearful and happy expressions (Morris et al., 1996). Results of this study showed increased left amygdala activity in response to faces morphed to show higher intensity of fear, and decreased activity in response to faces showing higher intensity of happiness. These authors further showed that greater amygdala activity while subjects were viewing fearful faces was associated with greater activity in an area of visual cortex, whereas reduced amygdala activity during the viewing of happy faces was associated with reduced visual cortical activity (Morris et al., 1998). These data, and more recent research (Richardson, Strange, & Dolan, 2004; Vuilleumier, Richardson, Armony, Driver, & Dolan, 2004), indicate that the amygdala has a modulatory influence on other areas of the brain during the processing of social and emotional stimuli. These findings, along with those from neurophysiological studies of primates, indicate the central position that the amygdala occupies in the processing of social stimuli. It receives processed information via pathways from cortical regions, such as the superior temporal sulcus (Amaral, Price, Pitkanen, & Carmichael, 1992), but it also feeds back to higher-level visual cortex in response to socially salient information (Morris et al., 1998).

The face is a primary source of social information for primates, but other bodily expressions can also signal the social and emotional state of others (Atkinson, Dittrich, Gemmell, & Young, 2004). Several studies have shown amygdala activity to social signals arising from body expressions (Bonda, Petrides, Ostry, & Evans, 1996; de Gelder, Snyder, Greve, Gerard, & Hadjikhani, 2004; Hadjikhani & de Gelder, 2003). In this work, subjects were presented with images of actors showing bodily expressions of fear, compared to expressions of happiness and nonemotional expressions (de Gelder et al., 2004). Importantly, the facial expressions of the actors depicted in the stimuli were blurred, to control for effects of facial expression on neural activity. Results of these studies showed activity in a network of regions, including the amygdala and fusiform cortex, in the processing of bodily emotional expressions. The amygdala was especially responsive to bodily expressions of fear. This work suggests that the amygdala is not merely sensitive to social signals from the face, but also to other channels of expression, such as those emanating from body posture (although see Adolphs & Tranel, 2003, for a discussion of the pattern of emotion recognition from bodily responses after amygdala damage).

Just as much of the work on the neural response to social stimuli has focused on facial signals, much of the work on the role of the amygdala in processing social stimuli in primates has focused on the visual domain. By contrast, work in other animals has sampled other sensory domains, such as olfaction (Knuepfer, Eismann, Schutze, Stumpf, & Stock, 1995) and audition (Gil-da-Costa et al., 2004; LeDoux, Farb, & Ruggiero, 1990). We note that the relative importance of the visual environment in guiding primate behavior has probably placed selection pressure on the neural structures involved in visual processing. The results of functional neuroimaging studies of the neural response to social stimuli indicate that the amygdala may show a preferential response to social stimuli presented in the visual domain. This could be due to a sampling bias, though, because research on social sounds and smells is less commonly reported than that focusing on visual social signals. In fact, several studies have shown pronounced amygdala responses to odorants (Gottfried, O'Doherty, & Dolan, 2002; Savic, Gulyas, Larsson, & Roland, 2000; Zald & Pardo, 1997); however, the social effects of odorants on human behavior remain unclear (Preti & Wysocki, 1999).

Research on the role of the human amygdala in the realm of auditory social processing has produced mixed results. Work in this area has used two different types of stimuli: nonverbal vocalizations, and affective prosody of spoken words and sentences. Several studies have shown that the amygdala responds to vocal nonverbal emotional expressions, such as screaming and crying (Morris, Scott, & Dolan, 1999; Phillips et al., 1998; Sander & Scheich, 2001). These findings complement results from a study showing impaired recognition of nonverbal emotional expressions in a patient with bilateral amygdala damage (Scott et al., 1997). Studies examining the neural response to another auditory expression of emotion, affective prosody, have not generally reported amygdala activity (Buchanan et al., 2000; Wildgruber et al., 2004; Wildgruber, Pihan, Ackermann, Erb, & Grodd, 2002). Similarly, two studies have shown normal recognition of affective prosody after bilateral amygdala damage (Adolphs & Tranel, 1999; Anderson & Phelps, 1998b). The results of these studies suggest that the amygdala may be a necessary component in the processing of nonverbal social information, but that it does not play an integral role in the processing of the affective inflection of spoken language. It may be that the amygdala is responsive to nonverbal auditory stimuli that are more intense and phylogenetically older, such as screams and crying; by contrast, the affective intonation of spoken language may be processed more by cortical regions and less by the amygdala. The distinction between effects of verbal and nonverbal auditory social cues on amygdala activity has not been systematically addressed, however. In spite of the lack of amygdala involvement in the processing of affective prosody, two studies have shown amygdala activity in response to cross-modal presentations of face and voice, wherein amygdala activity is greatest when face and voice both express fear (Dolan, Morris, & de Gelder, 2001; Ethofer et al., 2006). This work supports findings from animal research describing a role for the amygdala in the binding of information across sensory modalities (Murray & Mishkin, 1985; although see Nahm, Tranel, Damasio, & Damasio, 1993, for an exception).

ANATOMY AND NEUROPSYCHOLOGY OF HUMAN AMYGDALA DAMAGE

Although several psychiatric illnesses are thought to involve pathology in the amygdala, overt neurological damage to this structure is not all that common. Posttraumatic stress disorder, the other anxiety disorders, schizophrenia, depression, and autism have all been linked to amygdala pathology (Aggleton, 1992, 2000). On the basis of functional imaging studies, the evidence for amygdala dysfunction in mood disorders is fairly strong (Davidson & Irwin, 1999; Drevets, 2000); however, it leaves open the question of whether such functional abnormality in fact arises from pathology within the amygdala, or is a consequence of pathology elsewhere that has a distal effect on amygdala function. One model of phobias, for instance, is that there is abnormal prefrontal regulation of amygdala function, resulting in an inability to down-regulate amygdala activity as a function of the context in which a stimulus occurs. Similar distal effects on evoked amygdala activation may account for many of the abnormal blood-oxygenation-level-dependent (BOLD) responses in cognitive activation studies that have been reported in a variety of other psychiatric illnesses. In autism, histological and volumetric MRI studies have found abnormal amygdala cell density or volume through development—providing perhaps a stronger link directly to the amygdala as a possible source of pathology in this disorder, and a basis for explaining abnormal amygdala activation in people with autism in fMRI studies. Nonetheless, insofar as autism is a developmental disorder, even these findings leave open the question of primary pathology in the brain.

The most common neurological cause of amygdala damage is medial temporal lobe epilepsy. Depending on the severity and years of duration of the epilepsy, medial temporal lobe sclerosis can damage structures in the medial temporal lobe that include the amygdala (and prominently also the hippocampus). A fairly common elective surgery for the treatment of medically refractory epilepsy is neurosurgical temporal lobectomy. This also results in variable damage to the amygdala, depending on clinical criteria and the particular approach of the surgeon. In some cases resection of the amygdala is complete, whereas in others there is only damage to adjacent white matter. In all these cases, however, the damage is unilateral and is never selective to the amygdala. Nonetheless, unilateral amygdala damage resulting from temporal lobectomy accounts for by far the largest sample of neurological subjects with amygdala damage (Plate 13.1a in color insert).

Less common is bilateral damage to the medial temporal lobe resulting from encephalitis. Limbic encephalitis and herpes simplex encephalitis are two examples of inflammatory illnesses that can disproportionately damage the medial temporal lobe, and generally do so bilaterally (Plate 13.1b). When severe, such encephalitis can result in complete bilateral destruction of the amygdala; however, it is never selective, typically involving adjacent hippocampal, entorhinal, and parahippocampal regions, and consequently resulting in a dense amnesic syndrome that makes interpretation of the patients' performances on many experimental tasks a challenge.

There are a very few cases of neurological patients who have relatively selective damage to the amygdala. In such patients, the vagaries of a stroke, epilepsy, or surgery result in damage that is relatively restricted to the amygdala on one side or even bilaterally to some extent. One such important patient is S. P., who has been studied in detail by Phelps and colleagues (Anderson & Phelps, 1998a, 2000, 2001). Another is D. R. who has been studied by Young and colleagues (Calder, Young, Perrett, Etcoff, & Rowland, 1996; Young et al., 1995). The most neuroanatomically selective lesion cases can arise in extremely rare individuals who have Urbach–Wiethe disease. This disease, also called lipoid proteinosis, is due to a mutation in the gene coding for extracellular matrix protein 1 and shows an autosomal recessive inheritance pattern (Hamada et al., 2002). Roughly half of the affected individuals have calcifications of medial temporal lobe structures, usually bilateral and often encompassing the amygdala, entorhinal cortex, and surrounding white matter (Hofer, 1973). Little is known about the developmental time course of these calcifications, or about the cellular processes that result in calcification. There appears to be an early developmental calcification of vasculature in the affected structures, followed by atrophy. Several such patients have been studied by Markowitsch and colleagues, who have documented some progression in the disease, and consequences for emotion and memory processing (Babinsky et al., 1993; Markowitsch et al., 1994; Siebert, Markowitsch, & Bartel, 2003).

We have studied two patients with Urbach–Wiethe disease, S. M. (Adolphs, Damasio, Tranel, Cooper, & Damasio, 2000; Tranel & Hyman, 1990) and A. P. Both patients are female; at this writing, S. M. is 40 years old, and A. P. is 19 years old. Although we do not know the exact onset of their amygdala lesions, both patients presented with bilateral, fairly symmetrical, and relatively restricted lesions to the amygdala when we first scanned them (in her early 20s for S. M. and at age 14 for A. P.), and their neuroanatomy has been stable since. Their lesions are portrayed in panels c and d of Plate 13.1 (in color insert); Plates 13.2 (in color insert) and 13.3 (in color insert) provide further views of A. P.'s lesions. We are conducting additional studies of these rare patients—using high-angular-resolution diffusion-weighted imaging to generate probabilistic maps of anatomical connectivity; using magnetic resonance spectroscopy to examine abnormal metabolites in the region of the lesion, as well as in distal targets of the amygdala; and using cognitive activation studies (echo planar imaging [EPI] with BOLD contrast). For the latter, it is important also to document the possible distortions of the magnetic field that could result from the different magnetic susceptibility of the calcifications in the amygdala compared to surrounding tissue. As shown in Plate 13.2, however, this appears to be a nearly negligible effect, thus perhaps making it possible to examine functional activity even in close proximity to the lesion.

Neuropsychological Profiles of S. M. and A. P.

S. M.'s neuropsychological profile has been described in detail elsewhere (Adolphs & Tranel, 2000; Tranel & Hyman, 1990), and is updated and summarized in Table 13.1. The neuropsychological profile of A. P. has not been published before. S. M. has 12 years of formal schooling and lives independently. A. P. is currently enrolled in college. Both patients are fully right-handed (+100 on the Geschwind–Oldfield questionnaire). We briefly summarize the neuropsychological profiles of the two patients below; Table 13.1 provides quantitative information.

Behavioral Observations

In all testing sessions in our laboratory, S. M. and A. P. have been alert, fully oriented, and entirely cooperative. Their attention and cognitive stamina are intact. S. M.'s interpersonal behavior has been remarkable for a somewhat coquettish, disinhibited style, and this has remained constant across the years. She tends to be very friendly with experimenters and other laboratory personnel, and she has a very comfortable, "hands-on" style of interaction that goes somewhat beyond the norm for conventional U.S. Midwestern culture. However, her behavior is not inappropriate, and she is capable of focusing on specific task and situational demands. It is important to emphasize that S. M. does not exhibit true features of the classic Klüver–Bucy syndrome (Klüver & Bucy, 1937). A. P.'s presentation is reminiscent of S. M.'s, but her interpersonal behavior is less disinhibited. She is friendly and cooperative, and very open and forthcoming in her social interactions. Her parents have noted that

TABLE 13.1. Neuropsychological Profiles for S. M. and A. P.

Test/function	Score/result	
	S. M.	A. P.
Part A: Intellect and academic achievement		
Wechsler Adult Intelligence Scale (WAIS-R for S. M., WAIS-III for A. P.) (age-corrected scaled scores)		
Verbal IQ	86	92
Information	8	10
Digit Span	9	10
Vocabulary	7	10
Arithmetic	6	9
Comprehension	7	9
Similarities	10	8
Performance IQ	95	106
Picture Completion	10	8
Picture Arrangement	14	8
Block Design	9	13
Object Assembly	7	10
Digit Symbol–Coding	7	13
Full Scale IQ	88	98
Wide Range Achievement Test (WRAT-R for S. M., WRAT-III for A. P.) (standard scores)		
Reading	79	113
Spelling	91	118
Arithmetic	72	102
Part B: Memory		
Wechsler Memory Scale—Revised (indexes)		
Verbal Memory Index	90	—
Visual Memory Index	93	—
General Memory Index	89	—
Attention/Concentration Index	87	—
Delayed Recall Index	88	—
Rey Auditory–Verbal Learning Test (AVLT) (# words recalled/15)		
Trial 1	5	6
Trial 2	9	10
Trial 3	11	11
Trial 4	14	13
Trial 5	13	15
30-minute delayed recall	10	12
30-minute delayed recognition (#/30)	29	30
Benton Visual Retention Test		
Number correct (maximum = 10)	5	10
Number errors	7	t0
Complex Figure Test (30-minute recall)	14/36	28/36

(continued)

TABLE 13.1. *(continued)*

Test/function	S. M.	A. P.
	Score/result	

Part C: Speech and linguistic functions

Speech	Hoarse	Hoarse
Fluency	Normal	Normal
Paraphasias	None	None
Articulation	Normal	Normal
Prosody	Normal	Normal

Linguistic functions		
Boston Naming Test	47/60	46/60
Sentence repetition	15th %ile	—
Reading comprehension 9/10	—	
Writing	Normal	Normal
Controlled Oral Word Association Test	3rd %ile	3rd %ile
Token Test	44/44	—

Part D: Visuoperceptual and visuoconstructional functions

Facial Recognition Test	90th %ile	85th %ile
Judgment of Line Orientation	22nd %ile	>74th %ile
Hooper Visual Organization Test	25.5/30	24/30
Complex Figure Test (copy)	32/36	36/36

Drawing to dictation		
Clock	Normal	Normal
House	Normal	Normal
Person	Normal	Normal
Three-dimensional block construction	29/29	—

Grooved Pegboard Test		
Right hand	5th %ile	37th %ile
Left hand	9th %ile	38th %ile

Part E. Executive control and related functions

Wisconsin Card Sorting Test		
Number Correct	68	73
Errors	27th %ile	25th %ile
Perseverative responses	53rd %ile	32nd %ile
Nonperseverative errors	18th %ile	58th %ile
Perseverative errors	84th %ile	8th %ile
Number of categories	6 (>16th %ile)	6 (>16th %ile)

Trail-Making Test		
Part A	45	54
Part B	35	42

(continued)

TABLE 13.1. *(continued)*

Test/function	Score/result	
	S. M.	A. P.
Tower of Hanoi		
(# moves; means for age-matched controls in brackets)		
Trial 1 [80.6]	120	120
Trial 2 [61.4]	97	53
Trial 3 [63.6]	57	61
Trial 4 [59.8]	88	120
Tower of London		
Minimum moves	86	—
Excess moves	20	—
% above optimal strategy	23	—

Part F: Standardized personality assessment

Minnesota Multiphasic Personality Inventory (MMPI-2 for S. M., MMPI-A for A. P.)
(*T*-scores)

	S. M.	A. P.
Scale *L*	66	58
Scale *F*	48	42
Scale *K*	59	57
Scale 1	72	46
Scale 2	51	46
Scale 3	68	48
Scale 4	75	41
Scale 5	66	59
Scale 6	56	41
Scale 7	67	43
Scale 8	68	45
Scale 9	53	39
Scale 0	49	34

Part G: Further tests of social function

Bar-On Emotional Quotient Inventory, short form
(*z*-scores)

	S. M.	A. P.
TRA (Intrapersonal)	−0.7	0.07
TER (Interpersonal)	0.6	−0.02
SMS (Stress Management)	−0.3	1.0
AS (Adaptability)	−0.8	0.3
GMS (General Mood)	−0.5	−0.9
PIS (Positive Impression)	−1.2	0.2
EQ (Total Emotional Quotient)	−0.8	−0.1
Endler Multidimensional Anxiety Scales (nonsocial anxiety)	All in the normal range	All in the normal range
Endler Multidimensional Anxiety Scales (social anxiety)	All in the normal range	All in the normal range

(continued)

TABLE 13.1. *(continued)*

Test/function	Score/result	
	S. M.	A. P.
Social Problem Solving Inventory, Revised (z-scores)		
PPO	0.4	−0.5
NPO	−0.1	−0.3
PDF	−1.2	0.2
GAS	0.5	0.1
DM	−1.0	0.3
SIV	−0.8	−0.1
RPS	−0.7	0.1
ICS	0.8	−1.8
AS	0.1	−0.8
RAW (overall score)	−0.3	1.0
NEO Personality Inventory (z-scores)		
Neuroticism	−0.6	−0.1
Extraversion	2.0	−2.0
Openness	0.5	1.1
Agreeableness	−0.8	−1.0
Conscientiousness	−1.4	0.5

she tends to "trust" people too easily, and the parents have made an effort to teach her to be more wary of strangers. A. P.'s behavior in the laboratory setting is entirely appropriate. We discuss the "social cognition" of the patients in more detail in the next section.

Intellect and Academic Achievement

Part A of Table 13.1 presents data from the Wechsler Adult Intelligence Scale (WAIS) and the Wide Range Achievement Test (WRAT). S. M.'s IQ scores have remained stable across time. Her intellectual abilities range from the lower end of the average range to the upper end of the low average range—within typical expectations, given her educational and occupational background. Academic achievement skills range from average (spelling) to borderline (reading, arithmetic), commensurate with her educational background. A. P.'s intellectual abilities fall mainly in the average range, although a couple of her WAIS Performance subtest scores are high average (Block Design, Digit Symbol–Coding). All of the IQ scores for A. P. are in the average range. A. P. scored in the high average range on the Reading and Spelling subtests of the WRAT, and in the average range on the Arithmetic subtest. Like S. M., A. P. shows no indication of defects on any of the intellectual and achievement subtests.

Memory

Performances on various memory tests for the two patients are enumerated in Part B of Table 13.1. S. M.'s performances on all various components of the Wechsler Memory Scale—Revised are fully within normal expectations. As judged from the Rey Auditory–Verbal Learning Test (AVLT), S. M.'s ability to acquire and retain verbal information is intact. The same is true of A. P., who had a perfect 15/15 score on Trial 5 of the AVLT, and a perfect delayed recognition score of 30/30. S. M. has a mild weakness in the domain of nonverbal, visual memory (Benton Visual Retention Test, Complex Figure Test recall), which has characterized her profile over many years and has remained stable across time. A. P. scored perfectly on the Benton Visual Retention Test, and her performance on the Complex Figure Test recall is normal. Overall, both patients demonstrate essentially normal ability to acquire and retain declarative information, although S. M. may have a mild weakness for nonverbal, visuospatial material.

Speech and Linguistic Function

The findings for speech and linguistic function assessment are enumerated in Part C of Table 13.1. Both patients have markedly hoarse speech, characteristic of persons with Urbach–Wiethe disease (and both patients have had multiple vocal cord operations). With this exception, the speech of both patients is normal in every respect: Fluency, articulation, and prosody are intact, and there are no paraphasic errors. Linguistic functioning is also intact in both patients. However, both patients performed defectively (3rd percentile) on the Controlled Oral Word Association Test, which could suggest an "executive functioning" defect (see below).

Visuoperceptual and Visuoconstructional Functions

Part D of Table 13.1 enumerates data for tests of visuoperceptual, visuospatial, and visuoconstructional functioning in the two patients. For both patients, these abilities are essentially intact across the board (although S. M.'s psychomotor skills, as indexed by the Grooved Pegboard Test, are somewhat weak). These are important findings, especially in the realm of visual perception, and it is worth reiterating that there is no indication that the patients suffer from any type of basic visual information-processing disturbance that might contribute to their many defective performances on tests of facial emotion recognition and other related experiments reviewed elsewhere in this chapter.

Executive Control and Related Functions

Data for executive control and related functions are enumerated in Part E of Table 13.1. Both patients produced normal performances on the Wisconsin

Card Sorting Test and on the Trail-Making Test. By contrast, both of them demonstrated some difficulty with the Tower of Hanoi task, and as noted above, both produced relatively poor performances on the Controlled Oral Word Association Test. Thus the data hint at some mild "executive functioning" defects—something we have noted previously for S. M.

Personality Assessment

Part F of Table 13.1 summarizes the *T*-scores from the Minnesota Multiphasic Personality Inventory (MMPI), a standard measure of personality and psychopathology. The important conclusion to be drawn from these data is that neither S. M. nor A. P. evidences any form of significant psychopathology. The profiles are not suggestive, nor is there any evidence from their everyday lives, of a formal psychiatric diagnosis. Neither patient has ever manifested clinically significant depression or anxiety.

Further Tests of Social Functioning

Additional test scores are summarized under Part G of Table 13.1, all in *z*-scores from published norms. Again, what is most notable here is that neither patient's scores are abnormal, and in those cases where there might be a trend toward abnormality, they often go in opposite directions. In particular, there is no evidence of impairment on the Bar-On Emotional Quotient Inventory or on measures of anxiety, including social anxiety. Consistent with the results from the MMPI given in Part F, there is no evidence of psychopathology from the NEO Personality Inventory.

SOCIAL COGNITION
FOLLOWING AMYGDALA DAMAGE

Our earlier work and considerable work by others suggested the view that the amygdala is "specialized" for processing information about fear. Amygdala lesions resulted in a disproportionate impairment in the recognition of fear from facial expressions, compared to other emotions (Adolphs, Tranel, Damasio, & Damasio, 1994; Calder, Young, Rowland, & Perrett, 1996), and viewing facial expressions of fear resulted in amygdala activation in healthy individuals (Morris et al., 1996; Whalen et al., 2001). Although it is now clear that the amygdala is not so specialized for fear, but processes a broader range of emotions, it remains the case that S. M. is much more impaired in recognizing fear from facial expressions than in recognizing other emotions. Patient S. M. has been especially informative here because of the specificity of both her lesion and her impairment (Adolphs et al., 2000; Tranel & Hyman, 1990; see Plate 13.1d in color insert). On a series of tasks, S. M. has shown disproportionate impairment in recognizing the intensity of fear from faces (Adolphs et al., 1994). When asked to rate the intensity of fear and of other emotions in facial expressions, S. M. was relatively selectively impaired in regard to faces showing fear, with a much slighter impairment also in conceptually related emotions, such as surprise and anger. In addition, it was found that S. M. was impaired in her ability to judge the level of arousal of emotions with negative valence (unpleasant emotions), including fear, anger, disgust, and sadness. Since fear is normally judged to be one of the most arousing unpleasant emotions, S. M.'s impairment may be disproportionate to fear for this reason.

The amygdala's role is not limited to making judgments about basic emotions, but includes a role in making social judgments. This fact was already suggested by earlier studies in nonhuman primates (Kling & Brothers, 1992; Klüver & Bucy, 1937; Rosvold, Mirsky, & Pribram, 1954), which demonstrated impaired social behavior after amygdala damage. It has been corroborated in recent times by studying monkeys with more selective amygdala lesions, and by using more sophisticated ways of assessing social behavior (Emery & Amaral, 1999; Emery et al., 2001); it has also been shown now in humans. Building on these findings, some recent studies suggest a general role for the amygdala in so-called "theory-of-mind" abilities—the collection of abilities whereby we humans attribute internal mental states, intentions, desires, and emotions to other people (Baron-Cohen et al., 2000; Fine, Lumsden, & Blair, 2001). Relatedly, the amygdala shows differential habituation of activation to faces of people of a different race from the viewer (Hart et al., 2000), and amygdala activation has been found to correlate with race stereotypes of which the viewer may be unaware (Phelps et al., 2000). However, the amygdala's role in processing information about race is still unclear: Other brain regions, in extrastriate visual cortex, are also activated differentially as a function of race (Golby, Gabrieli, Chiao, & Eberhardt, 2001), and lesions of the amygdala do not appear to impair race judgments (Phelps, Cannistraci, & Cunningham, 2003).

In studies using faces as stimuli, we found that subjects with bilateral amygdala damage were also impaired in judging the untrustworthiness of faces from their appearance. Although they were able to judge trustworthy-looking faces normally, both in terms of the absolute ratings these faces were given and in terms of their relative rank order, subjects with bilateral amygdala damage failed to rate normally those faces that are normally judged to look the least trustworthy (Adolphs, Tranel, & Damasio, 1998). The impairment consisted of two components: a general positive bias for rating faces normally judged to look untrustworthy, and an inability to rank or discriminate those faces in terms of their perceived trustworthiness. The finding was followed up by a functional imaging study, which corroborated the basic finding: Activation of the amygdala was correlated with the judged untrustworthiness of the face. That study also found activation to perceived untrustworthiness in the insula, and it was able to show that amygdala activation to untrustworthy faces held even when other factors were minimized: The stimuli were all direct gaze, all faces were male, and emotion ratings were used as covariates in the analysis (Winston, Strange, O'Doherty, & Dolan, 2002).

Another study examined recognition of social emotion in individuals with amygdala damage, using a set of stimuli developed by Baron-Cohen for research into theory-of-mind abilities in people with autism. When shown faces that signal complex and social mental states, patients with bilateral amygdala damage performed disproportionately worse than comparison subjects (Adolphs, Tranel, & Baron-Cohen, 2002). Furthermore, the impairment held when just the eye region of the faces was shown, consistent with the idea that the eyes signal considerable social information that depends on the amygdala for its processing.

Although we will come back to the role of specific facial features, such as the eyes, it is worth noting a study in which the importance of the face, relative to other visual information, was examined. S. M.'s inability to recognize fear (as well as the impairments of other subjects with unilateral and bilateral amygdala damage) was relatively specific to faces, as opposed to other contextual visual information (Adolphs & Tranel, 2003). In that experiment, subjects were presented with scenes showing people that included facial expressions, as well as with the same scenes with the faces erased. Whereas nondisabled subjects' performance accuracy in judging the emotion decreased when the faces were erased (as one would predict, given that the face is a potent source of social information), the performance of subjects with amygdala damage did not suffer the same decrement. Indeed, for negative emotions, subjects with bilateral amygdala damage performed better when they were shown the stimuli with the faces erased than when the faces were present—presumably indicating that when the faces were present, they attempted to recognize them but got them wrong (Figure 13.1).

One interpretation of the data, and one that is still likely to be part of the story, proposed that the amygdala would link two kinds of representations: a visual representation of the other person's face one is viewing; and a somatic representation that would simultaneously represent one's own emotional response to seeing the person's face, as well as the presumed emotional state of that person (Adolphs, 2002). This link effected by the amygdala could be fairly direct (via direct projections from the amygdala to the insula, an interoceptive somatosensory cortex), or more indirect (via first eliciting an actual emotional response in the viewer's body that could then subsequently be represented in structures like the insula). There are now several studies indicating that the observation of another person's emotional state recruits structures like the insula (Jackson, Meltzoff, & Decety, 2005; Singer et al., 2004), which is also involved in representing one's own somatic states. Interestingly, the insula has been hypothesized (Craig, 2002; Damasio, 1999) and recently shown (Critchley, Wiens, Rotshtein, Oehman, & Dolan, 2004) to be associated with the conscious experience of one's own body state. This suggests that one person's knowledge of another person's emotional state through

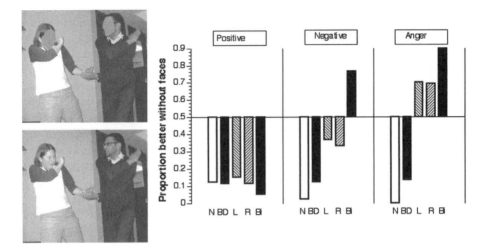

FIGURE 13.1. Recognition of emotion from emotional scenes with facial expressions or with erased faces. *Left:* Examples of the stimuli. *Right:* Performance accuracy in recognizing basic emotions. Bars going downward represent better accuracy on scenes with faces; bars going upward represent better accuracy on scenes with faces erased. Data are broken down for positive emotions, negative emotions, and anger. N, healthy comparison subjects; BD, brain-damaged subjects with no amygdala damage; L, R, subjects with unilateral left or right amygdala damage from surgical temporal lobectomy; Bi, subjects with complete bilateral amygdala damage. From Adolphs and Tranel (2003). Copyright 2003 by Elsevier. Reprinted by permission.

simulation of his or her presumed somatic state relies on a simulation that is explicit, in the sense of providing conscious access to the emotion being simulated. That is, the simulation mechanism through which one infers another person's emotion is empathic: It involves actually feeling (aspects of) the emotion of the other person.

In one study from our laboratory, we found evidence supporting a role for simulation in emotion recognition (Adolphs et al., 2000). In a lesion study of 108 patients with focal brain damage, it was found that lesions in right somatosensory cortices (including the insula) were associated with impairments in the ability to recognize emotion from other people's facial expressions. One interpretation of the findings was as follows: In order to trigger an image of the somatosensory state associated with an emotion, a viewer uses structures that link perception of the stimulus (the facial expression seen) to a somatic response (or directly to the representation thereof). One route for triggering such an emotional response to viewing another person's expression in the first place would be structures such as the amygdala.

This account of how one person might infer another's emotional state via an essentially simulation-based mechanism (Goldman & Sripada, 2005) has turned out to be an incomplete picture. A key recent insight has been that the generative nature of cognition is driven not only by the inferences made once sensory information has been perceived; it is driven also by the possibility of discovering new information in the environment in the first place. We humans explore our environment, and we actively seek out social information. This idea was borne out in a more recent study (Adolphs et al., 2005) of Patient S. M., who, as discussed above, is impaired in the ability to use information from a diagnostic facial feature—the eye region of the face. To establish this, we used a new technique to assess the use of visual information from faces (Gosselin & Schyns, 2001, 2002). The method is called "bubbles" and addresses an important open question: What is it about certain faces that makes them look fearful? This method, akin to reverse correlation, randomly samples a stimulus space to extract those components of the space that drive behavioral discrimination. We used a three-dimensional search space for faces: the two dimensions (x, y) of the image plane, plus a dimension of spatial frequency into which the face has been decomposed (Figure 13.2). Thus a given trial shows only randomly revealed areas of the face at each spatial frequency band, determined by the number of bubbles (e.g., the sample stimulus shown at the far bottom right of Plate 13.4 in color insert). The more bubbles there are, the more area of the face is revealed to a viewer. The viewer then makes a judgment based on what is revealed. Regressing performance across all the trials (the dependent measure) onto the bubbles masks used in each trial (the predictor variables) yields a z-score for each sampled region of the image space. The entire image search space can then be statistically thresholded to reveal those portions of the image search space at which there was a significant association between the part of the face that was revealed and performance accuracy.

In order to visualize this statistically thresholded search space, it is superimposed on a face base image (one of the images that was sampled in the first place). The result is what is shown in Plate 13.4a: Those regions of the face that are visible are the portions of the face search space within which there was a statistically reliable association (at $p < .05$) between showing that region

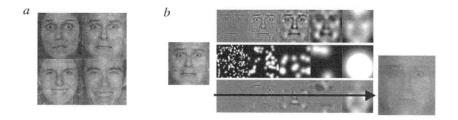

FIGURE 13.2. Construction of "bubbles" stimuli. (a) Four initial faces were normalized and (b) sampled at five bands of spatial frequencies to yield the final stimuli that subjects saw (far bottom right). Total bubbles provided were adjusted online to maintain performance throughout the task at 75% correct. From Adolphs et al. (2005). Copyright 2005 by the Nature Publishing Group. Reprinted by permission.

and the viewer's performance accuracy in classifying the stimulus as "happy" or "afraid." One interpretation of Plate 13.4a (in color insert) is that it depicts the visual information that viewers rely on to make judgments about the face. We found that S.M. failed to use the eye region of faces effectively in order to discriminate fear (Plate 13.4a).

These findings fit well with other results showing amygdala activation to fearful eyes (Morris, deBonis, & Dolan, 2002), or only to the briefly presented whites of eyes (Whalen et al., 2004). A further role for the amygdala in processing aspects of faces comes from studies of the interaction between facial emotion and eye gaze. The direction of eye gaze in other individuals' faces is an important source of information about their emotional state, intention, and likely future behavior. Eye gaze is a key social signal in many species (Emery, 2000), especially apes and humans, whose white sclera makes the pupil more easily visible and permits better discrimination of gaze. Human viewers make preferential fixations onto the eye region of others' faces (Janik, Wellens, Goldberg, & Dell'Osso, 1978)—a behavior that appears early in development and may contribute to the socioemotional impairments seen in such developmental disorders as autism (Baron-Cohen, 1995). Eyes signal important information about emotional states, and there is evidence from functional imaging studies that at least some of this processing recruits the amygdala (Baron-Cohen et al., 1999; Kawashima et al., 1999; Wicker, Perrett, Baron-Cohen, & Decety, 2003). The interaction between facial emotion and direction of eye gaze has been explored only very recently. It was found that direct gaze facilitated processing of approach-oriented emotions such as anger, whereas averted gaze facilitated the processing of avoidance-oriented emotions such as fear (Adams, Gordon, Baird, Ambady, & Kleck, 2003), and that this processing facilitation correlated with increased activation of the amygdala in a functional imaging study (Adams & Kleck, 2003).

In fact, we found that the deficit was even more basic: The reason why S. M. did not use information about the eye region effectively was that she did not fixate the eye region in the first place (Plate 13.4b). This finding is based on her eye-tracking performance during an emotion judgment task, to assess where she directed her gaze when viewing face stimuli. We instructed S. M. to direct her gaze onto the eyes of other people's faces, and found that this manipulation temporarily allowed her to generate a normal performance on a fear recognition task in which she was otherwise severely impaired. We could thus trace a causal chain from an impaired inclination spontaneously to fixate the eyes in other people's faces, to an impaired ability to make use of information from the eye region of faces, to our earlier reported impairments in judgments about the emotional and social nature of those faces (Adolphs et al., 1994, 1998).

It is worth noting two key further results from the study of patient S. M. described above (Adolphs et al., 2005). S. M. failed to fixate the eyes in any face, not just facial expressions of fear. In fact, she simply failed to explore faces in general, which included a failure to direct her gaze toward the eye region. We have attributed the finding that this general impairment resulted in a relatively specific impairment in fear recognition to the further fact that the eye region of the face is in fact the most diagnostic for signaling fear, rather than other emotions, on our discrimination task (Smith, Cottrell, Gosselin, & Schyns, 2005). Interestingly, unpublished data indicate that S. M. does fixate the eye region when the faces are shown inverted (Adolphs, Buchanan, & Tranel, unpublished data). So, while the brain does not first need to know that a face is showing fear in order for the impaired eye fixations to occur, it apparently does need to know that the stimulus is a face.

A second point worth noting is that the explicit instruction to fixate the eyes in faces, while rescuing S. M.'s impaired recognition of fear, did so only transiently (as long as that block of the experiment lasted). When later asked to view faces, S. M. spontaneously reverted to her lack of exploration of the face, and once again showed impaired fear recognition. One reason why the improvement was not more permanent may well be that S. M. was unaware that she failed to fixate the eyes, as she was unaware that her performance in fear recognition was impaired. This raises further questions: Why did she not ask about her performance? Why did she not notice that she failed to fixate the eyes? These questions point toward a broader interpretation of the impairment: S. M., as a result of damage to her amygdala, lacks a normal mechanism to explore the environment. One aspect of this impairment is a failure to fixate the eyes in faces, to explore them normally with her gaze. Another aspect of the impairment in this particular experiment was a failure to question what was going on in any way, or to monitor her own performance during the experiment. In both instances, there remains a passive ability to process sensory information, but the instrumental component of seeking out such information in the first place has been severely compromised. This interpretation is related to other proposals of amygdala function in social exploration (Sander et al., 2003) and stimulus disambiguation (Whalen, 1998), and fits also with the known role of the amygdala in modulating attention in both animals (Holland & Gallagher, 1999) and humans (Anderson & Phelps, 2001; Vuilleumier, Armony, Driver, & Dolan, 2001). It raises important open questions: Can the amygdala's role in decision making be formalized as a role in exploring new choice options? Is its role disproportionate for exploring social options, or does it play an entirely domain-general role in exploring options regardless of their social nature (Adolphs, 2003)?

It has been well established that the amygdala is critical for processing various aspects of emotion, and in particular for perceiving negative emotions such as fear. One question that has remained unanswered, though, is whether S. M. has a normal phenomenological experience of emotion, especially negative emotion. To explore this, we designed a study in which two experienced clinical psychologists who were not provided any background information regarding S. M. conducted interviews with her (Tranel, Gullickson, Koch, & Adolphs, 2006). The psychologists were asked to interview S. M. to determine whether she exhibited any psychopathology, with a special eye toward her emotional phenomenology. Both of them reached the conclusion that S. M. expressed a normal range of affect and emotion, and neither felt that she warranted a formal psychiatric diagnosis. However, they both noted that S. M. was remarkably dispassionate when relating highly emotional and traumatic life experiences, and they noted that she did not seem to have a normal sense of distrust and "danger." Indeed, to the psychologists, S. M. came across as a "survivor"—as being "resilient" and even "heroic" in the way she had dealt with adversity in her life. In full light, however, these observations reflect the fact that S. M. is missing from her phenomenology of life some of the deepest negative emotions, in a manner that parallels her defect in perceiving such emotions in external stimuli. These findings have interesting parallels with recent animal work (cf. Bauman et al., 2004b), and they provide valuable insights into the emotional life of an individual with complete bilateral amygdala damage.

AN INTEGRATIVE MODEL FOR THE SOCIAL FUNCTIONS OF THE HUMAN AMYGDALA

In this chapter, we have provided evidence for a model of amygdala function in social processing. On the basis of previous work suggesting a role for the amygdala in processing ambiguity and/or relevance (Sander et al., 2003; Whalen, 1998), we suggest that the social environment constitutes an especially ambiguous set of stimuli, and that the amygdala is critically involved in the disambiguation of such sets of stimuli. This model provides a parsimonious account of data from lesion studies of nonhuman primates and humans, as well as from neurophysiology and functional neuroimaging studies. The framework treats the amygdala as making a contribution to the motivation to seek out certain stimuli, or certain features of stimuli, at the expense of others. This role may well be analogous to a filter (enabling an individual to disregard information that is irrelevant), and it may also involve actively seeking out information. Together, these components can specify what is salient in the environment—what needs to be paid attention to, what should be assigned priority for further processing, and what stimuli have a premium on behavioral modulation.

The prediction and comprehension of others' behavior are clearly extremely important aspects of social functioning. There are any number of ways that conspecifics—whether they are rhesus monkey cage mates or coworkers in an office—may behave. The accurate recognition of conspecific behavior may proceed without explicit awareness in healthy individuals. An inability to understand the ambiguous behavior of others could produce profound deficits in social functioning, as evidenced by monkeys with early-onset bilateral amygdala damage. The altered affiliation and social withdrawal behaviors of these animals may reflect the inability to make sense of socially relevant situations without a functioning amygdala. It is perhaps no surprise, then, that one of the hallmarks of proper social development is a predictable (unambiguous) relationship between a mother and infant (Bowlby, 1969). The descriptions of monkeys with neonatal amygdala lesions demonstrate abnormal relationships between infants and mothers initially, and this abnormality is later evidenced between these infants and their peers (Bauman et al., 2004a, 2004b). It is an intriguing possibility that such altered relationships between mothers and amygdala-damaged infants set the stage for later abnormalities in social behavior.

The instrumental role for the amygdala in seeking out potentially relevant social information we have sketched above needs, of course, to be situated with the amygdala as one component in a distributed neural system. Given the evidence for fast subcortical visual inputs to the amygdala (Johnson, 2005), as well as slower but more fine-grained visual information conveyed through cortical routes (Amaral et al., 1992), an important open question concerns the point in time at which the amygdala comes into play. There are rapid visually evoked responses even to fairly complex social scenes (Oya, Kawasaki, Howard, & Adolphs, 2002), demonstrating that at least some superordinate categorization of such stimuli in terms of their social meaning can occur within about 120 msec. One possibility is that the amygdala's modulation of eye movements and visual attention, perhaps in part via its projections back to visual cortices, comes into play very early and depends largely on subcortical visual inputs. This would make it possible, in principle, for the amygdala to modulate visual attentional processing in visual cortices (Anderson & Phelps, 2001; Vuilleumier et al., 2004) at the earliest processing times—before the cortical information has even reached the amygdala. This attentional modulation at early processing times by the amygdala may then be followed by a longer-latency role, based on cortical visual inputs as well as contextual modulation and self-regulation, in which it triggers emotional responses and participates in a simulation-based reconstruction of social information. It would seem likely that these two components depend, moreover, on separate nuclei within the amygdala.

WHAT WE THINK

This chapter raises two potentially conflicting views. Clearly, the amygdala is important for aspects of social cognition and social behavior; equally clearly, it is involved in aspects of attention, emotion, and memory that have nothing at all to do with social behavior (e.g., fear conditioning). So does the amygdala contribute something essential that is specific to social cognition? If so, what?

As we speculate on answers to this question, two points are worth making. Given the many functions in which the amygdala has been implicated, and given that it consists of over a dozen nuclei in primates, it will participate in both social and nonsocial aspects of cognition and behavior. Nonetheless, the question above

remains: Are there some aspects of amygdala function that are socially specialized? The second point is that it is not clear that there is any aspect of social
cognition that does not have a nonsocial basis. Nonetheless, the question remains
whether certain features of social cognition make processing demands unlike those
posed by nonsocial stimuli.

Rather than trying to identify a single aspect of information processing that
might distinguish social cognition and the amygdala's role in it, we may do better to acknowledge that social cognition is distinguished by the sheer variety of
processes that come into play, and the way in which they need to be integrated.
We are reminded here of the hodological analysis of Young, Scannell, Burns, and
Blakemore (1994), which represents the amygdala as centrally connected in a multidimensional scaling representation. By modulating social cognition at the earliest
times as well as at later times, at attention, perception, memory, decision making,
and emotional reaction, the amygdala may be particularly well positioned to contribute what is the hallmark of social cognition: modulating all of cognition.

ACKNOWLEDGMENTS

We thank J. Michael Tyszka for help with the images shown in Plates 13.2 and 13.3,
and Hanna Damasio for help with the images shown in Plate 13.1.

REFERENCES

Adams, R. B., Gordon, H. L., Baird, A. A., Ambady, N., & Kleck, R. E. (2003). Effects
of gaze on amygdala sensitivity to anger and fear faces. *Science, 300,* 1536.
Adams, R. B., & Kleck, R. E. (2003). Perceived gaze direction and the processing of
facial displays of emotion. *Psychological Science, 14,* 644–647.
Adolphs, R. (2002). Recognizing emotion from facial expressions: Psychological and
neurological mechanisms. *Behavioral and Cognitive Neuroscience Reviews, 1,*
21–61.
Adolphs, R. (2003). Cognitive neuroscience of human social behavior. *Nature Reviews
Neuroscience, 4,* 165–178.
Adolphs, R., Damasio, H., Tranel, D., Cooper, G., & Damasio, A. R. (2000). A role
for somatosensory cortices in the visual recognition of emotion as revealed by
three-dimensional lesion mapping. *Journal of Neuroscience, 20*(7), 2683–2690.
Adolphs, R., Gosselin, F., Buchanan, T. W., Tranel, D., Schyns, P., & Damasio, A.
R. (2005). A mechanism for impaired fear recognition after amygdala damage.
Nature, 433, 68–72.
Adolphs, R., & Tranel, D. (1999). Intact recognition of emotional prosody following
amygdala damage. *Neuropsychologia, 37*(11), 1285–1292.
Adolphs, R., & Tranel, D. (2000). Emotion recognition and the human amygdala. In
J.P. Aggleton (Ed.), *The amygdala: A functional analysis* (2nd ed., pp. 587–630).
Oxford, UK: Oxford University Press. Pp. 587–630.
Adolphs, R., & Tranel, D. (2003). Amygdala damage impairs emotion recognition
from scenes only when they contain facial expressions. *Neuropsychologia,
41*(10), 1281–1289.

Adolphs, R., Tranel, D., & Baron-Cohen, S. (2002). Amygdala damage impairs recognition of social emotions from facial expressions. *Journal of Cognitive Neuroscience, 14*, 1264–1274.

Adolphs, R., Tranel, D., & Damasio, A. R. (1998). The human amygdala in social judgment. *Nature, 393*, 470–474.

Adolphs, R., Tranel, D., Damasio, H., & Damasio, A. (1994). Impaired recognition of emotion in facial expressions following bilateral damage to the human amygdala. *Nature, 372*, 669–672.

Aggleton, J. P. (Ed.). (1992). *The amygdala: Neurobiological aspects of emotion, memory, and mental dysfunction.* New York: Wiley-Liss.

Aggleton, J. P. (Ed.). (2000). *The amygdala: A functional analysis* (2nd ed.). Oxford, UK: Oxford University Press.

Amaral, D. G., Price, J. L., Pitkanen, A., & Carmichael, S. T. (1992). Anatomical organization of the primate amygdaloid complex. In J. P. Aggleton (Ed.), *The amygdala: Neurobiological aspects of emotion, memory, and mental dysfunction* (pp. 1–66). New York: Wiley-Liss.

Anderson, A. K., & Phelps, E. A. (1998a). *Bilateral amygdala damage impairs evaluation of facial but not vocal expressions of fear.* Paper presented at the annual meeting of the Cognitive Neuroscience Society, San Francisco.

Anderson, A. K., & Phelps, E. A. (1998b). Intact recognition of vocal expressions of fear following bilateral lesions of the human amygdala. *NeuroReport, 9*(16), 3607–3613.

Anderson, A. K., & Phelps, E. A. (2000). Expression without recognition: Contributions of the human amygdala to emotional communication. *Psychological Science, 11*(2), 106–111.

Anderson, A. K., & Phelps, E. A. (2001). Lesions of the human amygdala impair enhanced perception of emotionally salient events. *Nature, 411*, 305–309.

Atkinson, A. P., Dittrich, W. H., Gemmell, A. J., & Young, A. W. (2004). Emotion perception from dynamic and static body expressions in point-light and full-light displays. *Perception, 33*(6), 717–746.

Babinsky, R., Calabrese, P., Durwen, H. F., Markowitsch, H. J., Brechtelsbauer, D., Heuser, L., et al. (1993). The possible contribution of the amygdala to memory. *Behavioural Neurology, 6*, 167–170.

Baron-Cohen, S. (1995). *Mindblindness: An essay on autism and theory of mind.* Cambridge, MA: MIT Press.

Baron-Cohen, S., Ring, H. A., Bullmore, E. T., Wheelwright, S., Ashwin, C., & Williams, S. C. (2000). The amygdala theory of autism. *Neuroscience and Biobehavioral Reviews, 24*(3), 355–364.

Baron-Cohen, S., Ring, H. A., Wheelwright, S., Bullmore, E. T., Brammer, M. J., Simmons, A., et al. (1999). Social intelligence in the normal and autistic brain: An fMRI study. *European Journal of Neuroscience, 11*(6), 1891–1898.

Bauman, M. D., Lavenex, P., Mason, W. A., Capitanio, J. P., & Amaral, D. G. (2004a). The development of mother–infant interactions after neonatal amygdala lesions in rhesus monkeys. *Journal of Neuroscience, 24*(3), 711–721.

Bauman, M. D., Lavenex, P., Mason, W. A., Capitanio, J. P., & Amaral, D. G. (2004b). The development of social behavior following neonatal amygdala lesions in rhesus monkeys. *Journal of Cognitive Neuroscience, 16*(8), 1388–1411.

Bonda, E., Petrides, M., Ostry, D., & Evans, A. (1996). Specific involvement of human parietal systems and the amygdala in the perception of biological motion. *Journal of Neuroscience, 16*(11), 3737–3744.

Bowlby, J. (1969). *Attachment and loss: Vol. 1. Attachment.* London: Hogarth Press.

Brothers, L., & Ring, B. (1993). Mesial temporal neurons in the macaque monkey with responses selective for aspects of social stimuli. *Behavioural Brain Research, 57*(1), 53–61.

Brothers, L., Ring, B., & Kling, A. (1990). Response of neurons in the macaque amygdala to complex social stimuli. *Behavioural Brain Research, 41*(3), 199–213.

Brown, S., & Schafer, A. (1888). An investigation in the functions of the occipital and temporal lobes of the monkey's brain. *Philosophical Transactions of the Royal Society of London, 179,* 303–327.

Buchanan, T. W., & Adolphs, R. (2004). The neuroanatomy of emotional memory in humans. In D. Reisberg & P. Hertel (Eds.), *Memory and emotion* (pp. 42–75). New York: Oxford University Press.

Buchanan, T. W., Lutz, K., Mirzazade, S., Specht, K., Shah, N. J., Zilles, K., et al. (2000). Recognition of emotional prosody and verbal components of spoken language: an fMRI study. *Brain Research: Cognitive Brain Research, 9*(3), 227–238.

Calder, A. J., Young, A. W., Perrett, D. I., Etcoff, N. L., & Rowland, D. (1996). Categorical perception of morphed facial expressions. *Visual Cognition, 3,* 81–117.

Calder, A. J., Young, A. W., Rowland, D., & Perrett, D. I. (1996). Facial emotion recognition after bilateral amygdala damage: Differentially severe impairment of fear. *Cognitive Neuropsychology, 13,* 699–745.

Craig, A. D. (2002). How do you feel?: Interoception—the sense of the physiological condition of the body. *Nature Reviews Neuroscience, 3,* 655–666.

Critchley, H. D., Wiens, S., Rotshtein, P., Oehman, A., & Dolan, R. J. (2004). Neural systems supporting interoceptive awareness. *Nature Neuroscience, 7,* 189–195.

Damasio, A. R. (1999). *The feeling of what happens: Body and emotion in the making of consciousness.* New York: Harcourt, Brace.

Davidson, R. J., & Irwin, W. (1999). The functional neuroanatomy of emotion and affective style. *Trends in Cognitive Sciences, 3*(1), 11–21.

de Gelder, B., Snyder, J., Greve, D., Gerard, G., & Hadjikhani, N. (2004). Fear fosters flight: A mechanism for fear contagion when perceiving emotion expressed by a whole body. *Proceedings of the National Academy of Sciences USA, 101,* 16701–16706.

Dicks, D., Myers, R. E., & Kling, A. (1968). Uncus and amygdala lesions: Effects on social behavior in the free-ranging rhesus monkey. *Science, 165,* 69–71.

Dolan, R. J., Morris, J. S., & de Gelder, B. (2001). Crossmodal binding of fear in voice and face. *Proceedings of the National Academy of Sciences USA, 98,* 10006–10010.

Drevets, W. C. (2000). Neuroimaging studies of mood disorders. *Biological Psychiatry, 48,* 813–829.

Emery, N. J. (2000). The eyes have it: The neuroethology, function and evolution of social gaze. *Neuroscience and Biobehavioral Reviews, 24,* 581–604.

Emery, N. J., & Amaral, D. G. (1999). The role of the amygdala in primate social cognition. In R. D. Lane & L. Nadel (Eds.), *Cognitive neuroscience of emotion* (pp. 156–191). Oxford, UK: Oxford University Press.

Emery, N. J., Capitanio, J. P., Mason, W. A., Machado, C. J., Mendoza, S. P., & Amaral, D. G. (2001). The effects of bilateral lesions of the amygdala on dyadic social interactions in rhesus monkeys (*Macaca mulatta*). *Behavioral Neuroscience, 115*(3), 515–544.

Ethofer, T., Anders, S., Erb, M., Droll, C., Royen, L., Saur, R., et al. (2006). Impact of voice on emotional judgment of faces: An event-related fMRI study. *Human Brain Mapping, 27*(9), 707–714.

Fine, C., Lumsden, J., & Blair, R. J. R. (2001). Dissociation between `theory of mind' and executive functions in a patient with early left amygdala damage. *Brain, 124*, 287–298.

Fried, I., MacDonald, K. A., & Wilson, C. L. (1997). Single neuron activity in human hippocampus and amygdala during recognition of faces and objects. *Neuron, 18*(5), 753–765.

Gil-da-Costa, R., Braun, A., Lopes, M., Hauser, M. D., Carson, R. E., Herscovitch, P., et al. (2004). Toward an evolutionary perspective on conceptual representation: Species-specific calls activate visual and affective processing systems in the macaque. *Proceedings of the National Academy of Sciences USA, 101*, 17516–17521.

Golby, A. J., Gabrieli, J. D. E., Chiao, J. Y., & Eberhardt, J. L. (2001). Differential responses in the fusiform region to same-race and other-race faces. *Nature Neuroscience, 4*, 845–850.

Goldman, A. I., & Sripada, C. S. (2005). Simulationist models of face-based emotion recognition. *Cognition, 94*(3), 193–213.

Gosselin, F., & Schyns, P. G. (2001). Bubbles: A technique to reveal the use of information in recognition. *Vision Research, 41*, 2261–2271.

Gosselin, F., & Schyns, P. G. (2002). RAP: A new framework for visual categorization. *Trends in Cognitive Sciences, 6*, 70–78.

Gottfried, J. A., O'Doherty, J., & Dolan, R. J. (2002). Appetitive and aversive olfactory learning in humans studied using event-related functional magnetic resonance imaging. *Journal of Neuroscience, 22*, 10829–10837.

Hadjikhani, N., & de Gelder, B. (2003). Seeing fearful body expressions activates the fusiform cortex and amygdala. *Current Biology, 13*, 2201–2205.

Hamada, T., McLean, W. H., Ramsay, M., Ashton, G. H., Nanda, A., Jenkins, T., et al. (2002). Lipoid proteinosis maps to 1q21 and is caused by mutations in the extracellular matrix protein 1 gene (ECM1). *Human Molecular Genetics, 11*, 833–840.

Hart, A. J., Whalen, P. J., Shin, L. M., McInerney, S. C., Fischer, H., & Rauch, S. L. (2000). Differential response in the human amygdala to racial outgroup vs. ingroup face stimuli. *NeuroReport, 11*, 2351–2355.

Hofer, P.-A. (1973). Urbach–Wiethe disease: A review. *Acta Dermato-Venereologica, 53*, 5–52.

Holland, P. C., & Gallagher, M. (1999). Amygdala circuitry in attentional and representational processes. *Trends in Cognitive Sciences, 3*(2), 65–73.

Jackson, P. L., Meltzoff, A. N., & Decety, J. (2005). How do we perceive the pain of others?: A window into the neural processes involved in empathy. *NeuroImage, 24*(3), 771–779.

Janik, S. W., Wellens, A. R., Goldberg, M. L., & Dell'Osso, L. F. (1978). Eyes as the center of focus in the visual examination of human faces. *Perceptual and Motor Skills, 47*, 857–858.

Johnson, M. H. (2005). Subcortical face processing. *Nature Reviews Neuroscience,* 6, 766–774.

Kawashima, R., Sugiura, M., Kato, T., Nakamura, A., Natano, K., Ito, K., et al. (1999). The human amygdala plays an important role in gaze monitoring. *Brain,* 122, 779–783.

Kling, A. S., & Brothers, L. A. (1992). The amygdala and social behavior. In J. P. Aggleton (Ed.), *The amygdala: Neurobiological aspects of emotion, memory, and mental dysfunction.* New York: Wiley-Liss.

Kling, A. S., Steklis, H. D., & Deutsch, S. (1979). Radiotelemetered activity from the amygdala during social interactions in the monkey. *Experimental Neurology,* 66(1), 88–96.

Klüver, H., & Bucy, P. C. (1937). "Psychic blindness" and other symptoms following bilateral temporal lobectomy in rhesus monkeys. *American Journal of Physiology,* 119, 352–353.

Knuepfer, M. M., Eismann, A., Schutze, I., Stumpf, H., & Stock, G. (1995). Responses of single neurons in amygdala to interoceptive and exteroceptive stimuli in conscious cats. *American Journal of Physiology,* 268(3, Pt. 2), R666–R675.

LeDoux, J. E., Farb, C. F., & Ruggiero, D. A. (1990). Topographic organization of neurons in the acoustic thalamus that project to the amygdala. *Journal of Neuroscience,* 10, 1043–1054.

Leonard, C. M., Rolls, E. T., Wilson, F. A., & Baylis, G. C. (1985). Neurons in the amygdala of the monkey with responses selective for faces. *Behavioural Brain Research,* 15(2), 159–176.

Lloyd, R. L., & Kling, A. S. (1991). Delta activity from amygdala in squirrel monkeys (*Saimiri sciureus*): Influence of social and environmental context. *Behavioral Neuroscience,* 105(2), 223–229.

Markowitsch, H. J., Calabrese, P., Wuerker, M., Durwen, H. F., Kessler, J., Babinsky, R., et al. (1994). The amygdala's contribution to memory: A study on two patients with Urbach–Wiethe disease. *NeuroReport,* 5, 1349–1352.

McGaugh, J. L., Cahill, L., & Roozendaal, B. (1996). Involvement of the amygdala in memory storage: Interaction with other brain systems. *Proceedings of the National Academy of Sciences USA,* 93, 13508–13514.

Morris, J. S., deBonis, M., & Dolan, R. J. (2002). Human amygdala responses to fearful eyes. *NeuroImage,* 17, 214–222.

Morris, J. S., Friston, K. J., Büchel, C., Frith, C. D., Young, A. W., Calder, A. J., et al. (1998). A neuromodulatory role for the human amygdala in processing emotional facial expressions. *Brain,* 121(Pt. 1), 47–57.

Morris, J. S., Frith, C. D., Perrett, D. I., Rowland, D., Young, A. W., Calder, A. J., et al. (1996). A differential neural response in the human amygdala to fearful and happy facial expressions. *Nature,* 383, 812–815.

Morris, J. S., Scott, S. K., & Dolan, R. J. (1999). Saying it with feeling: Neural responses to emotional vocalizations. *Neuropsychologia,* 37(10), 1155–1163.

Murray, E. A., & Mishkin, M. (1985). Amygdalectomy impairs crossmodal association in monkeys. *Science,* 228, 604–606.

Nahm, F. K. D., Tranel, D., Damasio, H., & Damasio, A. R. (1993). Cross-modal associations and the human amygdala. *Neuropsychologia,* 31, 727–744.

Oya, H., Kawasaki, H., Howard, M. A., & Adolphs, R. (2002). Electrophysiological responses in the human amygdala discriminate emotion categories of complex visual stimuli. *Journal of Neuroscience,* 22, 9502–9512.

Phelps, E. A., Cannistraci, C. J., & Cunningham, W. A. (2003). Intact performance on an indirect measure of race bias following amygdala damage. *Neuropsychologia, 41*, 203–209.

Phelps, E. A., O'Connor, K. J., Cunningham, W. A., Funayama, E. S., Gatenby, J. C., Gore, J. C., et al. (2000). Performance on indirect measures of race evaluation predicts amygdala activation. *Journal of Cognitive Neuroscience, 12*, 729–738.

Phillips, M. L., Young, A. W., Scott, S. K., Calder, A. J., Andrew, C., Giampietro, V., et al. (1998). Neural responses to facial and vocal expressions of fear and disgust. *Proceedings of the Royal Society of London, Series B, 265*, 1809–1817.

Preti, G., & Wysocki, C. J. (1999). Human pheromones: Releasers or primers—fact or myth. In R. E. Johnston, D. Muller-Schwarze, & P. Sorenson (Eds.), *Advances in chemical signals in vertebrates* (Vol. 8, pp. 315–331). New York: Plenum Press.

Richardson, M. P., Strange, B. A., & Dolan, R. J. (2004). Encoding of emotional memories depends on amygdala and hippocampus and their interactions. *Nature Neuroscience, 7*, 278–285.

Rosvold, H. E., Mirsky, A. F., & Pribram, K. (1954). Influence of amygdalectomy on social behavior in monkeys. *Journal of Comparative and Physiological Psychology, 47*, 173–178.

Sander, D., Grafman, J., & Zalla, T. (2003). The human amygdala: An evolved system for relevance detection. *Review of Neuroscience, 14*(4), 303–316.

Sander, K., & Scheich, H. (2001). Auditory perception of laughing and crying activates human amygdala regardless of attentional state. *Brain Research: Cognitive Brain Research, 12*(2), 181–198.

Savic, I., Gulyas, B., Larsson, M., & Roland, P. (2000). Olfactory functions are mediated by parallel and hierarchical processing. *Neuron, 26*(3), 735–745.

Scott, S. K., Young, A. W., Calder, A. J., Hellawell, D. J., Aggleton, J. P., & Johnson, M. (1997). Impaired auditory recognition of fear and anger following bilateral amygdala lesions. *Nature, 385*, 254–257.

Siebert, M., Markowitsch, H. J., & Bartel, P. (2003). Amygdala, affect and cognition: Evidence from 10 patients with Urbach–Wiethe disease. *Brain, 126*, 2627–2637.

Singer, T., Seymour, B., O'Doherty, J., Kaube, H., Dolan, R. J., & Frith, C. D. (2004). Empathy for pain involves the affective but not sensory components of pain. *Science, 303*, 1157–1162.

Smith, M. L., Cottrell, G. W., Gosselin, F., & Schyns, P. G. (2005). Transmitting and decoding facial expressions. *Psychological Science, 16*, 184–189.

Thompson, C. I., Bergland, R. M., & Towfighi, J. T. (1977). Social and nonsocial behaviors of adult rhesus monkeys after amygdalectomy in infancy or adulthood. *Journal of Comparative and Physiological Psychology, 91*(3), 533–548.

Tranel, D., Gullickson, G., Koch, M., & Adolphs, R. (2006). Altered experience of emotion following bilateral amygdala damage. *Cognitive Neuropsychiatry, 11*, 219–232.

Tranel, D., & Hyman, B. T. (1990). Neuropsychological correlates of bilateral amygdala damage. *Archives of Neurology, 47*(3), 349–355.

Vuilleumier, P., Armony, J. L., Driver, J., & Dolan, R. J. (2001). Effects of attention and emotion on face processing in the human brain: An event-related fMRI study. *Neuron, 30*, 829–841.

Vuilleumier, P., Richardson, M. P., Armony, J. L., Driver, J., & Dolan, R. J. (2004). Distant influences of amygdala lesion on visual cortical activation during emotional face processing. *Nature Neuroscience, 7*, 1271–1278.

318 HUMAN AMYGDALA FUNCTION

Weiskrantz, L. (1956). Behavioral changes associated with ablation of the amygdaloid complex in monkeys. *Journal of Comparative and Physiological Psychology, 49,* 381–391.

Whalen, P. J. (1998). Fear, vigilance, and ambiguity: Initial neuroimaging studies of the human amygdala. *Current Directions in Psychological Science, 7,* 177–188.

Whalen, P. J., Kagan, J., Cook, R. G., Davis, F. C., Kim, H., Polis, S., et al. (2004). Human amygdala responsivity to masked fearful eye whites. *Science, 306,* 2061.

Whalen, P. J., Shin, L. M., McInerney, S. C., Fischer, H., Wright, C. I., & Rauch, S. L. (2001). A functional MRI study of human amygdala responses to facial expressions of fear versus anger. *Emotion, 1,* 70–83.

Wicker, B., Perrett, D. I., Baron-Cohen, S., & Decety, J. (2003). Being the target of another's emotion: A PET study. *Neuropsychologia, 41,* 139–146.

Wildgruber, D., Hertrich, I., Riecker, A., Erb, M., Anders, S., Grodd, W., et al. (2004). Distinct frontal regions subserve evaluation of linguistic and emotional aspects of speech intonation. *Cerebral Cortex, 14*(12), 1384–1389.

Wildgruber, D., Pihan, H., Ackermann, H., Erb, M., & Grodd, W. (2002). Dynamic brain activation during processing of emotional intonation: Influence of acoustic parameters, emotional valence, and sex. *NeuroImage, 15*(4), 856–869.

Winston, J. S., Strange, B. A., O'Doherty, J., & Dolan, R. J. (2002). Automatic and intentional brain responses during evaluation of trustworthiness of faces. *Nature Neuroscience, 5*(3), 277–283.

Young, A. W., Aggleton, J. P., Hellawell, D. J., Johnson, M., Broks, P., & Hanley, J. R. (1995). Face processing impairments after amygdalotomy. *Brain, 118*(Pt. 1), 15–24.

Young, M. P., Scannell, J. W., Burns, G. A., & Blakemore, C. (1994). Analysis of connectivity: Neural systems in the cerebral cortex. *Review of Neuroscience, 5*(3), 227–250.

Zald, D. H., & Pardo, J. V. (1997). Emotion, olfaction, and the human amygdala: Amygdala activation during aversive olfactory stimulation. *Proceedings of the National Academy of Sciences USA, 94*(8), 4119–4124.

PART III

Human Amygdala Dysfunction

CHAPTER 14

The Human Amygdala
in Anxiety Disorders

*Lisa M. Shin, Scott L. Rauch, Roger K. Pitman,
and Paul J. Whalen*

As has been demonstrated by decades of research in the field of neuropsychology, our understanding of normal brain function can often be enhanced by studying patients in whom brain function and behavior go awry. In order to better understand the function of the healthy human amygdala, researchers have attempted to characterize how amygdala function may be altered in neuropsychiatric disease. Data indicating abnormal amygdala function in neuropsychiatric disease may also (1) inform neurocircuitry models of such disorders, (2) suggest neurotransmitter systems to target via pharmacotherapy, and (3) assist in diagnosis or in the prediction of treatment response.

Over the past decade, neuroimaging techniques have been critical to assessing amygdala function in neuropsychiatric disease. In the current chapter, we first describe the basic paradigms used to study amygdala function in patients with anxiety disorders. Next, we review findings from studies using functional magnetic resonance imaging (fMRI), positron emission tomography (PET), single-photon emission computed tomography (SPECT), structural magnetic resonance imaging (MRI), and magnetic resonance spectroscopy (MRS) to assess the function, structure, and neurochemistry of the amygdala in posttraumatic stress disorder (PTSD), panic disorder (PD), social phobia (SP), and obsessive–compulsive disorder (OCD). In separate sections, we describe the symptoms of each disorder, as well as relevant neurocircuitry models. Finally, we offer a summary and discuss future possible directions of this research.

PARADIGMS

Several different functional neuroimaging paradigms have been used to assess brain function in anxiety disorders. Neutral state paradigms involve studying participants while they rest quietly or perform simple continuous performance tasks in the scanner. Such studies typically involve using PET or SPECT to measure regional cerebral blood flow or glucose metabolic rate. In this type of paradigm, data from patients and comparison subjects are directly compared. Neutral state paradigms have been used frequently to assess treatment-related changes in brain activity.

Symptom provocation paradigms involve studying patients during symptomatic and neutral states, which can be achieved via exposure to feared and neutral stimuli, respectively. Brain activation differences between conditions are assessed, and the resulting functional contrast images are then compared between patient and comparison groups. Correlations between activation in a given region and symptom severity can be assessed and are particularly helpful in determining the possible clinical relevance of a functional neuroimaging finding. Although most commonly conducted with PET and SPECT, this type of paradigm has also successfully been carried out with fMRI.

In cognitive activation studies, participants perform validated cognitive tasks that are designed to activate a priori regions of interest. The behavioral data (e.g., response times and accuracy) and activation in the region of interest (as well as in other regions) are compared between groups. For example, in order to examine amygdala function in anxiety and mood disorders, researchers have presented facial expressions (e.g., fearful vs. happy or angry vs. neutral) to patients and healthy comparison subjects. As noted above, correlations between symptom severity and degree of activation of a region of interest (e.g., the amygdala) may be particularly powerful demonstrations of the relevance of the functional neuroimaging finding to the clinical picture of the disorder in question.

NEUROIMAGING FINDINGS

Posttraumatic Stress Disorder

PTSD can occur in individuals who have experienced an event (or events) involving death or threat of death or serious injury and who have reacted with intense fear, helplessness or horror (American Psychiatric Association [APA], 2000). PTSD is marked by unwanted reexperiencing of the traumatic event, avoidance of traumatic reminders, emotional numbing, and hyperarousal (APA, 2000). This disorder may affect up to 14% of persons exposed to trauma (Breslau et al., 1998; Kessler, Sonnega, Bromet, Hughes, & Nelson, 1995), although prevalence rates can be even higher in some traumatized groups, such as Vietnam combat veterans and survivors of childhood sexual abuse (Ackerman, Newton, McPherson, Jones, & Dykman, 1998; Dohrenwend et al., 2006). Given the symptoms of hypervigilance, exaggerated startle, and intense distress in response to traumatic reminders, and considering the role of fear conditioning in PTSD, many researchers have hypothesized that the amygdala may be hyperresponsive in this disorder (e.g., Rauch, Shin, & Phelps, 2006; Shin, Rauch, & Pitman, 2006). According to one neurocircuitry model of PTSD, a hyperresponsive amygdala fails to be inhibited by a hyporesponsive medial prefrontal cortex (mPFC) (Rauch, Shin, Whalen, & Pitman, 1998). Similar models have been described elsewhere (Elzinga & Bremner, 2002; Hamner, Lorberbaum, & George, 1999; Layton & Krikorian, 2002).

Amygdala Function

Amygdala hyperresponsivity in PTSD has been observed during the presentation of idiographic traumatic narratives or cues (Driessen et al., 2004; Rauch et al., 1996; Shin et al., 2004), combat sounds (Liberzon et al., 1999; Pissiota et al., 2002), combat photographs (Hendler et al., 2003; Shin et al., 1997), and trauma-related words (Protopopescu et al., 2005). Exaggerated amygdala activation in PTSD also occurs in response to trauma-unrelated, emotional material, such as fearful facial expressions (Rauch et al., 2000; Shin et al., 2005; Williams et al., 2006), but not to trauma-unrelated aversive photographs in one study (Phan, Britton, Taylor, Fig, & Liberzon, 2006). Studies have also demonstrated heightened amygdala activity in the resting state (Chung et al., 2006), as well as during the performance of neutral, nonemotional auditory oddball and continuous performance tasks in PTSD (Bryant et al., 2005; Semple et al., 2000).

Importantly, amygdala activation has been shown to be positively correlated with PTSD symptom severity (Armony, Corbo, Clement, & Brunet, 2005; Protopopescu et al., 2005; Rauch et al., 1996; Shin et al., 2004) and self-reported anxiety (Fredrikson & Furmark, 2003; Pissiota et al., 2002) in several studies. Four studies have reported significant correlations between amygdala and mPFC activation (Gilboa et al., 2004; Shin et al., 2004, 2005; Williams et al., 2006), although the findings are mixed with regard to the direction of this correlation. Whether amygdala responses habituate normally in PTSD is currently unclear (Protopopescu et al., 2005; Shin et al., 2005; Williams et al., 2006); future research is very likely to address this issue further.

Given the important role of the amygdala in fear conditioning (see Öhman, Chapter 6, this volume), as well as evidence for heightened acquisition of conditioned fear in PTSD (Orr et al., 2000; Peri, Ben-Shakhar, Orr, & Shalev, 2000), researchers have become interested in studying amygdala function during fear conditioning and extinction in patients with PTSD (Rauch et al., 2006). One recent PET study has shown amygdala hyperresponsivity during the acquisition of fear conditioning in abuse survivors with PTSD, compared to healthy control subjects without abuse histories (Bremner et al., 2005). Future studies promise to extend this work by using fMRI and trauma-exposed comparison groups without PTSD.

We qualify the review above with a reminder that not all functional neuroimaging studies have found exaggerated amygdala activation in PTSD (Bremner, Innis, et al., 1997; Bremner, Narayan, et al., 1999; Bremner, Staib, et al., 1999; Lanius et al., 2001; Shin et al., 1999). Nonreplication of this finding may be attributable to poor temporal or spatial resolution (e.g., in SPECT or PET), inadequate symptom provocation, or Type II error associated with small sample sizes. Other potential contributors to interparticipant variability in amygdala activation may include variable symptom profiles (e.g., patients with predominant avoidance/numbing symptoms vs. reexperiencing/hyperarousal symptoms), differing degrees of regulatory input from the mPFC, and/or the presence of genetic variants (e.g., polymorphisms of the human serotonin transporter gene) (Furmark et al., 2004; Hariri et al., 2005; Pezawas et al., 2005). However, numerous functional neuroimaging studies of PTSD have provided compelling evidence in support of amygdala hyperresponsivity, as well as a positive relationship between amygdala activation and PTSD symptom severity.

Amygdala Structure and Neurochemistry

Relatively few studies have focused on examining amygdala volumes or neurochemistry in PTSD. One study reported smaller amygdala volumes in breast cancer survivors with intrusive recollections than in survivors without such recollections, although none of the participants met diagnostic criteria for PTSD (Matsuoka, Yamawaki, Inagaki, Akechi, & Uchitomi, 2003). Two studies found trends for smaller left amygdala volumes in patients with PTSD than in trauma-unexposed healthy comparison groups (Bremner, Randall, et al., 1997; Wignall et al., 2004; see also Karl et al., 2006). Most other studies that examined amygdala volumes found no significant differences between PTSD and comparison groups (Bonne et al., 2001; De Bellis, Hall, Boring, Frustaci, & Moritz, 2001; De Bellis et al., 2002; Fennema-Notestine, Stein, Kennedy, Archibald, & Jernigan, 2002; Gilbertson et al., 2002; Gurvits et al., 1996; Lindauer, Vlieger, et al., 2004). One recent study using PET and [¹¹C]carfentanil has reported diminished mu-opioid receptor binding in the extended amygdala in trauma-exposed individuals with versus without PTSD (Liberzon et al., 2007).

Morphometric studies have typically quantified total amygdala volume. However, the amygdala is composed of functionally distinct subnuclei (Davis & Whalen, 2001; LeDoux, 2000), and current techniques may be insensitive to differences therein. New techniques that enable the measurement of these subnuclei may reveal volumetric differences between groups. Additional research using larger cohorts and more uniform volumetric methodologies will be necessary before we can draw conclusions about amygdala structure and neurochemistry in PTSD and how those measures are related to amygdala function in this disorder.

Panic Disorder

A panic attack is an episode of intense fear and sympathetic nervous system arousal that occurs in the absence of true danger in the environment (APA, 2000). Panic attacks are fairly common in the general population, although the prevalence of PD is substantially lower (Kessler et al., 2006). Individuals who meet diagnostic criteria for PD experience recurrent, unexpected panic attacks, along with persistent concern about possible implications or consequences of the attacks (APA, 2000).

Neurocircuitry models of PD involve some of the same brain systems implicated in fear conditioning and PTSD (Coplan & Lydiard, 1998; Gorman, Kent, Sullivan, & Coplan, 2000; Rauch, Shin, & Wright, 2003). According to such models, the "fear network" (including the amygdala, hippocampus, thalamus, and brainstem structures) is hypersensitive. Furthermore, frontal and somatosensory cortices fail to provide top-down inhibitory input to the amygdala, leading to exaggerated amygdala activation and unnecessary activation of the entire fear network, resulting in a panic attack (Gorman et al., 2000). The functional neuroimaging literature on PD is relatively small, and evidence supporting amygdala hypersensitivity in this disorder is mixed.

Amygdala Function

Most neuroimaging studies of resting state in PD have reported abnormalities in hippocampal or parahippocampal blood flow and/or metabolic rates (Bisaga et al., 1998; De Cristofaro, Sessarego, Pupi, Biondi, & Faravelli, 1993; Nordahl et al., 1990, 1998). One recent PET study found greater resting glucose metabolism in the amygdala, as well as in hippocampus, thalamus, and brainstem, in patients with PD compared to healthy control subjects (Sakai et al., 2005). Amygdala glucose metabolism did not, however, change after effective treatment with cognitive-behavioral therapy (Sakai et al., 2006).

During pharmacologically induced anxiety/panic states, healthy individuals show robust amygdala activation (Benkelfat et al., 1995; Javanmard et al., 1999; Ketter et al., 1996; Servan-Schreiber, Perlstein, Cohen, & Mintun, 1998). In contrast, another study found relatively decreased amygdala activity during anticipatory anxiety in patients with PD compared to control participants (Boshuisen, Ter Horst, Paans, Reinders, & den Boer, 2002).

Several recent studies have assessed amygdala responses to the presentation of emotional stimuli in PD. In an emotional Stroop paradigm, patients with PD exhibited amygdala activation and slower color naming in response to panic-related words (van den Heuvel, Veltman, Groenewegen, Witter, et al., 2005). Thomas and colleagues (2001) found greater amygdala activation to fearful versus neutral faces in a mixed cohort of children with generalized anxiety disorder and PD than in children without anxiety disorders. In contrast, Pillay, Gruber, Rogowska, Simpson, and Yurgelun-Todd (2006) found less amygdala activation to overtly presented fearful facial expressions in patients with PD than in healthy control participants, although this finding could be attributed to treatment with antidepressant medication in the PD group (see Harmer, Mackay, Reid, Cowen, & Goodwin, 2006). Highlighting possible genetic contributions to amygdala activation, patients with PD who had the 5-HT1A x1019 GG genotype exhibited greater amygdala responses to (unmasked) happy faces than patients with the 5-HT1A x1019 CC/CG genotype (Domschke et al., 2006). This finding suggests that (1) variability in amygdala findings across studies of PD could be explained in part by variability in this or other genotypes, and (2) the presence of a particular genotype may be more predictive of amygdala activation than diagnostic status. Additional research is needed to assess these possibilities.

Amygdala Structure and Neurochemistry

Vythilingam and colleagues (2000) found reduced bilateral temporal lobe volumes in PD, although amygdala volumes were not reported. In addition, a small morphometric MRI study revealed smaller left temporal lobe volumes (and trends for smaller right temporal lobe and bilateral amygdala volumes) in patients with PD than in healthy comparison participants (Uchida et al., 2003). In a third study, bilateral amygdala volumes were smaller in patients with PD than in healthy participants (Massana et al., 2003). The findings remained significant when amygdala volumes were normalized using total intracranial volumes. Amygdala volumes were not significantly correlated with symptom severity measures.

Using MRS, Dager and colleagues have demonstrated widespread brain lactate increases during hyperventilation and lactate infusions in PD (Dager et al., 1995, 1999; Dager, Richards, Strauss, & Artru, 1997). In another MRS study, Massana and colleagues (2002) found reduced levels of creatine and phosphocreatine in the right medial temporal lobe (including the amygdala and part of the hippocampus) in PD—a finding that was interpreted as possibly representing a hypermetabolic state in the right medial temporal region. Interestingly, these investigators also reported a trend for reduced N-acetyl aspartate (NAA) in the right medial temporal lobe in PD, perhaps reflecting diminished neuronal integrity in that region. PET and SPECT studies designed to examine benzodiazepine receptor function have reported decreased gamma-aminobutyric acid (GABA)–benzodiazepine receptor binding in PD (Kaschka, Feistel, & Ebert, 1995; Malizia et al., 1998; Schlegel et al., 1994; but see also

Brandt et al., 1998), although most of these findings were not specific to the amygdala or medial temporal lobes.

Social Phobia

SP is characterized by a marked and persistent fear of social or performance situations involving possible scrutiny from others (APA, 2000). The fear of embarrassment can lead to avoidance of these situations and impairment in social, occupational, and academic realms. Several lines of evidence suggest a neurobiological basis for SP (Liebowitz, Ninan, Schneier, & Blanco, 2005; Mathew, Coplan, & Gorman, 2001; Stein, 1998), and the amygdala has been considered an important region of interest (Amaral, 2002). The results of recent functional neuroimaging studies have been supportive of this claim.

Amygdala Function

Several studies have examined amygdala function in SP during symptomatic states. Using PET, Tillfors and colleagues (2001) found greater amygdala activation during public versus private speaking in participants with SP than in healthy participants. In addition, amygdala responses in the SP group were positively correlated with self-reported fear increases. Using this same paradigm, Furmark and colleagues (2004) found that patients with SP who had a short allele of the serotonin transporter polymorphism exhibited greater amygdala responses during public versus private speaking, compared to patients with SP who had long alleles (Furmark et al., 2004). Exaggerated amygdala activation has also been reported during the anticipation of public speaking in patients with SP (Lorberbaum et al., 2004; Tillfors, Furmark, Marteinsdottir, & Fredrikson, 2002). Amygdala activation during public speaking in such patients appears to decrease with successful pharmacological treatment (Furmark et al., 2005). In contrast, one recent study found decreased amygdala activation during script-driven imagery of anxiety-provoking social situations and a mental arithmetic task in patients with SP (Kilts et al., 2006).

Several recent neuroimaging studies of SP have demonstrated exaggerated amygdala activation in response to facial expressions, including neutral (Birbaumer et al., 1998; Veit et al., 2002), angry (Phan, Fitzgerald, Nathan, & Tancer, 2006; Stein, Goldin, Sareen, Zorrilla, & Brown, 2002; Straube, Mentzel, & Miltner, 2005), contemptuous (Stein et al., 2002), disgusted (Phan, Fitzgerald, et al., 2006), fearful (Phan, Fitzgerald, et al., 2006), and even happy (Straube et al., 2005) expressions. Furthermore, amygdala activation to harsh (angry, fearful, disgusted) versus happy facial expressions is positively correlated with severity of social anxiety symptoms (Phan, Fitzgerald, et al., 2006). Interestingly, one report has described exaggerated amygdala responses to novel versus familiar (neutral) faces in adults who were categorized as behaviorally inhibited during their second year of life (Schwartz, Wright, Shin, Kagan, & Rauch, 2003). The results remained unchanged when two subjects with SP were removed from the analyses. Given that behavioral inhibition appears to be a risk factor for the development of SP, these findings suggest that exaggerated amygdala activation too may reflect a risk for, rather than a concomitant or consequence of, SP.

Two studies have used conditioning paradigms to study amygdala function in SP. Using fMRI, Schneider and colleagues (1999) paired neutral face stimuli (conditioned stimuli) with negative or neutral odors (unconditioned stimuli). In response to the neutral faces associated with the negative odor, the group with SP displayed signal increases within the amygdala and hippocampus, whereas the healthy comparison group displayed signal decreases in these same regions. In a differential conditioning paradigm using neutral faces as the conditioned stimuli (CS+ and CS–) and painful pressure as the unconditioned stimulus, Veit and colleagues (2002) found greater amygdala activation to all neutral faces during habituation in patients with SP than in comparison participants. No differential conditioning (in terms of skin conductance or amygdala activation to the CS+ versus CS–) was found in the patients with SP, perhaps due to the exaggerated amygdala responses during habituation and/ or to the very small number of patients studied ($n = 4$).

Amygdala Structure and Neurochemistry

We are aware of no structural MRI studies in the literature that have assessed amygdala volumes in SP. Although a few studies of neurochemistry and receptor function in SP have been conducted, they have generally reported results in regions other than the amygdala (Davidson et al., 1993; Phan et al., 2005; Tiihonen et al., 1997; Tupler et al., 1997). Thus, at the current time, little information is available concerning amygdala structure and neurochemistry in this disorder.

Obsessive–Compulsive Disorder

Symptoms of OCD include recurrent, unwanted thoughts or images that cause distress (obsessions), as well as excessive ritualistic behaviors or mental acts (compulsions) that are typically carried out in response to the obsessions (APA, 2000). Although anxiety is certainly a concomitant of OCD, data thus far suggest that the pathophysiology of OCD may be different from that of other anxiety disorders. A corticostriatothalamocortical model of OCD posits that the primary pathology is in the striatum (caudate nucleus), leading to inefficient gating in the thalamus (Rauch, Whalen, Dougherty, & Jenike, 1998). This may result in hyperactivity in both orbitofrontal cortex (which may correspond to intrusive thoughts) and anterior cingulate cortex (which may reflect nonspecific anxiety). Compulsions may recruit the inefficient striatum in order to achieve thalamic gating and neutralize obsessions and anxiety.

A few studies have reported abnormalities of amygdala structure and function in OCD.

Amygdala Function

The most commonly reported functional neuroimaging findings in OCD include abnormal orbitofrontal cortex, anterior cingulate cortex, and/or caudate activity (e.g., Baxter et al., 1987, 1988; Chen, Xie, Han, Cui, & Zhang, 2004; Fitzgerald et al., 2005; Nakao et al., 2005a; Nordahl et al., 1989; Rauch et al., 1994, 1997; Saxena et al., 2004; Swedo et al., 1989; van den Heuvel, Veltman, Groenewegen, Cath, et al., 2005), which declines after treatment (Baxter et al., 1992; Nakao et al., 2005b; Perani et al., 1995; Saxena et al., 2002; Schwartz, Stoessel, Baxter, Martin, & Phelps, 1996; Swedo et al., 1992). Only a few studies have demonstrated functional abnormalities in the amygdala in OCD.

Van Laere and colleagues (2006) reported a trend toward increased glucose metabolism during rest in the left amygdala in OCD, which was normalized after electrostimulation in the anterior capsule. Two studies have reported enhanced amygdala activation in response to contamination-related stimuli (Breiter et al., 1996; van den Heuvel et al., 2004), and one study found sensitization in the right amygdala during symptom provocation over time (van den Heuvel et al., 2004). However, the majority of symptom provocation and resting state studies, as well as one recent study that used fearful facial expressions as stimuli (Cannistraro et al., 2004), have found no evidence of exaggerated amygdala activation in OCD.

Amygdala Structure and Neurochemistry

Most structural MRI studies of OCD have reported volumetric abnormalities in the striatum (Robinson et al., 1995; Rosenberg et al., 1997), thalamus (Atmaca et al., 2006; Gilbert et al., 2000; Rosenberg, Benazon, Gilbert, Sullivan, & Moore, 2000), orbitofrontal cortex (Kang et al., 2004; Pujol et al., 2004; Valente et al., 2005), or anterior cingulate cortex (Valente et al., 2005). Two recent MRI studies found reduced amygdala volumes in OCD (Pujol et al., 2004; Szeszko et al., 1999), although other studies have reported evidence of greater left amygdala volumes (Kwon et al., 2003) or amygdala volumetric asymmetries (left > right) in OCD (Szeszko et al., 2004).

Several MRS studies of OCD have reported reduced NAA concentrations in the thalamus (Fitzgerald, Moore, Paulson, Stewart, & Rosenberg, 2000), striatum (Bartha et al., 1998; Ebert et al., 1997), and anterior cingulate (Ebert et al., 1997), as well as increased glutamatergic concentrations in the striatum (Moore, MacMaster, Stewart, & Rosenberg, 1998; Rosenberg, MacMaster, et al., 2000), but no such findings have been reported in the amygdala. Finally, serotonin transporter availability in limbic regions, including the amygdala, appears to be normal in OCD (Simpson et al., 2003).

SUMMARY AND CONCLUSIONS

The literature reviewed above suggests that the amygdala may be hyperresponsive in PTSD, and that amygdala activation is positively related to PTSD symptom severity. Evidence for exaggerated amygdala responsivity in SP and PD is increasing, although the findings are still mixed for PD. Additional cognitive activation studies that more directly assess amygdala function in those disorders are warranted. In contrast, there is relatively little evidence that the amygdala plays a major role in the pathophysiology of OCD.

These findings suggest that OCD may be neurobiologically distinct from the other anxiety disorders considered here. The similar results in PTSD, PD, and SP may challenge the diagnostic specificity of amygdala hyperresponsivity. We hasten to note that despite apparent similarities in amygdala hyperresponsivity across these three disorders, the literature is presently small, and differential activation in other brain regions may still distinguish the disorders. For example, a robust finding in PTSD has been hyporesponsivity in the mPFC (Bremner, Narayan, et al., 1999; Bremner, Staib, et al., 1999; Bremner et al., 2004; Britton, Phan, Taylor, Fig, & Liberzon, 2005; Lanius et al., 2001, 2002; Lindauer, Booij, et al., 2004; Shin et al., 1999, 2001, 2004, 2005; Williams et al., 2006; Yang, Wu, Hsu, & Ker, 2004), and inverse correlations between mPFC activity and PTSD symptoms have been reported (Britton et al., 2005; Shin et al., 2004, 2005; Williams et al., 2006). PTSD could differ from SP, for example, on the basis of responsivity in mPFC or the interaction between amygdala and mPFC. Cognitive activation studies directly comparing SP, PD, and PTSD are needed to address these specificity issues.

Exciting recent studies have reported that a variant of the serotonin transporter gene is associated with exaggerated amygdala activity, both in healthy individuals and in patients with anxiety disorders (Furmark et al., 2004; Hariri et al., 2005; Pezawas et al., 2005). In addition, adults classified as behaviorally inhibited at an early age appear to have exaggerated amygdala activation to novel faces (Schwartz et al., 2003) and a greater risk for developing SP (Biederman et al., 2001) and social anxiety (Schwartz, Snidman, & Kagan, 1999). Findings such as these raise the issue of whether amygdala hyperresponsivity may be a risk factor for the development of anxiety disorders, rather than a marker of the disorders themselves. Twin and/or longitudinal studies will be needed in order to address this issue.

Enthusiasm regarding the neuroimaging findings reviewed above must be tempered by an acknowledgement of the limitations of this type of research. The spatial resolution of functional neuroimaging techniques such as PET and SPECT limits precise neuroanatomical localization. Even fMRI does not permit the type of localization to which neuroanatomists are accustomed. Both PET and fMRI are limited in temporal resolution as well. Measuring the time course of brain responses to stimuli is critical for studying the flow of information in the brain (e.g., bottom-up vs. top-down). Unfortunately, the neuroimaging methods that have the best temporal resolution (e.g., electro-encephalography and magnetoencephalography) also have the most difficulty detecting deep subcortical structures such as the amygdala.

Methodology, including data acquisition parameters, cognitive paradigms, and data-analytic techniques, may vary widely across neuroimaging studies, sometimes making findings across studies difficult to reconcile. With regard to PTSD, much research has been conducted on adult samples of patients with chronic PTSD; future research is needed to determine whether brain abnormalities differ between acute and chronic PTSD and between childhood-onset and adult-onset PTSD. Regarding PD, functional neuroimaging data acquired during panic attacks may be affected by hyperventilation-induced hypocapnia and resulting blood flow changes. Cognitive activation paradigms (that are not likely to result in panic attacks) may be especially useful in the examination of amygdala function in PD. Across the anxiety disorders, comorbidity (especially with depression) is common. Although a few past studies have attempted to assess the effect of this potentially confounding factor, future research ought to directly compare patient groups with and without comorbidity. Finally, the relationship between amygdala volume and function has not been assessed in anxiety disorders, and future research will need to address that issue (Drevets, 2001).

WHAT WE THINK

The amygdala is responsive to predictors of threat, particularly potential predictors whose contingency with threatening outcomes is currently underdetermined (i.e., predictive ambiguity or uncertainty) (Davis & Whalen, 2001; Holland & Gallagher, 1999; Kapp, Whalen, Supple, & Pascoe, 1992; Whalen, 1998). In such situations, the amygdala calls upon sensory cortical regions to facilitate further environmental information processing. In this way, the amygdala determines the organism's overall level of vigilance, thereby facilitating learning about the potential threat and/or resolving the predictive uncertainty. Ordinarily this function is adaptive, because it initiates the gathering of further information, eventually leading to the selection of an appropriate response. However, the amygdala appears to be maladaptively hyperresponsive in patients with anxiety disorders, such as PTSD. Indeed, patients with PTSD are hypervigilant and physiologically reactive to reminders of past traumatic events, even when no current threat is present. Importantly, amygdala responsivity is greater among patients with more severe PTSD symptoms, suggesting that amygdala function is closely tied to the clinical presentation of this disorder.

Although amygdala hyperresponsivity may mediate some of the symptoms of PTSD, it is unlikely to be the only brain structure involved in the pathophysiology of this disorder. The mPFC, which plays a critical role in retaining extinction of conditioned fear (Milad & Quirk, 2002; Quirk, Russo, Barron, & Lebron, 2000) and is reciprocally connected to the amygdala, shows diminished function in PTSD (Shin et al., 2006). Thus impaired function of the mPFC may be associated with a failure to inhibit the amygdala and may lead to or further exacerbate amygdala hyper-responsivity in PTSD.

To what extent amygdala hyperresponsivity in PTSD can be explained by diminished top-down inhibition by the mPFC versus exaggerated bottom-up sensitivity of the amygdala remains to be determined. The most parsimonious explanation for exaggerated amygdala responsivity in PTSD may be impaired top-down inhibition by the mPFC. This hypothesis is consistent with findings of diminished anterior cingulate volumes in PTSD (Kitayama, Quinn, & Bremner, 2006; Rauch, Shin, Segal, et al., 2003; Woodward et al., 2006; Yamasue et al., 2003). Alternatively, PTSD could be associated with a combination of exaggerated bottom-up responsivity in the amygdala and deficient top-down inhibition by the mPFC; the latter may further increase the already exaggerated amygdala responses.

REFERENCES

Ackerman, P. T., Newton, J. E., McPherson, W. B., Jones, J. G., & Dykman, R. A. (1998). Prevalence of post traumatic stress disorder and other psychiatric diagnoses in three groups of abused children (sexual, physical, and both). *Child Abuse and Neglect, 22*, 759–774.

Amaral, D. G. (2002). The primate amygdala and the neurobiology of social behavior: Implications for understanding social anxiety. *Biological Psychiatry, 51*, 11–17.

American Psychiatric Association (APA). (2000). *Diagnostic and statistical manual of mental disorders* (4th ed., text rev.). Washington, DC: Author.

Armony, J. L., Corbo, V., Clement, M. H., & Brunet, A. (2005). Amygdala response in patients with acute PTSD to masked and unmasked emotional facial expressions. *American Journal of Psychiatry, 162*, 1961–1963.

Atmaca, M., Yildirim, B. H., Ozdemir, B. H., Aydin, B. A., Tezcan, A. E., & Ozler, A. S. (2006). Volumetric MRI assessment of brain regions in patients with refractory obsessive–compulsive disorder. *Progress in Neuropsychopharmacology and Biological Psychiatry, 30*, 1051–1057.

Bartha, R., Stein, M. B., Williamson, P. C., Drost, D. J., Neufeld, R. W., Carr, T. J., et al. (1998). A short echo 1H spectroscopy and volumetric MRI study of the corpus striatum in patients with obsessive–compulsive disorder and comparison subjects. *American Journal of Psychiatry, 155*, 1584–1591.

Baxter, L. R., Jr., Phelps, M. E., Mazziotta, J. C., Guze, B. H., Schwartz, J. M., & Selin, C. E. (1987). Local cerebral glucose metabolic rates in obsessive–compulsive disorder: A comparison with rates in unipolar depression and in normal controls. *Archives of General Psychiatry, 44*, 211–218.

Baxter, L. R., Jr., Schwartz, J. M., Bergman, K. S., Szuba, M. P., Guze, B. H., Mazziotta, J. C., et al. (1992). Caudate glucose metabolic rate changes with both drug and behavior therapy for obsessive–compulsive disorder. *Archives of General Psychiatry, 49*, 681–689.

Baxter, L. R., Jr., Schwartz, J. M., Mazziotta, J. C., Phelps, M. E., Pahl, J. J., Guze, B. H., et al. (1988). Cerebral glucose metabolic rates in nondepressed patients with obsessive–compulsive disorder. *American Journal of Psychiatry, 145*, 1560–1563.

Benkelfat, C., Bradwejn, J., Meyer, E., Ellenbogen, M., Milot, S., Gjedde, A., et al. (1995). Functional neuroanatomy of CCK4-induced anxiety in normal healthy volunteers. *American Journal of Psychiatry, 152*, 1180–1184.

Biederman, J., Hirshfeld-Becker, D. R., Rosenbaum, J. F., Herot, C., Friedman, D.,

Snidman, N., et al. (2001). Further evidence of association between behavioral inhibition and social anxiety in children. *American Journal of Psychiatry, 158,* 1673–1679.

Birbaumer, N., Grodd, W., Diedrich, O., Klose, U., Erb, M., Lotze, M., et al. (1998). fMRI reveals amygdala activation to human faces in social phobics. *NeuroReport, 9,* 1223–1226.

Bisaga, A., Katz, J. L., Antonini, A., Wright, C. E., Margouleff, C., Gorman, J. M., et al. (1998). Cerebral glucose metabolism in women with panic disorder. *American Journal of Psychiatry, 155,* 1178–1183.

Bonne, O., Brandes, D., Gilboa, A., Gomori, J. M., Shenton, M. E., Pitman, R. K., et al. (2001). Longitudinal MRI study of hippocampal volume in trauma survivors with PTSD. *American Journal of Psychiatry, 158,* 1248–1251.

Boshuisen, M. L., Ter Horst, G. J., Paans, A. M., Reinders, A. A., & den Boer, J. A. (2002). rCBF differences between panic disorder patients and control subjects during anticipatory anxiety and rest. *Biological Psychiatry, 52,* 126–135.

Brandt, C. A., Meller, J., Keweloh, L., Hoschel, K., Staedt, J., Munz, D., et al. (1998). Increased benzodiazepine receptor density in the prefrontal cortex in patients with panic disorder. *Journal of Neural Transmission, 105,* 1325–1333.

Breiter, H. C., Rauch, S. L., Kwong, K. K., Baker, J. R., Weisskoff, R. M., Kennedy, D. N., et al. (1996). Functional magnetic resonance imaging of symptom provocation in obsessive–compulsive disorder. *Archives of General Psychiatry, 53,* 595–606.

Bremner, J. D., Innis, R. B., Ng, C. K., Staib, L. H., Salomon, R. M., Bronen, R. A., et al. (1997). Positron emission tomography measurement of cerebral metabolic correlates of yohimbine administration in combat-related posttraumatic stress disorder. *Archives of General Psychiatry, 54,* 246–254.

Bremner, J. D., Narayan, M., Staib, L. H., Southwick, S. M., McGlashan, T., & Charney, D. S. (1999). Neural correlates of memories of childhood sexual abuse in women with and without posttraumatic stress disorder. *American Journal of Psychiatry, 156,* 1787–1795.

Bremner, J. D., Randall, P., Vermetten, E., Staib, L., Bronen, R. A., Mazure, C., et al. (1997). Magnetic resonance imaging-based measurement of hippocampal volume in posttraumatic stress disorder related to childhood physical and sexual abuse: A preliminary report. *Biological Psychiatry, 41,* 23–32.

Bremner, J. D., Staib, L. H., Kaloupek, D., Southwick, S. M., Soufer, R., & Charney, D. S. (1999). Neural correlates of exposure to traumatic pictures and sound in Vietnam combat veterans with and without posttraumatic stress disorder: A positron emission tomography study. *Biological Psychiatry, 45,* 806–816.

Bremner, J. D., Vermetten, E., Schmahl, C., Vaccarino, V., Vythilingam, M., Afzal, N., et al. (2005). Positron emission tomographic imaging of neural correlates of a fear acquisition and extinction paradigm in women with childhood sexual-abuse-related post-traumatic stress disorder. *Psychological Medicine, 35,* 791–806.

Bremner, J. D., Vermetten, E., Vythilingam, M., Afzal, N., Schmahl, C., Elzinga, B., et al. (2004). Neural correlates of the classic color and emotional Stroop in women with abuse-related posttraumatic stress disorder. *Biological Psychiatry, 55,* 612–620.

Breslau, N., Kessler, R. C., Chilcoat, H. D., Schultz, L. R., Davis, G. C., & Andreski, P. (1998). Trauma and posttraumatic stress disorder in the community: The 1996 Detroit Area Survey of Trauma. *Archives of General Psychiatry, 55,* 626–632.

Britton, J. C., Phan, K. L., Taylor, S. F., Fig, L. M., & Liberzon, I. (2005). Corticolimbic blood flow in posttraumatic stress disorder during script-driven imagery. *Biological Psychiatry, 57*, 832–840.

Bryant, R. A., Felmingham, K. L., Kemp, A. H., Barton, M., Peduto, A. S., Rennie, C., et al. (2005). Neural networks of information processing in posttraumatic stress disorder: A functional magnetic resonance imaging study. *Biological Psychiatry, 58*, 111–118.

Cannistraro, P. A., Wright, C. I., Wedig, M. M., Martis, B., Shin, L. M., Wilhelm, S., et al. (2004). Amygdala responses to human faces in obsessive–compulsive disorder. *Biological Psychiatry, 56*, 916–920.

Chen, X. L., Xie, J. X., Han, H. B., Cui, Y. H., & Zhang, B. Q. (2004). MR perfusion-weighted imaging and quantitative analysis of cerebral hemodynamics with symptom provocation in unmedicated patients with obsessive–compulsive disorder. *Neuroscience Letters, 370*, 206–211.

Chung, Y. A., Kim, S. H., Chung, S. K., Chae, J. H., Yang, D. W., Sohn, H. S., et al. (2006). Alterations in cerebral perfusion in posttraumatic stress disorder patients without re-exposure to accident-related stimuli. *Clinical Neurophysiology, 117*, 637–642.

Coplan, J. D., & Lydiard, R. B. (1998). Brain circuits in panic disorder. *Biological Psychiatry, 44*, 1264–1276.

Dager, S. R., Friedman, S. D., Heide, A., Layton, M. E., Richards, T., Artru, A., et al. (1999). Two-dimensional proton echo-planar spectroscopic imaging of brain metabolic changes during lactate-induced panic. *Archives of General Psychiatry, 56*, 70–77.

Dager, S. R., Richards, T., Strauss, W., & Artru, A. (1997). Single-voxel 1H-MRS investigation of brain metabolic changes during lactate-induced panic. *Psychiatry Research, 76*, 89–99.

Dager, S. R., Strauss, W. L., Marro, K. I., Richards, T. L., Metzger, G. D., & Artru, A. A. (1995). Proton magnetic resonance spectroscopy investigation of hyperventilation in subjects with panic disorder and comparison subjects. *American Journal of Psychiatry, 152*, 666–672.

Davidson, J. R., Krishnan, K. R., Charles, H. C., Boyko, O., Potts, N. L., Ford, S. M., et al. (1993). Magnetic resonance spectroscopy in social phobia: Preliminary findings. *Journal of Clinical Psychiatry, 54*(Suppl.), 19–25.

Davis, M., & Whalen, P. J. (2001). The amygdala: Vigilance and emotion. *Molecular Psychiatry, 6*, 13–34.

De Bellis, M. D., Hall, J., Boring, A. M., Frustaci, K., & Moritz, G. (2001). A pilot longitudinal study of hippocampal volumes in pediatric maltreatment-related posttraumatic stress disorder. *Biological Psychiatry, 50*, 305–309.

De Bellis, M. D., Keshavan, M. S., Shifflett, H., Iyengar, S., Beers, S. R., Hall, J., et al. (2002). Brain structures in pediatric maltreatment-related posttraumatic stress disorder: A sociodemographically matched study. *Biological Psychiatry, 52*, 1066–1078.

De Cristofaro, M. T., Sessarego, A., Pupi, A., Biondi, F., & Faravelli, C. (1993). Brain perfusion abnormalities in drug-naive, lactate-sensitive panic patients: A SPECT study. *Biological Psychiatry, 33*, 505–512.

Dohrenwend, B. P., Turner, J. B., Turse, N. A., Adams, B. G., Koenen, K. C., & Marshall, R. (2006). The psychological risks of Vietnam for U.S. veterans: A revisit with new data and methods. *Science, 313*, 979–982.

Domschke, K., Braun, M., Ohrmann, P., Suslow, T., Kugel, H., Bauer, J., et al. (2006). Association of the functional –1019C/G 5-HT 1A polymorphism with prefrontal cortex and amygdala activation measured with 3 T fMRI in panic disorder. *International Journal of Neuropsychopharmacology, 9,* 349–355.

Drevets, W. C. (2001). Integration of structural and functional imaging. In D. Dougherty & S. L. Rauch (Eds.), *Psychiatric neuroimaging research: Contemporary strategies* (pp. 249–290). Washington, DC: American Psychiatric Press.

Driessen, M., Beblo, T., Mertens, M., Piefke, M., Rullkoetter, N., Silva-Saavedra, A., et al. (2004). Posttraumatic stress disorder and fMRI activation patterns of traumatic memory in patients with borderline personality disorder. *Biological Psychiatry, 55,* 603–611.

Ebert, D., Speck, O., Konig, A., Berger, M., Hennig, J., & Hohagen, F. (1997). 1H-magnetic resonance spectroscopy in obsessive–compulsive disorder: Evidence for neuronal loss in the cingulate gyrus and the right striatum. *Psychiatry Research, 74,* 173–176.

Elzinga, B. M., & Bremner, J. D. (2002). Are the neural substrates of memory the final common pathway in posttraumatic stress disorder (PTSD)? *Journal of Affective Disorders, 70,* 1–17.

Fennema-Notestine, C., Stein, M. B., Kennedy, C. M., Archibald, S. L., & Jernigan, T. L. (2002). Brain morphometry in female victims of intimate partner violence with and without posttraumatic stress disorder. *Biological Psychiatry, 52,* 1089–1101.

Fitzgerald, K. D., Moore, G. J., Paulson, L. A., Stewart, C. M., & Rosenberg, D. R. (2000). Proton spectroscopic imaging of the thalamus in treatment-naive pediatric obsessive–compulsive disorder. *Biological Psychiatry, 47,* 174–182.

Fitzgerald, K. D., Welsh, R. C., Gehring, W. J., Abelson, J. L., Himle, J. A., Liberzon, I., et al. (2005). Error-related hyperactivity of the anterior cingulate cortex in obsessive–compulsive disorder. *Biological Psychiatry, 57,* 287–294.

Fredrikson, M., & Furmark, T. (2003). Amygdaloid regional cerebral blood flow and subjective fear during symptom provocation in anxiety disorders. *Annals of the New York Academy of Sciences, 985,* 341–347.

Furmark, T., Appel, L., Michelgard, A., Wahlstedt, K., Ahs, F., Zancan, S., et al. (2005). Cerebral blood flow changes after treatment of social phobia with the neurokinin-1 antagonist GR205171, citalopram, or placebo. *Biological Psychiatry, 58,* 132–142.

Furmark, T., Tillfors, M., Garpenstrand, H., Marteinsdottir, I., Langstrom, B., Oreland, L., et al. (2004). Serotonin transporter polymorphism related to amygdala excitability and symptom severity in patients with social phobia. *Neuroscience Letters, 362,* 189–192.

Gilbert, A. R., Moore, G. J., Keshavan, M. S., Paulson, L. A., Narula, V., MacMaster, F. P., et al. (2000). Decrease in thalamic volumes of pediatric patients with obsessive–compulsive disorder who are taking paroxetine. *Archives of General Psychiatry, 57,* 449–456.

Gilbertson, M. W., Shenton, M. E., Ciszewski, A., Kasai, K., Lasko, N. B., Orr, S. P., et al. (2002). Smaller hippocampal volume predicts pathologic vulnerability to psychological trauma. *Nature Neuroscience, 5,* 1242–1247.

Gilboa, A., Shalev, A. Y., Laor, L., Lester, H., Louzoun, Y., Chisin, R., et al. (2004). Functional connectivity of the prefrontal cortex and the amygdala in posttraumatic stress disorder. *Biological Psychiatry, 55,* 263–272.

Gorman, J. M., Kent, J. M., Sullivan, G. M., & Coplan, J. D. (2000). Neuroanatomical hypothesis of panic disorder, revised. *American Journal of Psychiatry, 157,* 493–505.

Gurvits, T. V., Shenton, M. E., Hokama, H., Ohta, H., Lasko, N. B., Gilbertson, M. W., et al. (1996). Magnetic resonance imaging study of hippocampal volume in chronic, combat-related posttraumatic stress disorder. *Biological Psychiatry, 40,* 1091–1099.

Hamner, M. B., Lorberbaum, J. P., & George, M. S. (1999). Potential role of the anterior cingulate cortex in PTSD: Review and hypothesis. *Depression and Anxiety, 9,* 1–14.

Hariri, A. R., Drabant, E. M., Munoz, K. E., Kolachana, B. S., Mattay, V. S., Egan, M. F., et al. (2005). A susceptibility gene for affective disorders and the response of the human amygdala. *Archives of General Psychiatry, 62,* 146–152.

Harmer, C. J., Mackay, C. E., Reid, C. B., Cowen, P. J., & Goodwin, G. M. (2006). Antidepressant drug treatment modifies the neural processing of nonconscious threat cues. *Biological Psychiatry, 59,* 816–820.

Hendler, T., Rotshtein, P., Yeshurun, Y., Weizmann, T., Kahn, I., Ben-Bashat, D., et al. (2003). Sensing the invisible: Differential sensitivity of visual cortex and amygdala to traumatic context. *NeuroImage, 19,* 587–600.

Holland, P. C., & Gallagher, M. (1999). Amygdala circuitry in attentional and representational processes [Review]. *Trends in Cognitive Science, 3,* 65–73.

Javanmard, M., Shlik, J., Kennedy, S. H., Vaccarino, F. J., Houle, S., & Bradwejn, J. (1999). Neuroanatomic correlates of CCK-4-induced panic attacks in healthy humans: A comparison of two time points. *Biological Psychiatry, 45,* 872–882.

Kang, D. H., Kim, J. J., Choi, J. S., Kim, Y. I., Kim, C. W., Youn, T., et al. (2004). Volumetric investigation of the frontal–subcortical circuitry in patients with obsessive–compulsive disorder. *Journal of Neuropsychiatry and Clinical Neurosciences, 16,* 342–349.

Kapp, B. S., Whalen, P. J., Supple, W. F., & Pascoe, J. P. (1992). Amygdaloid contributions to conditioned arousal and sensory information processing. In J. P. Aggleton (Ed.), *The amygdala: Neurobiological aspects of emotion, memory, and mental dysfunction* (pp. 229–254). New York: Wiley-Liss.

Karl, A., Schaefer, M., Malta, L. S., Dorfel, D., Rohleder, N., & Werner, A. (2006). A meta-analysis of structural brain abnormalities in PTSD. *Neuroscience and Biobehavioral Reviews, 30,* 1004–1031.

Kaschka, W., Feistel, H., & Ebert, D. (1995). Reduced benzodiazepine receptor binding in panic disorders measured by iomazenil SPECT. *Journal of Psychiatric Research, 29,* 427–434.

Kessler, R. C., Chiu, W. T., Jin, R., Ruscio, A. M., Shear, K., & Walters, E. E. (2006). The epidemiology of panic attacks, panic disorder, and agoraphobia in the National Comorbidity Survey replication. *Archives of General Psychiatry, 63,* 415–424.

Kessler, R. C., Sonnega, A., Bromet, E., Hughes, M., & Nelson, C. B. (1995). Posttraumatic stress disorder in the National Comorbidity Survey. *Archives of General Psychiatry, 52,* 1048–1060.

Ketter, T. A., Andreason, P. J., George, M. S., Lee, C., Gill, D. S., Parekh, P. I., et al. (1996). Anterior paralimbic mediation of procaine-induced emotional and psychosensory experiences. *Archives of General Psychiatry, 53,* 59–69.

Kilts, C. D., Kelsey, J. E., Knight, B., Ely, T. D., Bowman, F. D., Gross, R. E., et al. (2006). The neural correlates of social anxiety disorder and response to pharmacotherapy. *Neuropsychopharmacology, 31,* 2243–2253.

Kitayama, N., Quinn, S., & Bremner, J. D. (2006). Smaller volume of anterior cingulate cortex in abuse-related posttraumatic stress disorder. *Journal of Affective Disorders, 90,* 171–174.

Kwon, J. S., Shin, Y. W., Kim, C. W., Kim, Y. I., Youn, T., Han, M. H., et al. (2003). Similarity and disparity of obsessive–compulsive disorder and schizophrenia in MR volumetric abnormalities of the hippocampus–amygdala complex. *Journal of Neurology, Neurosurgery and Psychiatry, 74,* 962–964.

Lanius, R. A., Williamson, P., Boksman, K., Densmore, M., Gupta, M., Neufeld, R., et al. (2002). Brain activation during script-driven imagery induced dissociative responses in PTSD: A functional magnetic resonance imaging investigation. *Biological Psychiatry, 52,* 305–311.

Lanius, R. A., Williamson, P. C., Densmore, M., Boksman, K., Gupta, M. A., Neufeld, R. W., et al. (2001). Neural correlates of traumatic memories in posttraumatic stress disorder: A functional MRI investigation. *American Journal of Psychiatry, 158,* 1920–1922.

Layton, B., & Krikorian, R. (2002). Memory mechanisms in posttraumatic stress disorder. *Journal of Neuropsychiatry and Clinical Neurosciences, 14,* 254–261.

LeDoux, J. E. (2000). Emotion circuits in the brain. *Annual Review of Neuroscience, 23,* 155–184.

Liberzon, I., Taylor, S. F., Amdur, R., Jung, T. D., Chamberlain, K. R., Minoshima, S., et al. (1999). Brain activation in PTSD in response to trauma-related stimuli. *Biological Psychiatry, 45,* 817–826.

Liberzon, I., Taylor, S. F., Phan, K. L., Britton, J. C., Fig, L. M., Bueller, J. A., et al. (2007). Altered central mu-opioid receptor binding after psychological trauma. *Biological Psychiatry, 61,* 1030–1038.

Liebowitz, M. R., Ninan, P. T., Schneier, F. R., & Blanco, C. (2005). Integrating neurobiology and psychopathology into evidence-based treatment of social anxiety disorder. *CNS Spectrums, 10*(Suppl. 13), 1–11.

Lindauer, R. J., Booij, J., Habraken, J. B., Uylings, H. B., Olff, M., Carlier, I. V., et al. (2004). Cerebral blood flow changes during script-driven imagery in police officers with posttraumatic stress disorder. *Biological Psychiatry, 56,* 853–861.

Lindauer, R. J., Vlieger, E. J., Jalink, M., Olff, M., Carlier, I. V., Majoie, C. B., et al. (2004). Smaller hippocampal volume in Dutch police officers with posttraumatic stress disorder. *Biological Psychiatry, 56,* 356–363.

Lorberbaum, J. P., Kose, S., Johnson, M. R., Arana, G. W., Sullivan, L. K., Hamner, M. B., et al. (2004). Neural correlates of speech anticipatory anxiety in generalized social phobia. *NeuroReport, 15,* 2701–2705.

Malizia, A. L., Cunningham, V. J., Bell, C. J., Liddle, P. F., Jones, T., & Nutt, D. J. (1998). Decreased brain GABA(A)-benzodiazepine receptor binding in panic disorder: Preliminary results from a quantitative PET study. *Archives of General Psychiatry, 55,* 715–720.

Massana, G., Gasto, C., Junque, C., Mercader, J. M., Gomez, B., Massana, J., et al. (2002). Reduced levels of creatine in the right medial temporal lobe region of panic disorder patients detected with (1)H magnetic resonance spectroscopy. *NeuroImage, 16,* 836–842.

Massana, G., Serra-Grabulosa, J. M., Salgado-Pineda, P., Gasto, C., Junque, C., Massana, J., et al. (2003). Amygdalar atrophy in panic disorder patients detected by volumetric magnetic resonance imaging. *NeuroImage, 19*, 80–90.

Mathew, S. J., Coplan, J. D., & Gorman, J. M. (2001). Neurobiological mechanisms of social anxiety disorder. *American Journal of Psychiatry, 158*, 1558–1567.

Matsuoka, Y., Yamawaki, S., Inagaki, M., Akechi, T., & Uchitomi, Y. (2003). A volumetric study of amygdala in cancer survivors with intrusive recollections. *Biological Psychiatry, 54*, 736–743.

Milad, M. R., & Quirk, G. J. (2002). Neurons in medial prefrontal cortex signal memory for fear extinction. *Nature, 420*, 70–74.

Moore, G. J., MacMaster, F. P., Stewart, C., & Rosenberg, D. R. (1998). Case study: Caudate glutamatergic changes with paroxetine therapy for pediatric obsessive–compulsive disorder. *Journal of the American Academy of Child and Adolescent Psychiatry, 37*, 663–667.

Nakao, T., Nakagawa, A., Yoshiura, T., Nakatani, E., Nabeyama, M., Yoshizato, C., et al. (2005a). A functional MRI comparison of patients with obsessive–compulsive disorder and normal controls during a Chinese character Stroop task. *Psychiatry Research, 139*, 101–114.

Nakao, T., Nakagawa, A., Yoshiura, T., Nakatani, E., Nabeyama, M., Yoshizato, C., et al. (2005b). Brain activation of patients with obsessive–compulsive disorder during neuropsychological and symptom provocation tasks before and after symptom improvement: A functional magnetic resonance imaging study. *Biological Psychiatry, 57*, 901–910.

Nordahl, T. E., Benkelfat, C., Semple, W. E., Gross, M., King, A. C., & Cohen, R. M. (1989). Cerebral glucose metabolic rates in obsessive compulsive disorder. *Neuropsychopharmacology, 2*, 23–28.

Nordahl, T. E., Semple, W. E., Gross, M., Mellman, T. A., Stein, M. B., Goyer, P., et al. (1990). Cerebral glucose metabolic differences in patients with panic disorder. *Neuropsychopharmacology, 3*, 261–272.

Nordahl, T. E., Stein, M. B., Benkelfat, C., Semple, W. E., Andreason, P., Zametkin, A., et al. (1998). Regional cerebral metabolic asymmetries replicated in an independent group of patients with panic disorders. *Biological Psychiatry, 44*, 998–1006.

Orr, S. P., Metzger, L. J., Lasko, N. B., Macklin, M. L., Peri, T., & Pitman, R. K. (2000). De novo conditioning in trauma-exposed individuals with and without posttraumatic stress disorder. *Journal of Abnormal Psychology, 109*, 290–298.

Perani, D., Colombo, C., Bressi, S., Bonfanti, A., Grassi, F., Scarone, S., et al. (1995). [18F]FDG PET study in obsessive–compulsive disorder: A clinical/metabolic correlation study after treatment. *British Journal of Psychiatry, 166*, 244–250.

Peri, T., Ben-Shakhar, G., Orr, S. P., & Shalev, A. Y. (2000). Psychophysiologic assessment of aversive conditioning in posttraumatic stress disorder. *Biological Psychiatry, 47*, 512–519.

Pezawas, L., Meyer-Lindenberg, A., Drabant, E. M., Verchinski, B. A., Munoz, K. E., Kolachana, B. S., et al. (2005). 5-HTTLPR polymorphism impacts human cingulate–amygdala interactions: A genetic susceptibility mechanism for depression. *Nature Neuroscience, 8*, 828–834.

Phan, K. L., Britton, J. C., Taylor, S. F., Fig, L. M., & Liberzon, I. (2006). Corticolimbic blood flow during nontraumatic emotional processing in posttraumatic stress disorder. *Archives of General Psychiatry, 63*, 184–192.

Phan, K. L., Fitzgerald, D. A., Cortese, B. M., Seraji-Bozorgzad, N., Tancer, M. E., & Moore, G. J. (2005). Anterior cingulate neurochemistry in social anxiety disorder: 1H-MRS at 4 Tesla. *NeuroReport, 16,* 183–186.

Phan, K. L., Fitzgerald, D. A., Nathan, P. J., & Tancer, M. E. (2006). Association between amygdala hyperactivity to harsh faces and severity of social anxiety in generalized social phobia. *Biological Psychiatry, 59,* 424–429.

Pillay, S. S., Gruber, S. A., Rogowska, J., Simpson, N., & Yurgelun-Todd, D. A. (2006). fMRI of fearful facial affect recognition in panic disorder: The cingulate gyrus–amygdala connection. *Journal of Affective Disorders, 94,* 173–181.

Pissiota, A., Frans, O., Fernandez, M., von Knorring, L., Fischer, H., & Fredrikson, M. (2002). Neurofunctional correlates of posttraumatic stress disorder: A PET symptom provocation study. *European Archives of Psychiatry and Clinical Neuroscience, 252,* 68–75.

Protopopescu, X., Pan, H., Tuescher, O., Cloitre, M., Goldstein, M., Engelien, W., et al. (2005). Differential time courses and specificity of amygdala activity in posttraumatic stress disorder subjects and normal control subjects. *Biological Psychiatry, 57,* 464–473.

Pujol, J., Soriano-Mas, C., Alonso, P., Cardoner, N., Menchon, J. M., Deus, J., et al. (2004). Mapping structural brain alterations in obsessive–compulsive disorder. *Archives of General Psychiatry, 61,* 720–730.

Quirk, G. J., Russo, G. K., Barron, J. L., & Lebron, K. (2000). The role of ventromedial prefrontal cortex in the recovery of extinguished fear. *Journal of Neuroscience, 20,* 6225–6231.

Rauch, S. L., Jenike, M. A., Alpert, N. M., Baer, L., Breiter, H. C., Savage, C. R., et al. (1994). Regional cerebral blood flow measured during symptom provocation in obsessive–compulsive disorder using oxygen 15-labeled carbon dioxide and positron emission tomography. *Archives of General Psychiatry, 51,* 62–70.

Rauch, S. L., Savage, C. R., Alpert, N. M., Dougherty, D., Kendrick, A., Curran, T., et al. (1997). Probing striatal function in obsessive–compulsive disorder: A PET study of implicit sequence learning. *Journal of Neuropsychiatry and Clinical Neurosciences, 9,* 568–573.

Rauch, S. L., Shin, L. M., & Phelps, E. A. (2006). Neurocircuitry models of posttraumatic stress disorder and extinction: Human neuroimaging research—past, present, and future. *Biological Psychiatry, 60,* 376–382.

Rauch, S. L., Shin, L. M., Segal, E., Pitman, R. K., Carson, M. A., McMullin, K., et al. (2003). Selectively reduced regional cortical volumes in post-traumatic stress disorder. *NeuroReport, 14,* 913–916.

Rauch, S. L., Shin, L. M., Whalen, P. J., & Pitman, R. K. (1998). Neuroimaging and the neuroanatomy of PTSD. *CNS Spectrums, 3*(Suppl. 2), 30–41.

Rauch, S. L., Shin, L. M., & Wright, C. I. (2003). Neuroimaging studies of amygdala function in anxiety disorders. *Annals of the New York Academy of Sciences, 985,* 389–410.

Rauch, S. L., van der Kolk, B. A., Fisler, R. E., Alpert, N. M., Orr, S. P., Savage, C. R., et al. (1996). A symptom provocation study of posttraumatic stress disorder using positron emission tomography and script-driven imagery. *Archives of General Psychiatry, 53,* 380–387.

Rauch, S. L., Whalen, P., Dougherty, D., & Jenike, M. (1998). Neurobiological models of obsessive compulsive disorders. In M. Jenike, L. Baer, & W. Minichiello

(Eds.), *Obsessive–compulsive disorders: Practical management* (pp. 222–253). St. Louis, MO: Mosby.

Rauch, S. L., Whalen, P. J., Shin, L. M., McInerney, S. C., Macklin, M. L., Lasko, N. B., et al. (2000). Exaggerated amygdala response to masked facial stimuli in posttraumatic stress disorder: A functional MRI study. *Biological Psychiatry, 47*, 769–776.

Robinson, D., Wu, H., Munne, R. A., Ashtari, M., Alvir, J. M., Lerner, G., et al. (1995). Reduced caudate nucleus volume in obsessive–compulsive disorder. *Archives of General Psychiatry, 52*, 393–398.

Rosenberg, D. R., Benazon, N. R., Gilbert, A., Sullivan, A., & Moore, G. J. (2000). Thalamic volume in pediatric obsessive–compulsive disorder patients before and after cognitive behavioral therapy. *Biological Psychiatry, 48*, 294–300.

Rosenberg, D. R., Keshavan, M. S., O'Hearn, K. M., Dick, E. L., Bagwell, W. W., Seymour, A. B., et al. (1997). Frontostriatal measurement in treatment-naive children with obsessive–compulsive disorder. *Archives of General Psychiatry, 54*, 824–830.

Rosenberg, D. R., MacMaster, F. P., Keshavan, M. S., Fitzgerald, K. D., Stewart, C. M., & Moore, G. J. (2000). Decrease in caudate glutamatergic concentrations in pediatric obsessive–compulsive disorder patients taking paroxetine. *Journal of the American Academy of Child and Adolescent Psychiatry, 39*, 1096–1103.

Sakai, Y., Kumano, H., Nishikawa, M., Sakano, Y., Kaiya, H., Imabayashi, E., et al. (2005). Cerebral glucose metabolism associated with a fear network in panic disorder. *NeuroReport, 16*, 927–931.

Sakai, Y., Kumano, H., Nishikawa, M., Sakano, Y., Kaiya, H., Imabayashi, E., et al. (2006). Changes in cerebral glucose utilization in patients with panic disorder treated with cognitive-behavioral therapy. *NeuroImage, 33*, 218–226.

Saxena, S., Brody, A. L., Ho, M. L., Alborzian, S., Maidment, K. M., Zohrabi, N., et al. (2002). Differential cerebral metabolic changes with paroxetine treatment of obsessive–compulsive disorder vs. major depression. *Archives of General Psychiatry, 59*, 250–261.

Saxena, S., Brody, A. L., Maidment, K. M., Smith, E. C., Zohrabi, N., Katz, E., et al. (2004). Cerebral glucose metabolism in obsessive–compulsive hoarding. *American Journal of Psychiatry, 161*, 1038–1048.

Schlegel, S., Steinert, H., Bockisch, A., Hahn, K., Schloesser, R., & Benkert, O. (1994). Decreased benzodiazepine receptor binding in panic disorder measured by iomazenil-SPECT: A preliminary report. *European Archives of Psychiatry and Clinical Neuroscience, 244*, 49–51.

Schneider, F., Weiss, U., Kessler, C., Muller-Gartner, H. W., Posse, S., Salloum, J. B., et al. (1999). Subcortical correlates of differential classical conditioning of aversive emotional reactions in social phobia. *Biological Psychiatry, 45*, 863–871.

Schwartz, C. E., Snidman, N., & Kagan, J. (1999). Adolescent social anxiety as an outcome of inhibited temperament in childhood. *Journal of the American Academy of Child and Adolescent Psychiatry, 38*, 1008–1015.

Schwartz, C. E., Wright, C. I., Shin, L. M., Kagan, J., & Rauch, S. L. (2003). Inhibited and uninhibited infants "grown up": Adult amygdalar response to novelty. *Science, 300*, 1952–1953.

Schwartz, J. M., Stoessel, P. W., Baxter, L. R., Jr., Martin, K. M., & Phelps, M. E. (1996). Systematic changes in cerebral glucose metabolic rate after successful behavior modification treatment of obsessive–compulsive disorder. *Archives of General Psychiatry, 53*, 109–113.

Semple, W. E., Goyer, P. F., McCormick, R., Donovan, B., Muzic, R. F., Jr., Rugle, L., et al. (2000). Higher brain blood flow at amygdala and lower frontal cortex blood flow in PTSD patients with comorbid cocaine and alcohol abuse compared with normals. *Psychiatry, 63*, 65–74.

Servan-Schreiber, D., Perlstein, W. M., Cohen, J. D., & Mintun, M. (1998). Selective pharmacological activation of limbic structures in human volunteers: A positron emission tomography study. *Journal of Neuropsychiatry and Clinical Neurosciences, 10*, 148–159.

Shin, L. M., Kosslyn, S. M., McNally, R. J., Alpert, N. M., Thompson, W. L., Rauch, S. L., et al. (1997). Visual imagery and perception in posttraumatic stress disorder: A positron emission tomographic investigation. *Archives of General Psychiatry, 54*, 233–241.

Shin, L. M., McNally, R. J., Kosslyn, S. M., Thompson, W. L., Rauch, S. L., Alpert, N. M., et al. (1999). Regional cerebral blood flow during script-driven imagery in childhood sexual abuse-related PTSD: A PET investigation. *American Journal of Psychiatry, 156*, 575–584.

Shin, L. M., Orr, S. P., Carson, M. A., Rauch, S. L., Macklin, M. L., Lasko, N. B., et al. (2004). Regional cerebral blood flow in amygdala and medial prefrontal cortex during traumatic imagery in male and female Vietnam veterans with PTSD. *Archives of General Psychiatry, 61*, 168–176.

Shin, L. M., Rauch, S. L., & Pitman, R. K. (2006). Amygdala, medial prefrontal cortex, and hippocampal function in PTSD. *Annals of the New York Academy of Sciences, 1071*, 67–79.

Shin, L. M., Whalen, P. J., Pitman, R. K., Bush, G., Macklin, M. L., Lasko, N. B., et al. (2001). An fMRI study of anterior cingulate function in posttraumatic stress disorder. *Biological Psychiatry, 50*, 932–942.

Shin, L. M., Wright, C. I., Cannistraro, P. A., Wedig, M. M., McMullin, K., Martis, B., et al. (2005). A functional magnetic resonance imaging study of amygdala and medial prefrontal cortex responses to overtly presented fearful faces in posttraumatic stress disorder. *Archives of General Psychiatry, 62*, 273–281.

Simpson, H. B., Lombardo, I., Slifstein, M., Huang, H. Y., Hwang, D. R., Abi-Dargham, A., et al. (2003). Serotonin transporters in obsessive–compulsive disorder: A positron emission tomography study with [(11)C]McN 5652. *Biological Psychiatry, 54*, 1414–1421.

Stein, M. B. (1998). Neurobiological perspectives on social phobia: from affiliation to zoology. *Biological Psychiatry, 44*, 1277–1285.

Stein, M. B., Goldin, P. R., Sareen, J., Zorrilla, L. T., & Brown, G. G. (2002). Increased amygdala activation to angry and contemptuous faces in generalized social phobia. *Archives of General Psychiatry, 59*, 1027–1034.

Straube, T., Mentzel, H. J., & Miltner, W. H. (2005). Common and distinct brain activation to threat and safety signals in social phobia. *Neuropsychobiology, 52*, 163–168.

Swedo, S. E., Pietrini, P., Leonard, H. L., Schapiro, M. B., Rettew, D. C., Goldberger, E. L., et al. (1992). Cerebral glucose metabolism in childhood-onset obsessive-compulsive disorder: Revisualization during pharmacotherapy. *Archives of General Psychiatry, 49*, 690–694.

Swedo, S. E., Schapiro, M. B., Grady, C. L., Cheslow, D. L., Leonard, H. L., Kumar, A., et al. (1989). Cerebral glucose metabolism in childhood-onset obsessive-compulsive disorder. *Archives of General Psychiatry, 46,* 518–523.

Szeszko, P. R., MacMillan, S., McMeniman, M., Lorch, E., Madden, R., Ivey, J., et al. (2004). Amygdala volume reductions in pediatric patients with obsessive-compulsive disorder treated with paroxetine: Preliminary findings. *Neuropsychopharmacology, 29,* 826–832.

Szeszko, P. R., Robinson, D., Alvir, J. M., Bilder, R. M., Lencz, T., Ashtari, M., et al. (1999). Orbital frontal and amygdala volume reductions in obsessive–compulsive disorder. *Archives of General Psychiatry, 56,* 913–919.

Thomas, K. M., Drevets, W. C., Dahl, R. E., Ryan, N. D., Birmaher, B., Eccard, C. H., et al. (2001). Amygdala response to fearful faces in anxious and depressed children. *Archives of General Psychiatry, 58,* 1057–1063.

Tiihonen, J., Kuikka, J., Bergstrom, K., Lepola, U., Koponen, H., & Leinonen, E. (1997). Dopamine reuptake site densities in patients with social phobia. *American Journal of Psychiatry, 154,* 239–242.

Tillfors, M., Furmark, T., Marteinsdottir, I., & Fredrikson, M. (2002). Cerebral blood flow during anticipation of public speaking in social phobia: A PET study. *Biological Psychiatry, 52,* 1113–1119.

Tillfors, M., Furmark, T., Marteinsdottir, I., Fischer, H., Pissiota, A., Langstrom, B., et al. (2001). Cerebral blood flow in subjects with social phobia during stressful speaking tasks: A PET study. *American Journal of Psychiatry, 158,* 1220–1226.

Tupler, L. A., Davidson, J. R., Smith, R. D., Lazeyras, F., Charles, H. C., & Krishnan, K. R. (1997). A repeat proton magnetic resonance spectroscopy study in social phobia. *Biological Psychiatry, 42,* 419–424.

Uchida, R. R., Del-Ben, C. M., Santos, A. C., Araujo, D., Crippa, J. A., Guimaraes, F. S., et al. (2003). Decreased left temporal lobe volume of panic patients measured by magnetic resonance imaging. *Brazilian Journal of Medical and Biological Research, 36,* 925–929.

Valente, A. A., Jr., Miguel, E. C., Castro, C. C., Amaro, E., Jr., Duran, F. L., Buchpiguel, C. A., et al. (2005). Regional gray matter abnormalities in obsessive-compulsive disorder: A voxel-based morphometry study. *Biological Psychiatry, 58,* 479–487.

van den Heuvel, O. A., Veltman, D. J., Groenewegen, H. J., Cath, D. C., van Balkom, A. J., van Hartskamp, J., et al. (2005). Frontal–striatal dysfunction during planning in obsessive–compulsive disorder. *Archives of General Psychiatry, 62,* 301–309.

van den Heuvel, O. A., Veltman, D. J., Groenewegen, H. J., Dolan, R. J., Cath, D. C., Boellaard, R., et al. (2004). Amygdala activity in obsessive–compulsive disorder with contamination fear: A study with oxygen-15 water positron emission tomography. *Psychiatry Research, 132,* 225–237.

van den Heuvel, O. A., Veltman, D. J., Groenewegen, H. J., Witter, M. P., Merkelbach, J., Cath, D. C., et al. (2005). Disorder-specific neuroanatomical correlates of attentional bias in obsessive–compulsive disorder, panic disorder, and hypochondriasis. *Archives of General Psychiatry, 62,* 922–933.

Van Laere, K., Nuttin, B., Gabriels, L., Dupont, P., Rasmussen, S., Greenberg, B. D., et al. (2006). Metabolic imaging of anterior capsular stimulation in refractory obsessive–compulsive disorder: A key role for the subgenual anterior cingulate and ventral striatum. *Journals of Nuclear Medicine, 47,* 740–747.

Veit, R., Flor, H., Erb, M., Hermann, C., Lotze, M., Grodd, W., & et al. (2002). Brain circuits involved in emotional learning in antisocial behavior and social phobia in humans. *Neuroscience Letters, 328,* 233–236.

Vythilingam, M., Anderson, E. R., Goddard, A., Woods, S. W., Staib, L. H., Charney, D. S., et al. (2000). Temporal lobe volume in panic disorder: A quantitative magnetic resonance imaging study. *Psychiatry Research, 99,* 75–82.

Whalen, P. J. (1998). Fear, vigilance, and ambiguity: Initial neuroimaging studies of the human amygdala. *Current Directions in Psychological Science, 6,* 178–188.

Wignall, E. L., Dickson, J. M., Vaughan, P., Farrow, T. F., Wilkinson, I. D., Hunter, M. D., et al. (2004). Smaller hippocampal volume in patients with recent-onset posttraumatic stress disorder. *Biological Psychiatry, 56,* 832–836.

Williams, L. M., Kemp, A. H., Felmingham, K., Barton, M., Olivieri, G., Peduto, A., et al. (2006). Trauma modulates amygdala and medial prefrontal responses to consciously attended fear. *NeuroImage, 29,* 347–357.

Woodward, S. H., Kaloupek, D. G., Streeter, C. C., Martinez, C., Schaer, M., & Eliez, S. (2006). Decreased anterior cingulate volume in combat-related PTSD. *Biological Psychiatry, 59,* 582–587.

Yamasue, H., Kasai, K., Iwanami, A., Ohtani, T., Yamada, H., Abe, O., et al. (2003). Voxel-based analysis of MRI reveals anterior cingulate gray-matter volume reduction in posttraumatic stress disorder due to terrorism. *Proceedings of the National Academy of Sciences USA, 100,* 9039–9043.

Yang, P., Wu, M. T., Hsu, C. C., & Ker, J. H. (2004). Evidence of early neurobiological alternations in adolescents with posttraumatic stress disorder: A functional MRI study. *Neuroscience Letters, 370,* 13–18.

CHAPTER 15

The Human Amygdala in Schizophrenia

Daphne J. Holt and Mary L. Phillips

ABNORMAL EMOTIONAL INFORMATION PROCESSING AND AMYGDALA FUNCTION IN SCHIZOPHRENIA

A characteristic feature of schizophrenia is impaired interpersonal function, with social/occupational dysfunction forming one of the diagnostic criteria for the disorder (American Psychiatric Association, 2000). However, the specific changes in emotional and social-cognitive processing that underlie this impairment have not been fully identified. Some theories of abnormal emotional information processing in schizophrenia have emphasized abnormally increased attention to threatening stimuli (Locascio & Snyder, 1975), particularly in individuals with persecutory delusions. Other theories have emphasized the presence of an abnormal reasoning style, with a tendency for individuals with schizophrenia—again, particularly those with delusions—to adopt an information-processing style of "jumping to conclusions" rather than reappraisal (Huq, Garety, & Hemsley, 1988). More recently, a "vigilance–avoidance" attentional style has been proposed, in which persecutory-themed symptoms of schizophrenia are associated with a "subjective expectation" of threat, coupled with a withdrawal from such stimuli (Green & Phillips, 2004).

These theories point to abnormal function in neural systems associated with appraisal of emotional stimuli, including threatening (or potentially threatening) stimuli in individuals with schizophrenia. As a key component of this neural system (Davis & Whalen, 2001; Phillips, Drevets, Rauch, & Lane, 2003a), the amygdala would be an obvious focus for studies examining the neural systems underlying emotion perception in schizophrenia.

344

In addition to psychotic symptoms (hallucinations and delusions), schizophrenia is characterized by negative symptoms (including affective flattening and anhedonia); disorganization (disordered speech and odd behavior); and cognitive deficits, which have been increasingly recognized as conferring substantial functional disability, particularly deficits in emotional perception and social cognition (Hooker & Park, 2002). Thus the impaired interpersonal functioning characteristic of schizophrenia may be closely linked to deficits in social cognition. Distinct and possibly independent abnormalities in emotional perception and brain function may contribute to these different symptom domains of schizophrenia.

In this chapter, we describe the evidence for abnormal amygdala function in individuals with schizophrenia. First, we examine findings from studies employing an indirect measure of amygdala function: the ability to correctly identify emotionally salient stimuli. Second, we examine findings from neuroimaging studies in which direct measures of amygdala structure and function have been obtained in individuals with schizophrenia and compared with those of healthy individuals. We also describe evidence gathered in individuals with schizophrenia for abnormalities in the hippocampus and parahippocampal gyrus, which are closely connected to the amygdala and are important components of the neural system for stimulus appraisal. We conclude by suggesting that a combination of functional abnormalities in the amygdala and these additional regions may underlie the changes in emotional perception and the associated symptoms in schizophrenia.

DO INDIVIDUALS WITH SCHIZOPHRENIA SHOW ABNORMAL EMOTION IDENTIFICATION?

Evidence from Studies Examining Labeling of Facial Expressions

Facial expressions are among the most socially salient of all stimuli. It is therefore not surprising that impaired processing of facial expressions has been postulated to underlie the social-communicative problems in individuals with schizophrenia. Numerous studies have indeed demonstrated facial expression recognition deficits in schizophrenia (for reviews, see Edwards, Jackson, & Pattison, 2002; Mandal, Pandey, & Prasad, 1998; Morrison, Bellack, & Mueser, 1988). According to some authors, the facial affect recognition deficit varies, depending on the phase of illness (Mueser, Penn, Blanchard, & Bellack, 1997): Some studies report greater deficits in chronic than in acute stages of illness (e.g., Kucharska-Pietura, David, Masiak, & Phillips, 2005). Other findings suggest, however, that emotion identification deficits are present from the onset of the disorder (Edwards, Pattison, Jackson, & Wales, 2001), or that social dysfunction and emotional disturbance may even predate disease onset (Baum & Walker, 1995; Cannon, Mednick, & Parnas, 1990; Walker, Grimes, Davis, & Smith, 1993). Emotion identification difficulties have been recently reported to have a significant impact on social functioning in schizophrenia (Hooker & Park, 2002; Kee, Green, Mintz, & Brekke, 2003).

Studies directly addressing the specificity of this deficit have compared the performance of individuals with schizophrenia and those with mood disorders, demonstrating a greater overall impairment in schizophrenia, with no significant difference between individuals with mood disorders and healthy comparison individuals (Feinberg, Rifkin, Schaffer, & Walker, 1986; Loughland, Williams, & Gordon, 2002). It should also be noted, however, that some studies have indicated abnormal facial affect recognition in persons with depression versus healthy individuals (Gur et al., 1992; Surguladze et al., 2004). Furthermore, it remains unclear whether the emotion identification deficit in schizophrenia represents a generalized performance deficit (Archer, Hay, & Young, 1992; Feinberg et al., 1986; Johnston, Katsikitis, & Carr, 2001; Kerr & Neale, 1993; Kohler, Bilker, Hagendoorn, Gur, & Gur, 2000; Sachs, Steger-Wuchse, Kryspin-Exner, Gur, & Katschnig, 2004; Salem, Kring, & Kerr, 1996; Whittaker, Deakin, & Tomenson, 2001), or a more specific emotion identification deficit (e.g., Borod, Martin, Alpert, Brozgold, & Welkowitz, 1993; Hall et al., 2004; Heimberg, Gur, Erwin, Shtasel, & Gur, 1992; Penn et al., 2000; Silver, Shlomo, Turner, & Gur, 2002; Walker, McGuire, & Betts, 1984).

With regard to the emotion recognition deficit in schizophrenia, there have also been reports indicating an emotion specificity of this deficit, particularly for negative facial expressions (An et al., 2003; Bell, Bryson, & Lysaker, 1997; Borod et al., 1993; Davis & Gibson, 2000; Kline, Smith, & Ellis, 1992; Kucharska-Pietura, David, Dropko, & Klimkowski, 2002; Mandal & Palchoudhury, 1985; Muzekari & Bates, 1977; Pilowsky & Bassett, 1980), such as fear (Evangeli & Broks, 2000), disgust (Mandal, 1987), and sadness (Silver et al., 2002). Other findings indicate a misattribution of negative emotion labels to neutral faces in individuals with schizophrenia (Kohler et al., 2003).

Some studies have associated facial expression recognition deficits with specific symptoms. For example, because delusions are often associated clinically with a tendency to misattribute emotional significance to emotionally neutral or ambiguous information, it has been proposed that delusions arise from a fundamental abnormality in the assignment of emotional meaning to stimuli in the environment (Holt, Titone, et al., 2006; Kapur, 2003).

Evidence from Studies Examining Emotion Labeling of Word Stimuli

Studies using word stimuli have also found that patients with schizophrenia who have delusions are highly sensitive to the emotional content of words. Relative to patients without delusions, patients with delusions have been found to pay more attention to threat-related (Bentall & Kaney, 1989; Fear, Sharp, & Healy, 1996) or generally affect-laden (Kinderman, 1994; Rossell, Shapleske,

& David, 2000) words. Also, patients with persecutory delusions demonstrate higher rates of recall of threat-related words (Bentall, Kaney, & Bowen-Jones, 1995) and propositions (Kaney, Wolfenden, Dewey, & Bentall, 1992) than nondelusional patients do; this suggests that the neural mechanism mediating preferential encoding of emotional over nonemotional information in healthy individuals (Dolan, 2002; Hamann, 2001) is overactive in delusions.

In a study in which participants explicitly evaluated the emotional salience of words, patients with schizophrenia who had active delusions, relative to those without delusions and to healthy subjects, were more likely to classify neutral words as unpleasant (Holt, Titone, et al., 2006). This tendency was correlated with severity of delusional ideation, but not with the severity of hallucinations or depressive symptoms. Taken together, these observations suggest that patients with delusions may be hypervigilant for potentially emotionally salient information in the environment, and consequently may misassign emotional meaning to ambiguous or neutral stimuli.

DO INDIVIDUALS WITH SCHIZOPHRENIA SHOW ABNORMAL APPRAISAL OF EMOTIONAL STIMULI?: EVIDENCE FROM VISUAL SCANPATH STUDIES

Measurement of visual scanpaths allows the direct monitoring of attention to visual stimuli. It not only permits investigators to determine the location of foci of attention on the stimulus, but also provides information about the overall visual appraisal style of the individual. For example, studies employing visual scanpath measurements to examine visual attention to facial stimuli have demonstrated an avoidance of salient facial features and a restricted visual scanning style for emotional faces in individuals with schizophrenia, relative to healthy comparison subjects (Loughland et al., 2002; Streit, Wolwer, & Gaebel, 1997). Other studies have demonstrated similar patterns of abnormal visual attention in delusional patients viewing different facial identities (Phillips & David, 1997, 1998). Green, Williams, and Davidson (2003) found in individuals with persecutory delusions a marked tendency to attend to *less* threatening facial expressions. These findings were interpreted as evidence of increased sensitivity to threat and subsequent threat avoidance in this population, consistent with the vigilance–avoidance model of schizophrenia (Green & Phillips, 2004).

Findings from studies measuring visual attention to other types of emotional stimuli (e.g., pictures of social scenes) have also demonstrated increased visual attention to neutral, but not to overly threatening, components of these scenes in schizophrenia with persecutory delusions (Phillips, Senior, & David, 2000). These findings further suggest that the psychotic symptoms of schizophrenia may be associated with an increased perception of threat from inappropriate stimuli, such as those classified as neutral by healthy individuals.

348   HUMAN AMYGDALA DYSFUNCTION

THE NEURAL BASIS OF ABNORMAL
EMOTION PROCESSING IN SCHIZOPHRENIA

Evidence from Structural Neuroimaging Studies
of the Medial Temporal Lobe in Schizophrenia

It has long been proposed that the medial temporal lobe (which includes the amygdala, hippocampus, and parahippocampal gyrus) represents the neural generator of psychosis (Bogerts, 1997). This hypothesis was based on the early observation that epileptic seizures with foci in the medial temporal lobe are often accompanied by psychotic symptoms, such as hallucinations and delusions (Gaitatzis, Trimble, & Sander, 2004; Kanner, 2004). However, it has been difficult to identify the abnormality within the medial temporal lobe in schizophrenia. Several meta-analyses of structural neuroimaging studies in schizophrenia have shown evidence for volume reductions of both the amygdala and hippocampus of 4–10% (Honea, Crow, Passingham, & Mackay, 2005; Lawrie & Abukmeil, 1998; Nelson, Saykin, Flashman, & Riordan, 1998; Wright et al., 2000), mirroring findings of postmortem studies. Also, several studies have found volume reductions in the amygdalohippocampal complex in individuals at high risk for schizophrenia, including the offspring (Keshavan et al., 2002) and first-degree relatives (Lawrie, Whalley, Job, & Johnstone, 2003) of patients with schizophrenia, and in individuals with schizotypal personality disorder (Suzuki et al., 2005). These findings suggest that reduced medial temporal lobe volumes may represent a genetically mediated risk factor for schizophrenia. One study reported a bilateral reduction in amygdala volume in neuroleptic-naive, first-episode patients (Joyal et al., 2003), indicating that decreased amygdala volume in schizophrenia is unlikely to represent a consequence of treatment with antipsychotic medications.

Several recent studies, however, have not confirmed these earlier findings. A meta-analysis of morphometric studies of patients with a first episode of schizophrenia found evidence for bilateral volume reduction of the hippocampus, but no evidence for reduced amygdala volume (Vita, De Peri, Silenzi, & Dieci, 2006). Also, a large cross-sectional study of medial temporal lobe volumes in (1) individuals at risk for developing psychosis, (2) patients with a first episode of affective psychosis, (3) patients with a first episode of schizophrenia, and (4) patients with chronic schizophrenia found no changes in any group other than the second one, which showed amygdala enlargement; hippocampal volume reductions were shown only in the first-episode and chronic patients, not in the schizophreniform or at-risk subjects (Velakoulis et al., 2006). Another study of schizophrenia and comparison subjects who were drawn from a population-based birth cohort found no evidence for hippocampal or amygdala volume reduction in patients with chronic schizophrenia (Tanskanen et al., 2005). A small study also found no between-group differences in amygdala volume in a comparison of patients with schizophrenia and healthy subjects after intracranial volume normalization was performed; however, in this study, the regional diffusional anisotropy of the amygdala was smaller in the patients than in the controls (Kalus et al., 2005). Possible confounding factors in these studies include illness duration, which in one study correlated inversely with amygdala gray matter density (Hulshoff Pol et al., 2001); gender, as amygdala volume reductions in schizophrenia may occur more frequently in males than in females (Gur et al., 2000); and methodological differences among studies (variability in methods used to delineate the amygdalohippocampal boundary, and inconsistent use of whole-brain volume corrections). In one study, amygdala volumes of patients and healthy subjects predicted performance on an emotional learning task (Exner, Boucsein, Degner, Irle, & Weniger, 2004), suggesting that amygdala volume reductions are associated with emotional perception deficits in schizophrenia.

Evidence from Functional Neuroimaging Studies of the Medial Temporal Lobe

Functional neuroimaging studies using positron emission tomography (PET) and functional magnetic resonance imaging (fMRI) have sought to identify the neural basis of the observed abnormalities in identification and appraisal of emotional stimuli in schizophrenia. Evidence has accumulated to suggest that the different components of the medial temporal lobe, including the amygdala, hippocampus, and parahippocampal gyrus, interact during the encoding and retrieval of the emotional meaning of stimuli encountered in the environment. Studies in healthy subjects have shown that the amygdala and hippocampus are both activated during the successful encoding of emotionally salient information (Dolcos, LaBar, & Cabeza, 2004; Kensinger & Corkin, 2004; Maratos, Dolan, Morris, Henson, & Rugg, 2001; Smith, Dolan, Henson, & Rugg, 2004) and the viewing of emotional facial expressions (R. C. Gur et al., 2002; Williams et al., 2001). The amygdala and hippocampus may influence one another during emotional processing via reciprocal projections (Krettek & Price, 1977; Pitkänen, Pikkarainen, Nurminen, & Ylinen, 2000). The hippocampus has been proposed to be involved in the resolution of conflicts between expectations and current perceptions (Gray, 1998; Gray et al., 1995)—that is, the integration of the assigned value of incoming information with the stored context that has been built up during previous experience. Also, the parahippocampal gyrus has multiple direct connections with the hippocampus and amygdala, and is involved in novelty detection (Schroeder et al., 2004), episodic and spatial memory (Malkova & Mishkin, 2003; Tsukiura et al., 2002) and context appraisal (Sacchetti, Lorenzini, Baldi, Tassoni, & Bucherelli, 1999). Thus dysfunction of the medial temporal lobe in schizophrenia could lead to misassignment of salience to nonsalient stimuli and to impaired retrieval of the previously learned value of objects or events.

Studies conducted to date suggest that medial temporal lobe function in schizophrenia is complex; similar to the pattern of cognitive impairment in schizophrenia, distinct components of emotional processing appear to be differentially affected by the disorder. Differences in experimental design across studies (which may be sensitive to different stages of emotional appraisal) have led to reports of reduced, unchanged, and elevated medial temporal lobe activity during emotional processing in individuals with schizophrenia, relative to healthy comparison subjects. Below we summarize the findings of these studies, and then present one model of abnormal medial temporal lobe and emotional function in schizophrenia.

Studies That Showed *Reduced* Medial Temporal Lobe Responses

To date, 13 functional neuroimaging studies (11 using fMRI and 2 using [^{15}O] PET) have shown evidence for abnormal reductions in amygdala activity in patients with schizophrenia, relative to healthy controls. In 9 of these studies, subjects performed a cognitive task (an explicit affect judgment or gender discrimination task) (R. E. Gur et al., 2002, 2007; Hempel, Hempel, Schonknecht, Stippich, & Schroder, 2003; Johnston, Stojanov, Devir, & Schall, 2005; Phillips et al., 1999; Williams et al., 2004, 2007) or underwent mood induction (Habel et al., 2004; Schneider et al., 1998) while viewing emotional facial expressions. Also, in 3 studies, subjects performed cognitive tasks while viewing emotionally salient pictures (Paradiso et al., 2003; Takahashi et al., 2004; Taylor, Liberzon, Decker, & Koeppe, 2002). Of these 13 studies, 6 (R. E. Gur et al., 2002, 2007; Hempel et al., 2003; Paradiso et al., 2003; Takahashi et al., 2004; Williams et al., 2007) reported reduced activity of the hippocampus as well as the amygdala in the patient group. The majority of these studies used one of two designs: (1) a comparison of responses to emotional stimuli (faces or pictures) to responses to neutral stimuli (Das et al., 2007; Hempel et al., 2003; Paradiso et al., 2003; Phillips et al., 1999; Takahashi et al., 2004; Taylor et al., 2002; Williams et al., 2007); or (2) a comparison of responses to emotional facial expressions during an explicit emotional judgment or mood induction task to responses to the same stimuli during a gender discrimination task (R. E. Gur et al., 2002; Habel et al., 2004; Schneider et al., 1998).

Given that all of these studies were conducted with medicated patients, it is possible that treatment with antipsychotic medication played a role in these findings. However, although there is evidence that antipsychotic treatment inhibits amygdala function (Greba, Gifkins, & Kokkinidis, 2001; Pezze & Feldon, 2004), one study demonstrated diminished amygdala activity during sad mood induction in unaffected brothers of individuals with schizophrenia, relative to healthy subjects without such relatives (Habel et al., 2004)—suggesting that functional impairment of the amygdala could represent a marker of genetic vulnerability to schizophrenia.

Studies That Showed *Increased* Medial Temporal Lobe Responses

Three studies have reported increased responses of the amygdala in patients with schizophrenia, relative to healthy controls, in response to happy (Kosaka et al., 2002), fearful (Gur et al., 2007; Holt, Kunkel, et al., 2006), and neutral

(Holt, Kunkel, et al., 2006) facial expressions. Unlike the studies that found decreased amygdala responses to emotional facial expressions in schizophrenia, the baseline, comparator condition in two of these studies (Holt, Kunkel, et al., 2006; Kosaka et al., 2002) did not include faces. One study found elevated amygdala activation in patients relative to controls when fearful faces were incorrectly identified, but greater amygdala activation in controls relative to patients when fearful faces were correctly identified (Gur et al., 2007), suggesting that uncertainty about the emotion expressed by the faces may have led to elevated amygdala activation in the patients. In general, these studies that found abnormally increased medial temporal lobe activity in schizophrenia were minimally demanding from a cognitive standpoint, with an easy task that both groups performed at ceiling levels (Gur et al., 2007; Kosaka et al., 2002), or no task at all (Holt, Kunkel, et al., 2006). Also, one of these studies and three additional studies found increased hippocampal and/or parahippocampal gyral responses to emotional (Holt et al., 2005; Holt, Kunkel, et al., 2006; Russell et al., 2007) and neutral or less fearful (Holt, Kunkel, et al., 2006; Surguladze et al., 2006) facial expressions in patients relative to healthy subjects, supporting the notion that a number of regions within the medial temporal lobe may be involved in the generation of abnormal emotional appraisals in schizophrenia.

Studies That Showed *Normal* Medial Temporal Lobe Responses

Two functional neuroimaging studies failed to detect differences between healthy participants and patients with schizophrenia in amygdala activity when responses to emotional facial expressions (Holt, Kunkel, et al., 2006) or emotional pictures (Taylor, Phan, Britton, & Liberzon, 2005) were compared with responses to neutral stimuli of the same category.

Studies That Showed Subtype- or Symptom-Specific Effects

Patients with schizophrenia with prominent psychotic symptoms (paranoid subtype) have shown diminished amygdala responses to fearful facial expressions, relative to patients without paranoia (Williams et al., 2004, 2007) and healthy control subjects (Phillips et al., 1999; Williams et al., 2004). Given that in these studies, amygdala responses to fearful faces were compared with responses to neutral faces, abnormally elevated amygdala responses to neutral facial expressions in the paranoid patients may have contributed to these results. Consistent with this possibility is a parallel finding in one of these studies (Williams et al., 2004) of greater autonomic responding (higher number of skin conductance responses) to neutral facial expressions, as well as to fearful expressions, in the patients than in the controls. Similarly, a finding of a positive correlation between the magnitude of parahippocampal gyral responses to neutral facial expressions and severity of psychosis (Surguladze et al., 2006) supports this interpretation. Also, positive correlations between

(1) amygdala responses to sad facial expressions and thought disorder severity (Schneider et al., 1998); (2) amygdala responses to dynamic representations of decreasing rather than increasing fearful facial expressions and levels of positive psychotic symptoms (Russell et al., 2007); and (3) amygdala responses to neutral pictures (and, to a lesser extent, to unpleasant pictures) and levels of psychotic symptoms (Taylor et al., 2002) provide additional evidence for a direct link between amygdala responsivity to nonthreatening stimuli and psychosis severity.

SUMMARY AND OVERALL MODEL

Studies examining emotion labeling in patients with schizophrenia show evidence for an attentional bias toward potential threat and attribution of threat to ambiguous or even neutral stimuli. Visual scanpath studies provide evidence of both an avoidance of visual attention to overtly threatening stimuli and relative increases in visual attention to more neutral components of a stimulus. The functional neuroimaging studies discussed above provide parallel, paradoxical findings regarding the processing of threat-related information in patients with schizophrenia, in that many suggest *decreased* rather than increased amygdala activity to explicitly negative emotional stimuli. Of the studies showing increases in amygdala, hippocampal, and parahippocampal gyral activity in schizophrenia, many of these increases in neural activity were to the *less negative or neutral* stimuli in the study, rather than the negative stimuli.

The tendency of patients with schizophrenia to label neutral stimuli as negative, together with findings of an increase in amygdala activity to the less negative or neutral stimuli in a given experimental context rather than to the explicitly negative stimuli, suggests dysfunctional rather than decreased amygdala activity per se. In these studies, abnormal *increases* in amygdala activity occurred to stimuli other than those depicting prototypical displays of fear. These findings suggest that a response bias in the amygdala to potentially *ambiguous*, rather than explicitly threatening, stimuli may be present in patients with schizophrenia, particularly in those individuals with positive symptoms or persecutory delusions (Phillips, Drevets, Rauch, & Lane, 2003b). Visual scanpath studies provide parallel findings of relative increases in attention to more neutral components of a complex stimulus in patients with delusions (Phillips et al., 2000).

These findings indicate the presence of an abnormal appraisal process, such that sustained attention may occur to ambiguous (i.e., potentially threatening) rather than to overtly threatening stimuli in individuals with schizophrenia—particularly in those with persecutory delusions. If this is the case, then we would expect to observe increased activity in other regions linked functionally with the amygdala during the response to less negative versus more negative emotional stimuli. Consistent with this are findings of increased hippocampal and parahippocampal gyral activity to neutral stimuli in patients with schizophrenia, particularly in those with positive symptoms. Thus the coordinated activity of the amygdala, hippocampus and parahippocampal gyrus may therefore be disrupted in schizophrenia, leading to abnormal assignment of salience to ambiguous, potentially threatening stimuli in the environment.

Findings from the studies of emotion labeling, visual scanpaths, and neuroimaging reviewed in this chapter therefore suggest the following:

1. Patients with schizophrenia show impaired recognition and increased avoidance of threatening stimuli, and reduced medial temporal lobe responses to explicitly negative stimuli.
2. An attentional bias toward threatening stimuli is present in some such patients, particularly in those with positive symptoms.
3. Individuals with positive or persecutory-themed symptoms of schizophrenia show a tendency to mislabel neutral or ambiguous stimuli as threatening, and to exhibit increased medial temporal lobe activity to neutral or ambiguous stimuli.

These findings can be incorporated into an overall model proposing that early hypervigilance for threat is accompanied by a more sustained avoidance and withdrawal from threatening stimuli and contexts in schizophrenia (Green & Phillips, 2004). This early, increased vigilance to threatening stimuli may be accompanied by a corresponding increase in medial temporal lobe activity. However, increases in medial temporal lobe activity may be detectable only under certain experimental conditions—for example, in functional neuroimaging studies that focus on early responses to stimuli by using short stimulus durations and/or event-related designs. Consistent with this possibility is the finding of greater amygdala activation in patients with schizophrenia than in healthy controls during the *initial* presentation of fearful and neutral facial expressions (Holt, Kunkel, et al., 2006).

The subsequent avoidance of, and withdrawal from, threatening stimuli may be associated with *decreased* rather than increased medial temporal lobe activity, and with corresponding diminished attention to threatening stimuli or stimulus components. This pattern of an initial increase, coupled with a more sustained decrease, in activity of the medial temporal lobe during emotional processing in schizophrenia may result from distinct effects of the illness on automatic versus controlled emotional appraisal mechanisms (LeDoux, 2000). In schizophrenia, fast, automatic emotional appraisal processes may be intact or hyperresponsive, while strategic, controlled emotional appraisal may be impaired to a greater extent, leading to a failure to effectively regulate automatic emotional responses to environmental stimuli.

These distinct abnormalities in automatic and controlled emotional appraisal processes could result from disrupted interactions among the amygdala, hippocampus, and parahippocampal gyrus (as well as interactions with other closely connected regions, such as the medial prefrontal cortex, posterior cingulate gyrus, and midbrain). Such disruptions may lead to elevated responses to neutral stimuli in patients with schizophrenia, particularly in those with positive symptoms, and to abnormal attribution of salience to otherwise neutral or ambiguous information.

WHAT WE THINK

The complex nature of abnormalities in emotional processing in schizophrenia, and their potential relationships to concurrent abnormalities in cognitive and sensory function, highlights the importance of careful study design and characterization of study participants (in particular, attention to heterogeneity within groups of participants diagnosed with schizophrenia). The possibility that the changes in brain function during emotional processing in schizophrenia are highly dynamic in nature— with an initial hyperresponsivity followed by hyporesponsivity of medial temporal lobe structures—can be evaluated further by using techniques with high levels of temporal sensitivity, such as electroencephalography and magnetoencephalography, in combination with those with high spatial resolution, such as fMRI. Also, the identification of disrupted interactions among components of the medial temporal lobe in schizophrenia will require a more complete understanding of the functional relationships among these structures in healthy individuals. Ultimately, studies that combine behavioral and neuroimaging methods, and that include detailed assessments of the symptomatic state of the patients studied, will bring us closer to a quantitative understanding of the function of the amygdala and other areas of the medial temporal lobe in individuals with schizophrenia.

REFERENCES

American Psychiatric Association. (2000). *Diagnostic and statistical manual of mental disorders* (4th ed., text rev.). Washington, DC: Author.

An, S. K., Lee, S. J., Lee, C. H., Cho, H. S., Lee, P. G., Lee, C. I., et al. (2003). Reduced P3 amplitudes by negative facial emotional photographs in schizophrenia. *Schizophrenia Research, 64,* 125–135.

Archer, J., Hay, D. C., & Young, A. W. (1992). Face processing in psychiatric conditions. *British Journal of Clinical Psychology, 31*(Pt. 1), 45–61.

Baum, K. M., & Walker, E. F. (1995). Childhood behavioral precursors of adult symptom dimensions in schizophrenia. *Schizophrenia Research, 16,* 111–120.

Bell, M., Bryson, G., & Lysaker, P. (1997). Positive and negative affect recognition in schizophrenia: A comparison with substance abuse and normal control subjects. *Psychiatry Research, 73,* 73–82.

Bentall, R. P., & Kaney, S. (1989). Content specific information processing and persecutory delusions: An investigation using the emotional Stroop test. *British Journal of Medical Psychology, 62*(Pt. 4), 355–364.

Bentall, R. P., Kaney, S., & Bowen-Jones, K. (1995). Persecutory delusions and recall of threat-related, depression-related, and neutral words. *Cognitive Therapy and Research, 19,* 445–457.

Bogerts, B. (1997). The temporolimbic system theory of positive schizophrenic symptoms. *Schizophrenia Bulletin, 23*, 423–435.

Borod, J. C., Martin, C. C., Alpert, M., Brozgold, A., & Welkowitz, J. (1993). Perception of facial emotion in schizophrenic and right brain-damaged patients. *Journal of Nervous and Mental Disease, 181*, 494–502.

Cannon, T. D., Mednick, S. A., & Parnas, J. (1990). Antecedents of predominantly negative- and predominantly positive-symptom schizophrenia in a high-risk population. *Archives of General Psychiatry, 47*, 622–632.

Das, P., Kemp, A. H., Flynn, G., Harris, A. W., Liddell, B. J., Whitford, T. J., et al. (2007). Functional disconnections in the direct and indirect amygdala pathways for fear processing in schizophrenia. *Schizophrenia Research, 90*, 284–294.

Davis, M., & Whalen, P. J. (2001). The amygdala: Vigilance and emotion. *Molecular Psychiatry, 6*, 13–34.

Davis, P. J., & Gibson, M. G. (2000). Recognition of posed and genuine facial expressions of emotion in paranoid and nonparanoid schizophrenia. *Journal of Abnormal Psychology, 109*, 445–450.

Dolan, R. J. (2002). Emotion, cognition, and behavior. *Science, 298*, 1191–1194.

Dolcos, F., LaBar, K. S., & Cabeza, R. (2004). Interaction between the amygdala and the medial temporal lobe memory system predicts better memory for emotional events. *Neuron, 42*, 855–863.

Edwards, J., Jackson, H. J., & Pattison, P. E. (2002). Emotion recognition via facial expression and affective prosody in schizophrenia: A methodological review. *Clinical Psychology Review, 22*, 789–832.

Edwards, J., Pattison, P. E., Jackson, H. J., & Wales, R. J. (2001). Facial affect and affective prosody recognition in first-episode schizophrenia. *Schizophrenia Research, 48*, 235–253.

Evangeli, M., & Broks, M. E. (2000). Face processing in schizophrenia: Parallels with the effects of amygdala damage. *Cognitive Neuropsychiatry, 5*, 81–104.

Exner, C., Boucsein, K., Degner, D., Irle, E., & Weniger, G. (2004). Impaired emotional learning and reduced amygdala size in schizophrenia: A 3-month follow-up. *Schizophrenia Research, 71*, 493–503.

Fear, C., Sharp, H., & Healy, D. (1996). Cognitive processes in delusional disorders. *British Journal of Psychiatry, 168*, 61–67.

Feinberg, T. E., Rifkin, A., Schaffer, C., & Walker, E. (1986). Facial discrimination and emotional recognition in schizophrenia and affective disorders. *Archives of General Psychiatry, 43*, 276–279.

Gaitatzis, A., Trimble, M. R., & Sander, J. W. (2004). The psychiatric comorbidity of epilepsy. *Acta Neurologica Scandinavica, 110*, 207–220.

Gray, J. A. (1998). Integrating schizophrenia. *Schizophrenia Bulletin, 24*, 249–266.

Gray, J. A., Joseph, M. H., Hemsley, D. R., Young, A. M., Warburton, E. C., Boulenguez, P., et al. (1995). The role of mesolimbic dopaminergic and retrohippocampal afferents to the nucleus accumbens in latent inhibition: Implications for schizophrenia. *Behavioural Brain Research, 71*, 19–31.

Greba, Q., Gifkins, A., & Kokkinidis, L. (2001). Inhibition of amygdaloid dopamine D2 receptors impairs emotional learning measured with fear-potentiated startle. *Brain Research, 899*, 218–226.

Green, M. J., & Phillips, M. L. (2004). Social threat perception and the evolution of paranoia. *Neuroscience and Biobehavioral Reviews, 28*, 333–342.

Green, M. J., Williams, L. M., & Davidson, D. (2003). Visual scanpaths to threat-related faces in deluded schizophrenia. *Psychiatry Research*, 119, 271–285.

Gur, R. C., Erwin, R. J., Gur, R. E., Zwil, A. S., Heimberg, C., & Kraemer, H. C. (1992). Facial emotion discrimination: II. Behavioral findings in depression. *Psychiatry Research*, 42, 241–251.

Gur, R. C., Schroeder, L., Turner, T., McGrath, C., Chan, R. M., Turetsky, B. I., et al. (2002). Brain activation during facial emotion processing. *NeuroImage*, 16, 651–662.

Gur, R. E., Loughead, J., Kohler, C. G., Elliott, M. A., Lesko, K., Ruparel, K., et al. (2007). Limbic activation associated with misidentification of fearful faces and flat affect in schizophrenia. *Archives of General Psychiatry*, 64, 1356–1366.

Gur, R. E., McGrath, C., Chan, R. M., Schroeder, L., Turner, T., Turetsky, B. I., et al. (2002). An fMRI study of facial emotion processing in patients with schizophrenia. *American Journal of Psychiatry*, 159, 1992–1999.

Gur, R. E., Turetsky, B. I., Cowell, P. E., Finkelman, C., Maany, V., Grossman, R. I., et al. (2000). Temporolimbic volume reductions in schizophrenia. *Archives of General Psychiatry*, 57, 769–775.

Habel, U., Klein, M., Shah, N. J., Toni, I., Zilles, K., Falkai, P., et al. (2004). Genetic load on amygdala hypofunction during sadness in nonaffected brothers of schizophrenia patients. *American Journal of Psychiatry*, 161, 1806–1813.

Hall, J., Harris, J. M., Sprengelmeyer, R., Sprengelmeyer, A., Young, A. W., Santos, I. M., et al. (2004). Social cognition and face processing in schizophrenia. *British Journal of Psychiatry*, 185, 169–170.

Hamann, S. (2001). Cognitive and neural mechanisms of emotional memory. *Trends in Cognitive Sciences*, 5, 394–400.

Heimberg, C., Gur, R. E., Erwin, R. J., Shtasel, D. L., & Gur, R. C. (1992). Facial emotion discrimination: III. Behavioral findings in schizophrenia. *Psychiatry Research*, 42, 253–265.

Hempel, A., Hempel, E., Schonknecht, P., Stippich, C., & Schroder, J. (2003). Impairment in basal limbic function in schizophrenia during affect recognition. *Psychiatry Research*, 122, 115–124.

Holt, D. J., Kunkel, L., Weiss, A. P., Goff, D. C., Wright, C. I., Shin, L. M., et al. (2006). Increased medial temporal lobe activation during the passive viewing of emotional and neutral facial expressions in schizophrenia. *Schizophrenia Research*, 82, 153–162.

Holt, D. J., Titone, D., Long, L. S., Goff, D. C., Cather, C., Rauch, S. L., et al. (2006). The misattribution of salience in delusional patients with schizophrenia. *Schizophrenia Research*, 83, 247–256.

Holt, D. J., Weiss, A. P., Rauch, S. L., Wright, C. I., Zalesak, M., Goff, D. C., et al. (2005). Sustained activation of the hippocampus in response to fearful faces in schizophrenia. *Biological Psychiatry*, 57, 1011–1019.

Honea, R., Crow, T. J., Passingham, D., & Mackay, C. E. (2005). Regional deficits in brain volume in schizophrenia: A meta-analysis of voxel-based morphometry studies. *American Journal of Psychiatry*, 162, 2233–2245.

Hooker, C., & Park, S. (2002). Emotion processing and its relationship to social functioning in schizophrenia patients. *Psychiatry Research*, 112, 41–50.

Hulshoff Pol, H. E., Schnack, H. G., Mandl, R. C., van Haren, N. E., Koning, H., Collins, D. L., et al. (2001). Focal gray matter density changes in schizophrenia. *Archives of General Psychiatry*, 58, 1118–1125.

Huq, S. F., Garety, P. A., & Hemsley, D. R. (1988). Probabilistic judgements in deluded and non-deluded subjects. *Quarterly Journal of Experimental Psychology A*, *40*, 801–812.

Johnston, P. J., Katsikitis, M., & Carr, V. J. (2001). A generalised deficit can account for problems in facial emotion recognition in schizophrenia. *Biological Psychology*, *58*, 203–227.

Johnston, P. J., Stojanov, W., Devir, H., & Schall, U. (2005). Functional MRI of facial emotion recognition deficits in schizophrenia and their electrophysiological correlates. *European Journal of Neuroscience*, *22*, 1221–1232.

Joyal, C. C., Laakso, M. P., Tiihonen, J., Syvalahti, E., Vilkman, H., Laakso, A., et al. (2003). The amygdala and schizophrenia: A volumetric magnetic resonance imaging study in first-episode, neuroleptic-naive patients. *Biological Psychiatry*, *54*, 1302–1304.

Kalus, P., Slotboom, J., Gallinat, J., Federspiel, A., Gralla, J., Remonda, L., et al. (2005). New evidence for involvement of the entorhinal region in schizophrenia: A combined MRI volumetric and DTI study. *NeuroImage*, *24*, 1122–1129.

Kaney, S., Wolfenden, M., Dewey, M. E., & Bentall, R. P. (1992). Persecutory delusions and recall of threatening propositions. *British Journal of Clinical Psychology*, *31*(Pt. 1), 85–87.

Kanner, A. M. (2004). Recognition of the various expressions of anxiety, psychosis, and aggression in epilepsy. *Epilepsia*, *45*(Suppl. 2), 22–27.

Kapur, S. (2003). Psychosis as a state of aberrant salience: A framework linking biology, phenomenology, and pharmacology in schizophrenia. *American Journal of Psychiatry*, *160*, 13–23.

Kee, K. S., Green, M. F., Mintz, J., & Brekke, J. S. (2003). Is emotion processing a predictor of functional outcome in schizophrenia? *Schizophrenia Bulletin*, *29*, 487–497.

Kensinger, E. A., & Corkin, S. (2004). Two routes to emotional memory: Distinct neural processes for valence and arousal. *Proceedings of the National Academy of Sciences USA*, *101*, 3310–3315.

Kerr, S. L., & Neale, J. M. (1993). Emotion perception in schizophrenia: Specific deficit or further evidence of generalized poor performance? *Journal of Abnormal Psychology*, *102*, 312–318.

Keshavan, M. S., Dick, E., Mankowski, I., Harenski, K., Montrose, D. M., Diwadkar, V., et al. (2002). Decreased left amygdala and hippocampal volumes in young offspring at risk for schizophrenia. *Schizophrenia Research*, *58*, 173–183.

Kinderman, P. (1994). Attentional bias, persecutory delusions and the self-concept. *British Journal of Medical Psychology*, *67*(Pt. 1), 53–66.

Kline, J. S., Smith, J. E., & Ellis, H. C. (1992). Paranoid and nonparanoid schizophrenic processing of facially displayed affect. *Journal of Psychiatric Research*, *26*, 169–182.

Kohler, C. G., Bilker, W., Hagendoorn, M., Gur, R. E., & Gur, R. C. (2000). Emotion recognition deficit in schizophrenia: Association with symptomatology and cognition. *Biological Psychiatry*, *48*, 127–136.

Kohler, C. G., Turner, T. H., Bilker, W. B., Brensinger, C. M., Siegel, S. J., Kanes, S. J., et al. (2003). Facial emotion recognition in schizophrenia: Intensity effects and error pattern. *American Journal of Psychiatry*, *160*, 1768–1774.

Kosaka, H., Omori, M., Murata, T., Iidaka, T., Yamada, H., Okada, T., et al. (2002).

Differential amygdala response during facial recognition in patients with schizophrenia: An fMRI study. *Schizophrenia Research, 57,* 87–95.

Krettek, J. E., & Price, J. L. (1977). Projections from the amygdaloid complex and adjacent olfactory structures to the entorhinal cortex and to the subiculum in the rat and cat. *Journal of Comparative Neurology, 172,* 723–752.

Kucharska-Pietura, K., David, A. S., Dropko, P., & Klimkowski, M. (2002). The perception of emotional chimeric faces in schizophrenia: Further evidence of right hemisphere dysfunction. *Neuropsychiatry, Neuropsychology, and Behavioral Neurology, 15,* 72–78.

Kucharska-Pietura, K., David, A. S., Masiak, M., & Phillips, M. L. (2005). Perception of facial and vocal affect by people with schizophrenia in early and late stages of illness. *British Journal of Psychiatry, 187,* 523–528.

Lawrie, S. M., & Abukmeil, S. S. (1998). Brain abnormality in schizophrenia: A systematic and quantitative review of volumetric magnetic resonance imaging studies. *British Journal of Psychiatry, 172,* 110–120.

Lawrie, S. M., Whalley, H. C., Job, D. E., & Johnstone, E. C. (2003). Structural and functional abnormalities of the amygdala in schizophrenia. *Annals of the New York Academy of Sciences, 985,* 445–460.

LeDoux, J. E. (2000). Emotion circuits in the brain. *Annual Review of Neuroscience, 23,* 155–184.

Locascio, J. J., & Snyder, C. R. (1975). Selective attention to threatening stimuli and field independence as factors in the etiology of paranoid behavior. *Journal of Abnormal Psychology, 84,* 637–643.

Loughland, C. M., Williams, L. M., & Gordon, E. (2002). Visual scanpaths to positive and negative facial emotions in an outpatient schizophrenia sample. *Schizophrenia Research, 55,* 159–170.

Malkova, L., & Mishkin, M. (2003). One-trial memory for object–place associations after separate lesions of hippocampus and posterior parahippocampal region in the monkey. *Journal of Neuroscience, 23,* 1956–1965.

Mandal, M. K. (1987). Decoding of facial emotions, in terms of expressiveness, by schizophrenics and depressives. *Psychiatry, 50,* 371–376.

Mandal, M. K., & Palchoudhury, S. (1985). Decoding of facial affect in schizophrenia. *Psychological Reports, 56,* 651–652.

Mandal, M. K., Pandey, R., & Prasad, A. B. (1998). Facial expressions of emotions and schizophrenia: A review. *Schizophrenia Bulletin, 24,* 399–412.

Maratos, E. J., Dolan, R. J., Morris, J. S., Henson, R. N., & Rugg, M. D. (2001). Neural activity associated with episodic memory for emotional context. *Neuropsychologia, 39,* 910–920.

Morrison, R. L., Bellack, A. S., & Mueser, K. T. (1988). Deficits in facial-affect recognition and schizophrenia. *Schizophrenia Bulletin, 14,* 67–83.

Mueser, K. T., Penn, D. L., Blanchard, J. J., & Bellack, A. S. (1997). Affect recognition in schizophrenia: A synthesis of findings across three studies. *Psychiatry, 60,* 301–308.

Muzekari, L. H., & Bates, M. E. (1977). Judgment of emotion among chronic schizophrenics. *Journal of Clinical Psychology, 33,* 662–666.

Nelson, M. D., Saykin, A. J., Flashman, L. A., & Riordan, H. J. (1998). Hippocampal volume reduction in schizophrenia as assessed by magnetic resonance imaging: A meta-analytic study. *Archives of General Psychiatry, 55,* 433–440.

Paradiso, S., Andreasen, N. C., Crespo-Facorro, B., O'Leary, D. S., Watkins, G. L.,

Boles Ponto, L. L., et al. (2003). Emotions in unmedicated patients with schizophrenia during evaluation with positron emission tomography. *American Journal of Psychiatry, 160*, 1775–1783.

Penn, D. L., Combs, D. R., Ritchie, M., Francis, J., Cassisi, J., Morris, S., et al. (2000). Emotion recognition in schizophrenia: Further investigation of generalized versus specific deficit models. *Journal of Abnormal Psychology, 109*, 512–516.

Pezze, M. A., & Feldon, J. (2004). Mesolimbic dopaminergic pathways in fear conditioning. *Progress in Neurobiology, 74*, 301–320.

Phillips, M. L., & David, A. S. (1997). Visual scan paths are abnormal in deluded schizophrenics. *Neuropsychologia, 35*, 99–105.

Phillips, M. L., & David, A. S. (1998). Abnormal visual scan paths: A psychophysiological marker of delusions in schizophrenia. *Schizophrenia Research, 29*, 235–245.

Phillips, M. L., Drevets, W. C., Rauch, S. L., & Lane, R. (2003a). Neurobiology of emotion perception: I. The neural basis of normal emotion perception. *Biological Psychiatry, 54*, 504–514.

Phillips, M. L., Drevets, W. C., Rauch, S. L., & Lane, R. (2003b). Neurobiology of emotion perception: II. Implications for major psychiatric disorders. *Biological Psychiatry, 54*, 515–528.

Phillips, M. L., Senior, C., & David, A. S. (2000). Perception of threat in schizophrenics with persecutory delusions: An investigation using visual scan paths. *Psychological Medicine, 30*, 157–167.

Phillips, M. L., Williams, L., Senior, C., Bullmore, E. T., Brammer, M. J., Andrew, C., et al. (1999). A differential neural response to threatening and non-threatening negative facial expressions in paranoid and non-paranoid schizophrenics. *Psychiatry Research, 92*, 11–31.

Pilowsky, I., & Bassett, D. (1980). Schizophrenia and the response to facial emotions. *Comprehensive Psychiatry, 21*, 236–244.

Pitkänen, A., Pikkarainen, M., Nurminen, N., & Ylinen, A. (2000). Reciprocal connections between the amygdala and the hippocampal formation, perirhinal cortex, and postrhinal cortex in rat: A review. *Annals of the New York Academy of Sciences, 911*, 369–391.

Rossell, S. L., Shapleske, J., & David, A. S. (2000). Direct and indirect semantic priming with neutral and emotional words in schizophrenia: Relationship to delusions. *Cognitive Neuropsychiatry, 5*, 271–292.

Russell, T. A., Reynaud, E., Kucharska-Pietura, K., Ecker, C., Benson, P. J., Zelaya, F., et al. (2007). Neural responses to dynamic expressions of fear in schizophrenia. *Neuropsychologia, 45*(1), 107–123.

Sacchetti, B., Lorenzini, C. A., Baldi, E., Tassoni, G., & Bucherelli, C. (1999). Auditory thalamus, dorsal hippocampus, basolateral amygdala, and perirhinal cortex role in the consolidation of conditioned freezing to context and to acoustic conditioned stimulus in the rat. *Journal of Neuroscience, 19*, 9570–9578.

Sachs, G., Steger-Wuchse, D., Kryspin-Exner, I., Gur, R. C., & Katschnig, H. (2004). Facial recognition deficits and cognition in schizophrenia. *Schizophrenia Research, 68*, 27–35.

Salem, J. E., Kring, A. M., & Kerr, S. L. (1996). More evidence for generalized poor performance in facial emotion perception in schizophrenia. *Journal of Abnormal Psychology, 105*, 480–483.

Schneider, F., Weiss, U., Kessler, C., Salloum, J. B., Posse, S., Grodd, W., et al. (1998).

Differential amygdala activation in schizophrenia during sadness. *Schizophrenia Research, 34,* 133–142.

Schroeder, U., Hennenlotter, A., Erhard, P., Haslinger, B., Stahl, R., Lange, K. W., et al. (2004). Functional neuroanatomy of perceiving surprised faces. *Human Brain Mapping, 23,* 181–187.

Silver, H., Shlomo, N., Turner, T., & Gur, R. C. (2002). Perception of happy and sad facial expressions in chronic schizophrenia: Evidence for two evaluative systems. *Schizophrenia Research, 55,* 171–177.

Smith, A. P., Henson, R. N., Dolan, R. J., & Rugg, M. D. (2004). fMRI correlates of the episodic retrieval of emotional contexts. *NeuroImage, 22,* 868–878.

Streit, M., Wolwer, W., & Gaebel, W. (1997). Facial-affect recognition and visual scanning behaviour in the course of schizophrenia. *Schizophrenia Research, 24,* 311–317.

Surguladze, S., Russell, T., Kucharska-Pietura, K., Travis, M. J., Giampietro, V., David, A. S., et al. (2006). A reversal of the normal pattern of parahippocampal response to neutral and fearful faces is associated with reality distortion in schizophrenia. *Biological Psychiatry, 60(5),* 423–431.

Surguladze, S. A., Young, A. W., Senior, C., Brebion, G., Travis, M. J., & Phillips, M. L. (2004). Recognition accuracy and response bias to happy and sad facial expressions in patients with major depression. *Neuropsychology, 18,* 212–218.

Suzuki, M., Zhou, S. Y., Takahashi, T., Hagino, H., Kawasaki, Y., Niu, L., et al. (2005). Differential contributions of prefrontal and temporolimbic pathology to mechanisms of psychosis. *Brain, 128,* 2109–2122.

Takahashi, H., Koeda, M., Oda, K., Matsuda, T., Matsushima, E., Matsuura, M., et al. (2004). An fMRI study of differential neural response to affective pictures in schizophrenia. *NeuroImage, 22,* 1247–1254.

Tanskanen, P., Veijola, J. M., Piippo, U. K., Haapea, M., Miettunen, J. A., Pyhtinen, J., et al. (2005). Hippocampus and amygdala volumes in schizophrenia and other psychoses in the Northern Finland 1966 birth cohort. *Schizophrenia Research, 75,* 283–294.

Taylor, S. F., Liberzon, I., Decker, L. R., & Koeppe, R. A. (2002). A functional anatomic study of emotion in schizophrenia. *Schizophrenia Research, 58,* 159–172.

Taylor, S. F., Phan, K. L., Britton, J. C., & Liberzon, I. (2005). Neural response to emotional salience in schizophrenia. *Neuropsychopharmacology, 30,* 984–995.

Tsukiura, T., Fujii, T., Takahashi, T., Xiao, R., Sugiura, M., Okuda, J., et al. (2002). Medial temporal lobe activation during context-dependent relational processes in episodic retrieval: An fMRI study. Functional magnetic resonance imaging. *Human Brain Mapping, 17,* 203–213.

Velakoulis, D., Wood, S. J., Wong, M. T., McGorry, P. D., Yung, A., Phillips, L., et al. (2006). Hippocampal and amygdala volumes according to psychosis stage and diagnosis: A magnetic resonance imaging study of chronic schizophrenia, first-episode psychosis, and ultra-high-risk individuals. *Archives of General Psychiatry, 63,* 139–149.

Vita, A., De Peri, L., Silenzi, C., & Dieci, M. (2006). Brain morphology in first-episode schizophrenia: A meta-analysis of quantitative magnetic resonance imaging studies. *Schizophrenia Research, 82,* 75–88.

Walker, E., McGuire, M., & Bettes, B. (1984). Recognition and identification of facial stimuli by schizophrenics and patients with affective disorders. *British Journal of Clinical Psychology, 23*(Pt. 1), 37–44.

Walker, E. F., Grimes, K. E., Davis, D. M., & Smith, A. J. (1993). Childhood precursors of schizophrenia: Facial expressions of emotion. *American Journal of Psychiatry, 150*, 1654–1660.

Whittaker, J. F., Deakin, J. F., & Tomenson, B. (2001). Face processing in schizophrenia: Defining the deficit. *Psychological Medicine, 31*, 499–507.

Williams, L. M., Das, P., Harris, A. W., Liddell, B. B., Brammer, M. J., Olivieri, G., et al. (2004). Dysregulation of arousal and amygdala–prefrontal systems in paranoid schizophrenia. *American Journal of Psychiatry, 161*, 480–489.

Williams, L. M., Das, P., Liddell, B. J., Olivieri, G., Peduto, A. S., David, A. S., et al. (2007). Fronto-limbic and autonomic disjunctions to negative emotion distinguish schizophrenia subtypes. *Psychiatry Research, 155*, 29–44.

Williams, L. M., Phillips, M. L., Brammer, M. J., Skerrett, D., Lagopoulos, J., Rennie, C., et al. (2001). Arousal dissociates amygdala and hippocampal fear responses: Evidence from simultaneous fMRI and skin conductance recording. *NeuroImage, 14*, 1070–1079.

Wright, I. C., Rabe-Hesketh, S., Woodruff, P. W., David, A. S., Murray, R. M., & Bullmore, E. T. (2000). Meta-analysis of regional brain volumes in schizophrenia. *American Journal of Psychiatry, 157*, 16–25.

CHAPTER 16

The Human Amygdala in Autism

Cynthia Mills Schumann and David G. Amaral

A utism spectrum disorders are a group of neurodevelopmental disorders with varying degrees of behavioral impairment. The cause(s) of these disorders are unknown, and the neuropathology has not yet been clearly established. According to the *Diagnostic and Statistical Manual of Mental Disorders*, fourth edition, text revision (DSM-IV-TR), which includes the autism spectrum in its category of "pervasive developmental disorders," diagnosis is based on detecting behavioral impairments in three categories: (1) social and emotional reciprocity; (2) communication and language development; and (3) stereotyped, repetitive behaviors and interests (American Psychiatric Association [APA], 2000). As toddlers, children with autism may display unusual affective behavior, lack of interest in family members, poor eye contact, and lack of response to name (Dawson, 1999; Werner, Dawson, Osterling, & Dinno, 2000). Since Leo Kanner (1943) initially described autism over 60 years ago, the definition of the autism spectrum has evolved and now encompasses a wide range of severity of social and emotional abnormalities, with varying levels of cognitive and linguistic functioning. The spectrum ranges from lower-functioning autism with mental retardation, to higher-functioning autism with normal IQ, to Asperger syndrome with normal to high IQ and relatively normal language development. (For the sake of simplicity, we use "autism" in this chapter as a term for the entire spectrum, unless specific points on the spectrum are meant.) Comorbid conditions are present at all points on the spectrum and include epilepsy, anxiety, gastrointestinal and gross motor problems, and the inability to modulate sensory input. Although Kanner's (1943) original report provided a detailed description of the social impairments seen in autism, he also emphasized that his cohort of children exhibited substantial anxious behavior. The presence of anxiety has been noted in descriptions of autism (APA, 2000; Wing, 1976), and several studies suggest that anxiety is a common feature (e.g., Muris, Steerneman, Merckelbach, Holdrinet, & Meesters, 1998).

Since autism includes impairments in different domains of behavior, it is likely that its pathophysiology involves several brain regions. Circuits implicated in the regulation of social and emotional behavior, including regions such as the amygdala and orbitofrontal cortex, were among the first to be implicated in autism (Damasio & Maurer, 1978; DeLong, 1992). In the following sections, we review the various lines of evidence supporting the notion that the amygdala is pathological in autism. We then discuss the functional implications of this pathology as it relates to the behavioral impairments associated with autism spectrum disorders.

EVIDENCE THAT THE AMYGDALA IS PATHOLOGICAL IN AUTISM

Postmortem Studies

Bauman and Kemper (1985, 1994) were the first to report abnormalities in the microscopic organization of the amygdala in postmortem cases of autism. Their initial report was of a 29-year-old male with autism, seizure disorder, and mental retardation, compared to a 25-year-old typically developing control male (Bauman & Kemper, 1985). Nissl-stained whole-brain serial sections from the man with autism and the control subject were viewed side by side under a microscope at the same magnification. Density measures were made in the central part of each cytoarchitectonic region. Bauman and Kemper observed increased cell-packing density in the central, medial, and cortical nuclei (40%, 28%, and 35%, respectively) in the man with autism. They also noted that cell size in these areas was reduced. The basal, lateral, and accessory basal nuclei showed less consistent differences.

Kemper and Bauman (1993) followed up their initial case study with five additional cases of autism (four males and one female), ages 9, 10, 12, 22, and 28. Nissl-stained sections of brain tissue from these individuals were compared to sections from age-matched controls, and corresponding areas were again viewed side by side under a microscope. Qualitative observations indicated that neurons in the amygdala of the individuals with autism appeared unusually small and more densely packed than in those of age-matched controls. This was most pronounced in the cortical, medial, and central nuclei, whereas the lateral nucleus generally appeared to be comparable to that of controls. Kemper and Bauman suggested that densely packed amygdala neurons may be manifested during an early stage of maturation, a time at which the neuronal size and complexity of neuropil have not reached adult levels. These changes could result from a curtailment of normal maturation.

The results of Bauman and Kemper are complicated by the fact that four of the six cases also had a seizure disorder. Studies focusing on cases of epilepsy without autism indicate a reduction in amygdala volume of 10–30%, with neuronal cell loss reported in the lateral and basal nuclei (Pitkänen, Tuuanen, Kalviainen, Partanen, & Salmenpera, 1998). In addition, recent studies have raised methodological concerns about the interpretation of density measurements as an indication of neuropathology. Tissue undergoes variable shrinkage during processing, and the only way to unambiguously interpret pathological changes in cell number or density is to estimate actual neuron number in the entire amygdala.

We recently carried out a study using unbiased stereological methods to estimate the number of neurons in the autistic amygdala (Schumann & Amaral, 2006). The goal of our study was to measure neuronal number, regional volume, neuronal density, and mean neuronal cross-sectional area in the entire amygdaloid complex and in individual nuclei in postmortem cases of autism without seizure disorder, compared to typically developing age-matched controls. The intact amygdala was collected from one brain hemisphere in each of 9 males with autism and 10 age-matched control males (10–44 years of age at death). A principle of design-based stereological techniques is that the entire area of interest must be reliably sampled. Prior to initiating our study of the cases with autism, we extensively defined the borders of the amygdaloid complex in the 10 control cases (Schumann & Amaral, 2005). We then outlined the amygdaloid complex on every 100-µm Nissl section in which it was present (approximately 20–25 sections per case), while remaining unaware of the cases' status (autism vs. control). The amygdaloid complex was further partitioned into five subdivisions: (1) lateral nucleus, (2) basal nucleus, (3) accessory basal nucleus, (4) central nucleus, and (5) remaining nuclei (Figure 16.1).

We counted neurons in the total amygdala and each of the five subdivisions, using the optical fractionator technique (West, Slomianka, & Gundersen, 1991). The major finding was that the total autistic amygdala and the lateral nucleus had significantly fewer neurons than those of controls (Plate 16.1 in color insert). We did not find increased neuronal density, as Bauman and Kemper (1985, 1994) had previously reported.

What might account for the lower number of neurons in the autistic amygdala? Two possible hypotheses are these: (1) Fewer neurons are generated during early development; or (2) a normal or even excessive number of neurons are generated initially, but some of these subsequently degenerate during adulthood. Unfortunately, there is currently no evidence enabling us to support or reject either of these possibilities. The resolution of this issue would require similar postmortem stereological studies of the amygdala in younger individuals with autism. It is interesting to note, however, that structural magnetic resonance imaging (MRI) studies of young children with autism (see below) indicate that the amygdala is larger than normal (Mosconi et al., 2005; Schumann et al., 2004; Sparks et al., 2002), whereas studies carried out in older adolescents and adults suggest a normal or even smaller amygdala (Ayl-

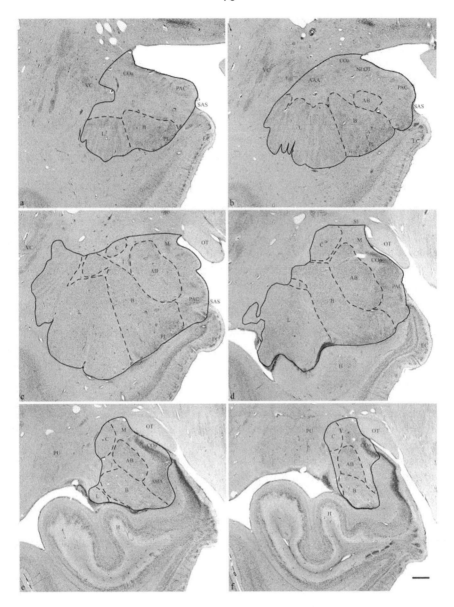

FIGURE 16.1. Lateral view of the left hemisphere of the brain displaying the cuts made to obtain a tissue block of the intact amygdala. Scale bar: 1 cm. AB, accessory basal nucleus; B, basal nucleus; C, central nucleus; EC, entorhinal cortex; I, intercalated nuclei; L, lateral nucleus; M, medial nucleus; OT, optic tract; PAC, peri-amygdaloid cortex; PL, paralaminar nucleus; SAS, semiannular sulcus; VC, ventral claustrum. From Schumann and Amaral (2005). Copyright 2005 by John Wiley & Sons, Inc. Reprinted by permission.

ward et al., 1999; Nacewicz et al., 2006; Pierce, Muller, Ambrose, Allen, & Courchesne, 2001). This raises the prospect that the amygdala has a normal or perhaps even increased number of neurons in early postnatal life, and that a degenerative process takes place at some later time.

Structural Imaging Studies

Until recently, structural MRI studies painted an unclear and inconsistent picture of the amygdala in autism. Some studies reported decreased volume (Aylward et al., 1999; Pierce et al., 2001); others found increased volume (Howard et al., 2000; Mosconi et al., 2005; Schumann et al., 2004; Sparks et al., 2002); and still others found no difference in volume (Haznedar et al., 2000; Schumann et al., 2004) in individuals with autism. These studies varied in the age groups studied, diagnostic and exclusionary criteria, and neuroanatomical methods for defining the amygdala on MRI scans.

Sparks and colleagues (2002) were the only group to measure the volume of the amygdala in young children (36–56 months of age). They found that in males with autism, the amygdala was larger by 16% on the right and 13% on the left, relative to that of controls. The right amygdala enlargement in these children was associated with more severe social and communication impairments, as assessed by the Autism Diagnostic Interview—Revised (Lord, Rutter, & Le Couteur, 1994). Larger right amygdala volume was also predictive of poorer social and communication abilities at 6 years of age (Munson et al., 2006).

We recently carried out a study in order to (1) compare volume measurements of the amygdala in children across the autistic spectrum (Plate 16.2 in color insert), and (2) attempt to reconcile the contradictory results of previously published MRI studies (Schumann et al., 2004). The volume of the amygdala was measured in 85 male children 7–18 years of age in four diagnostic groups: low-functioning autism, high-functioning autism, Asperger syndrome, and age-matched typically developing controls (Plate 16.3 in color insert). One striking finding was that the amygdala in the typically developing male children increased in size by approximately 40% from 8 to 18 years of age. This finding is consistent with studies from Giedd and colleagues (Giedd, 1997; Giedd et al., 1996), who reported a 50% increase in volume from 4 to 18 years of age in males, but not females. However, we found that the children with autism did not undergo this same pattern of development (Plate 16.3).

The amygdala in our young children 8–12 years of age with autism was initially larger than that of the controls by approximately 15%. We found a significant difference in amygdala volume in children with both low- and high-functioning autism, indicating that the difference was related to autism rather than to mental retardation. This enlargement was not paralleled by an overall enlarged brain, because there was no difference in total cerebral volume in this age range. Studies from other groups are now confirming this finding of a larger amygdala in very young children. Mosconi and colleagues (2005) measured the amygdala in children 18–35 months of age and found that even at this early stage of development, the amygdala was enlarged by 16% in toddlers diagnosed with autism.

Our study did not find a difference in the volume of the amygdala between children with autism and typically developing controls ages 13–18 years. Thus the amygdala is initially larger than normal in the children with autism, but does not undergo the same age-related increase in volume that takes place in typically developing children. The recent findings from our laboratory and others help to explain the variability in reports from previous MRI studies of individuals with autism. In younger children, the amygdala is larger in those with autism than in age-matched typically developing controls (Mosconi et al., 2005; Schumann et al., 2004; Sparks et al., 2002). However, studies focusing primarily on older adolescents, adults, or a wide age range of subjects have found no difference in (Haznedar et al., 2000), or potentially smaller (Aylward et al., 1999; Nacewicz et al., 2006; Pierce et al., 2001), amygdala volumes in individuals with autism (Figure 16.2).

Although we found that the amygdala of older children with autism are approximately the same size as those of younger children, we would predict that the abnormal developmental time course should result in fundamental abnormalities in the neuroanatomical and functional organization of the amygdala in individuals with autism. These differences are likely to persist into adulthood.

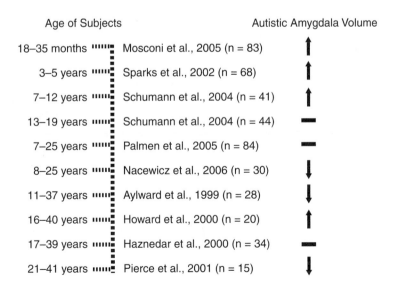

FIGURE 16.2. Reports on volumes of the amygdala in subjects with autism relative to typically developing controls by age.

NORMAL AND PATHOLOGICAL FUNCTION OF THE AMYGDALA

Patients with Amygdala Lesions

Human patients with amygdala lesions are rare, but provide invaluable insight into the clinical and behavioral implications of a pathological amygdala. As discussed elsewhere in this book (see Buchanan, Tranel, & Adolphs, Chapter 13), an exceptional subject, patient S. M., is one of the most extensively studied individuals with a selective and complete bilateral amygdala lesion (Adolphs, Tranel, Damasio, & Damasio, 1994; Bechara et al., 1995). Despite her lack of amygdala function, S. M.'s social behavior remains relatively intact. However, human patients with damage to the amygdala, including S. M., display deficits in fear conditioning (Bechara et al., 1995; LaBar, LeDoux, Spencer, & Phelps, 1995) and recognizing emotions in facial expressions, primarily fear (Adolphs et al., 1994; Adolphs, Tranel, Damasio, & Damasio, 1995; Bechara et al., 1995).

The role of the amygdala in processing stimuli related to potential threat may extend to complex judgments on the basis of which individuals approach or trust other people. Patients with bilateral amygdala damage, including S. M., are impaired in judging the trustworthiness of another person from viewing a photo of that person's face (Adolphs, Tranel, & Damasio, 1998). The patients judged the people in the photos as more trustworthy and more approachable than did normal viewers. Recently, Adolphs and colleagues (2005) found that S. M. is impaired in her ability to make normal use of information from the eye region of the face when judging emotions, and that the eyes may be the most notable feature for identifying emotions, such as fear.

Patients with amygdala lesions and individuals with autism share some common deficits. Although patients with amygdala lesions are clearly not autistic, Adolphs, Sears, and Piven (2001) found that individuals with autism perform similarly to patients with amygdala lesions in judging people to be more trustworthy and more approachable than normal individuals. Pelphrey and colleagues (2002) found that, similar to patients with amygdala lesions, individuals with autism are impaired in identifying anger and fear from faces, but only mildly impaired at identifying happy, disgusted, sad, and surprised faces. Commonalities among individuals with amygdala lesions, such as patient S. M., and those with autism also extend beyond the processing of faces. Typically developing individuals will attribute social meaning to ambiguous, moving geometric shapes that appear to have goal-directed movement and intentions (i.e., the social attribution task) (Heider & Simmel, 1944). Klin (2000) found that individuals with autism provide narrations similar to those of patient S. M., which are limited to strictly physical, asocial, and geometric terms (Heberlein & Adolphs, 2004).

Animal Models of Amygdala Function

Several laboratories have utilized animal models to examine the role of the amygdala in social behavior and emotional processing, which are some of the core deficits of autism. Early amygdala lesion studies in nonhuman adult primates observed profound behavioral abnormalities (i.e., the Klüver–Bucy syndrome), including an inability to judge the significance of a stimulus and an overall lack of emotional response (Klüver & Bucy, 1939). The inability of amygdala-lesioned monkeys to interact within a social context observed in these and subsequent studies led to the proposal that the amygdala is essential for the interpretation and production of species-typical social behavior. Our laboratory investigated the impact of selective bilateral amygdala lesions on adult primate social behavior (Emery et al., 2001) and found that animals with amygdala lesions were not socially withdrawn; indeed, they engaged in increased levels of social interaction. We raised the possibility that the amygdala is a critical neural structure for restraining social behavior until an adequate assessment of the intentions and disposition of a novel social partner can be made. This conclusion was substantiated by Málková, Barrow, Lower, and Gales (2003), who found that intra-amygdala infusion of the gamma-aminobutyric acid$_A$ (GABA$_A$) antagonist bicuculline, which effectively disinhibits the amygdala by blocking the inhibitory affect of GABA, resulted in decreased social contact, a complete loss of social play, and an increase in active withdrawal in monkeys.

Bachevalier (1994) evaluated the effects of early amygdala damage by lesioning the amygdala in monkeys within the first postnatal month of life. At 6 months of age, the amygdala-lesioned infants showed a reduction in social interactions, compared to the controls (Newman & Bachevalier, 1997). Given that impaired social communication and a lack of social interest are hallmarks of autism, Bachevalier (1994, 2000) proposed that lesions of the medial temporal lobe, specifically the amygdala, might provide an animal model of autism.

Bauman and colleagues (Bauman, Lavenex, Mason, Capitanio, & Amaral, 2004a, 2004b; Prather et al., 2001) in our laboratory have carried out a series of experiments to evaluate the effects of early amygdala damage by producing selective ibotenic acid lesions in the amygdala of socially reared rhesus monkeys, beginning at 2 weeks of age. We predicted that if the amygdala is a core component of the social brain and the primary structure responsible for social deficits in autism, then removal of the amygdala early in development would profoundly alter fundamental features of social behavior. The amygdala-lesioned infants showed no differences in mother–infant interactions at 3 months of age, and they continued to develop a species-typical repertoire of social behavior after being weaned from their mothers (Bauman et al., 2004b). These findings indicate that a functional amygdala is not needed to develop fundamental aspects of social behavior. One striking finding was that the amygdala-lesioned subjects displayed inappropriate fear behaviors and produced fear behaviors more frequently during social interactions with both novel and familiar social partners (Bauman et al., 2004b).

As discussed elsewhere in this book, there is an abundance of evidence from animal studies (Davis, Walker, & Myers, 2003; LeDoux, 2000) to implicate the amygdala in the detection of danger, as well as in the production of fear and anxiety. In rodents, the acquisition of conditioned fear involves sensory input into the lateral nucleus of the amygdala, which in turn excites neurons in the central nucleus and evokes a fear response via the brainstem and hypothalamus (LeDoux, Iwata, Cicchetti, & Reis, 1988). Lesions of the lateral nucleus in rodents interferes with conditioned fear learning (Campeau & Davis, 1995; LeDoux, Cicchetti, Xagoraris, & Romanski, 1990), and lesions to the central nucleus interfere with the expression of the conditioned fear response (Gentile, Jarrell, Teich, McCabe, & Schneiderman, 1986; Hitchcock & Davis, 1986; Iwata, LeDoux, Meeley, Arneric, & Reis, 1986). As discussed above, damage to the amygdala produces abnormal fear behavior, and infant macaque monkeys without an amygdala demonstrate an impaired ability to evaluate dangerous versus benign stimuli (Bauman et al., 2004b). Therefore, our laboratory has proposed that through its mediation of fear, the amygdala plays a modulatory, rather than an essential, role in the development of social behavior (Amaral, Bauman, & Schumann, 2003; Bauman et al., 2004b).

Normal Function of the Human Amygdala from Functional MRI Studies

As reviewed extensively elsewhere in this book, several functional imaging studies have investigated the role of the typically developing amygdala in brain function. Facial expressions are among the most replicable elicitors of human amygdala activation, particularly facial expressions depicting fear (Breiter et al., 1996; Canli, Sivers, Whitfield, Gotlib, & Gabrieli, 2002; Morris et al., 1996, 1998). Viewing fearful eyes alone is sufficient to evoke increased amygdala activity (Morris, deBonis, & Dolan, 2002). Other facial expressions depicting negative emotions, such as disgust (Phillips et al., 1997), anger (Morris et al., 1998), and sadness (Blair, Morris, Frith, Perrett, & Dolan, 1999), activate the amygdala. There are reports that highly positive emotions (e.g., sexual arousal) (Breiter et al., 1996; Canli et al., 2002) can activate the amygdala, but not as consistently as fearful expressions. Recent evidence indicates that slight differences in the stimuli, such as direction of eye gaze, alter the response of the amygdala to different emotional expressions (Adams, Gordon, Baird, Ambady, & Kleck, 2003). These findings have led to the hypothesis that fearful facial expressions may serve as a warning of potential danger, and that the function of the amygdala is to constantly monitor the environment for danger and modulate levels of vigilance (Davis & Whalen, 2001; Whalen et al., 1998). Amygdala activation is not limited to evaluating facial expressions in human subjects, but is also activated when subjects are undergoing fear conditioning (Büchel, Morris, Dolan, & Friston, 1998; Cheng, Knight, Smith, Stein, & Helmstetter, 2003; LaBar, Gatenby, Gore, LeDoux, & Phelps, 1998), viewing pictures of phobia-related stimuli (Dilger et al., 2003), anticipating aversive stimuli (e.g., shock) (Phelps et al., 2001), and viewing threatening and fearful nonsocial stimuli (Hariri, Mattay, Tessitore, Fera, & Weinberger, 2003). These findings support the hypothesis that the amygdala primarily serves as a detector of danger, which in humans may be more robust in situations with a social component (such as judging the trustworthiness of another person) (Winston, Strange, O'Doherty, & Dolan, 2002).

Functional Studies of the Amygdala in Autism

Functional neuroimaging studies have indicated that individuals with autism spectrum disorders show abnormal patterns of amygdala activation in response to social stimuli. Adults with high-functioning autism or Asperger syndrome demonstrate deficits in the ability to judge from images of another person's eyes what that person might be thinking (Baron-Cohen, Jolliffe, Mortimore, & Robertson, 1997). When combined with functional imaging, this task revealed that control subjects activated the amygdala and superior temporal gyrus when inferring the mental or emotional state of another person. In contrast, individuals with autism or Asperger syndrome activated the frontotemporal regions, but not the amygdala, when making social inferences from the eyes (Baron-Cohen et al., 1999). Pierce and colleagues (2001) found that the amygdala was activated when typically developing individuals viewed unfamiliar faces, but was not activated in individuals with autism during this task. Children and adolescents with autism spectrum disorders showed abnormal amygdala activation while matching faces by emotion and assigning a label to facial expressions (Wang, Dapretto, Hariri, Sigman, & Bookheimer, 2004). Children in the control group showed more amygdala activation when matching faces by emotion than when assigning a verbal label, but the children with autism spectrum disorders did not demonstrate this pattern of task-dependent amygdala modulation.

One caveat to interpreting findings from face-processing studies is that subjects with autism are reluctant to make eye contact, and there is some controversy as to whether they are actually examining the face in a manner similar to that of controls (Davidson & Slagter, 2000). In fact, persons with autism show abnormal visual scanpaths during eye-tracking studies when viewing faces, typically spending little time on core social features such as the eyes (Klin, Jones, Schultz, Volkmar, & Cohen, 2002; Pelphrey et al., 2002). It is unclear whether these findings represent active avoidance of the eye region, potentially involving the amygdala, or a more global lack of social interest or motivation. An emerging hypothesis is that the amygdala may play a role in mediating or directing visual attention to the eyes (Adolphs et al., 2005; Grelotti, Gauthier, & Schultz, 2002; Schultz, 2005). Pierce, Haist, Sedaghat, and Courchesne (2004) found that when subjects with autism viewed familiar faces, they were able to activate the amygdala appropriately in response to familiar and unfamiliar faces, suggesting that the familiar faces may have enhanced motivation or attention to all of the stimuli.

Although inattention to faces, particularly the eye region, is an early and consistent symptom of autism, little is known regarding the underlying cause(s) of this abnormal pattern of social attention. One possibility is that children with autism simply lack social motivation and thus lack interest in attending to the face. An alternative view is that individuals with autism perceive social interactions as threatening, and therefore avoid socialization as a means of alleviating the fear triggered by social encounters. Indeed, one study of typically developing children found that children who were physiologically aroused by a distressing film were more likely to avert their gaze from the stimulus (Fabes, Eisenberg, & Eisenbud, 1993). It is plausible that children with autism utilize a similar strategy of gaze aversion in response to arousing social stimuli. Given the amygdala's role in fear and anxiety, one would predict heightened amygdala activation during eye contact in persons with autism if they found the eye contact aversive. Dalton and colleagues (2005) recently carried out a series of studies utilizing functional imaging and eye-tracking technology simultaneously while showing subjects familiar and unfamiliar faces. They found that the amount of time persons with autism spent looking at the eye region of the face was strongly positively correlated with amygdala activation, but that this was not so in typically developing control subjects. The subjects with autism also showed greater left amygdala activation relative to controls in response to unfamiliar faces, and greater right amygdala activation in response to both familiar and unfamiliar faces. This suggests a heightened emotional, or even fearful, response when individuals with autism look at other persons' eyes, regardless of whether they are familiar or unfamiliar. Nacewicz and colleagues (2006) recently found that individuals with autism (8–25 years of age) who had smaller amygdala were also slower to distinguish emotional from neutral expressions and showed least fixation on the eye regions of the face. These same individuals were also the most socially impaired in early childhood.

Recently, Ashwin, Baron-Cohen, Wheelwright, O'Riordan, and Bullmore (2007) found that during the perception of fearful faces, patients with Asperger syndrome showed less activation in the left amygdala than did controls. However, these results may again be due to the abnormal way in which individuals with autism view faces. Spezio, Adolphs, Hurley, and Piven (2007) confirmed that participants with autism showed less fixation on the eyes and mouth, but also a greater tendency to saccade away from the eyes when information was present in those regions. This study provides insight into the aberrant manner in which people with autism view faces, which is likely to influence face processing and subsequent functional imaging study results. Additional studies would benefit from measuring the physiological responses associated with arousal and anxiety (increased heart rate, skin response, etc.) during face processing in individuals with autism.

CONCLUSIONS

We carried out a series of studies to determine whether the amygdala is pathological in autism. We found that the amygdala undergoes an abnormal pattern of development in individuals with autism, which includes precocious early enlargement in childhood and a reduced number of neurons in adulthood. The amygdala evidently undergoes an abnormal pattern of structural development, but the cause(s) and behavioral ramifications of this abnormality, as well as its possible contribution to the symptoms of autism, are less clear.

Baron-Cohen and colleagues (2000) proposed that pathology of the amygdala is responsible for the behavioral impairments in individuals with autism. However, as discussed above and elsewhere, recent evidence indicates that the amygdala plays a modulatory role in social behavior, but is not essential for producing a normal repertoire of social behavior and therefore cannot be solely responsible for the severe social impairments in autism. It is evident that both animal and human subjects with lesions of the amygdala are capable of producing species-typical social behavior. Therefore, it is unlikely that hypofunction of the amygdala in autism is responsible for the core deficits in social interaction.

However, converging neurobiological evidence from both human and animal models indicates that the amygdala plays an essential role in regulating fear behaviors, which may in turn mediate social processing (Adolphs, 2003). As discussed in detail above, the amygdala is activated while a person is gauging potentially threatening stimuli that contribute to social perception of the environment, such as judging personality characteristics from pictures of faces (Adolphs et al., 1998; Baron-Cohen et al., 1999; Winston et al., 2002). The role of the normally functioning amygdala may be to evaluate the potential danger of a stimulus in the environment and to generate the appropriate physiological and emotional response. Then, depending on the context, this response may either inhibit or facilitate both social and nonsocial interactions. A hyperresponsive amygdala could lead to withdrawal from social and emotional interactions.

In Kanner's (1943) original description of autism, he noted unusual fear or anxiety in several of his young patients. Insistence on sameness leads children with autism to become greatly distressed by changes, and often to demand consistency in the sequence of events. Kanner noted that although many individuals with autism learn to tolerate changes in routine and interactions with other people in their environment as adults, these interruptions cause a great deal of anxiety in young children with autism. Social interactions with other people are an unwelcome intrusion. When social interaction is forced upon such a child, Kanner observed that the child, with a great deal of anxiety, will either ignore the person attempting to interact or quickly answer to end the intrusion. This aspect of autism, although consistently described by parents (Wing, 1976) and included as a feature in the DSM-IV-TR (APA, 2000), has not been extensively studied (Gillott, Furniss, & Walter, 2001; Muris et al., 1998).

It is plausible that pathology of the amygdala may alter the ability to correctly evaluate both social and nonsocial stimuli in the environment, and thus to produce an appropriate response. In individuals with autism, this pathology may contribute to the comorbid symptoms of anxiety. Muris and colleagues (1998) examined the presence of co-occurring anxiety symptoms in 44 children diagnosed with autism or pervasive developmental disorders. Using parental report, they found that 84% of the children met criteria for at least one anxiety disorder. Gillott and colleagues (2001) compared children with high-functioning autism to typically developing children on measures of anxiety and social worry. The children with autism were found to be significantly more anxious on both indices. Similarly, Kim, Szatmari, Bryson, Streiner, and Wilson (2000) evaluated the prevalence of anxiety and mood problems in 59 children with high-functioning autism or Asperger syndrome, reporting that these children were at greater risk for mood and anxiety problems than the general population. In addition, recent studies have found that amygdala enlargement is associated with more severe anxiety (Juranek et al., 2006) and worse social communication skills in children with autism (Munson et al., 2006)

One intriguing hypothesis to explain the initial overgrowth in volume of the amygdala in early childhood, followed by a reduction in the number of neurons in adulthood, in individuals with autism is that of "allostatic overload" (McEwen, 2004; McEwen & Lasley, 2003)—the possibility that a biological defect inherent to autism leads to the production of a larger and more active amygdala (Nacewicz et al., 2006). The more active amygdala produces a heightened level of fear and anxiety typical of autism (Muris et al., 1998), as well as a heightened and chronic stress response. Over time, the heightened stress response could possibly have damaging effects, leading to the loss of neurons and a smaller amygdala. This hypothesis remains speculative at present. Younger persons with autism need to be evaluated with postmortem stereological techniques, to determine at what stage of development the loss of neurons occurs.

Thus, based on our current knowledge of amygdala function and pathology, it is plausible that abnormal amygdala development contributes to abnormal fear and anxiety processing in children with autism, which may in turn exacerbate the hallmark feature of social avoidance. The amygdala, with its dense reciprocal connections with the visual stream (Amaral & Price, 1984), modulates many levels of visual processing, which in turn may influence the development of early preference for faces seen in typical newborns (Johnson, Dziurawiec, Ellis, & Morton, 1991). Schultz (2005) suggests that abnormalities in the amygdala in autism, and diminished attention to faces at an early age (Osterling & Dawson, 1994), may be the first in a cascade of problems that lead to later emotional and social impairments. However, it is clear that the amygdala is not the only structure responsible for the behavioral impairments of autism spectrum disorders, and that many other areas of the brain need to be explored. The amygdala is just one of several structures that work in parallel to produce normal social cognition, one of the core impairments in autism. The amygdala, when presented with a socially demanding situation, will evaluate and allocate resources to those stimuli that pose a potential threat. Such structures as the fusiform gyrus, frontal cortex, cingulate cortex, somatosensory cortex, and superior temporal gyrus also have specialized roles in the broader system of social behavior (Adolphs, 2001), and the detection of potential neuropathology in these regions is an important direction for future study.

WHAT WE THINK

There is now compelling evidence that the amygdala is pathological in autism spectrum disorders. The amygdala undergoes an abnormal pattern of structural development in individuals with autism, which includes precocious early enlargement in childhood and a reduced number of neurons in adulthood. What is the implication of this pathology for the symptomatology of autism? The pathological amygdala has been proposed by some to be responsible for the core deficit of social behavior in people with autism. However, both animals and rare human subjects with bilateral amygdala damage do not show gross impairments in generating appropriate species-specific social responses. These findings indicate that the amygdala plays a modulatory role in social behavior, but is not essential for producing a normal repertoire of social behavior. Therefore, the amygdala cannot be solely responsible for the severe social impairments displayed by individuals with autism. The one consistent and robust feature of animals and humans with a dysfunctional amygdala is impairment in the danger detection system. We suggest that the role of a normally functioning amygdala is to constantly monitor the environment, evaluate the potential danger of a stimulus, and generate appropriate physiological and emotional responses. This function may extend to situations with a social component, such as directing visual attention to the eyes or judging the trustworthiness of another person. We propose that a pathological amygdala in individuals with autism should lead them to perceive social interactions as threatening, and therefore to avoid eye contact and socialization as a means of alleviating the anxiety triggered by social encounters, further exacerbating their social isolation. This scenario raises the need for better assessment and treatment of comorbid psychopathology, particularly anxiety, in autism spectrum disorders.

REFERENCES

Adams, R. B., Jr., Gordon, H. L., Baird, A. A., Ambady, N., & Kleck, R. E. (2003). Effects of gaze on amygdala sensitivity to anger and fear faces. *Science, 300,* 1536.

Adolphs, R. (2001). The neurobiology of social cognition. *Current Opinion in Neurobiology, 11,* 231–239.

Adolphs, R. (2003). Cognitive neuroscience of human social behaviour. *Nature Reviews Neuroscience, 4,* 165–178.

Adolphs, R., Gosselin, F., Buchanan, T. W., Tranel, D., Schyns, P., & Damasio, A. R. (2005). A mechanism for impaired fear recognition after amygdala damage. *Nature, 433,* 68–72.

Adolphs, R., Sears, L., & Piven, J. (2001). Abnormal processing of social information from faces in autism. *Journal of Cognitive Neuroscience, 13,* 232–240.

Adolphs, R., Tranel, D., & Damasio, A. R. (1998). The human amygdala in social judgment. *Nature, 393,* 470–474.

Adolphs, R., Tranel, D., Damasio, H., & Damasio, A. (1994). Impaired recognition of emotion in facial expressions following bilateral damage to the human amygdala. *Nature, 372,* 669–672.

Adolphs, R., Tranel, D., Damasio, H., & Damasio, A. R. (1995). Fear and the human amygdala. *Journal of Neuroscience, 15,* 5879–5891.

Amaral, D. G., Bauman, M. D., & Schumann, C. M. (2003). The amygdala and autism: Implications from non-human primate studies. *Genes, Brain, and Behavior, 2,* 295–302.

Amaral, D. G., & Price, J. L. (1984). Amygdalo-cortical projections in the monkey (*Macaca fascicularis*). *Journal of Comparative Neurology, 230,* 465–496.

American Psychiatric Association (APA). (2000). *Diagnostic and statistical manual of mental disorders* (4th ed., text rev.) Washington, DC: Author.

Ashwin, C., Baron-Cohen, S., Wheelwright, S., O'Riordan, M., & Bullmore, E. T. (2007). Differential activation of the amygdala and the `social brain' during fearful face-processing in Asperger syndrome. *Neuropsychologia, 45,* 2–14.

Aylward, E. H., Minshew, N. J., Goldstein, G., Honeycutt, N. A., Augustine, A. M., Yates, K. O., et al. (1999) MRI volumes of amygdala and hippocampus in non-mentally retarded autistic adolescents and adults. *Neurology, 53,* 2145–2150.

Bachevalier, J. (1994). Medial temporal lope structures and autism: A review of clinical and experimental findings. *Neuropsychologia, 32,* 627–648.

Bachevalier, J. (2000). The amygdala, social cognition, and autism. In J. P. Aggleton (Ed.), *The amygdala: A functional analysis* (2nd ed., pp. 509–543). Oxford, UK: Oxford University Press.

Baron-Cohen, S., Jolliffe, T., Mortimore, C., & Robertson, M. (1997). Another advanced test of theory of mind: Evidence from very high functioning adults with autism or Asperger syndrome. *Journal of Child Psychology and Psychiatry, 38,* 813–822.

Baron-Cohen, S., Ring, H. A., Bullmore, E. T., Wheelwright, S., Ashwin, C., & Williams, S. C. (2000). The amygdala theory of autism. *Neuroscience and Biobehavioral Reviews, 24,* 355–364.

Baron-Cohen, S., Ring, H. A., Wheelwright, S., Bullmore, E. T., Brammer, M. J., Simmons, A., et al. (1999). Social intelligence in the normal and autistic brain: An fMRI study. *European Journal of Neuroscience, 11,* 1891–1898.

Bauman, M., & Kemper, T. L. (1985). Histoanatomic observations of the brain in early infantile autism. *Neurology, 35,* 866–874.

Bauman, M., & Kemper, T. L. (1994), Neuroanatomic observations of the brain in autism. In M. Bauman & T. L. Kemper (Eds.), *The neurobiology of autism* (pp. 119–145). Baltimore: Johns Hopkins University Press.

Bauman, M. D., Lavenex, P., Mason, W. A., Capitanio, J. P., & Amaral, D. G. (2004a). The development of mother–infant interactions after neonatal amygdala lesions in rhesus monkeys. *Journal of Neuroscience, 24,* 711–721.

Bauman, M. D., Lavenex, P., Mason, W. A., Capitanio, J. P., & Amaral, D. G. (2004b). The development of social behavior following neonatal amygdala lesions in rhesus monkeys. *Journal of Cognitive Neuroscience, 16,* 1388–1411.

Bechara, A., Tranel, D., Damasio, H., Adolphs, R., Rockland, C., & Damasio, A. R. (1995). Double dissociation of conditioning and declarative knowledge relative to the amygdala and hippocampus in humans. *Science, 269,* 1115–1118.

Blair, R. J., Morris, J. S., Frith, C. D., Perrett, D. I., & Dolan, R. J. (1999). Dissociable neural responses to facial expressions of sadness and anger. *Brain, 122*(Pt. 5), 883–893.

Breiter, H. C., Etcoff, N. L., Whalen, P. J., Kennedy, W. A., Rauch, S. L., Buckner, R. L., et al. (1996). Response and habituation of the human amygdala during visual processing of facial expression. *Neuron, 17,* 875–887.

Büchel, C., Morris, J., Dolan, R. J., & Friston, K. J. (1998). Brain systems mediating aversive conditioning: An event-related fMRI study. *Neuron, 20,* 947–957.

Campeau, S., & Davis, M. (1995). Involvement of subcortical and cortical afferents to the lateral nucleus of the amygdala in fear conditioning measured with fear-potentiated startle in rats trained concurrently with auditory and visual conditioned stimuli. *Journal of Neuroscience, 15,* 2312–2327.

Canli, T., Sivers, H., Whitfield, S. L., Gotlib, I. H., & Gabrieli, J. D. (2002). Amygdala response to happy faces as a function of extraversion. *Science, 296,* 2191.

Cheng, D. T., Knight, D. C., Smith, C. N., Stein, E. A., & Helmstetter, F. J. (2003). Functional MRI of human amygdala activity during Pavlovian fear conditioning: Stimulus processing versus response expression. *Behavioral Neuroscience, 117,* 3–10.

Dalton, K. M., Nacewicz, B. M., Johnstone, T., Schaefer, H. S., Gernsbacher, M. A., Goldsmith, H. H., et al. (2005). Gaze fixation and the neural circuitry of face processing in autism. *Nature Neuroscience, 8,* 519–526.

Damasio, A. R., & Maurer, R. G (1978). A neurological model for childhood autism. *Archives of Neurology, 35,* 777–786.

Davidson, R. J., & Slagter, H. A. (2000). Probing emotion in the developing brain: Functional neuroimaging in the assessment of the neural substrates of emotion in normal and disordered children and adolescents. *Mental Retardation and Developmental Disabilities Research Reviews, 6,* 166–170.

Davis, M., Walker, D. L., & Myers, K. M. (2003). Role of the amygdala in fear extinction measured with potentiated startle. *Annals of the New York Academy of Sciences, 985,* 218–232.

Davis, M., & Whalen, P. J. (2001). The amygdala: Vigilance and emotion. *Molecular Psychiatry, 6,* 13–34.

Dawson, G. (1999). Autism or a related developmental disability. *Journal of Autism and Developmental Disorders, 29,* 97.

DeLong, G. R. (1992). Autism, amnesia, hippocampus, and learning. *Neuroscience and Biobehavioral Reviews, 16,* 63–70.

Dilger, S., Straube, T., Mentzel, H. J., Fitzek, C., Reichenbach, J. R., Hecht, H., et al. (2003). Brain activation to phobia-related pictures in spider phobic humans: An event-related functional magnetic resonance imaging study. *Neuroscience Letters, 348,* 29–32.

Emery, N. J., Capitanio, J. P., Mason, W. A., Machado, C. J., Mendoza, S. P., & Amaral, D. G. (2001). The effects of bilateral lesions of the amygdala on dyadic social interactions in rhesus monkeys (*Macaca mulatta*). *Behavioral Neuroscience, 115,* 515–544.

Fabes, R. A., Eisenberg, N., & Eisenbud, L. (1993). Behavioral and physiological correlates of children's reactions to others in distress. *Developmental Psychology, 29,* 655–663.

Gentile, C. G., Jarrell, T. W., Teich, A., McCabe, P. M., & Schneiderman, N. (1986). The role of amygdaloid central nucleus in the retention of differential Pavlovian conditioning of bradycardia in rabbits. *Behavioural Brain Research, 20,* 263–273.

Giedd, J. N. (1997). Normal development. *Child and Adolescent Psychiatric Clinics of North America, 6,* 265–282.

Giedd, J. N., Vaituzis, A. C., Hamburger, S. D., Lange, N., Rajapakse, J. C., Kaysen, D., et al. (1996). Quantitative MRI of the temporal lobe, amygdala, and hippocampus in normal human development: Ages 4–18 years. *Journal of Comparative Neurology, 366,* 223–230.

Gillott, A., Furniss, F., & Walter, A. (2001). Anxiety in high-functioning children with autism. *Autism, 5,* 277–286.

Grelotti, D. J., Gauthier, I., & Schultz, R. T. (2002). Social interest and the development of cortical face specialization: What autism teaches us about face processing. *Developmental Psychobiology, 40,* 213–225.

Griffin, G. A., & Harlow, H. F. (1966). Effects of three months of total social deprivation on social adjustment and learning in the rhesus monkey. *Child Development, 37,* 533–547.

Hariri, A. R., Mattay, V. S., Tessitore, A., Fera, F., & Weinberger, D. R. (2003). Neocortical modulation of the amygdala response to fearful stimuli. *Biological Psychiatry, 53,* 494–501.

Haznedar, M. M., Buchsbaum, M. S., Wei, T. C., Hof, P. R., Cartwright, C., Bienstock, C. A., et al. (2000). Limbic circuitry in patients with autism spectrum disorders studied with positron emission tomography and magnetic resonance imaging. *American Journal of Psychiatry, 157,* 1994–2001.

Heberlein, A. S., & Adolphs, R. (2004). Impaired spontaneous anthropomorphizing despite intact perception and social knowledge. *Proceedings of the National Academy of Sciences USA, 101,* 7487–7491.

Heider, F., & Simmel, M. (1944). An experimental study of apparent behavior. *American Journal of Psychology, 57,* 243–259.

Hitchcock, J., & Davis, M. (1986). Lesions of the amygdala, but not of the cerebellum or red nucleus, block conditioned fear as measured with the potentiated startle paradigm. *Behavioral Neuroscience, 100,* 11–22.

Howard, M. A., Cowell, P. E., Boucher, J., Broks, P., Mayes, A., Farrant A, et al. (2000). Convergent neuroanatomical and behavioural evidence of an amygdala hypothesis of autism. *NeuroReport, 11,* 2931–2935.

Iwata, J., LeDoux, J. E., Meeley, M. P., Arneric, S., & Reis, D. J. (1986). Intrinsic neurons in the amygdaloid field projected to by the medial geniculate body mediate emotional responses conditioned to acoustic stimuli. *Brain Research, 383,* 195–214.

Johnson, M. H., Dziurawiec, S., Ellis, H., & Morton, J. (1991). Newborns' preferential tracking of face-like stimuli and its subsequent decline. *Cognition, 40,* 1–19.

Juranek, J., Filipek, P. A., Berenji, G. R., Modahl, C., Osann, K., & Spence, M. A. (2006). Association between amygdala volume and anxiety level: Magnetic resonance imaging (MR) study in autistic children. *Journal of Child Neurology, 21*(12), 1051–1058.

Kanner, L. (1943). Autistic disturbances of affective contact. *Nervous Child, 2,* 217–250.

Kemper, T. L., & Bauman, M. L. (1993). The contribution of neuropathologic studies to the understanding of autism. *Neurologic Clinics, 11,* 175–187.

Kim, J. A., Szatmari, P., Bryson, S. E., Streiner, D. L., & Wilson, F. J. (2000). The prevalence of anxiety and mood problems among children with autism and Asperger syndrome. *Autism, 4,* 117–132.

Klin, A. (2000). Attributing social meaning to ambiguous visual stimuli in higher-functioning autism and Asperger syndrome: The Social Attribution Task. *Journal of Child Psychology and Psychiatry, 41,* 831–846.

Klin, A., Jones, W., Schultz, R., Volkmar, F., & Cohen, D. (2002). Visual fixation patterns during viewing of naturalistic social situations as predictors of social competence in individuals with autism. *Archives of General Psychiatry, 59,* 809–816.

Klüver, H., & Bucy, P. (1939). Preliminary analysis of functioning of the temporal lobes in monkeys. *Archives of Neurology and Psychiatry, 42,* 979–1000.

LaBar, K. S., Gatenby, J. C., Gore, J. C., LeDoux, J. E., & Phelps, E. A. (1998). Human amygdala activation during conditioned fear acquisition and extinction: A mixed-trial fMRI study. *Neuron, 20,* 937–945.

LaBar, K. S., LeDoux, J. E., Spencer, D. D., & Phelps, E. A. (1995). Impaired fear conditioning following unilateral temporal lobectomy in humans. *Journal of Neuroscience, 15,* 6846–6855.

LeDoux, J. E. (2000). Emotion circuits in the brain. *Annual Review of Neuroscience, 23,* 155–184.

LeDoux, J. E., Cicchetti, P., Xagoraris, A., & Romanski, L. M. (1990). The lateral amygdaloid nucleus: Sensory interface of the amygdala in fear conditioning. *Journal of Neuroscience, 10,* 1062–1069.

LeDoux, J. E., Iwata, J., Cicchetti, P., & Reis, D. J. (1988). Different projections of the central amygdaloid nucleus mediate autonomic and behavioral correlates of conditioned fear. *Journal of Neuroscience, 8,* 2517–2529.

Lord, C., Rutter, M., & Le Couteur, A. (1994). Autism Diagnostic Interview—Revised: A revised version of a diagnostic interview for caregivers of individuals with possible pervasive developmental disorders. *Journal of Autism and Developmental Disorders, 24,* 659–685.

Málková, L., Barrow, K. V., Lower, L. L., & Gales, K. (2003). Decreased social interactions in monkeys after unilateral blockade of GABA$_A$ receptors in the basolateral amygdala. *Annals of the New York Academy of Sciences, 985,* 540–541.

McEwen, B. S. (2004). Protection and damage from acute and chronic stress: Allostasis and allostatic overload and relevance to the pathophysiology of psychiatric disorders. *Annals of the New York Academy of Sciences, 1032,* 1–7.

McEwen, B. S., & Lasley, E. N. (2003). Allostatic load: When protection gives way to damage. *Advances in Mind–Body Medicine, 19,* 28–33.

Morris, J. S., deBonis, M., & Dolan, R. J. (2002). Human amygdala responses to fearful eyes. *NeuroImage, 17,* 214–222.

Morris, J. S., Friston, K. J., Büchel, C., Frith, C. D., Young, A. W., Calder, A. J., et al. (1998). A neuromodulatory role for the human amygdala in processing emotional facial expressions. *Brain, 121*(Pt. 1), 47–57.

Morris, J. S., Frith, C. D., Perrett, D. I., Rowland, D., Young, A. W., Calder, A. J., et al. (1996). A differential neural response in the human amygdala to fearful and happy facial expressions. *Nature, 383,* 812–815.

Mosconi, M., Cody, H., Poe, M., Joshi, S., Peterson, S., & Piven, J. (2005). *Amygdala and hippocampal enlargement in young children with autism.* Paper presented at the International Meeting for Autism Research, Boston.

Munson, J., Dawson, G., Abbott, R., Faja, S., Webb, S. J., Friedman, S. D., et al. (2006). Amygdalar volume and behavioral development in autism. *Archives of General Psychiatry, 63,* 686–693.

Muris, P., Steerneman, P., Merckelbach, H., Holdrinet, I., & Meesters, C. (1998). Comorbid anxiety symptoms in children with pervasive developmental disorders. *Journal of Anxiety Disorders, 12,* 387–393.

Nacewicz, B. M., Dalton, K. M., Johnstone, T., Long, M. T., McAuliff, E. M., Oakes, T. R., et al. (2006). Amygdala volume and nonverbal social impairment in adolescent and adult males with autism. *Archives of General Psychiatry, 63,* 1417–1428.

Newman, J. D., & Bachevalier, J. (1997). Neonatal ablations of the amygdala and inferior temporal cortex alter the vocal response to social separation in rhesus macaques. *Brain Research, 758,* 180–186.

Osterling, J., & Dawson, G. (1994). Early recognition of children with autism: A study of first birthday home videotapes. *Journal of Autism and Developmental Disorders, 24,* 247–257.

Palmen, S. J., Durston, S., Nederveen, H., & Van Engeland, H. N. (2006). No evidence for preferential involvement of medial temporal lobe structures in high-functioning autism. *Psychological Medicine, 36*(6), 827–834.

Pelphrey, K. A., Sasson, N. J., Reznick, J. S., Paul, G., Goldman, B. D., & Piven, J. (2002). Visual scanning of faces in autism. *Journal of Autism and Developmental Disorders, 32,* 249–261.

Phelps, E. A., O'Connor, K. J., Gatenby, J. C., Gore, J. C., Grillon, C., & Davis, M. (2001). Activation of the left amygdala to a cognitive representation of fear. *Nature Neuroscience, 4,* 437–441.

Phillips, M. L., Young, A. W., Senior, C., Brammer, M., Andrew, C., Calder, A. J., et al. (1997). A specific neural substrate for perceiving facial expressions of disgust. *Nature, 389,* 495–498.

Pierce, K., Haist, F., Sedaghat, F., & Courchesne, E. (2004). The brain response to personally familiar faces in autism: Findings of fusiform activity and beyond. *Brain, 127,* 2703–2716.

Pierce, K., Muller, R. A., Ambrose, J., Allen, G., & Courchesne, E. (2001). Face processing occurs outside the fusiform "face area" in autism: Evidence from functional MRI. *Brain, 124,* 2059–2073.

Pitkänen, A., Tuunanen, J., Kalviainen, R., Partanen, K., & Salmenpera, T. (1998). Amygdala damage in experimental and human temporal lobe epilepsy. *Epilepsy Research, 32,* 233–253.

Prather, M. D., Lavenex, P., Mauldin-Jourdain, M. L., Mason, W. A., Capitanio, J. P., Mendoza, S. P., et al. (2001). Increased social fear and decreased fear of objects in monkeys with neonatal amygdala lesions. *Neuroscience, 106,* 653–658.

Schultz, R. T. (2005). Developmental deficits in social perception in autism: The role of the amygdala and fusiform face area. *International Journal of Developmental Neuroscience, 23,* 125–141.

Schumann, C. M., & Amaral, D. G. (2005). Stereological estimation of the number of neurons in the human amygdaloid complex. *Journal of Comparative Neurology, 491,* 320–329.

Schumann, C. M., & Amaral, D. G. (2006). Stereological analysis of amygdala neuron number in autism. *Journal of Neuroscience, 26,* 7674–7679.

Schumann, C. M., Hamstra, J., Goodlin-Jones, B. L., Lotspeich, L. J., Kwon, H.,

Buonocore, M. H., et al. (2004). The amygdala is enlarged in children but not adolescents with autism; the hippocampus is enlarged at all ages. *Journal of Neuroscience, 24,* 6392–6401.

Sparks, B. F., Friedman, S. D., Shaw, D. W., Aylward, E. H., Echelard, D., Artru, A. A., et al. (2002). Brain structural abnormalities in young children with autism spectrum disorder. *Neurology, 59,* 184–192.

Spezio, M. L., Adolphs, R., Hurley, R. S., & Piven, J. (2007). Abnormal use of facial information in high-functioning autism. *Journal of Autism and Developmental Disorders, 37*(5), 929–939.

Wang, A. T., Dapretto, M., Hariri, A. R., Sigman, M., & Bookheimer, S. Y. (2004) Neural correlates of facial affect processing in children and adolescents with autism spectrum disorder. *Journal of the American Academy of Child and Adolescent Psychiatry, 43,* 481–490.

Werner, E., Dawson, G., Osterling, J., & Dinno, N. (2000). Brief report: Recognition of autism spectrum disorder before one year of age: A retrospective study based on home videotapes. *Journal of Autism and Developmental Disorders, 30,* 157–162.

West, M. J., Slomianka, L., & Gundersen, H. J. (1991). Unbiased stereological estimation of the total number of neurons in the subdivisions of the rat hippocampus using the optical fractionator. *Anatomical Record, 231,* 482–497.

Whalen, P. J., Rauch, S. L., Etcoff, N. L., McInerney, S. C., Lee, M. B., & Jenike, M. A. (1998). Masked presentations of emotional facial expressions modulate amygdala activity without explicit knowledge. *Journal of Neuroscience, 18,* 411–418.

Wing, L. (1976). Diagnosis, clinical description and prognosis. In L. Wing (Ed.), *Early childhood autism* (pp. 15–48). Oxford, UK: Pergamon Press.

Winston, J. S., Strange, B. A., O'Doherty, J., & Dolan, R. J. (2002). Automatic and intentional brain responses during evaluation of trustworthiness of faces. *Nature Neuroscience, 5,* 277–283.

CHAPTER 17

The Human Amygdala in Normal Aging and Alzheimer's Disease

Christopher I. Wright

GENERAL INTRODUCTION AND NOMENCLATURE ISSUES

The purpose of this chapter is to give an overview of the current state of knowledge on amygdala structure and function in healthy human aging and in Alzheimer's disease (AD). Alterations of the amygdala with aging have recently received renewed attention, particularly given the "graying" of the North American population and the increasing prevalence of late-life neuropsychiatric disorders. AD is the most common neurodegenerative disorder of aging. Although the classic clinical hallmarks of AD relate to memory loss or amnesia, behavioral and neuropsychiatric disturbances are very common, even early in the clinical disease course. These latter symptoms are often the most distressing to families and patients, increase the probability that the disease may progress, and are frequently the reasons why patients are institutionalized. As reviewed below, there is significant neuropathological involvement of the amygdala in AD. However, there are gaps in our understanding of how this may contribute to the neuropsychiatric symptoms of the disease.

Though most studies use fairly consistent boundaries for defining the major nuclei of the amygdala, several different nomenclatures are used. The cortical (Co), medial (Me), lateral (La), and central (Ce) amygdala nuclei, and the amygdalocortical transition area (ATA), are treated similarly in most works (see Figure 17.1). Although subregions within these nuclei have been

Nuclear Divisions of the Amygdala

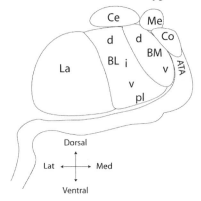

FIGURE 17.1. *Divisions of the human amygdala.* A schematic representation of the major amygdala nuclei from the human brain. A single coronally oriented section is shown for purposes of illustration. Included are the lateral neucleus (La), the baso-lateral nucleus (BL), the basomedial nucleus (BM), the central nucleus (Ce), the corti-cal nucleus (Co), the medial nucleus (Me), and the amygdalocortical transition area (ATA). Dorsal (d), intermediate (i), ventral (v), and paralaminar (pl) portions of the BL are indicated, as are the dorsal and ventral portions of the BM. There is a decrease in neuron perikaryon size from dorsal to ventral in the BL and BM. Although additional nuclei and subdivisions have been described, only those most relevant to the current topic have been included. The orientation of the slice is as indicated.

described, they are treated as unitary structures in this chapter, because sig-nificant subregional effects in aging and AD have not been described. For the basal nuclear complex, the nomenclature is more variable, and subregional differences in aging and AD are clearly present. In this chapter, the nomen-clature of De Olmos (2003) is followed throughout (see also Amaral, Price, Pitkänen, & Carmichael, 1992; Johnston, 1923) to enable clear comparisons among studies in regard to this nuclear complex. Thus the accessory basal nucleus of Lauer (1945) is designated the basomedial nucleus (BM), while the medial basal nucleus of Crosby and Humphrey (1941) is considered to be the ventral extension of the basolateral (BL) nucleus (Figure 17.1). Within these regions, further distinctions are made when they are relevant to the regional age- or AD-related effects. In particular, within the BL, dorsal (d), intermedi-ate (i), and ventral (v) regions are distinguished on the basis of cell size, with larger cells in the BLdi and smaller cells in the BLv. A superficial extension inferior to the BLv is also recognized, called the paralaminar region (BLpl). Dorsal (d) and ventral (v) parts of the BM can also be distinguished on the basis of larger neurons in BMd than in the BMv (see also Amaral et al., 1992). Because data on the anterior amygdaloid area and extended amygdala are limited, these divisions are not a focus of this chapter.

THE AMYGDALA IN NORMAL AGING

Structural Changes

Although relatively few studies have concentrated on the effects of healthy aging on amygdala volume, the available research suggests fairly modest atrophy—on the order of 2–20%, depending on the study (Herzog & Kemper, 1980; Laakso, Partanen, et al., 1995; Mu, Xie, Wen, Weng, & Shuyun, 1999; Smith et al., 1999; Wedig, Rauch, Albert, & Wright, 2005; Wright, Wedig, Williams, Rauch, & Albert, 2006). For this chapter (Figure 17.2), I have pooled structural data from past (Wedig et al., 2005; Wright, Feczko, Dickerson, & Williams, 2007; Wright, Wedig, et al., 2006; Wright, Williams, 2006; Wright, Dickerson, Feczko, Negeira, & Williams, 2007; Wright, Feczko, et al., 2007) and current MRI studies of young and elderly subjects, and found total average amygdala volumes to be 7% smaller in the elderly adults (volume: $M = 1596$ mm^3, $SD = 241$ mm^3) than in the young adults (volume: $M = 1724$ mm^3, $SD = 269$ mm^3). After adjustments for intracranial volumes, the volume difference between groups was 4%. No effects of gender or hemisphere that differed with aging were found, in line with the results of earlier studies (Mu et al., 1999; Pruessner, Collins, Pruessner, & Evans, 2001). Amygdala volume differences with age appear to be greatest after 60, and significant differences in volume have been described between subject groups in the later decades of life (Jack et al., 1997; Mu et al., 1999; Pruessner et al., 2001).

The sources of amygdala atrophy in healthy aging are poorly understood. One small study (comparing four younger and four older individuals) indicated that there were differences in amygdala nuclei with regard to aging,

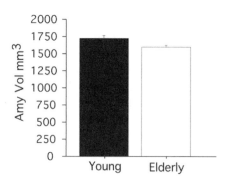

FIGURE 17.2. *Amygdala volume differences with aging.* Mean amygdala volumes (average of left and right combined) in a cohort of healthy young ($n = 56$) and elderly ($n = 58$) subjects, demonstrating modest between-group size differences. The small bars show one standard error.

with the Ce and Co demonstrating the greatest atrophy, whereas the Me and ventral BM exhibited stable or slightly increased volume (Herzog & Kemper, 1980). Cell-packing density in that study followed a similar pattern in these subnuclei, suggesting variable changes in neuron versus neuropil loss; however, this interpretation must be considered with caution, as absolute neuron numbers were not calculated and these neural components were not separately analyzed.

Neurochemical Changes

A small number of works have examined neurochemical alterations in the amygdala with healthy aging. One positron emission tomography (PET) study demonstrated preserved serotonin (5-hydroxytryptamine, or 5-HT) binding in the amygdala with aging (Andersson, Sundman, & Marcusson, 1992). A separate PET study of the amygdala cholinergic system showed decreased muscarinic receptor binding *in vivo* (Whitehouse & Au, 1986) in young versus elderly subjects, while a study of postmortem tissue demonstrated stable amygdala choline acetyltransferase (ChAT) and acetylcholinesterase (AChE) levels in middle-aged and elderly individuals (Emre, Heckers, Mash, Geula, & Mesulam, 1993). PET studies of the dopaminergic system show modest changes (7%) in dopamine (DA) D2 and D3 receptor density from ages 19 to 74 (Kaasinen et al., 2000); D1 receptors appear to remain stable after 40 years of age, though decreases occur in the initial decades of life (Cortes, Gueye, Pazos, Probst, & Palacios, 1989). The causes and consequences of these changes remain poorly understood, but they may relate to the structural changes described above, or to the differences in amygdala function with aging that have received recent attention.

Functional Changes

Although the amygdala in young healthy adults is responsive to a fairly vast array of emotional stimuli and situations (e.g., Anderson & Phelps, 2001; Breiter et al., 1996; Dubois et al., 1999; Gur et al., 2002; Hadjikhani & de Gelder, 2003; Hariri, Bookheimer, & Mazziotta, 2000; Irwin et al., 1996; Lane et al., 1997; Morris, deBonis, & Dolan, 2002; Morris et al., 1996; Morris, Öhman, & Dolan, 1998; Phan et al., 2004; Phelps, Delgado, Nearing, & LeDoux, 2004; Phelps et al., 2001; Phillips et al., 2001; Royet et al., 2000; Schwartz et al., 2003; Whalen et al., 1998, 2001, 2004; Wright et al., 2001, 2003; Wright, Martis, Shin, Fischer, & Rauch, 2002; Zald, Lee, Fluegel, & Pardo, 1998; Zald & Pardo, 1997), this does not appear to be the case in healthy aging. Recent functional imaging studies over the past few years suggest that the amygdala in elderly versus young adults has smaller or weaker responses to certain negative emotional stimuli (Fischer et al., 2005; Gunning-Dixon et al., 2003; Iidaka et al., 2002; Tessitore et al.,

2005). Recent experiments in our laboratory (Plate 17.1 in color insert, top panels) and in others (Williams et al., 2006) suggest that these differences begin in middle age. This relative lack of amygdala activation to negative emotional stimuli with aging does not appear to be a consequence of vascular or other generic age-related factors. In fact, robust and similar amygdala activation in young and elderly adults has been observed in studies using paradigms involving novel and age in-group faces (Wright, Dickerson, et al., 2007; Wright, Wedig, et al., 2006; Wright et al., in press) (Plate 17.2 in color insert). Furthermore, though there is evidence that in certain cases positive emotional stimuli do not appear to activate the amygdala in elderly versus young adults (Gunning-Dixon et al., 2003; Iidaka et al., 2002), in other settings viewing positive pictures or faces does leads to greater amygdala activation to positive versus negative stimuli in elderly than in young subjects (Mather et al., 2004; Williams et al., 2006).

Understanding these differences between amygdala responses to positive pictures and to positive faces is important, particularly in the context of "socioemotional selectivity theory," a major theory of aging. This theory posits that social decisions, via enhanced emotional regulation, are redirected in order to maximize the emotional meaning of life (Carstensen, Isaacowitz, & Charles, 1999). This leads to a smaller but more satisfying social circle with aging, along with a shift in focus from negative to positive emotions that has been called the "positivity effect" (Carstensen, Pasupathi, Mayr, & Nesselroade, 2000; Gross et al., 1997; Lang & Carstensen, 1994; Lang, Staudinger, & Carstensen, 1998; Lansford, Sherman, & Antonucci, 1998). Thus a shift in amygdala responsiveness from negative to positive stimuli with aging could be a neural correlate of this positivity effect in aging. However, unaccounted influences of stimulus type, novelty, functional magnetic resonance imaging (fMRI) methodology, or personality may also explain these apparently discordant results. For example, the amygdala response to positive stimuli found in one study (Mather et al., 2004) could have been obtained because the positive scenes used were more novel or arousing than pictures of positive faces used in other studies (Gunning-Dixon et al., 2003; Iidaka et al., 2002). This effect in the studies of faces may have been exacerbated by the fact that only one class of positive stimuli was used (happy facial expressions), whereas several classes of negative stimuli (e.g., expressions of disgust, anger, fear, and sadness) were used. Because the amygdala is known to habituate rapidly—an effect that is generally preserved with normal aging (Wedig et al., 2005)—there may have been greater habituation to the positive than to the negative stimuli in those studies. Other possible explanations for these differences include inaccuracies in anatomically registering the amygdala in elderly adults (Vandenbroucke et al., 2004), leading to overall negative results in the amygdala, or low levels of extraversion in the elderly versus young groups, which could have led to a lack of amygdala responses to positive stimuli (Canli, Sivers, Whitfield, Gotlib, & Gabrieli, 2002). Future work controlling and examining these factors will be of great interest.

THE AMYGDALA IN AD

Neuropathological Involvement of the Amygdala

In his initial case, Alois Alzheimer (1907) identified abnormal nerve cells and fiber clusters in the cerebral cortex of a 55-year-old woman with a progressive dementia, using then-new silver-staining methods at autopsy. These findings, now considered the hallmark neuropathological lesions of AD, are known as neurofibrillary tangles (NFTs) and neuritic plaques (NPs). The beta amyloid protein, a major component of the NPs, is currently thought to play a central pathophysiological role in the disease (Selkoe, 2003). NFTs, which are found in neurons and composed primarily of anomalous cytoskeletal proteins such as phosphorylated tau (Brion, 1998), may also be of relevance for AD pathophysiology (Iqbal et al., 2005). A third important histopathological feature of AD is the presence of neuropil threads (NTs); these are primarily dendrites of NFT-containing neurons that also have neurofibrillary pathology (Braak & Braak, 1988; Braak, Braak, Grundke-Iqbal, & Iqbal, 1986). NFTs, NTs, and NPs are selectively distributed in neocortical and subcortical regions, depending on the clinical stage of AD. Definitive diagnosis of AD rests upon postmortem findings of a specific distribution and number of these lesions (Hyman, 1997; Khachaturian, 1985).

Involvement of the amygdala in AD neuropathology was initially noted in the first half of the 20th century (Brockhaus, 1938; Grünthal, 1926). Tomlinson (1979) concluded that the amygdala is the brain region most severely affected by NPs and NFTs in AD and in normal aging. Subsequent work generally confirms these observations, and it is clear that, after the entorhinal cortex and hippocampus, the amygdala is one of the initial brain regions involved in AD pathology (Braak & Braak, 1991, 1997, 1998; Haroutunian et al., 1999; Mesulam, 2000; Mielke et al., 1996). This is not only the case in the earliest phases of clinical dementia, but also in the setting of memory impairment without dementia (i.e., mild cognitive impairment, or MCI) (Jicha et al., 2006; Markesbery et al., 2006; Mesulam, 2000; Petersen et al., 2006). Even cognitively normal elderly individuals often display NFTs and NPs in the amygdala (Davis, Schmitt, Wekstein, & Markesbery, 1999; Haroutunian et al., 1998, 1999; Knopman et al., 2003; Mesulam, 2000), suggesting that some of the above-noted age-associated changes in amygdala structure and function may be related to subclinical AD pathology. The number of NFTs in the amygdala correlates with the number in the neocortex (Esiri, Pearson, Steele, Bowen, & Powell, 1990). The number of NPs increases in the amygdala as the disease progresses—a relationship that may be more variable with NFTs (Tsuchiya & Kosaka, 1990). NTs are also present in the amygdala, and it appears that the majority are not related to nearby NFT-containing neurons, suggesting that NTs may disrupt local and long-distance circuitry in the amygdala (Schmidt, Murray, & Trojanowski, 1993).

The distribution of AD pathology within the amygdala is regionally selective (Figure 17.3), but studies suggest individual variability in the precise pat-

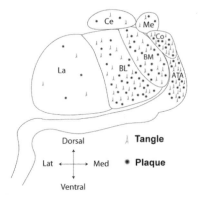

FIGURE 17.3. *Regional distribution of AD pathology in the amygdala.* Summary depiction of the approximate regional and nuclear distribution of neuritic plaques and neurofibrillary tangles in the amygdala in AD. As described in more detail in the text, there is greater involvement of the medial part of the amygdala than of lateral parts, and within the BL there is greater involvement ventrally than dorsally. For illustrative purposes, similar numbers of plaques and tangles are shown, but the precise relationship may vary according to the disease stage and specific study.

terns of nuclear and subnuclear involvement. In this regard, it should be noted that many of the neuropathological studies investigating NFT and NP distribution in AD examined relatively few subjects, with different stages of clinical disease severity and duration. In addition, the types of amyloid plaques enumerated by different authors may vary. Some include diffuse plaques (thought to be earlier or more benign lesions), whereas others limit the analyses to cored neuritic plaques (a later plaque form indicative of greater neuronal damage). All these factors probably contribute to some of the differences among the studies reviewed below.

Two early reports indicated that the medial half of the amygdala exhibited greater AD pathology than its lateral half (Corsellis, 1970; Hirano & Zimmerman, 1962). Subsequent studies examining the regional localization of AD pathology at higher resolution confirmed this global finding and extended it to specific amygdala subnuclei (Brashear, Godec, & Carlsen, 1988; Hopper & Vogel, 1976; Jamada & Mehraein, 1968; Kromer Vogt, Hyman, Van Hoesen, & Damasio, 1990; Tsuchiya & Kosaka, 1990; Unger, Lapham, McNeill, Eskin, & Hamill, 1991; Unger, McNeill, Lapham, & Hamill, 1988). Overall, as summarized in Figure 17.3, these works point to the greatest involvement by NFTs and NPs in the Co and ATA; intermediate involvement of the basal nuclei (including BL and BM); and the least involvement of the Ce and La nuclei (Brady & Mufson, 1990; Hopper & Vogel, 1976; Jamada & Mehraein, 1968; Tsuchiya & Kosaka, 1990; Unger et al., 1988, 1991). Of note, the Me and Co are often included together as the corticomedial nucleus (CoMe) (Corsellis, 1970; Hopper & Vogel, 1976; Unger et al., 1988, 1991), but studies examining these nuclei separately suggest that involvement of the Me is much less than that of the Co (Kromer Vogt et al., 1990; Tsuchiya & Kosaka, 1990).

The patterns of neuropathological involvement of the basal nuclei appear to be the most complex of all the amygdala nuclei. This complexity relates not only to the localization of pathology within specific subsectors of the basal nucleus, but possibly also to the extent that these subsectors are affected by NFTs or NPs. The literature to date suggests that the BM, BLv, and BLpl have higher concentrations of AD pathology than the intermediate and dorsal regions of the BL (Kromer Vogt et al., 1990; Tsuchiya & Kosaka, 1990; Unger et al., 1991; Van Hoesen, Augustinack, & Redman, 1999). This probably holds true for the presence of both NFTs and NPs. However, some works indicate different regional variations in NFT and NP distribution and density (Brady & Mufson, 1990; Kromer Vogt et al., 1990; Van Hoesen et al., 1999), whereas others report no clear relationships (Unger et al., 1991). These discrepancies may relate to individual variability, or to the fact that the histopathological and clinical severity of the disease differentially influences detection of NFTs and NPs (Tsuchiya & Kosaka, 1990; Unger et al., 1991). Although greater amygdala pathology has been linked to global measures of clinical AD severity (Bierer et al., 1995; Haroutunian et al., 1998, 1999), explaining some of this variance, the specific functional consequences of AD pathology in the amygdala are underexplored. For example, it would be of substantial clinical interest to know whether the extent of regional histopathology in the amygdala relates to specific neuropsychiatric symptoms in AD or MCI, but such work has not yet been reported.

Few studies have examined the regional distribution of NTs in the amygdala. However, experiments utilizing antibodies to paired helical filaments (e.g., Alz-50) suggest greater involvement by abnormal cytoskeletal proteins in the ventromedial (vs. dosolateral) amygdala, including the Co, ATA, and PL BL (Benzing, Ikonomovic, Brady, Mufson, & Armstrong, 1993; Unger et al., 1988, 1991). This partially mirrors the global distribution of NFTs and NPs.

Structural Changes

Significant decreases in the volume of the amygdala occur in AD relative to healthy aging. Both neuroimaging studies *in vivo* (Cuenod et al., 1993; Ishii et al., 2005; Jack et al., 1997; Laakso, Partanen, et al., 1995; Laakso, Soininen, et al., 1995; O'Brien et al., 1997; Smith et al., 1999) and postmortem neuropathological studies (Herzog & Kemper, 1980; Scott, DeKosky, & Scheff, 1991) suggest a 14–60% or greater loss of amygdala volume in AD. The extent of volume loss has been related to the clinical severity of the disease (Jack et al., 1997; Tsuchiya & Kosaka, 1990). Consistent with the fact that the findings of atrophy in mild AD are more variable, some studies have found significant differences relative to normal aging (Cuenod et al., 1993; Jack et al., 1997), but others have not (Laakso, Partanen, et al., 1995; Laakso, Soininen, et al., 1995). Of note, a few investigations suggest that amygdala volume losses have important clinical consequences: They may be related to deficits in emotional memory (Mori et al., 1999) and the presence of noncognitive or behavioral symptoms in AD (Martinez-Castillo, Arrazola, Fernandez, Maestu, & Ortiz, 2001; Smith et al., 1999).

The sources of amygdala volume reductions include losses of neurons, glia, and neuropil. Studies on amygdala cell-packing density have been equivocal, with one study showing a decrease (Herzog & Kemper, 1980), but another showing an increase (Scott, DeKosky, Sparks, Knox, & Scheff, 1992) in this measure. This may be because neuronal packing densities are dependent on the extent of volume loss relative to neuronal loss, and therefore may differ according to the stage or duration of the disease, or to the specific cases studied. Studies of absolute neuron number are more reliable and have consistently indicated significant (50–60%) neuronal losses that are directly related to the clinical stage of the disease (Scott et al., 1992; Tsuchiya & Kosaka, 1990; Vereecken, Vogels, & Nieuwenhuys, 1994). These works also demonstrate selective shrinkage or loss of large neurons, with relative preservation of small neurons (Scott et al., 1992; Tsuchiya & Kosaka, 1990; Vereecken et al., 1994). In addition, significant (small and large) glial cell loss has been described in AD (Scott et al., 1992). Furthermore, neuropil loss appears to contribute to amygdala volume reductions as much as neuronal losses do (Scott et al., 1992).

As with the histopathological hallmarks of AD, the volume and neuronal losses in the amygdala are regionally variable. Only two studies have examined volume differences in detail (Herzog & Kemper, 1980; Scott et al., 1991). Taken together, these works suggest that the Me, Co, Ce, and La are similarly affected in a moderate to severe fashion, and that there is greater volume loss in dorsal relative to ventral parts of the BL and perhaps BM (Figure 17.4). However, there are several notable discrepancies between these two studies. Although the relative patterns mentioned were similar within each study, total

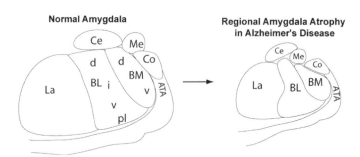

FIGURE 17.4. *Regional atrophy of the amygdala in AD.* Schematic depiction of the regional volume loss within the amygdala. There is generalized atrophy in addition to selective volume losses, particularly in the dorsal portions of the BL and BM.

and regional amygdala volume losses differed substantially between the studies. For example, total amygdala volume loss was 55% in one study (Scott et al., 1991), but only 26% in the other (Herzog & Kemper, 1980). Likewise, the range of subnuclear atrophy was 21–71% (Scott et al., 1991) versus 14–38% (Herzog & Kemper, 1980). Furthermore, the dorsal (large-celled) BM was much more severely affected than the ventral (small-celled) BM in the study of Scott and colleagues (1991), whereas there were similar extents of volume loss in these regions in Herzog and Kemper's (1980) study.

The results of these two studies were also discrepant with respect to the differences in regional cell-packing density. The work of Herzog and Kemper (1980) indicated the greatest *decreases* (35–52%) in cell-packing density in the central, cortical, and medial nuclei, with lesser *decreases* (16–32%) in the BL, BM, and La. A gradient of cell-packing density loss in the basal nuclei was also evident in that study, with the least losses in BLpl and ventral BM, but greater losses in more dorsal parts of the BL and BM. In contrast, Scott and colleagues' (1991) study indicated an approximately 35% *increase* in packing density in both the dorsal parts of the BL (BLdi) and the Co, which were the two areas examined in that study. There are several possible sources for the differences in the results of these two studies. As noted above, packing densities depend on the extent of volume loss relative to neuronal loss, and may differ according to disease stage or duration, or to the specific cases studied. The total brain weights for controls and patients with AD were very similar between the two studies, suggesting a similar stage of overall pathological involvement. However, the mean duration of illness was different between the two studies, as were tissue preparation methods. These factors may have additionally contributed to the differences between these studies.

The findings of regional differences in amygdala neuronal losses in AD (Figure 17.5) are also somewhat variable, and again few studies have examined this directly. Vereecken and colleagues (1994) reported that total neuron number loss was greatest (70%) in the BM and BLv, followed by (55–60%) the Co, BLdi, ATA, and centromedial nuclei (which they combined as one structure), with the least loss (38–39%) in the La and BLpl. The work of Tsuchiya and Kosaka (1990), though semiquantitative in nature, was in accordance with this general pattern, except that severe neuronal losses were noted in the La (which was not the case in the study of Vereecken et al., 1994). The work of Scott and colleagues (1991) reported only selected portions of the BL and Co and found similar neuronal losses in the large-celled dorsal parts of the BL and the Co (though there was greater glial cell loss in the BLdi than in the Co). Overall, the suggestion is that the ventral BL and BM are most severely affected by neuron loss, with intermediate losses in the Co; the lowest losses in the BLdi, Ce, Me, and BLpl; and the loss in the La varying from mild to severe (Figure 17.5).

When the regional localization of NPs and NFTs in the amygdala of patients with AD is considered with respect to the cell and volume loss, no clear direct correspondence among all three factors is apparent. For example,

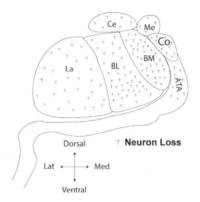

FIGURE 17.5. *Regional neuron loss in amygdala in AD.* Schematic depiction of regional neuron losses within the amygdala. Neuron losses are most severe in the ventral portions of the BL and throughout the BM, moderate in the Co and dorsal BL, and mild in the remaining regions.

the BLv has a greater burden of AD neuropathology and neuronal loss than the BLdi, but the BLdi has greater volume loss than the BLv. This suggests perhaps an inverse relationship between AD histopathology and atrophy/cell loss in these areas. Likewise, the La and Ce have a relatively low neuropathological burden, but may have fairly prominent volume and cell loss. The correspondence between neuropathological involvement and neuron/volume loss is most direct in the Co and Me nuclei, where these factors seem to correspond best. The precise reasons for these differences remain to be explored. Factors such as differential losses of neurons versus glia, or of cell bodies versus neuropil, are possible explanations. For example, losses of glial cells and intrinsic (e.g., from the La) or extrinsic (e.g., from the frontotemporal cortex) afferent projections to dorsal parts of the BL may result in greater volume reductions than in the ventral parts of the BL, where neuronal loss or shrinkage leads to relatively less atrophy in the setting of tissue displacement by abundant AD histopathology (i.e., NPs and NFTs). The differences in volume and cell loss may also be related to neuron size differences between various nuclei. The larger neurons of the dorsal BL and BM may project to several sites far outside the amygdala (prefrontal cortex and occipototemporal cortex) and to sites where significant AD pathology is present (hippocampus and entorhinal cortex) (Amaral, Behniea, & Kelly, 2003; Amaral & Price, 1984; Amaral et al., 1992; Barbas & De Olmos, 1990; Stefanacci & Amaral, 2002). In the presence of relatively light local AD histopathology, distant deafferentation could lead to cell body shrinkage of these larger cells without death, resulting in greater atrophy relative to neuron loss. Beyond these cytoarchitectural and hodological contributions to volume loss, differences in specific types of clinical symptoms could contribute to variability and are often not accounted for. In this regard, it would be of interest to know whether the presence of neuropsychiatric symptoms (e.g., anxiety or agitation) is related to the involvement of certain subnuclei or to specific cellular or extracellular changes.

Neurochemical Changes

Degeneration of the basal forebrain cholinergic system is one of the earliest and best-described neurotransmitter changes in AD. Likewise, the most published data about neurochemical changes in the amygdala in AD relates to decrements in various cholinergic markers. Several PET studies have demonstrated decreased AChE in the amygdala in patients with AD (Herholz et al., 2004; Shinotoh et al., 2000a, 2000b, 2003). This occurs in both early- and late-onset disease (Shinotoh et al., 2000a), and is correlated with cognitive functioning as measured by the Mini-Mental State Exam (Shinotoh et al., 2003). Neuropathological studies also reveal significant and parallel reductions in both AChE and ChAT in the amygdala in AD (Emre et al., 1993; Esiri et al., 1990; Unger et al., 1988). The Co, BM, and La exhibit greater losses of cholinergic nervous system markers than the BL and Ce, suggesting regionally selective effects (Emre et al., 1993; Unger et al., 1988). However, the nature of the link between regional amygdala burden of NFT and NP pathology on the one hand, and AChE and ChAT loss on the other, is uncertain. Several studies suggest that there may be an inverse relationship between NFT/NP pathology and cholinergic losses in the amygdala, with areas having the greatest concentration of cholinergic markers being the ones least affected by AD histopathology (Emre et al., 1993; Kromer Vogt et al., 1990; Unger et al., 1988).

It is also well established that most of the widely projecting neurotransmitter systems are damaged by AD pathology. Similarly, the available evidence suggests that several neurotransmitter systems are affected in the amygdala in addition to the cholinergic system. Although there are significant losses of terminals containing 5-HT and its metabolite 5-hydroxyindoleacetic acid in the amygdala in AD (Arai, Kosaka, & Iizuka, 1984; Burke et al., 1990; Yates, Simpson, & Gordon, 1986), 5-HT receptor losses are more variable. For example, 5-HT_3 receptor density is preserved in AD (Barnes, Costall, Naylor, Williams, & Wischik, 1990), whereas 5-HT_2 receptors appear to be lost earlier in the disease, with 5-HT_1 receptor losses occurring later in the disease (Cross et al., 1984). Studies of the dopaminergic system are variable, with one study showing depletion of DA and its metabolite homovanillic acid in the amygdala (Joyce, Kaeger, Ryoo, & Goldsmith, 1993), while another did not (Nazarali & Reynolds, 1992). Depletion of DA D2 receptors has been reported in AD, with the greatest losses in the BL (Joyce et al., 1993). Noradrenergic neurotransmitter changes occur in the amygdala in AD, and two studies have reported low norepinephrine (NE) levels in patients with AD versus controls (Arai et al., 1984; Hoogendijk et al., 1999), but one did not (Nazarali & Reynolds, 1992). One study (Hoogendijk et al., 1999) examined NE and its metabolite, 3-methoxy-4-hydroxyphenylglycol (MHPG), finding a high MHPG-to-NE ratio (suggesting higher NE metabolism) in patients with

AD relative to controls. There are a few reports suggesting involvement of multiple local-circuit neurotransmitters/neuropeptides or metabolites in the amygdala of AD as well. For example, decreased somatostatin, neurotensin, neuropeptide Y, the enkephalins, and opioid receptors have been described in AD (Barg et al., 1993; Benzing, Mufson, & Armstrong, 1993; Rinne et al., 1993; Unger et al., 1988). Likewise, N-acetyl aspartate and N-acetyl aspartyl-glutamate are also reduced in the amygdala (Jaarsma, Veenma-van der Duin, & Korf, 1994). The functional and clinical consequences of these various neurotransmitter changes are poorly understood, but recent functional neuroimaging studies suggest that the activity of the amygdala is significantly altered in AD.

Functional Changes

Despite the substantial literature on neuropathological, morphometric, and neurotransmitter effects of AD on the amygdala, relatively few reports have focused on changes in amygdala function that occur with AD. Several single-photon emission tomography (SPECT) studies have indicated decreased amygdala perfusion in AD (Callen, Black, & Caldwell, 2002; Johnson et al., 2001; Soininen et al., 1995; Tanaka et al., 1998). This finding is corroborated by a PET study demonstrating decreased amygdala glucose metabolism in AD relative to normal aging and MCI (Cao et al., 2002). An additional resting regional cerebral blood flow study using SPECT suggests that amygdala activity decreases as the clinical severity of AD increases (Kogure et al., 1999). Two PET studies using activation procedures (i.e., memory tasks) demonstrated functional changes in the amygdala in patients with AD relative to controls, but results were disparate. One study showed a decreased amygdala metabolic rate during a verbal memory task in patients with AD relative to controls (Valladares-Neto et al., 1995); the other demonstrated increased activity during a face memory task in the patient population relative to controls (Grady, Furey, Pietrini, Horwitz, & Rapoport, 2001). The reason for the differences between these two studies is uncertain, but possibilities include differences in disease severity or duration, the extent of amygdala atrophy, or the memory task utilized.

Using fMRI, my colleagues and I have recently started to examine amygdala activity in mild AD during viewing of human facial expressions (Wright, Dickerson, et al., 2007) (Plate 17.3 in color insert). To enable detection of amygdala responses in the elderly participants, the same paradigm comparing familiar neutral and novel fearful stimuli was used as in Plate 17.1 (in color insert) (Wright, Wedig, et al., 2006). This work indicates that the amygdala in patients with mild AD, relative to elderly controls, is excessively responsive to both familiar neutral and novel fearful faces. We did not observe significant between-group differences in the differential response (i.e., amygdala responses for novel fearful faces vs. familiar neutral faces were similar between the two groups). This suggests that the pathological changes in mild AD lead to exaggerated, stimulus-nonspecific amygdala activation. One possible mechanism for these findings is that a general reduction in habituation occurs, leading to greater responses to the face stimuli in AD than in normal aging. However, an examination of habituation to the face stimuli in the patients with AD versus the elderly controls suggested that hyperactivation was the mechanism underlying the exaggerated amygdala responses in the patients. Of note, the group effects described above were regionally selective, as they were not found in the calcarine cortex. Furthermore, the exaggerated amygdala activity to the familiar neutral (but not novel fearful) faces was positively correlated with specific clinical measures of behavioral symptoms in AD, including irritability and agitation. This suggests that exaggerated responses to familiar, nonemotional stimuli in particular are an indicator of clinically relevant amygdala dysfunction in mild AD. This study highlights the potential relevance of investigating the relationships between clinical symptoms and amygdala physiology in AD.

CONCLUDING REMARKS ON AD AND THE AMYGDALA

How can sense be made of the variable literature on the distribution of AD histopathology, atrophy, and neuronal loss in the amygdala? A small number of studies suggest that some of this variability is related to the clinical severity of the disease or to the noncognitive or behavioral symptoms of AD. It is likely that further research involving more refined clinical–pathological correlations will help to explain some of the discrepant findings. Furthermore, such work will be important for enhancing our understanding of the neuropsychiatric symptoms of AD, which have ineffective and potentially harmful treatments, but serious consequences for the patient and family. Additional basic research examining how the various cellular (neuronal and glial) and neuropil components relate to atrophy and to the presence of NFTs and NPs may also help to elucidate the regionally variable relationships of these factors in the amygdala. Finally, further functional imaging studies in AD will be essential for understanding how the activity of the amygdala relates to the neuropsychiatric symptoms of the disorder. If preliminary work suggesting that specific aspects of amygdala activity relate to particular behavioral symptoms is replicated, it may be possible to establish surrogate markers for future clinical trials targeting these specific symptoms.

WHAT I THINK

What are the possible mechanisms for the differences in amygdala responses to emotional stimuli with aging? It is well established that specific regions of the amygdala and the medial prefrontal cortex (PFC) are interconnected (Carmichael & Price, 1995; Pandya, Van Hoesen, & Mesulam, 1981). From animal data, it appears that the medial PFC can regulate the responses of the amygdala—so-called "top-down" regulation. Furthermore, studies of humans indicate a reciprocal relationship between the activities of the medial PFC and amygdala activity (e.g., Beauregard, Levesque, & Bourgouin, 2001; Kim, Somerville, Johnstone, Alexander, & Whalen, 2003; Shin et al., 2005). My colleagues and I therefore hypothesized that there might be lesser medial PFC activity, but greater amygdala activity in the young, with the opposite pattern in older subjects (i.e., greater medial PFC activity, but less amygdala activity). We examined this prediction, using a cohort of young and middle-aged subjects (see Plate 17.1 in color insert, bottom panels). As described at the beginning of this chapter, there was decreased activation in the amygdala in the middle-aged relative to the young participants for the contrast between fearful and neutral faces, but the medial PFC activation showed the anticipated *opposite* pattern. Specifically, the young subjects had reduced activations (in fact, deactivations were present) in the medial PFC to the fearful–neutral faces contrast, in comparison with the middle-aged subjects (where activations were present). These findings are consistent with the recent work of others (Williams et al., 2006) and suggest that differences in medial PFC–amygdala interactions with aging may result in the decreased amygdala responses to negative versus neutral stimuli that have been observed with aging. This is particularly interesting to consider, given that recent morphometric studies indicate preservation, or even enlargement, of the medial PFC with aging (Grieve, Clark, Williams, Peduto, & Gordon, 2005; Salat et al., 2004), suggesting that enhanced top-down control with aging may have an anatomical signature in the medial PFC.

ACKNOWLEDGMENTS

This work was supported in part by National Institute of Mental Health Grant No. K23MH64806 and National Institute on Aging Grant No. R01AG030311 to Christopher I. Wright, as well as resource grants to the Martinos Center for Biomedical Imaging from the National Center for Research Resources (No. P41-RR14075), and the Mental Illness and Neuroscience Discovery Institute.

REFERENCES

Alzheimer, A. (1907). Ueber eine eigenartige erkrankung der hirnrinde. *Allgemeine Zeitschrift für Psychiatrie und Psychisch-Gerichtliche Medizin, 64*, 146–148.

Amaral, D. G., Behniea, H., & Kelly, J. L. (2003). Topographic organization of projections from the amygdala to the visual cortex in the macaque monkey. *Neuroscience, 118*(4), 1099–1120.

Amaral, D. G., & Price, J. L. (1984). Amygdalo-cortical projections in the monkey (*Macaca fascicularis*). *Journal of Comparative Neurology, 230*(4), 465–496.

Amaral, D. G., Price, J. L., Pitkänen, A., & Carmichael, S. T. (1992). Anatomic organization of the primate amygdala. In J. P. Aggleton (Ed.), *The amygdala: Neurobiological aspects of emotion, memory, and mental dysfunction* (pp. 1–66). New York: Wiley-Liss.

Anderson, A. K., & Phelps, E. A. (2001). Lesions of the human amygdala impair enhanced perception of emotionally salient events. *Nature, 411*, 305–309.

Andersson, A., Sundman, I., & Marcusson, J. (1992). Age stability of human brain 5-HT terminals studied with [³H]paroxetine binding. *Gerontology, 38*(3), 127–132.

Arai, H., Kosaka, K., & Iizuka, R. (1984). Changes of biogenic amines and their metabolites in postmortem brains from patients with Alzheimer-type dementia. *Journal of Neurochemistry, 43*(2), 388–393.

Barbas, H., & De Olmos, J. (1990). Projections from the amygdala to basoventral and mediodorsal prefrontal regions in the rhesus monkey. *Journal of Comparative Neurology, 300*(4), 549–571.

Barg, J., Belcheva, M., Rowinski, J., Ho, A., Burke, W. J., Chung, H. D., et al. (1993). Opioid receptor density changes in Alzheimer amygdala and putamen. *Brain Research, 632*(1–2), 209–215.

Barnes, N. M., Costall, B., Naylor, R. J., Williams, T. J., & Wischik, C. M. (1990). Normal densities of 5-HT3 receptor recognition sites in Alzheimer's disease. *NeuroReport, 1*(3–4), 253–254.

Beauregard, M., Levesque, J., & Bourgouin, P. (2001). Neural correlates of conscious self-regulation of emotion. *Journal of Neuroscience, 21*(18), RC165.

Benzing, W. C., Ikonomovic, M. D., Brady, D. R., Mufson, E. J., & Armstrong, D. M. (1993). Evidence that transmitter-containing dystrophic neurites precede paired helical filament and Alz-50 formation within senile plaques in the amygdala of nondemented elderly and patients with Alzheimer's disease. *Journal of Comparative Neurology, 334*(2), 176–191.

Benzing, W. C., Mufson, E. J., & Armstrong, D. M. (1993). Immunocytochemical distribution of peptidergic and cholinergic fibers in the human amygdala: Their depletion in Alzheimer's disease and morphologic alteration in non-demented elderly with numerous senile plaques. *Brain Research, 625*(1), 125–138.

Bierer, L. M., Hof, P. R., Purohit, D. P., Carlin, L., Schmeidler, J., Davis, K. L., et al. (1995). Neocortical neurofibrillary tangles correlate with dementia severity in Alzheimer's disease. *Archives of Neurology, 52*(1), 81–88.

Braak, H., & Braak, E. (1988). Neuropil threads occur in dendrites of tangle-bearing nerve cells. *Neuropathology and Applied Neurobiology, 14*(1), 39–44.

Braak, H., & Braak, E. (1991). Neuropathological stageing of Alzheimer-related changes. *Acta Neuropathologica (Berlin), 82*(4), 239–259.

Braak, H., & Braak, E. (1997). Diagnostic criteria for neuropathologic assessment of Alzheimer's disease. *Neurobiology of Aging, 18*(4, Suppl.), S85–S88.

Braak, H., & Braak, E. (1998). Evolution of neuronal changes in the course of Alzheimer's disease. *Journal of Neural Transmission, 53*(Suppl.), 127–140.

Braak, H., Braak, E., Grundke-Iqbal, I., & Iqbal, K. (1986). Occurrence of neuropil threads in the senile human brain and in Alzheimer's disease: A third location of paired helical filaments outside of neurofibrillary tangles and neuritic plaques. *Neuroscience Letters, 65*(3), 351–355.

Brady, D. R., & Mufson, E. J. (1990). Amygdaloid pathology in Alzheimer's disease: Qualitative and quantitative analysis. *Dementia, 1*, 5–17.

Brashear, H. R., Godec, M. S., & Carlsen, J. (1988). The distribution of neuritic plaques and acetylcholinesterase staining in the amygdala in Alzheimer's disease. *Neurology, 38*(11), 1694–1699.

Breiter, H. C., Etcoff, N. L., Whalen, P. J., Kennedy, W. A., Rauch, S. L., Buckner, R. L., et al. (1996). Response and habituation of the human amygdala during visual processing of facial expression. *Neuron, 17*(5), 875–887.

Brion, J. P. (1998). Neurofibrillary tangles and Alzheimer's disease. *European Neurology, 40*(3), 130–140.

Brockhaus, H. (1938). Zur anatomie des mendelkerngebietes. *Journal of Psychology and Neurology, 49,* 1–36.

Burke, W. J., Park, D. H., Chung, H. D., Marshall, G. L., Haring, J. H., & Joh, T. H. (1990). Evidence for decreased transport of tryptophan hydroxylase in Alzheimer's disease. *Brain Research, 537*(1–2), 83–87.

Callen, D. J., Black, S. E., & Caldwell, C. B. (2002). Limbic system perfusion in Alzheimer's disease measured by MRI-coregistered HMPAO SPECT. *European Journal of Nuclear Medicine and Molecular Imaging, 29*(7), 899–906.

Canli, T., Sivers, H., Whitfield, S. L., Gotlib, I. H., & Gabrieli, J. D. (2002). Amygdala response to happy faces as a function of extraversion. *Science, 296,* 2191.

Cao, Q., Jiang, K., Liu, Y., Zhang, M., Xiao, S., Zuo, C., et al. (2002). [The comparison of the regional cerebral metabolism rate of glucose in Alzheimer's disease with mild cognitive impairment]. *Zhonghua Yi Xue Za Zhi, 82*(23), 1613–1616.

Carmichael, S. T., & Price, J. L. (1995). Limbic connections of the orbital and medial prefrontal cortex in macaque monkeys. *Journal of Comparative Neurology, 363*(4), 615–641.

Carstensen, L. L., Isaacowitz, D. M., & Charles, S. T. (1999). Taking time seriously: A theory of socioemotional selectivity. *American Psychologist, 54*(3), 165–181.

Carstensen, L. L., Pasupathi, M., Mayr, U., & Nesselroade, J. R. (2000). Emotional experience in everyday life across the adult life span. *Journal of Personality and Social Psychology, 79*(4), 644–655.

Corsellis, J. A. N. (1970). The limbic areas in Alzheimer's disease and in other conditions associated with dementia. In G. E. W. Wolstenholme & M. O'Connor (Eds.), *Alzheimer's disease* (pp. 37–50). London: Churchill.

Cortes, R., Gueye, B., Pazos, A., Probst, A., & Palacios, J. M. (1989). Dopamine receptors in human brain: Autoradiographic distribution of d1 sites. *Neuroscience, 28*(2), 263–273.

Crosby, E. C., & Humphrey, T. (1941). Studies on the vertebrate telencephalon: II. The nuclear pattern of the anterior olfactory nucleus, tuberculum olfactorium and amygdaloid complex in man. *Journal of Comparative Neurology, 74,* 309–352.

Cross, A. J., Crow, T. J., Ferrier, I. N., Johnson, J. A., Bloom, S. R., & Corsellis, J. A. (1984). Serotonin receptor changes in dementia of the Alzheimer type. *Journal of Neurochemistry, 43*(6), 1574–1581.

Cuenod, C. A., Denys, A., Michot, J. L., Jehenson, P., Forette, F., Kaplan, D., et al. (1993). Amygdala atrophy in Alzheimer's disease: An *in vivo* magnetic resonance imaging study. *Archives of Neurology, 50*(9), 941–945.

Davis, D. G., Schmitt, F. A., Wekstein, D. R., & Markesbery, W. R. (1999). Alzheimer neuropathologic alterations in aged cognitively normal subjects. *Journal of Neuropathology and Experimental Neurology, 58*(4), 376–388.

De Olmos, J. (2003). Amygdaloid nuclear gray complex. In G. Paxinos & J. K. Mai (Eds.), *The human nervous system* (pp. 739–868). London: Academic Press.

Dubois, S., Rossion, B., Schiltz, C., Bodart, J. M., Michel, C., Bruyer, R., et al. (1999). Effect of familiarity on the processing of human faces. *NeuroImage, 9*(3), 278–289.

Emre, M., Heckers, S., Mash, D. C., Geula, C., & Mesulam, M. M. (1993). Cholinergic innervation of the amygdaloid complex in the human brain and its alterations in old age and Alzheimer's disease. *Journal of Comparative Neurology, 336*(1), 117–134.

Esiri, M. M., Pearson, R. C., Steele, J. E., Bowen, D. M., & Powell, T. P. (1990). A quantitative study of the neurofibrillary tangles and the choline acetyltransferase activity in the cerebral cortex and the amygdala in Alzheimer's disease. *Journal of Neurology, Neurosurgery and Psychiatry, 53*(2), 161–165.

Fischer, H., Sandblom, J., Gavazzeni, J., Fransson, P., Wright, C. I., & Backman, L. (2005). Age-differential patterns of brain activation during perception of angry faces. *Neuroscience Letters, 386*(2), 99–104.

Grady, C. L., Furey, M. L., Pietrini, P., Horwitz, B., & Rapoport, S. I. (2001). Altered brain functional connectivity and impaired short-term memory in Alzheimer's disease. *Brain, 124*(Pt. 4), 739–756.

Grieve, S. M., Clark, C. R., Williams, L. M., Peduto, A. J., & Gordon, E. (2005). Preservation of limbic and paralimbic structures in aging. *Human Brain Mapping, 25*(4), 391–401.

Gross, J. J., Carstensen, L. L., Pasupathi, M., Tsai, J., Skorpen, C. G., & Hsu, A. Y. (1997). Emotion and aging: Experience, expression, and control. *Psychology and Aging, 12*(4), 590–599.

Grünthal, E. (1926). Uber die Alzheimersche krankheit-Eine histopatholosich studie. *Zeitschrift Gesamte Neurologie und Psychiatrie, 101,* 128–157.

Gunning-Dixon, F. M., Gur, R. C., Perkins, A. C., Schroeder, L., Turner, T., Turetsky, B. I., et al. (2003). Age-related differences in brain activation during emotional face processing. *Neurobiology of Aging, 24*(2), 285–295.

Gur, R. C., Schroeder, L., Turner, T., McGrath, C., Chan, R. M., Turetsky, B. I., et al. (2002). Brain activation during facial emotion processing. *NeuroImage, 16*(3, Pt. 1), 651–662.

Hadjikhani, N., & de Gelder, B. (2003). Seeing fearful body expressions activates the fusiform cortex and amygdala. *Current Biology, 13,* 2201–2205.

Hariri, A. R., Bookheimer, S. Y., & Mazziotta, J. C. (2000). Modulating emotional responses: Effects of a neocortical network on the limbic system. *NeuroReport, 11*(1), 43–48.

Haroutunian, V., Perl, D. P., Purohit, D. P., Marin, D., Khan, K., Lantz, M., et al. (1998). Regional distribution of neuritic plaques in the nondemented elderly and subjects with very mild Alzheimer disease. *Archives of Neurology, 55*(9), 1185–1191.

Haroutunian, V., Purohit, D. P., Perl, D. P., Marin, D., Khan, K., Lantz, M., et al. (1999). Neurofibrillary tangles in nondemented elderly subjects and mild Alzheimer disease. *Archives of Neurology, 56*(6), 713–718.

Herholz, K., Weisenbach, S., Zundorf, G., Lenz, O., Schroder, H., Bauer, B., et al. (2004). *In vivo* study of acetylcholine esterase in basal forebrain, amygdala, and cortex in mild to moderate Alzheimer disease. *NeuroImage, 21*(1), 136–143.

Herzog, A. G., & Kemper, T. L. (1980). Amygdaloid changes in aging and dementia. *Archives of Neurology, 37*(10), 625–629.

Hirano, A., & Zimmerman, H. M. (1962). Alzheimer's neurofibrillary changes: A topographic study. *Archives of Neurology, 7,* 227–242.

Hoogendijk, W. J., Feenstra, M. G., Botterblom, M. H., Gilhuis, J., Sommer, I. E., Kamphorst, W., et al. (1999). Increased activity of surviving locus ceruleus neurons in Alzheimer's disease. *Annals of Neurology, 45*(1), 82–91.

Hopper, M. W., & Vogel, F. S. (1976). The limbic system in Alzheimer's disease: A neuropathologic investigation. *American Journal of Pathology, 85*(1), 1–20.

Hyman, B. T. (1997). The neuropathological diagnosis of Alzheimer's disease: Clinical–pathological studies. *Neurobiology of Aging, 18*(4, Suppl.), S27–S32.

Iidaka, T., Okada, T., Murata, T., Omori, M., Kosaka, H., Sadato, N., et al. (2002). Age-related differences in the medial temporal lobe responses to emotional faces as revealed by fMRI. *Hippocampus, 12*(3), 352–362.

Iqbal, K., Alonso Adel, C., Chen, S., Chohan, M. O., El-Akkad, E., Gong, C. X., et al. (2005). Tau pathology in Alzheimer disease and other tauopathies. *Biochimica et Biophysica Acta, 1739*(2–3), 198–210.

Irwin, W., Davidson, R. J., Lowe, M. J., Mock, B. J., Sorenson, J. A., & Turski, P. A. (1996). Human amygdala activation detected with echo-planar functional magnetic resonance imaging. *NeuroReport, 7*(11), 1765–1769.

Ishii, K., Sasaki, H., Kono, A. K., Miyamoto, N., Fukuda, T., & Mori, E. (2005). Comparison of gray matter and metabolic reduction in mild Alzheimer's disease using FDG-PET and voxel-based morphometric MR studies. *European Journal of Nuclear Medicine and Molecular Imaging, 32*(8), 959–963.

Jaarsma, D., Veenma-van der Duin, L., & Korf, J. (1994). N-acetylaspartate and N-acetylaspartylglutamate levels in Alzheimer's disease post-mortem brain tissue. *Journal of the Neurological Sciences, 127*(2), 230–233.

Jack, C. R., Jr., Petersen, R. C., Xu, Y. C., Waring, S. C., O'Brien, P. C., Tangalos, E. G., et al. (1997). Medial temporal atrophy on MRI in normal aging and very mild Alzheimer's disease. *Neurology, 49*(3), 786–794.

Jamada, M., & Mehraein, P. (1968). [Distribution of senile changes in the brain: The part of the limbic system in Alzheimer's disease and senile dementia]. *Archiv für Psychiatrie und Nervenkrankheit, 211*(3), 308–324.

Jicha, G. A., Parisi, J. E., Dickson, D. W., Johnson, K., Cha, R., Ivnik, R. J., et al. (2006). Neuropathologic outcome of mild cognitive impairment following progression to clinical dementia. *Archives of Neurology, 63*(5), 674–681.

Johnson, K. A., Lopera, F., Jones, K., Becker, A., Sperling, R., Hilson, J., et al. (2001). Presenilin-1-associated abnormalities in regional cerebral perfusion. *Neurology, 56*(11), 1545–1551.

Johnston, J. B. (1923). Further contributions to the study of the evolution of the forebrain. *Journal of Comparative Neurology, 35*, 337–381.

Joyce, J. N., Kaeger, C., Ryoo, H., & Goldsmith, S. (1993). Dopamine D2 receptors in the hippocampus and amygdala in Alzheimer's disease. *Neuroscience Letters, 154*(1–2), 171–174.

Kaasinen, V., Vilkman, H., Hietala, J., Nagren, K., Helenius, H., Olsson, H., et al. (2000). Age-related dopamine D2/D3 receptor loss in extrastriatal regions of the human brain. *Neurobiology of Aging, 21*(5), 683–688.

Khachaturian, Z. S. (1985). Diagnosis of Alzheimer's disease. *Archives of Neurology, 42*(11), 1097–1105.

Kim, H., Somerville, L. H., Johnstone, T., Alexander, A. L., & Whalen, P. J. (2003). Inverse amygdala and medial prefrontal cortex responses to surprised faces. *NeuroReport, 14*(18), 2317–2322.

Knopman, D. S., Parisi, J. E., Salviati, A., Floriach-Robert, M., Boeve, B. F., Ivnik, R. J., et al. (2003). Neuropathology of cognitively normal elderly. *Journal of Neuropathology and Experimental Neurology, 62*(11), 1087–1095.

Kogure, D., Matsuda, H., Ohnishi, T., Kunihiro, T., Uno, M., Asada, T., et al. (1999). [Longitudinal evaluation of early dementia of Alzheimer type using brain perfusion SPECT]. *Kaku Igaku, 36*(2), 91–101.

Kromer Vogt, L. J., Hyman, B. T., Van Hoesen, G. W., & Damasio, A. R. (1990). Pathological alterations in the amygdala in Alzheimer's disease. *Neuroscience, 37*(2), 377–385.

Laakso, M. P., Partanen, K., Lehtovirta, M., Hallikainen, M., Hanninen, T., Vainio, P., et al. (1995). MRI of amygdala fails to diagnose early Alzheimer's disease. *NeuroReport, 6*(17), 2414–2418.

Laakso, M. P., Soininen, H., Partanen, K., Helkala, E. L., Hartikainen, P., Vainio, P., et al. (1995). Volumes of hippocampus, amygdala and frontal lobes in the MRI-based diagnosis of early Alzheimer's disease: Correlation with memory functions. *Journal of Neural Transmission: Parkinson Disease and Dementia Section, 9*(1), 73–86.

Lane, R. D., Reiman, E. M., Bradley, M. M., Lang, P. J., Ahern, G. L., Davidson, R. J., et al. (1997). Neuroanatomical correlates of pleasant and unpleasant emotion. *Neuropsychologia, 35*(11), 1437–1444.

Lang, F. R., & Carstensen, L. L. (1994). Close emotional relationships in late life: Further support for proactive aging in the social domain. *Psychology and Aging, 9*(2), 315–324.

Lang, F. R., Staudinger, U. M., & Carstensen, L. L. (1998). Perspectives on socioemotional selectivity in late life: How personality and social context do (and do not) make a difference. *Journal of Gerontology, Series B, 53*(1), 21–29.

Lansford, J. E., Sherman, A. M., & Antonucci, T. C. (1998). Satisfaction with social networks: An examination of socioemotional selectivity theory across cohorts. *Psychology and Aging, 13*(4), 544–552.

Lauer, E. W. (1945). The nuclear pattern and fiber connections of certain telencephalix structures in the macaque. *Journal of Comparative Neurology, 154*, 215–254.

Markesbery, W. R., Schmitt, F. A., Kryscio, R. J., Davis, D. G., Smith, C. D., & Wekstein, D. R. (2006). Neuropathologic substrate of mild cognitive impairment. *Archives of Neurology, 63*(1), 38–46.

Martinez-Castillo, E., Arrazola, J., Fernandez, A., Maestu, F., & Ortiz, T. (2001). [Atrophy of the amygdala complex and neuropsychiatric expression of Alzheimer's disease]. *Revista de Neurologia, 33*(5), 477–482.

Mather, M., Canli, T., English, T., Whitfield, S., Wais, P., Ochsner, K., et al. (2004). Amygdala responses to emotionally valenced stimuli in older and younger adults. *Psychological Science, 15*(4), 259–263.

Mesulam, M. (2000). *Principles of behavioral and cognitive neurology*. Oxford, UK: Oxford University Press.

Mielke, R., Schroder, R., Fink, G. R., Kessler, J., Herholz, K., & Heiss, W. D. (1996). Regional cerebral glucose metabolism and postmortem pathology in Alzheimer's disease. *Acta Neuropathologica (Berlin), 91*(2), 174–179.

Mori, E., Ikeda, M., Hirono, N., Kitagaki, H., Imamura, T., & Shimomura, T. (1999). Amygdalar volume and emotional memory in Alzheimer's disease. *American Journal of Psychiatry, 156*(2), 216–222.

Morris, J. S., deBonis, M., & Dolan, R. J. (2002). Human amygdala responses to fearful eyes. *NeuroImage, 17*(1), 214–222.

Morris, J. S., Frith, C. D., Perrett, D. I., Rowland, D., Young, A. W., Calder, A. J., et al. (1996). A differential neural response in the human amygdala to fearful and happy facial expressions. *Nature, 383*, 812–815.

Morris, J. S., Öhman, A., & Dolan, R. J. (1998). Conscious and unconscious emotional learning in the human amygdala. *Nature, 393*, 467–470.

Mu, Q., Xie, J., Wen, Z., Weng, Y., & Shuyun, Z. (1999). A quantitative MR study of the hippocampal formation, the amygdala, and the temporal horn of the lateral ventricle in healthy subjects 40 to 90 years of age. *American Journal of Neuroradiology, 20*(2), 207–211.

Nazarali, A. J., & Reynolds, G. P. (1992). Monoamine neurotransmitters and their metabolites in brain regions in Alzheimer's disease: A postmortem study. *Cellular and Molecular Neurobiology, 12*(6), 581–587.

O'Brien, J. T., Desmond, P., Ames, D., Schweitzer, I., Chiu, E., & Tress, B. (1997). Temporal lobe magnetic resonance imaging can differentiate Alzheimer's disease from normal ageing, depression, vascular dementia and other causes of cognitive impairment. *Psychological Medicine, 27*(6), 1267–1275.

Pandya, D. N., Van Hoesen, G. W., & Mesulam, M. M. (1981). Efferent connections of the cingulate gyrus in the rhesus monkey. *Experimental Brain Research, 42*(3–4), 319–330.

Petersen, R. C., Parisi, J. E., Dickson, D. W., Johnson, K. A., Knopman, D. S., Boeve, B. F., et al. (2006). Neuropathologic features of amnestic mild cognitive impairment. *Archives of Neurology, 63*(5), 665–672.

Phan, K. L., Taylor, S. F., Welsh, R. C., Ho, S. H., Britton, J. C., & Liberzon, I. (2004). Neural correlates of individual ratings of emotional salience: A trial-related fMRI study. *NeuroImage, 21*(2), 768–780.

Phelps, E. A., Delgado, M. R., Nearing, K. I., & LeDoux, J. E. (2004). Extinction learning in humans: Role of the amygdala and vmPFC. *Neuron, 43*(6), 897–905.

Phelps, E. A., O'Connor, K. J., Gatenby, J. C., Gore, J. C., Grillon, C., & Davis, M. (2001). Activation of the left amygdala to a cognitive representation of fear. *Nature Neuroscience, 4*(4), 437–441.

Phillips, M. L., Medford, N., Young, A. W., Williams, L., Williams, S. C., Bullmore, E. T., et al. (2001). Time courses of left and right amygdalar responses to fearful facial expressions. *Human Brain Mapping, 12*(4), 193–202.

Pruessner, J. C., Collins, D. L., Pruessner, M., & Evans, A. C. (2001). Age and gender predict volume decline in the anterior and posterior hippocampus in early adulthood. *Journal of Neuroscience, 21*(1), 194–200.

Rinne, J. O., Lonnberg, P., Marjamaki, P., Molsa, P., Sako, E., & Paljarvi, L. (1993). Brain methionine- and leucine-enkephalin receptors in patients with dementia. *Neuroscience Letters, 161*(1), 77–80.

Royet, J. P., Zald, D., Versace, R., Costes, N., Lavenne, F., Koenig, O., et al. (2000). Emotional responses to pleasant and unpleasant olfactory, visual, and auditory stimuli: A positron emission tomography study. *Journal of Neuroscience, 20*, 7752–7759.

Salat, D. H., Buckner, R. L., Snyder, A. Z., Greve, D. N., Desikan, R. S., Busa, E., et al. (2004). Thinning of the cerebral cortex in aging. *Cerebral Cortex, 14*(7), 721–730.

Schmidt, M. L., Murray, J. M., & Trojanowski, J. Q. (1993). Continuity of neuropil threads with tangle-bearing and tangle-free neurons in Alzheimer disease cortex: A confocal laser scanning microscopy study. *Molecular and Chemical Neuropathology, 18*(3), 299–312.

Schwartz, C. E., Wright, C. I., Shin, L. M., Kagan, J., Whalen, P. J., McMullin, K. G., et al. (2003). Differential amygdalar response to novel versus newly familiar neutral faces: A functional MRI probe developed for studying inhibited temperament. *Biological Psychiatry, 53*(10), 854–862.

Scott, S. A., DeKosky, S. T., & Scheff, S. W. (1991). Volumetric atrophy of the amygdala in Alzheimer's disease: Quantitative serial reconstruction. *Neurology, 41*(3), 351–356.

Scott, S. A., DeKosky, S. T., Sparks, D. L., Knox, C. A., & Scheff, S. W. (1992). Amygdala cell loss and atrophy in Alzheimer's disease. *Annals of Neurology, 32*(4), 555–563.

Selkoe, D. J. (2003). Aging, amyloid, and Alzheimer's disease: A perspective in honor of Carl Cotman. *Neurochemical Research, 28*(11), 1705–1713.

Shin, L. M., Wright, C. I., Cannistraro, P. A., Wedig, M. M., McMullin, K., Martis, B., et al. (2005). A functional magnetic resonance imaging study of amygdala and medial prefrontal cortex responses to overtly presented fearful faces in posttraumatic stress disorder. *Archives of General Psychiatry, 62*(3), 273–281.

Shinotoh, H., Fukushi, K., Nagatsuka, S., Tanaka, N., Aotsuka, A., Ota, T., et al. (2003). The amygdala and Alzheimer's disease: Positron emission tomographic study of the cholinergic system. *Annals of the New York Academy of Sciences, 985*, 411–419.

Shinotoh, H., Namba, H., Fukushi, K., Nagatsuka, S., Tanaka, N., Aotsuka, A., et al. (2000a). Progressive loss of cortical acetylcholinesterase activity in association with cognitive decline in Alzheimer's disease: A positron emission tomography study. *Annals of Neurology, 48*(2), 194–200.

Shinotoh, H., Namba, H., Fukushi, K., Nagatsuka, S., Tanaka, N., Aotsuka, A., et al. (2000b). Brain acetylcholinesterase activity in Alzheimer disease measured by positron emission tomography. *Alzheimer Disease and Associated Disorders, 14*(Suppl. 1), S114–S118.

Smith, C. D., Malcein, M., Meurer, K., Schmitt, F. A., Markesbery, W. R., & Pettigrew, L. C. (1999). MRI temporal lobe volume measures and neuropsychologic function in Alzheimer's disease. *Journal of Neuroimaging, 9*(1), 2–9.

Soininen, H., Helkala, E. L., Kuikka, J., Hartikainen, P., Lehtovirta, M., & Riekkinen, P. J., Sr. (1995). Regional cerebral blood flow measured by 99MTC-HMPO SPECT differs in subgroups of Alzheimer's disease. *Journal of Neural Transmission: Parkinson Disease and Dementia Section, 9*(2–3), 95–109.

Stefanacci, L., & Amaral, D. G. (2002). Some observations on cortical inputs to the macaque monkey amygdala: An anterograde tracing study. *Journal of Comparative Neurology, 451*(4), 301–323.

Tanaka, S., Kawamata, J., Shimohama, S., Akaki, H., Akiguchi, I., Kimura, J., et al. (1998). Inferior temporal lobe atrophy and APOE genotypes in Alzheimer's disease: X-ray computed tomography, magnetic resonance imaging and XE-133 SPECT studies. *Dementia and Geriatric Cognitive Disorders, 9*(2), 90–98.

Tessitore, A., Hariri, A. R., Fera, F., Smith, W. G., Das, S., Weinberger, D. R., et al. (2005). Functional changes in the activity of brain regions underlying emotion processing in the elderly. *Psychiatry Research, 139*(1), 9–18.

Tomlinson, B. E. (1979). The ageing brain. In W. T. Smith & J. B. Cavanagh (Eds.), *Recent advances in neuropathology* (pp. 129–159). London: Churchill Livingstone.

Tsuchiya, K., & Kosaka, K. (1990). Neuropathological study of the amygdala in presenile Alzheimer's disease. *Journal of the Neurological Sciences, 100*(1–2), 165–173.

Unger, J. W., Lapham, L. W., McNeill, T. H., Eskin, T. A., & Hamill, R. W. (1991). The amygdala in Alzheimer's disease: Neuropathology and Alz 50 immunoreactivity. *Neurobiology of Aging, 12*(5), 389–399.

Unger, J. W., McNeill, T. H., Lapham, L. L., & Hamill, R. W. (1988). Neuropeptides and neuropathology in the amygdala in Alzheimer's disease: Relationship between somatostatin, neuropeptide Y and subregional distribution of neuritic plaques. *Brain Research, 452*(1–2), 293–302.

Valladares-Neto, D. C., Buchsbaum, M. S., Evans, W. J., Nguyen, D., Nguyen, P., Siegel, B. V., et al. (1995). EEG delta, positron emission tomography, and memory deficit in Alzheimer's disease. *Neuropsychobiology, 31*(4), 173–181.

Van Hoesen, G. W., Augustinack, J. C., & Redman, S. J. (1999). Ventromedial temporal lobe pathology in dementia, brain trauma, and schizophrenia. *Annals of the New York Academy of Sciences, 877*, 575–594.

Vandenbroucke, M. W., Goekoop, R., Duschek, E. J., Netelenbos, J. C., Kuijer, J. P., Barkhof, F., et al. (2004). Interindividual differences of medial temporal lobe activation during encoding in an elderly population studied by fMRI. *NeuroImage, 21*(1), 173–180.

Vereecken, T. H., Vogels, O. J., & Nieuwenhuys, R. (1994). Neuron loss and shrinkage in the amygdala in Alzheimer's disease. *Neurobiology of Aging, 15*(1), 45–54.

Wedig, M. M., Rauch, S. L., Albert, M. S., & Wright, C. I. (2005). Differential amygdala habituation to neutral faces in young and elderly adults. *Neuroscience Letters, 385*(2), 114–119.

Whalen, P. J., Kagan, J., Cook, R. G., Davis, F. C., Kim, H., Polis, S., et al. (2004). Human amygdala responsivity to masked fearful eye whites. *Science, 306*, 2061.

Whalen, P. J., Rauch, S. L., Etcoff, N. L., McInerney, S. C., Lee, M. B., & Jenike, M. A. (1998). Masked presentations of emotional facial expressions modulate amygdala activity without explicit knowledge. *Journal of Neuroscience, 18*(1), 411–418.

Whalen, P. J., Shin, L. M., McInerney, S. C., Fischer, H., Wright, C. I., & Rauch, S. L. (2001). A functional MRI study of human amygdala responses to facial expressions of fear versus anger. *Emotion, 1*(1), 70–83.

Whitehouse, P. J., & Au, K. S. (1986). Cholinergic receptors in aging and Alzheimer's disease. *Progress in Neuropsychopharmacology and Biological Psychiatry, 10*(3–5), 665–676.

Williams, L. M., Brown, K. J., Palmer, D., Liddell, B. J., Kemp, A. H., Olivieri, G., et al. (2006). The mellow years?: Neural basis of improving emotional stability over age. *Journal of Neuroscience, 26*, 6422–6430.

Wright, C. I., Dickerson, B. C., Feczko, E., Negeira, A., & Williams, D. (2007). A functional magnetic resonance imaging study of amygdala responses to human faces in aging and mild Alzheimer's disease. *Biological Psychiatry, 62*(12), 1388–1395.

Wright, C. I., Feczko, E., Dickerson, B., & Williams, D. (2007). Neuroanatomical correlates of personality in the elderly. *NeuroImage, 35*(1), 263–272.

Wright, C. I., Fischer, H., Whalen, P. J., McInerney, S. C., Shin, L. M., & Rauch, S. L. (2001). Differential prefrontal cortex and amygdala habituation to repeatedly presented emotional stimuli. *NeuroReport, 12*(2), 379–383.

Wright, C. I., Martis, B., Schwartz, C. E., Shin, L. M., Fischer, H. H., McMullin, K., et al. (2003). Novelty responses and differential effects of order in the amygdala, substantia innominata, and inferior temporal cortex. *NeuroImage, 18*(3), 660–669.

Wright, C. I., Martis, B., Shin, L. M., Fischer, H., & Rauch, S. L. (2002). Enhanced amygdala responses to emotional versus neutral schematic facial expressions. *NeuroReport, 13*(6), 785–790.

Wright, C. I., Negreira, A., Gold, A. L., Britton, J. C., Williams, D., & Feldman Barrett, L. (in press). Neural correlates of novelty and face-age effects in young and elderly adults. *NeuroImage.*

Wright, C. I., Wedig, M. M., Williams, D., Rauch, S. L., & Albert, M. S. (2006). Novel fearful faces activate the amygdala in healthy young and elderly adults. *Neurobiology of Aging, 27*(2), 361–374.

Wright, C. I., Williams, D., Feczko, E., Feldman Barrett, L., Dickerson, B. C., Schwartz, C. E., et al. (2006). Neuroanatomical correlates of extraversion and neuroticism. *Cerebral Cortex, 16*(12), 1809–1819.

Yates, C. M., Simpson, J., & Gordon, A. (1986). Regional brain 5-hydroxytryptamine levels are reduced in senile Down's syndrome as in Alzheimer's disease. *Neuroscience Letters, 65*(2), 189–192.

Zald, D. H., Lee, J. T., Fluegel, K. W., & Pardo, J. V. (1998). Aversive gustatory stimulation activates limbic circuits in humans. *Brain, 121*(Pt. 6), 1143–1154.

Zald, D. H., & Pardo, J. V. (1997). Emotion, olfaction, and the human amygdala: Amygdala activation during aversive olfactory stimulation. *Proceedings of the National Academy of Sciences USA, 94*(8), 4119–4124.

CHAPTER 18

The Genetic Basis
of Amygdala Reactivity

Ahmad R. Hariri and Daniel R. Weinberger

Individual differences in trait negative affect are important predictors of vulnerability for a wide spectrum of health-related disorders, including depression, anxiety, and cardiovascular disease. As such, identifying biological variables contributing to the emergence of such interindividual variability holds great potential for elucidating both the etiology and pathophysiology of these disorders. Moreover, certain biological variables may offer clinical utility by serving as predictive markers of increased disease risk. Converging evidence from research on rodents and nonhuman primates, as well as extensive human research, has implicated variability in serotonin (5-hydroxytryptamine, or 5-HT) neurotransmission as a key predictor of individual differences in multiple, overlapping behavioral constructs related to trait negative affect (Lucki, 1998; Manuck et al., 1998).

Research employing pharmacological challenge of the 5-HT system (via specific receptor agonism–antagonism or general reuptake blockade) has consistently illustrated that manipulations resulting in relatively increased postsynaptic 5-HT neurotransmission produce potentiated responses in affective neural circuitries, peripheral stress responses, and subjective negative affect (Bigos et al., in press; Burghardt, Bush, McEwen, & LeDoux, 2007; Burghardt, Sullivan, McEwen, Gorman, & LeDoux, 2004; Forster et al., 2006). These and other findings have subsequently spurred intensive efforts to identify genetic polymorphisms in 5-HT subsystems, which ultimately control the regulation of 5-HT neurotransmission as a function of both homeostatic drive and environmental feedback; as such, these polymorphisms may predict trait negative affect as well as differentiate relative risk for disease (Glatt & Freimer, 2002). In this chapter, we provide an overview of recent neuroimaging studies exploring the impact of genetically driven variability in the function of 5-HT (and related systems) on interindividual variability in human amygdala reactivity—a key neural component in the generation of physiological and behavioral arousal in response to environmental challenge.

THE SEROTONIN TRANSPORTER

Of particular importance in efforts to identify genetic polymorphisms in 5-HT subsystems that have an impact on trait negative affect and differentiate relative risk for disease has been the 5-HT transporter (5-HTT), which is responsible for the active clearance of synaptic 5-HT and thus for regulation of pre- and postsynaptic 5-HT receptor stimulation. In 1996, Lesch and colleagues identified a relatively common functional promoter polymorphism in the human 5-HTT gene (*SLC6A4*). The so-called 5-HTT gene-linked polymorphic region or 5-HTTLPR is typically defined by two variable-nucleotide tandem repeat elements: a short (S) allele comprising 14 copies of a 20- to 23-base-pair repeat unit, and a long (L) allele comprising 16 copies. Although initial *in vitro* (Lesch et al., 1996) and *in vivo* (Heinz et al., 2000) assays revealed relatively diminished 5-HTT density associated with the S allele, recent work has indicated that more complex mechanisms (e.g., regional up- and down-regulation of specific 5-HT receptors) and not altered 5-HTT density may mediate the long-term impact of 5-HTTLPR on 5-HT neurotransmission (Hariri & Holmes, 2006). Regardless of the underlying mechanisms of action, a modest association has been widely reported between the 5-HTTLPR S allele and relatively increased trait negative affect (Munafo, Clark, & Flint, 2005). Moreover, the 5-HTTLPR S allele has been associated with relatively increased risk for depression in the context of environmental adversity (Caspi et al., 2003)—a relationship that may be mediated by increased neuroticism, a psychometrically robust index of trait negative affect.

Functional magnetic resonance imaging (fMRI) studies have provided a unique understanding of how 5-HTTLPR may influence temperamental anxiety and risk for depression. In a landmark study, fMRI revealed that the reactivity of the amygdala to threat-related facial expressions was significantly exaggerated in carriers of the S allele (Hariri et al., 2002). Since this original study, there have been multiple replications of the association between the S allele and relatively increased amygdala reactivity in both healthy volunteers and patients with mood disorders (Munafo, Brown, & Hariri, 2008). In addition, the 5-HTTLPR S allele has been further linked with reduced gray matter volumes in, and functional coupling between, the amygdala and medial prefrontal cortex (Pezawas et al., 2005). As the magnitude of amygdala reactivity (as well as its functional coupling with medial prefrontal cortex) is associated with temperamental anxiety, these findings from imaging genetics suggest that the 5-HTTLPR S allele may be associated with increased risk for depression upon exposure to environmental stressors, because of its mediation of exaggerated corticolimbic reactivity to potential threat.

MONOAMINE OXIDASE A

To the extent that the effects of the 5-HTTLPR variant on corticolimbic development and function related to emotion processing are mediated by 5-HT, it would be expected that other genes related to 5-HT function would show similar effects on the function of this circuitry. 5-HT neurotransmission is also regulated through intracellular degradation via the metabolic enzyme monoamine oxidase A (MAO-A). A common genetic polymorphism in the MAO-A gene, resulting in a relatively low-activity enzyme, has been associated with increased risk for violent or antisocial behavior, as well as for depression and anxiety (Caspi et al., 2002; Kim-Cohen et al., 2006). Recent fMRI studies reported that the low-activity MAO-A allele is associated with relatively exaggerated amygdala reactivity and diminished prefrontal regulation of the amygdala (Buckholtz et al., 2008; Meyer-Lindenberg et al., 2006). The magnitude of functional coupling between these regions predicted levels of temperamental anxiety, suggesting that the genetic association between the MAO-A low-activity variant and abnormal behavior may be mediated through this circuit. Interestingly, both the 5-HTTLPR S allele and the MAO-A low-activity allele presumably result in relatively increased 5-HT signaling and exaggerated amygdala reactivity. As the directionality of these effects is consistent with animal studies documenting anxiogenic effects of 5-HT (Burghardt et al., 2004; Forster et al., 2006), as well as pharmacological neuroimaging studies demonstrating a potentiation of amygdala reactivity subsequent to acute 5-HT reuptake blockade (Bigos et al., in press), the imaging genetics data provide important insight into the neurobiological and behavioral effects of 5-HT.

TRYPTOPHAN HYDROXYLASE-2

Recent imaging genetics studies examining the impact of variation in 5-HT subsystems highlight the manner in which functional imaging and molecular genetics approaches can be reciprocally informative in advancing our understanding of the biological mechanisms of behavior. Tryptophan hydroxylase-2 (TPH2) is the rate-limiting enzyme in the synthesis of neuronal 5-HT and thus plays a key role in regulating 5-HT neurotransmission (Walther & Bader, 2003; Zhang, Beaulieu, Sotnikova, Gainetdinov, & Caron, 2004). A recent study found that a single-nucleotide polymorphism (SNP) in the regulatory region of the human TPH2 gene affects amygdala function. Specifically, the T allele of a common promoter polymorphism [G(–844)T] was associated with relatively exaggerated amygdala reactivity in comparison to the G allele (Brown et al., 2005). This report provides further insight into the biological significance of TPH2 in the human central nervous system, and furnishes a critical next step in our understanding of the importance of this newly identified second tryptophan hydroxylase isoform for human brain function. Moreover, it marks an important advance in the application of functional neuroimaging to the study of genes, brain, and behavior. In contrast to previous studies of genetic effects on brain function, where the molecular and cellular effects of the candidate variants had been demonstrated (e.g., 5-HTTLPR, MAO-A, catechol-O-methyltransferase, and brain-derived neurotrophic factor [BDNF]), these fMRI data provide the first evidence for potential functionality of a novel candidate polymorphism. In this way, the initial identification of a systems-level effect of a specific polymorphism provides impetus for the subsequent characterization of its functional effects at the molecular and cellular level. Building on this initial finding from imaging genetics (and a subsequent replication; Canli, Congdon, Gutknecht, Constable, & Lesch, 2005), a recent molecular study has demonstrated that the G(-844)T is in strong linkage with another promoter SNP that affects the transcriptional regulation of TPH2 and may affect enzyme availability and 5-HT biosynthesis (Chen, Vallender, & Miller, 2008). Such scientific reciprocity between imaging and molecular genetics illustrates how the contributions of variability in candidate neural systems to complex behaviors and emergent phenomena, possibly including psychiatric illnesses, can be understood from the perspective of their neurobiological origins.

BRAIN-DERIVED NEUROTROPHIC FACTOR

BDNF is a critical peptide neurotrophic factor involved in neuronal survival, differentiation, and synaptic plasticity (Binder & Scharfman, 2004). BDNF plays an important role in the expression of hippocampal and amygdala long-term potentiation during learning (Lu, Christian, & Lu, 2008; Rattiner, Davis, & Ressler, 2005). BDNF is also regulated by serotonergic signaling and is involved in the developmental sculpting of serotonergic innervation patterns (Luellen, Bianco, Schneider, & Andrews, 2007; Mossner et al., 2000). A popular theory about the efficacy of selective serotonin reuptake inhibitor antidepressant/antianxiety drugs is that they act via stimulation of BDNF expression (Bourin, David, Jolliet, & Gardier, 2002). The BNDF gene contains a common functional polymorphism: a valine (Val) to methionine (Met) substitution at codon 66 (Val66Met), which is associated with abnormal intracellular trafficking and regulated secretion of pro-BDNF, the precursor to functional BDNF (Egan et al., 2003). This SNP has also been associated with mood disorders and with anxious temperament (Hall, Dhilla, Charalambous, Gogos,

& Karayiorgou, 2003; Jian et al., 2005; Lam, Cheng, Hong, & Tsai, 2004; Lang et al., 2005; Strauss et al., 2004; Tsai, Hong, Yu, & Chen, 2004).

Because of the abundant expression of BDNF in hippocampus and its role in learning and memory, researchers have used neuroimaging to study it primarily in terms of hippocampal anatomy and memory processing. Consistent with the molecular effects of the Met66 allele, studies have documented relatively impaired episodic memory in human subjects carrying the Met66 allele (Egan et al., 2003). Converging evidence from several imaging genetics studies using different modalities suggests that the effects of Met66 on memory are mediated in part by its impact on hippocampal structure and function (Hariri et al., 2003; Pezawas et al., 2004). Most recently, a structural imaging genetics study revealed that the BDNF Val66Met can modulate the impact of the 5-HTTLPR short allele on corticolimbic circuitry. Specifically, the reduced amygdala gray matter volume typically associated with the 5-HTTLPR short allele was absent in subjects also possessing the BDNF Met66 allele (Pezawas et al., in press). The data suggest that the Met66 allele effectively blocks the relatively increased 5-HT stimulation of BDNF-mediated changes in brain morphology associated with the 5-HTTLPR short allele. As such, this functional genetic epistasis may partially account for the reduced risk of mood disorders associated with the BDNF Met66 allele.

NEUROPEPTIDE Y

In addition to 5-HT candidate genes, we have begun to explore the impact of genetic variation in neuropeptide Y (NPY), a 36-amino-acid peptide neurotransmitter that is an evolutionarily highly conserved molecular component of brain systems processing stress and emotion (Heilig & Widerlöv, 1990; Holmes, Heilig, Rupniak, Steckler, & Griebel, 2003). Anxiolytic-like effects of NPY have been reported in a wide range of pharmacologically validated animal models, and NPY release is profoundly induced by stress (Broqua, Wettstein, Rocher, Gauthier-Martin, & Junien, 1995; Heilig, Söderpalm, Engel, & Widerlöv, 1989; Heilig et al., 1993). In humans, both cerebrospinal fluid and plasma NPY levels correlate with anxiety and stress levels (Boulenger et al., 1996; Irwin et al., 1991; Widerlöv, Lindström, Wahlestedt, & Ekman, 1988). Recently, we demonstrated that the relatively common *NPY* diplotypes consistently predicted *NPY* messenger RNA in postmortem brain and lymphoblasts, as well as plasma concentrations of NPY (Zhou et al., 2008). Diplotype expression was inversely proportional to temperamental anxiety. Similar to the effect on trait anxiety, NPY diplotype predicted amygdala reactivity in gene–dosage (stepwise) fashion, with heterozygous individuals intermediate in activation. Importantly, the magnitude of amygdala activation predicts measures of temperamental anxiety in this sample. Together, the results suggest that NPY effects on temperamental anxiety are mediated in part through biased amygdala reactivity. In addition to these effects, task-related hippocampal activation was predicted by NPY diplotype. This finding is of interest because the functional interactions of the amygdala and hippocampus are critical for emotional memories, and long-lasting changes in hippocampal architecture are induced by stress.

SUMMARY AND FUTURE DIRECTIONS

This chapter has reviewed selected efforts to parse interindividual variability in human amygdala reactivity mediating emotion processing, based on common sequence variation in genes affecting key molecular systems (i.e., 5-HT, BDNF, and NPY) involved in regulating amygdala development and physiology. We have highlighted several recent studies in which genetic effects on brain function have been explored using neuroimaging—namely, imaging genetics (Hariri et al., 2006; Hariri & Weinberger, 2003). This work is just in its infancy, as the number of genes explored is very few, and the strategies for looking at gene effects in brain are relatively simplistic. Nevertheless, the studies cited provide compelling evidence that gene effects at the level of amygdala reactivity are much more robust (i.e., "penetrant") than those at the level of manifest emotional behaviors. This is consistent with the conclusion that genes related to affect, mood, and temperament are not encoding for behavior; rather, they influence the development and function of neural systems that mediate emotional experience and behavior. Emotional responses are complex and not the result of variation in any single gene. Future studies will emphasize interactions among genes, as well as interactions of genes with the environment. This is likely to add complexity but also improved resolution to the analyses.

Combining existing neuroimaging modalities is another important future direction for imaging genetics. Implementation of multimodal strategies is critical for identifying intermediate mechanisms mediating the effects of genetic polymorphisms on neural circuit function and related behaviors. The potential of multimodal neuroimaging was recently demonstrated in a study employing both positron emission tomography (PET) and fMRI to identify the impact of 5-HT$_{1A}$ autoreceptor regulation of 5-HT release on amygdala reactivity (Fisher et al., 2006). In the study, adult volunteers underwent [^{11}C] WAY100635 PET to determine 5-HT$_{1A}$ autoreceptor binding potential (an *in vivo* index of receptor density). During the same day, all subjects also underwent fMRI to determine the functional reactivity of the amygdala. Remarkably, the density of 5-HT$_{1A}$ autoreceptors accounted for 30–44% of the variability in amygdala reactivity. Downstream effects on 5-HT$_{1A}$ autoreceptors, notably reduced receptor density, have been hypothesized to mediate neural and behavioral changes associated with the 5-HTTLPR S allele. Thus these findings suggest that 5-HT$_{1A}$ autoreceptor regulation of corticolimbic circuitry represents a key molecular mechanism mediating the effects of the 5-HTTLPR (Fisher et al., 2006; Hariri & Fisher, 2007). Continued imaging genetics research at the interface of genes, brain, and behavior holds great promise in further explicating the neurobiological mechanisms through which variability in behavior emerges and affects risk for psychiatric disease in the context of environmental adversity.

WHAT WE THINK

As research in behavioral neuroscience has progressed in the last decades, there have been many important technological and methodological advances in the increasingly complimentary fields of molecular genetics and neuroimaging. These advances have facilitated fruitful collaboration across once disparate disciplines, with early results shedding new light on the mechanisms giving rise to individual differences in complex behaviors and related psychiatric disorders. At the leading edge of such efforts is imaging genetics, an experimental strategy for the effective integration of molecular genetics and neuroimaging technologies for the study of biological mechanisms mediating individual differences in behavior and related risk for psychiatric disorders. Imaging genetics studies have provided a more complex and nuanced understanding of the pathways and mechanisms through which the dynamic interplay of genes, brain, and environment shapes variability in behavior. The broader potential of imaging genetics is to inform risk and resiliency; however, this potential is likely to be realized only through an orchestrated application within longitudinal developmental studies and continued integration with basic animal research.

ACKNOWLEDGMENTS

Portions of this chapter are adapted from Hariri and Weinberger (2003), Hariri, Drabant, and Weinberger (2006), and Hariri and Fisher (2007). Copyright 2003 by Oxford University Press, 2006 by the Society of Biological Psychiatry, and 2007 by Future Medicine Ltd., respectively. Adapted by permission. This research was supported in part by National Institute of Mental Health Grant No. K01-MH072837 and by a Young Investigator Award from the National Alliance for Research on Schizophrenia and Depression to Ahmad R. Hariri.

REFERENCES

Bigos, K. L., Pollock, B. G., Aizenstein, H. J., Fisher, P. M., Bies, R. R., & Hariri, A. R. (in press). Acute 5-HT reuptake blockade potentiates human amygdala reactivity. *Neuropsychopharmacology.*

Binder, D. K., & Scharfman, H. E. (2004). Brain-derived neurotrophic factor. *Growth Factors, 22*(3), 123–131.

Boulenger, J. P., Jerabek, I., Jolicoeur, F. B., Lavallée, Y. J., Leduc, R., & Cadieux, A. (1996). Elevated plasma levels of neuropeptide Y in patients with panic disorder. *American Journal of Psychiatry, 153*(1), 114–116.

Bourin, M., David, D. J., Jolliet, P., & Gardier, A. (2002). [Mechanism of action of antidepressants and therapeutic perspectives]. *Therapie, 57*(4), 385–396.

Broqua, P., Wettstein, J. G., Rocher, M. N., Gauthier-Martin, B., & Junien, J. L. (1995). Behavioral effects of neuropeptide Y receptor agonists in the elevated plus-maze and fear-potentiated startle procedures. *Behavioural Pharmacology, 6*(3), 215–222.

Brown, S. M., Peet, E., Manuck, S. B., Williamson, D. E., Dahl, R. E., Ferrell, R. E., et al. (2005). A regulatory variant of the human tryptophan hydroxylase-2 gene biases amygdala reactivity. *Molecular Psychiatry, 10*(9), 805.

Buckholtz, J. W., Callicott, J. H., Kolachana, B., Hariri, A. R., Goldberg, T. E., Genderson, M., et al. (2008). Genetic variation in MAOA modulates ventromedial prefrontal circuitry mediating individual differences in human personality. *Molecular Psychiatry, 13*(3), 313–324.

Burghardt, N. S., Bush, D. E., McEwen, B. S., & LeDoux, J. E. (2007). Acute selective serotonin reuptake inhibitors increase conditioned fear expression: Blockade with a 5-HT(2C) receptor antagonist. *Biological Psychiatry, 62*(10), 1111–1118.

Burghardt, N. S., Sullivan, G. M., McEwen, B. S., Gorman, J. M., & LeDoux, J. E. (2004). The selective serotonin reuptake inhibitor citalopram increases fear after acute treatment but reduces fear with chronic treatment: A comparison with tianeptine. *Biological Psychiatry, 55*(12), 1171–1178.

Canli, T., Congdon, E., Gutknecht, L., Constable, R. T., & Lesch, K. P. (2005). Amygdala responsiveness is modulated by tryptophan hydroxylase-2 gene variation. *Journal of Neural Transmission, 112*, 1479–1485.

Caspi, A., McClay, J., Moffitt, T. E., Mill, J., Martin, J., Craig, I. W., et al. (2002). Role of genotype in the cycle of violence in maltreated children. *Science, 297*, 851–854.

Caspi, A., Sugden, K., Moffitt, T. E., Taylor, A., Craig, I. W., Harrington, H., et al. (2003). Influence of life stress on depression: Moderation by a polymorphism in the 5-HTT gene. *Science, 301*, 386–389.

Chen, G. L., Vallender, E. J., & Miller, G. M. (2008). Functional characterization of the human TPH2 5' regulatory region: Untranslated region and polymorphisms modulate gene expression *in vitro. Human Genetics, 122*(6), 645–657.

Egan, M. F., Kojima, M., Callicott, J. H., Goldberg, T. E., Kolachana, B. S., Bertolino, A., et al. (2003). The BDNF val66met polymorphism affects activity-dependent secretion of BDNF and human memory and hippocampal function. *Cell, 112*(2), 257–269.

Fisher, P. M., Meltzer, C. C., Ziolko, S. K., Price, J. C., Moses-Kolko, E. L., Berga, S. L., et al. (2006). Capacity for 5-HT$_{1A}$-mediated autoregulation predicts amygdala reactivity. *Nature Neuroscience, 9*, 1362–1363.

Forster, G. L., Feng, N., Watt, M. J., Korzan, W. J., Mouw, N. J., Summers, C. H., et al. (2006). Corticotropin-releasing factor in the dorsal raphe elicits temporally distinct serotonergic responses in the limbic system in relation to fear behavior. *Neuroscience, 141*(2), 1047–1055.

Glatt, C. E., & Freimer, N. B. (2002). Association analysis of candidate genes for neuropsychiatric disease: The perpetual campaign. *Trends in Genetics, 18*(6), 307–312.

Hall, D., Dhilla, A., Charalambous, A., Gogos, J. A., & Karayiorgou, M. (2003). Sequence variants of the brain-derived neurotrophic factor (BDNF) gene are strongly associated with obsessive–compulsive disorder. *American Journal of Human Genetics, 73*(2), 370–376.

Hariri, A. R., Drabant, E. M., & Weinberger, D. R. (2006). Imaging genetics: Perspectives from studies of genetically driven variation in serotonin function and corticolimbic affective processing. *Biological Psychiatry, 59*(10), 888–897.

Hariri, A. R., & Fisher, P. M. (2007). Regulation of corticolimbic reactivity via the 5-HT$_{1A}$ autoreceptor in the pathophysiology and treatment of depression. *Future Neurology, 2*(2), 121–124.

Hariri, A. R., Goldberg, T. E., Mattay, V. S., Kolachana, B. S., Callicott, J. H., Egan, M. F., et al. (2003). Brain-derived neurotrophic factor val66met polymorphism affects human memory-related hippocampal activity and predicts memory performance. *Journal of Neuroscience, 23*, 6690–6694.

Hariri, A. R., & Holmes, A. (2006). Genetics of emotional regulation: The role of the serotonin transporter in neural function. *Trends in Cognitive Science, 10*(4), 182–191.

Hariri, A. R., Mattay, V. S., Tessitore, A., Kolachana, B., Fera, F., Goldman, D., et al. (2002). Serotonin transporter genetic variation and the response of the human amygdala. *Science, 297*, 400–403.

Hariri, A. R., & Weinberger, D. R. (2003). Imaging genomics. *British Medical Bulletin, 65*, 259–270.

Heilig, M., McLeod, S., Brot, M., Heinrichs, S. C., Menzaghi, F., Koob, G. F., et al. (1993). Anxiolytic-like action of neuropeptide Y: Mediation by Y1 receptors in amygdala, and dissociation from food intake effects. *Neuropsychopharmacology, 8*(4), 357–363.

Heilig, M., Söderpalm, B., Engel, J. A., & Widerlöv, E. (1989). Centrally administered neuropeptide Y (NPY) produces anxiolytic-like effects in animal anxiety models. *Psychopharmacology, 98*(4), 524–529.

Heilig, M., & Widerlöv, E. (1990). Neuropeptide Y: An overview of central distribution, functional aspects, and possible involvement in neuropsychiatric illnesses. *Acta Psychiatrica Scandinavica, 82*(2), 95–114.

Heinz, A., Jones, D. W., Mazzanti, C., Goldman, D., Ragan, P., Hommer, D., et al. (2000). A relationship between serotonin transporter genotype and *in vivo* protein expression and alcohol neurotoxicity. *Biological Psychiatry, 47*(7), 643–649.

Holmes, A., Heilig, M., Rupniak, N. M., Steckler, T., & Griebel, G. (2003). Neuropeptide systems as novel therapeutic targets for depression and anxiety disorders. *Trends in Pharmacological Sciences, 24*(11), 580–588.

Irwin, M., Brown, M., Patterson, T., Hauger, R., Mascovich, A., & Grant, I. (1991). Neuropeptide Y and natural killer cell activity: Findings in depression and Alzheimer caregiver stress. *The FASEB Journal, 5*(15), 3100–3107.

Jiang, X., Xu, K., Hoberman, J., Tian, F., Marko, A. J., Waheed, J. F., et al. (2005). BDNF variation and mood disorders: A novel functional promoter polymorphism and Val66Met are associated with anxiety but have opposing effects. *Neuropsychopharmacology, 30*(7), 1353–1361.

Kim-Cohen, J., Caspi, A., Taylor, A., Williams, B., Newcombe, R., Craig, I. W., et al. (2006). MAOA, maltreatment, and gene–environment interaction predicting children's mental health: New evidence and a meta-analysis. *Molecular Psychiatry, 11*, 903–913.

Lam, P., Cheng, C. Y., Hong, C. J., & Tsai, S. J. (2004). Association study of a brain-derived neurotrophic factor (Val66Met) genetic polymorphism and panic disorder. *Neuropsychobiology, 49*(4), 178–181.

Lang, U. E., Hellweg, R., Kalus, P., Bajbouj, M., Lenzen, K. P., Sander, T., et al. (2005). Association of a functional BDNF polymorphism and anxiety-related personality traits. *Psychopharmacology, 130*(1), 95–99.

Lesch, K. P., Bengel, D., Heils, A., Sabol, S. Z., Greenberg, B. D., Petri, S., et al. (1996). Association of anxiety-related traits with a polymorphism in the serotonin transporter gene regulatory region. *Science, 274*, 1527–1531.

Lu, Y., Christian, K., & Lu, B. (2008). BDNF: A key regulator for protein synthesis-dependent LTP and long-term memory? *Neurobiology of Learning and Memory, 89*(3), 312–323.

Lucki, I. (1998). The spectrum of behaviors influenced by serotonin. *Biological Psychiatry, 44*(3), 151–162.

Luellen, B. A., Bianco, L. E., Schneider, L. M., & Andrews, A. M. (2007). Reduced brain-derived neurotrophic factor is associated with a loss of serotonergic innervation in the hippocampus of aging mice. *Genes, Brain, and Behavior, 6*, 482–490.

Manuck, S. B., Flory, J. D., McCaffery, J. M., Matthews, K. A., Mann, J. J., & Muldoon, M. F. (1998). Aggression, impulsivity, and central nervous system serotonergic responsivity in a nonpatient sample. *Neuropsychopharmacology, 19*(4), 287–299.

Meyer-Lindenberg, A., Buckholtz, J. W., Kolachana, B., Hariri, A. R., Pezawas, L., Blasi, G., et al. (2006). Neural mechanisms of genetic risk for impulsivity and violence in humans. *Proceedings of the National Academy of Sciences USA, 103*, 6269–6274.

Mossner, R., Daniel, S., Albert, D., Heils, A., Okladnova, O., Schmitt, A., et al. (2000). Serotonin transporter function is modulated by brain-derived neurotrophic factor (BDNF) but not nerve growth factor (NGF). *Neurochemistry International, 36*(3), 197–202.

Munafo, M. R., Brown, S. M., & Hariri, A. R. (2008). Serotonin transporter (5-HTTLPR) genotype and amygdala activation: A meta-analysis. *Biological Psychiatry, 63*(9), 852–857.

Munafo, M. R., Clark, T., & Flint, J. (2005). Does measurement instrument moderate the association between the serotonin transporter gene and anxiety-related personality traits?: A meta-analysis. *Molecular Psychiatry, 10*(4), 415–419.

Pezawas, L., Meyer-Lindenberg, A., Drabant, E. M., Verchinski, B. A., Munoz, K. E., Kolachana, B. S., et al. (2005). 5-HTTLPR polymorphism impacts human cingulate–amygdala interactions: A genetic susceptibility mechanism for depression. *Nature Neuroscience, 8*(6), 828–834.

Pezawas, L., Meyer-Lindenberg, A., Goldman, A. L., Verchinski, B. A., Chen, G., Kolachana, B. S., et al. (2008). Evidence of biologic epistasis between BDNF and SLC6A4 and implications for depression. *Molecular Psychiatry, 13*(7), 654, 709–716.

Pezawas, L., Verchinski, B. A., Mattay, V. S., Callicott, J. H., Kolachana, B. S., Straub, R. E., et al. (2004). The brain-derived neurotrophic factor val66met polymorphism and variation in human cortical morphology. *Journal of Neuroscience, 24*, 10099–10102.

Rattiner, L. M., Davis, M., & Ressler, K. J. (2005). Brain-derived neurotrophic factor in amygdala-dependent learning. *Neuroscientist, 11*(4), 323–333.

Strauss, J., Barr, C. L., George, C. J., King, N., Shaikh, S., Devlin, B., et al. (2004).

Association study of brain-derived neurotrophic factor in adults with a history of childhood onset mood disorder. *American Journal of Medical Genetics. Part B, Neuropsychiatric Genetics, 131*(1), 16–19.

Tsai, S. J., Hong, C. J., Yu, Y. W., & Chen, T. J. (2004). Association study of a brain-derived neurotrophic factor (BDNF) val66met polymorphism and personality trait and intelligence in healthy young females. *Neuropsychobiology, 49*(1), 13–16.

Walther, D. J., & Bader, M. (2003). A unique central tryptophan hydroxylase isoform. *Biochemical Pharmacology, 66*(9), 1673–1680.

Widerlöv, E., Lindström, L. H., Wahlestedt, C., & Ekman, R. (1988). Neuropeptide Y and peptide YY as possible cerebrospinal fluid markers for major depression and schizophrenia, respectively. *Journal of Psychiatric Research, 22*(1), 69–79.

Zhang, X., Beaulieu, J. M., Sotnikova, T. D., Gainetdinov, R. R., & Caron, M. G. (2004). Tryptophan hydroxylase-2 controls brain serotonin synthesis. *Science, 305,* 217.

Zhou, Z., Zhu, G., Hariri, A. R., Enoch, M. A., Scott, D., Sinha, R., et al. (2008). Genetic variation in human NPY expression affects stress response and emotion. *Nature, 452,* 997–1001.

Index

Page numbers followed by *f* indicate figure, *t* indicate table

Amygdala anatomy *(cont.)*
  nonhuman primates, 3–42
  organization and nomenclature, 44–45, 382–383
  rats versus humans, 267, 268*f*
  subdivisions and cytoarchitecture, 4–15
Amygdala damage/lesions
  and autism, 368
  emotional learning defects, 128–129
  emotional memory, 186–187
  fear conditioning, 128–130
  human studies, 161–165, 162*f*
  social function, 303–310
    animals, 290–292
  Urbach–Wiethe cases, 296–310
    social function, 303–310
Amygdala volume
  Alzheimer's disease, 389–392
  autism spectrum disorders, 366–367, 367*f*
    anxiety disorders link, 373–375
  normal aging, 384–385, 384*f*
  schizophrenia, 348–349
Amygdalocortical projections. *See* Prefrontal cortex–amygdala connections
Amygdalocortical transition area (ATA)
  Alzheimer's disease, 388–389, 388*f*, 391
  anatomy and nomenclature, 382–383, 383*f*
Amygdalohippocampal area (AHA)
  anatomy, 4, 7*f*, 8*f*, 10*f*, 15
  frontal cortex connections, 25, 25*f*
  schizophrenia, 348
  subcortical connections, 17–20
Amygdalohippocampal interactions
  emotional memory, 187, 188*f*, 194
  schizophrenia, 349
Amygdalohippocampectomy patients, 128–130
Amygdaloid complex. *See* Amygdala anatomy
Amygdalotomy, history, 158–159
Anatomy. *See* Amygdala anatomy
Angry faces processing
  versus fearful faces, 272–273, 272*f*
  ventral amygdala role, 272–273, 272*f*
Anisomycin, 213–214

Anterior amygdaloid area (AAA)
  anatomy, 4, 5*f*, 9*t*, 10*f*, 14
  frontal cortex connectivity, 25, 25*f*
  hippocampal connectivity, 28
  hypothalamic connectivity, 20
Anterior cortical nucleus (COa)
  anatomy, 4, 5*f*, 6*f*, 9*t*, 10*f*, 12–13
  connectivity, 17, 20, 22–23, 25, 25*f*
Anxiety disorders, 321–343
  attentional biases, 235
  and autism, 373–375
    amygdala neuropathology, 374–375
  basic paradigms, 322
  neuroimaging findings, 322–329
    limitations, 330–331
  See also specific disorders
Appraisal style
  schizophrenia, 347, 352–354
  visual scanpath studies, 347
Arousal
  attentional blink paradigm, 227–228
  dimensional approach, substrates, 277–279
  dorsal amygdala, 280
  emotional memory effects, 190–195
  and perception, 228
  valence difference/overlap, 276–277
Asperger syndrome
  fearful faces paradigm, 372
  social stimuli response, 371
Associative orienting
  and animal freezing response, 265–266
  predictive functon, 281
Attention, 220–249
  dimensional approach, substrates, 278
  dorsal amygdala, 279–280
  emotion interactions, 225–229, 226*f*, 233–240, 239*f*
  complementarity and independence, 233–236
  functional model, 238–240, 239*f*
  reflexive orienting, 236–238
  sensory processing pathways, 229–233, 230*f*
Attentional blink paradigm
  emotional facilitation, 226*f*, 227–228
  semantic processing, 228
Auditory cortex, amygdala connections, 230